ALZHEIMER'S DISEASE
The New **PREVENTION** Revolution

**BONUS!
Special Section on
Longevity!**

BRADFORD FRANK, MD, MPH, MBA

outskirtspress
DENVER, COLORADO

The opinions expressed in this manuscript are solely the opinions of the author and do not represent the opinions or thoughts of the publisher. The author has represented and warranted full ownership and/or legal right to publish all the materials in this book.

Alzheimer's Disease
The New Prevention Revolution
All Rights Reserved.
Copyright © 2015 Bradford Frank, MD, MPH, MBA
V3.0

Cover Photo © 2015 thinkstockphotos.com. All rights reserved - used with permission.

This book may not be reproduced, transmitted, or stored in whole or in part by any means, including graphic, electronic, or mechanical without the express written consent of the publisher except in the case of brief quotations embodied in critical articles and reviews.

Outskirts Press, Inc.
http://www.outskirtspress.com

ISBN: 978-1-4787-5853-2

Outskirts Press and the "OP" logo are trademarks belonging to Outskirts Press, Inc.

PRINTED IN THE UNITED STATES OF AMERICA

Dedication—

This book is dedicated to healthcare providers who care for those with Alzheimer's dementia. In conducting evaluations and providing care to thousands of patients with Alzheimer's dementia in nursing homes over the years, we have been impressed with the dedication, professionalism, and amazing quality of care that seems to be universal. This is not easy work, and we take this opportunity to thank you for your service.

Disclaimer

The information provided in this book is designed to provide helpful information on the subjects discussed. This book is not meant to be used, nor should it be used, to diagnose or treat any medical condition. For diagnosis or treatment of any medical problem, consult your own healthcare provider. The publisher and author are not responsible for any specific health or allergy needs that may require medical supervision and are not liable for any damages or negative consequences from any treatment, action, application or preparation, to any person reading or following the information in this book. References are provided for informational purposes only and do not constitute endorsement of any websites or other sources. Readers should be aware that the websites listed in this book may change.

CONTENTS

Chapter One: Introduction 1
    What Is Memory? 6
    Where In The Brain Is Memory Located? 9
Chapter Two: What is Alzheimer's Disease? 10
    Biochemistry 11
    Cost To The Nation 11
    2014 Costs of Alzheimer's = $214 Billion. 12
    Demographics 13
    Diagnosis 13
    Diagnostic Criteria 14
    Disease mechanism 14
    Impact on Caregivers 15
    Mortality 16
    Neuropathology 17
    Residential Care 17
    Women and Alzheimer's 18
    Ten warning signs of Alzheimer's disease 19
Chapter Three: Stages and Progression of Alzheimer's Disease .. 23
    Subjective Memory Impairment (SMI) 23
    Mild Cognitive Impairment, MCI 25
    Moderate AD 29
    Advanced AD 29
    "Sundowning" 30

Symptoms are not limited to but may include: 30
Lifespan with Alzheimer's Disease 32
Predicting Alzheimer's Disease 33
Early Onset Alzheimer Disease (EOAD) 36
Chapter Four: Possible Risk Factors for Alzheimer's 38
Alcohol Consumption 38
Anabolic Steroids 38
Antihistamines (and anticholinergics) 39
Adult Asthma 40
Benzodiazepine Use 41
Cancer 42
Diabetes 42
Educational Level 43
Electromagnetic Fields 43
Female Gender 45
Glaucoma 45
SATNAV or GPS 45
Gout 48
Heavy Metal Exposure 48
Herpes Simplex Virus (HSV) 52
Height 53
High Fat Diet 53
Inbreeding 54
Infections 54
Lack of Purpose in Life 56
Loneliness 57
Low Testosterone 57

- Mental Issues 58
- Obesity 59
- Osteoporosis 61
- Periodontitis 62
- Pesticides 64
- Pollution 66
- Relatives With Alzheimer's Disease 67
- Sleep Apnea 68
- Sleep Issues 68
- Smoking 70
- Stress 71
- Tooth Loss 72
- Traumatic Brain Injury (TBI) 72
- Use of Proton Pump Inhibitors 73
- Vascular and Cholesterol Risk 73

Chapter Five: Cause(s) and Pathology 78
- Introduction 78
- Arginine 79
- Genetics 80
- Cholinergic Hypothesis 80
- Amyloid Hypothesis 81
- Tau Hypothesis 82
- TDP-43 (A Protein) 83
- Homocysteine 83
- Inflammation 84
- Mitochondrial Dysfunction 88
- Diabetes 89

Other Hypotheses 94
Chapter Six: Differential Diagnosis of Alzheimer's Disease 96
Other Types of Dementia (DSM-V) 96
Depression 98
Delirium 98
Primary Progressive Aphasia 101
CADASIL (Cerebral Autosomal-Dominant Arteriopathy with Subcortical Infarcts and Leukoencephalopathy) 102
Binswanger's Disease 103
Progressive Supranuclear Palsy (PSP) 104
Why Early and Accurate Diagnosis is Important 104
Chapter Seven: Diagnosis 107
Introduction 107
Paper-and-Pencil Testing 110
ADCS Preclinical Alzheimer Cognitive Composite (ADCS-PACC) 110
Alzheimer Disease Assessment Scale-Cognitive Subscale (ADAS-Cog) 110
Alzheimer's Disease 8 Screening Questionnaire (AD8) 111
BIMS (Brief Interview for Mental Status) 111
Blessed Dementia Rating Scale (BDRS) 111
CFI (Cognitive Function Instrument) 112
Clinical Dementia Rating (CDR) 112
Clock Drawing Test (CDT) 113
Dementia Severity Rating Scale (DSRS) 114
Instrumental Activities of Daily Living (IADL) 114
MMSE (Mini-Mental State Exam) 115
Neuropsychological Testing 116

Clinical Evaluation 117
Depression Screening 118
Hamilton Depression Rating Scale (abbreviated HAM-D) 121
The Geriatric Depression Scale (GDS) 122
Cornell Scale for Depression in Dementia (CSDD) 122
Patient Health Questionnaire (PHQ-9) 123
Basic Blood Tests 123
Complete Metabolic Panel (CMP) 124
Complete Blood Count (CBC) 124
Lipid Profile or Panel (Cholesterol) 125
Vitamin D 125
Hemoglobin A_1C (HgbA_1C) 125
More Specialized Blood Tests 126
B12 126
C-reactive Protein (CRP) 127
Human immunodeficiency virus (HIV) 127
Homocysteine 127
Methylmalonic Acid 129
Thyroid Tests 129
Venereal Disease Research Laboratory test (VDRL) 129
Brain-derived neurotrophic factor (BDNF) 129
FDA Approves Blood Test That Gauges Heart Attack Risk 132
Specific Blood Tests for Alzheimer's Disease 133
Insulin Receptor Substrate-1 (IRS-1) 133
Platelet Proteins 134
CoQ10 Blood Levels 134
N-terminal pro-brain natriuretic peptide (NT-proBNP) 135

Tests Related to Abeta Amyloid and Tau Proteins 135
Immune Function and Oxidative Stress 136
Blood Test Panels 137
Genetic Testing 138
Cerebral Spinal Fluid (CSF) 142
CSF Amyloid Beta (Aß) and Tau 143
CSF Apolipoprotein E (ApoE) 145
CSF Endostatin 146
Neuroimaging (Brain Scans) 148
CT (Computed Tomography) Scan 149
MRI (Magnetic Resonance Imaging) 150
Positron Emission Tomography (PET) Scan 154
Magnetoencephalographic Imaging (MEGI) 157
EEG (Electroencephalogram) 158
Other Tests 160
Smell Test 160
Sleep Study 163
Virtual Reality 163
Gait & Balance Assessment 165
Life Space 165
Primitive Reflexes 166
Pulse Wave Velocity (PWV) 168
Retinal Assessment 169
Eye Movements 169
Volatile Organic Compounds (VOCs) 169
Transcranial Ultrasound 170
Event Related Potential P3 171

Chapter Eight: Treatment 172
  Introduction 172
  FDA-approved Medications 173
  Cholinergic Medications 174
  Cognex (tacrine) 177
  Aricept (donepezil) 178
  Exelon (rivastigmine) 179
  Reminyl (galantamine) 180
  NMDA (*N*-Methyl-D-aspartate) Medication 182
  Namenda XR (memantine) 182
  Combination Treatments 185
  Namzaric (donepezil + memantine) 185
  Medications Used for Agitation in Alzheimer's Patients 185
  "Mood Stabilizers" 186
  Second-generation or "Atypical" Antipsychotic Medications ... 186
  "Antidepressants" 189
  Benzodiazepines (Minor Tranquilizers) 192
  Other Medications for Agitation 193
  Nuedexta (dextromethorphan hydrobromide and
  quinidine sulfate) 193
  Medications Used for Inappropriate Sexual Behaviors 194
  Other Possible Treatments 198
  Cognitive Training & Mindfulness 198
  Neurosurgical Treatments 201
  Social Interaction 202
  Support Groups 202
  Tailored Lighting Intervention 204

Transcranial LED Therapy (TCLT) 204
Transcranial Stimulation 205
Reminiscence Therapy 205
Experimental Treatments 206
Antibodies and Immunotherapy 207
Diabetic Medications 211
Epigenetic Therapies 211
Hyperketonemia 212
Nanosolution 213
Nanotubes 214
Stem Cells 214
Ultrasound 215
Vaccines 216

Chapter Nine: Prevention 218
Introduction 218
FDA-approved Medications (Used "Off-label") 218
Antidepressants 221
SSRIs (Selective Serotonin Reuptake Inhibitors such as Celexa or citalopram; Zoloft or sertraline; Prozac, or fluoxetine; Lexapro, or escitalopram): 221
Celexa (citalopram; 5-20 mg in those 60 or older; up to 40 mg otherwise): 222
Prozac (fluoxetine; 5-80 mg) 224
Zoloft (Sertraline; 12.5-200 mg) 225
Fetzima (levomilnacipran; 20-120 mg) 226
Norepinephrine (a neurotransmitter): 226
Protriptyline (a tricyclic antidepressant or TCA) 227
Keppra (levetiracetam) 227

Lithium 227
Statins (HMG-CoA Reductase Inhibitors) 233
Anti-diabetic Medications 238
Metformin 242
Anti-inflammatory Medications 244
Cromolyn Sodium (disodium cromoglycate) 248
Anti-hypertensive Agents 248
Angiotensin-converting Enzyme (ACE) Inhibitors 250
Calcium-channel Blockers 251
Estrogens 252
Viagra (sildenafil) 254
Diets 255
Introduction 255
Meat Diet 257
Mediterranean and DASH Diets 259
Paleo Diet 263
Epigenetic Diet 265
Whole-food Diet 267
Ketogenic Diet 268
Fish Diet 268
Anti-Alzheimer's Diet 269
Healthy Lifestyle 271
Life Space 272
Mental Activities 273
Cognitive Training/Activity 273
Higher Education 275
Learning a Language 276

Meditation 277
Mindfulness 279
Physical Activity 280
Physical Activity Trackers 291
Supplements, Antioxidants, and Micronutrients 294
Caution 1 294
Caution 2 297
Introduction 305
A (Vitamin A; Retinol; Retinal; and Retinoic Acid; and β-carotene) 317
Acetyl-L-carnitine 319
Alpha-lipoic Acid 320
Ascorbic Acid (Vitamin C) 321
Ashwagandha (Withania somnifera) 322
B Vitamins 326
B12 (Vitamin B12) 328
Berberine 334
Black Pepper 336
Carotenoids (Including Lycopene, Lutein and Zeaxanthin) 336
Chia (*Salvia hispanica*) 340
Chinese Herbal Preparations 342
Coconut 344
Coffee 345
Coenzyme Q_{10} (CoQ10) 346
Curcumin (Turmeric) 349
D (Vitamin D) 351
E (Vitamin E) 354

Flavonoids and Polyphenols (Phytochemicals) 357
Folate (Folic Acid; Vitamin B$_9$) 363
Gelsolin 367
Ginkgo Biloba 368
Ginger 373
Ginseng 375
Grape Seed Extract (GSE) 378
Green (and Oolong, White, and Black) Tea 380
Hesperidin 386
Huperzine A (Hup A; Qian Ceng Ta) 387
Kale 390
Magnesium (Mg+) 393
Melatonin 395
N-acetyl cysteine (NAC) 401
Omega 3 Fatty Acids 402
Pomegranate Extract 409
Quercetin 413
Resveratrol 416
Rhodiola Rosea 423
Saffron (Crocus sativus L.) 427
Selenium 428
Souvenaid® 429
St John's Wort 432
Walnuts 435
Zinc 442
Other Prevention Programs 444
Introduction 444

Anti-Stress ... 445
Dental Care ... 446
Pets ... 447
Religion ... 447
Sleep ... 448
Social Relations ... 450
Chaper Ten: Longevity ... 452
Introduction ... 452
Definition of Aging ... 456
Definition of Longevity ... 459
Theories of Aging ... 460
Caloric Restriction ... 461
Exercise ... 465
Free Radical Theory of Aging ... 466
Genetics ... 467
Immunological Theory of Aging ... 469
Klotho ... 470
Mitochondrial Theory of Aging ... 471
Sirtuins ... 473
Telomere Length ... 475
Things That Predict Longevity ... 477
Introduction ... 477
Biomarkers & Genetics ... 479
Early-Life Nutrition ... 482
Exercise, Activity & Fitness Levels ... 482
Facial Scans ... 489
Fiber ... 491

Friend-rated Personality Traits	493
Handshake Strength	494
"Healthy" Diet	496
Heart Rate	496
Isolation	498
Matthew Effect	498
Mediterranean diet	500
Milk Consumption	501
Nut Consumption	503
Oral Health	504
Purpose in life	504
RDW (Red Blood Cell Distribution Width)	506
Real vs. Perceived Age	511
Sleep	512
Sun Activity When Born	513
Volatile Organic Compounds (VOCs)	515
Medications	515
Antidepressants	515
Angiotensin II Blockade	516
NSAIDS (Non-steroidal Anti-inflamatory Drugs)	516
Rapamycin	519
Senolytic Drugs	520
Metformin	520
Supplements & Vitamins	522
Introduction	522
Alpinia Zerumbet	527
D (Vitamin D)	529

Extra Virgin Olive Oil 530
Garlic 532
Resveratrol 533
Pomegranite Juice 539
Summary of Steps To Take 541
Basic Steps To Take: 541
Basic Things to Avoid: 543
Conclusion 544
Resources 546
Glossary 548
Index 574
References 580

An ounce of prevention is worth a pound of cure.

—Benjamin Franklin

CHAPTER ONE:
INTRODUCTION

From a scientific perspective, we truly live in exciting times. After spending hundreds of billions of dollars and through decades of effort, there are major discoveries being made across every field of science, but no more so than in the area of Alzheimer's disease (AD). Some of these discoveries are truly revolutionary, and we invite you to join with us in exploring them and spreading the word to your family, colleagues, and friends.

Alzheimer's disease is a devastating disorder that strikes 1 in 10 Americans over the age of 65, and almost half of all Americans over 85 years old. The odds of an individual developing AD double every five years after the age of 65. While it has become increasingly common to meet heart attack or cancer survivors, there are no Alzheimer's disease survivors.

The incidence of dementia is rapidly increasing in developed countries due to social and demographic changes. This trend is expected to worsen in the coming decades, with the number of cases possibly even tripling in the next twenty-five years. By 2034 it is forecast that five percent of the global population will be aged 85 years or over—approximately two and half fold increase on present day figures—which will inevitably lead to an increase in age-associated disorders such as Alzheimer's disease. Therefore Alzheimer's disease prevention is becoming a global health priority. Our knowledge of the process leading to the development of brain lesions that characterize AD has increased exponentially in recent years.

The number of patients with Alzheimer's disease is increasing worldwide, and available drugs have shown limited efficacy. Hence, preventive interventions and treatments for presymptomatic AD are currently considered very important. It is vitally important that we help people understand that taking appropriate action now can prevent or help to prevent Alzheimer's disease. Although there are no guarantees in life, there is compelling evidence that following the right steps can, if started early enough, prevent this dreaded disease. Contrary-wise, once Alzheimer's disease is present, the dietary, nutritional, and medication manipulations that can prevent it are no longer effective. To date, there is no treatment that cures Alzheimer's disease once the diagnosis is made. Eventually, there will be a cure for AD (as there will be for every other disease). Until then, we have to focus on prevention.

Attention, concentration, learning and memory are fundamental processes we use to adjust to environmental challenges, make decisions, and adapt. The aging process is associated with numerous problems or pathologies at the cellular and sub-cellular level. Decline or loss of brain functions, including learning and memory, is one of the most devastating and feared aspects of aging. However, normal aging of the brain does not result in major memory impairment. It is only Alzheimer's disease, or less common conditions, such as Parkinson's, Huntington's or vascular disease, that result in major brain dysfunction and memory loss. With rare exceptions, years of cellular, animal, and human research have failed to demonstrate beneficial effects of a multitude of vitamins, nutrients, dietary modifications or medications on the progression of AD, once symptoms are present. Fortunately, the story is very different when it comes to prevention.

For a nice video overview of Alzheimer's disease, that is a TED[1] presentation (What is Alzheimer's disease? – by Ivan Seah Yu Jun),

---

[1]TED (Technology, Entertainment and Design) is a nonprofit devoted to spreading ideas, usually in the form of short, powerful talks (18 minutes or less). TED began in 1984 as a conference where Technology, Entertainment and Design converged, and today covers almost all topics — from science to business to global issues — in more than 100 languages. Meanwhile, independently run TEDx events help share ideas in communities around the world.
TED is a global community, welcoming people from every discipline and culture who seek a deeper understanding of the world. We believe passionately in the power of

INTRODUCTION

referred to by Nancy Wurtzel on March 25, 2015, here is the web link: http://www.datingdementia.com/2015/03/25/ted-ed-alzheimers-tutorial/. Once on the web page, just scroll down to the video (3.50 minutes), or go to TED.com for the full presentation.

In addition to dietary, nutritional, and pharmacological (i.e. medications) interventions, it has become apparent that environmental and lifestyle factors, such as exercise and mental activity, can also play a role in prevention of AD.

We apologize ahead of time for the use of technical jargon. This book was written for those with inquiring minds, including scientists, doctors, nurses, other health professionals, and lay people. We have tried to summarize important findings for those less interested in the details and technical aspects of Alzheimer's disease.

As in all of life, nothing is perfect, including this book. This is the first edition, with many more to come. We look forward, with great anticipation, to receiving scientifically-based additions, corrections, and things that might be deleted. Please forward your comments and references to us. Contact information is available at the end of the book under Resources. Thank you in advance for your input. We are confident that future readers will appreciate it as much as we will.

Finally, while the main focus of this book is on the prevention of AD, we have included a bonus section on longevity, which is another area of intense research that is providing incredible insights into what can help us live longer and healthier.

NOTE: More than 800 scientific references reviewed for this work are available for further exploration in the Reference section at the end of the book. With the e-book, readers can double click on the reference

---

ideas to change attitudes, lives and, ultimately, the world. On TED.com, we're building a clearinghouse of free knowledge from the world's most inspired thinkers.
community of curious souls to engage with ideas and each other, both online and at TED and TEDx events around the world, all year long.

ALZHEIMER'S DISEASE

number which will take you to the actual scientific citation in the Reference section. If you want to read the full article abstract (summary), you can cut and then paste the citation in the search bar of the website Pubmed, where more than 20 million scientific articles are listed. Here is the link for Pubmed: http://www.ncbi.nlm.nih.gov/pubmed/ (or, just google "pubmed").

If you just want to look at the scientific reference citation, and then return to where you were in the e-book, just double click on the citation number in the Reference section and, in doing so, you will be able to jump back to your place in the book.

Or, if you prefer to skip this book altogether, you can just read the Institute of Medicine's (IOM)[1] report, Cognitive Aging: Progress in Understanding and Opportunities for Action[2], released April 14, 2015.

According to an article discussing the report:[1]

> Older adults can take action to combat the gradual decline in cognitive function that occurs naturally with age, the Institute of Medicine (IOM) says in a new report released today.

---

[1] The Institute of Medicine (IOM) is an American non-profit, non-governmental organization founded in 1970, under the congressional charter of the National Academy of Sciences. Its purpose is to provide national advice on issues relating to biomedical science, medicine, and health, and its mission to serve as adviser to the nation to improve health. It works outside the framework of the U.S. federal government to provide independent guidance and analysis and relies on a volunteer workforce of scientists and other experts, operating under a formal peer-review system. The Institute aims to provide unbiased, evidence-based, and authoritative information and advice concerning health and science policy to policy-makers, professionals, leaders in every sector of society, and the public at large.

[2] Summary available at:
http://www.iom.edu/Reports/2015/Cognitive-Aging.aspx?utm_source=feedburner&utm_medium=feed&utm_campaign=Feed percent3A+NewIomReports+ percent28New+IOM+Reports percent29).

INTRODUCTION

In the report, "Cognitive Aging: Progress in Understanding and Opportunities for Action," the IOM Committee on the Public Health Dimensions of Cognitive Aging advises that outside of the effects of neurologic disease, such as Alzheimer's disease, *individuals of all ages should take three steps to help promote cognitive health*:

- Be physically active.

- Reduce and manage cardiovascular disease risk factors, including high blood pressure, diabetes, and smoking.

- Regularly discuss and review with a healthcare professional health conditions and medications that might have a negative effect on cognitive function.

These three actions have the "best evidence" for promoting cognitive health in individuals of all ages, Kristin Yaffe, MD, committee vice chair, and professor of psychiatry, neurology, and epidemiology, University of California, San Francisco, said during a media briefing. Other actions the IOM says may promote cognitive health include the following:

- Being socially and intellectually active and continually seeking opportunities to learn.

- Getting adequate sleep and seeking professional treatment for sleep disorders, if needed.

- Taking steps to avoid a sudden acute decline in cognitive function (delirium) associated with medications or hospitalizations.

- Carefully evaluating products advertised to consumers to improve cognitive health, such as medications, nutritional supplements, and cognitive training.

"The brain ages in all of us, [but] there is a message of hope in this report. Actions can be taken" to promote brain health, said committee chair Daniel G. Blazer, MD, PhD, emeritus professor of psychiatry, Duke University Medical Center in Durham, North Carolina.

> *There is also only limited evidence on the benefits of vitamins and supplements to enhance cognition or prevent decline. The medical literature "does not convincingly support any vitamin supplement intervention to prevent cognitive decline," the report says.*
>
> *The IOM report was sponsored by the McKnight Brain Research Foundation, National Institutes of Health (National Institute of Neurological Disorders and Stroke and National Institute on Aging), Centers for Disease Control and Prevention, Retirement Research Foundation, and the AARP.*

So there you have it. According to the prestigious IOM, supported by all of the prestigious agencies listed above, there is also only limited evidence on the benefits of vitamins and supplements to enhance cognition or prevent decline. The medical literature "does not convincingly support any vitamin supplement intervention to prevent cognitive decline," the report says. So, no need to trouble oneself reviewing the 800+ scientific studies cited in this book, which show that there are GREAT benefits of vitamins and supplements to enhance cognition and prevent decline. You be the judge. Hopefully you will now understand why this book is so scientific and technical – to refute this crazy disinformation propagated by conservative, sclerotic, and dangerous organizations such as the "prestigious" IOM.

What Is Memory?

Memory is the process in which information is encoded, stored, and retrieved. Encoding allows information from the outside world to reach the five senses in the forms of chemical and physical stimuli. In this

INTRODUCTION

first stage the information must be changed so that it may be put into the encoding process. Storage is the second memory stage or process. This entails that information is maintained over periods of time. Finally, the third process is the retrieval of information that has been stored. Such information must be located and returned to the consciousness. Some retrieval attempts may be effortless due to the type of information, and other attempts to remember stored information may be more demanding for various reasons.

From an information processing perspective there are three main stages in the formation and retrieval of memory:

- Encoding or registration: receiving, processing and combining of received information.
- Storage: creation of a permanent record of the encoded information.
- Retrieval, recall or recollection: calling back the stored information in response to some cue for use in a process or activity.

Memory can be divided into three main types: sensory, short-term, and long-term.

Sensory memory holds sensory information for less than one second after an item is perceived. The ability to look at an item and remember what it looked like with just a split second of observation, or memorization, is the example of sensory memory. It is out of cognitive control and is an automatic response.

Short-term memory allows recall for a period of several seconds to a minute without rehearsal. Its capacity is also very limited: George A. Miller (1956), when working at Bell Laboratories, conducted experiments showing that the store of short-term memory was 7±2 items. Modern estimates of the capacity of short-term memory are lower, typically of the order of 4–5 items; however, memory capacity can be increased through a process called chunking. For example, in recalling a ten-digit telephone number, a person could chunk the digits into three groups: first, the area code (such as 123), then a three-digit chunk (456)

ALZHEIMER'S DISEASE

and lastly a four-digit chunk (7890). This method of remembering telephone numbers is far more effective than attempting to remember a string of 10 digits; this is because we are able to chunk the information into meaningful groups of numbers. This may be reflected in some countries in the tendency to display telephone numbers as several chunks of two to four numbers.

The storage in sensory memory and short-term memory generally has a strictly limited capacity and duration, which means that information is not retained indefinitely. By contrast, long-term memory can store much larger quantities of information for potentially unlimited duration (sometimes a whole life span). Its capacity is immeasurably large. For example, given a random seven-digit number we may remember it for only a few seconds before forgetting, suggesting it was stored in our short-term memory. On the other hand, we can remember telephone numbers for many years through repetition; this information is said to be stored in long-term memory.

Short-term memory is supported by transient patterns of neuronal communication, dependent on regions of the frontal lobe and the parietal lobe. Long-term memory, on the other hand, is maintained by more stable and permanent changes in neural connections widely spread throughout the brain. The hippocampus[1] is essential to the consolidation of information from short-term to long-term memory, although it does not seem to store information itself. Without the hippocampus, new memories are unable to be stored into long-term memory. You will be reading the word "hippocampus" throughout this book.

---

[1] The hippocampus is a major component of the brains of humans and other vertebrates. Humans and other mammals have two hippocampi, one in each side of the brain. It belongs to the limbic system and plays important roles in the consolidation of information from short-term memory to long-term memory and spatial navigation. The hippocampus is located under the cerebral cortex. When we think of memory, we often think of the hippocampus.

INTRODUCTION

Where In The Brain Is Memory Located?

Recognition tasks are often used to characterize and define the nature of memory deficits. Some experts believe that familiarity and recollection are independently involved in the recognition of previously encountered material and both contribute to successful recognition. Not to put too fine a point on it, researchers reviewed relevant literature on this topic and noted that, "...it has been suggested that perirhinal and entorhinal areas are selectively involved in familiarity-based recognition, while the hippocampus is associated with recollection. Interestingly, these regions are among the first to be targeted by neurofibrillary tangles, one of AD's neuropathological hallmarks. *Impairment in recognition performance can occur in the very early stages of AD, such as MCI.*"[2]

And, here is food for thought by Dr. Størmer, published in the November 2014 issue of Medical Hypotheses: "Human stem cells possess memory, and consequently all living human cells must have a memory system. How memory is stored in cells and organisms is an open question. Magnetite is perhaps the best candidate to be a universal memory molecule. Magnetite may give us a clue, because it is the Earth's most distributed and important magnetic material. It is found in living organisms with no known functions except for involvement in navigation in some organisms. In humans magnetite is found in the brain, heart, liver and spleen. Humans suffer from memory dysfunctions in many cases when iron is out of balance. Anomalous concentrations of magnetite is [sic] known to be associated with a neurodegenerative disorder like Alzheimer's disease."[3]

CHAPTER TWO:
WHAT IS ALZHEIMER'S DISEASE?

It was first described by, and later named after, German psychiatrist and pathologist Alois Alzheimer in 1906. Alzheimer's disease (AD), accounts for 60 percent to 70 percent of cases of dementia. Dementia is a broad category of brain diseases that cause a long term and often gradual decrease in the ability to think and remember such that a person's daily functioning is affected. AD is a chronic neurodegenerative[1] disease that usually starts slowly and gets worse over time.

The most common early symptom is difficulty in remembering recent events (short term memory loss). As the disease advances, symptoms can include: problems with language, disorientation (including easily getting lost), mood swings, loss of motivation, not managing self-care, and psychiatric issues, such as agitation or psychosis (hallucinations and/or delusions[2]). As a person's condition declines they often withdraw from family and society. Gradually, bodily functions are lost, ultimately leading to death. Although the speed of progression can vary, the average life expectancy following diagnosis is three to nine years.

---

[1]Neurodegeneration is the umbrella term for the progressive loss of structure or function of neurons (nerve cells), including death of neurons. Many neurodegenerative diseases including Parkinson's, Alzheimer's, and Huntington's occur as a result of neurodegenerative processes.

[2]One of the most common delusions is that someone is stealing from the person. Less commonly, the Capgras delusion (or Capgras syndrome) is a disorder in which a person holds that a friend, spouse, parent, or other close family member (or pet) has been replaced by an identical-looking impostor.

Biochemistry

Enzymes act on the APP (amyloid precursor protein) and cut it into fragments. The beta-amyloid fragment is crucial in the formation of senile plaques in Alzheimer's disease.

Alzheimer's disease has been identified as a *protein misfolding disease*, caused by plaque accumulation of abnormally folded amyloid beta and tau amyloid proteins in the brain. Plaques are made up of small peptides, 39–43 amino acids in length, called amyloid beta (A_β). A_β is a fragment from the larger amyloid precursor protein (APP). APP is a transmembrane protein that penetrates through the neuron's membrane. APP is critical to neuron growth, survival and post-injury repair. In Alzheimer's disease, an unknown enzyme in a proteolytic process causes APP to be divided into smaller fragments. One of these fragments gives rise to fibrils of amyloid beta, which then form clumps that deposit outside neurons in dense formations known as senile plaques.

AD is also considered a tauopathy due to abnormal aggregation of the tau protein. Every neuron has a cytoskeleton, an internal support structure partly made up of structures called microtubules. These microtubules act like tracks, guiding nutrients and molecules from the body of the cell to the ends of the axon and back. A protein called *tau* stabilizes the microtubules when phosphorylated, and is therefore called a microtubule-associated protein. In AD, tau undergoes chemical changes, becoming hyperphosphorylated; it then begins to pair with other threads, creating neurofibrillary tangles and disintegrating the neuron's transport system.

Cost To The Nation[1]

Alzheimer's disease is the most expensive condition in the nation. In 2014, the direct costs to American society of caring for those with Alz-

---

[1] According to the Alzheimer's Association (alz.org).

heimer's will total an estimated $214 billion, including $150 billion in costs to Medicare and Medicaid. Despite these staggering figures, Alzheimer's will cost an estimated $1.2 trillion (in today's dollars) in 2050.

2014 Costs of Alzheimer's = **$214 Billion.**

Nearly one in every five dollars spent by Medicare is on people with Alzheimer's or another dementia. The average per-person Medicare spending for those with Alzheimer's and other dementias is three times higher than for those without these conditions. The average per-person Medicaid spending for seniors with Alzheimer's and other dementias is nineteen times higher than average per-person Medicaid spending for all other seniors.

The financial toll of Alzheimer's on families rivals the costs to Medicaid. Total Medicaid spending for people with Alzheimer's disease is $37 billion and out-of-pocket spending for individuals with Alzheimer's and other dementias is estimated at $36 billion.

A new study published October 2014, "*'Informal Care' for Older Americans Tops $500B Annually,* Study Finds. The RAND Corp. study put a price tag on the time and wages that caregivers give up every year to help older people who need assistance in daily activities. Each year, people across the United States spend an estimated 30 billion hours caring for older relatives and friends, which costs $522 billion, according to new research. "Our findings provide a new and better estimate of the monetary value of the care that millions of relatives and friends provide to the nation's elderly," said study author, Amalavoyal Chari. "These numbers are huge and help put the enormity of this largely silent and unseen workforce into perspective."[4]

WHAT IS ALZHEIMER'S DISEASE?

Demographics[1]

An estimated 5.2 million Americans had Alzheimer's disease in 2014, including approximately 200,000 individuals younger than age 65 who have early-onset Alzheimer's disease (EOAD).

Almost two-thirds of American seniors living with Alzheimer's are women. Of the 5 million people age 65 and older with Alzheimer's in the United States, 3.2 million are women and 1.8 million are men.

The number of Americans with Alzheimer's disease and other dementias will escalate rapidly in coming years as the baby boom generation ages. By 2050, the number of people age 65 and older with Alzheimer's disease may nearly triple, from 5 million to as many as 16 million, barring the development of medical breakthroughs to prevent, slow or stop the disease.

Diagnosis

Alzheimer's disease is usually diagnosed based on the person's medical history, history from relatives, and behavioral observations. The presence of characteristic neurological and neuropsychological features and the absence of alternative conditions is supportive. Advanced medical imaging with computed tomography (CT) or magnetic resonance imaging (MRI), and with single-photon emission computed tomography (SPECT) or positron emission tomography (PET) can be used to help exclude other cerebral pathology or subtypes of dementia. Moreover, it may predict conversion from prodromal stages (mild cognitive impairment) to Alzheimer's disease.

Assessment of intellectual functioning including memory testing can further characterize the state of the disease. Medical organizations have created diagnostic criteria to ease and standardize the diagnostic process for practicing physicians. The diagnosis can be confirmed with

---

[1]According to the Alzheimer's Association (alz.org).

very high accuracy post-mortem (after death) when brain material is available and can be examined histologically.

Diagnostic Criteria

The National Institute of Neurological and Communicative Disorders and Stroke (NINCDS) and the Alzheimer's disease and Related Disorders Association (ADRDA, now known as the Alzheimer's Association) established the most commonly used NINCDS-ADRDA Alzheimer's Criteria for diagnosis in 1984, extensively updated in 2007. These criteria require that the presence of cognitive impairment, and a suspected dementia syndrome, be confirmed by neuropsychological testing for a clinical diagnosis of possible or probable AD. A histopathologic confirmation including a microscopic examination of brain tissue is required for a definitive diagnosis. Good statistical reliability and validity have been shown between the diagnostic criteria and definitive histopathological confirmation.

Eight cognitive domains are most commonly impaired in AD— memory, language, perceptual skills, attention, constructive abilities, orientation, problem solving and functional abilities. These domains are equivalent to the NINCDS-ADRDA Alzheimer's Criteria as listed in the Diagnostic and Statistical Manual of Mental Disorders (DSM-V) published by the American Psychiatric Association.

Disease mechanism

Exactly how disturbances of production and aggregation of the beta-amyloid peptide gives rise to the pathology of AD is not known. The amyloid hypothesis (discussed in more detail below) traditionally points to the accumulation of beta-amyloid peptides as the central event triggering neuron degeneration. Accumulation of aggregated amyloid fibrils, which are believed to be the toxic form of the protein responsible for disrupting the cell's calcium ion homeostasis, induces programmed cell death (apoptosis). It is also known that A_β selectively builds up in the mitochondria in the cells of Alzheimer's-affected brains, and it also inhibits certain enzyme functions and the utilization of glucose by neurons.

Various inflammatory processes (also discussed in more detail below) and cytokines[1] may also have a role in the pathology of Alzheimer's disease. Inflammation is a general marker of tissue damage in any disease, and may be either secondary to tissue damage in AD or a marker of an immunological response.

Alterations in the distribution of different neurotrophic factors and in the expression of their receptors such as the brain-derived neurotrophic factor (BDNF)[2] have been described in AD.

Impact on Caregivers[3]

In 2013, 15.5 million family and friends provided 17.7 billion hours of unpaid care to those with Alzheimer's and other dementias – care valued at $220.2 billion, which is nearly eight times the total revenue of McDonald's in 2012.

More than 60 percent of Alzheimer's and dementia caregivers are women.

---

[1]Cytokines are a broad and loose category of small proteins that are important in cell signaling. They are released by cells and affect the behavior of other cells. Cytokines include chemokines, interferons, interleukins, lymphokines, and tumour necrosis factor. They act through receptors, and are especially important in the immune system. They are important in health and disease, specifically in host responses to infection, immune responses, inflammation, trauma, sepsis, cancer, and reproduction.
[2]Brain-derived neurotrophic factor, also known as BDNF, is a protein. BDNF is a member of the neurotrophin family of growth factors, which are related to the canonical Nerve Growth Factor. Neurotrophic factors are found in the brain and the periphery. BDNF acts on certain neurons of the central nervous system and the peripheral nervous system, helping to support the survival of existing neurons, and encourage the growth and differentiation of new neurons and synapses. In the brain, it is active in the hippocampus, cortex, and basal forebrain—areas vital to learning, memory, and higher thinking,
[3]According to the Alzheimer's Association (alz.org).

ALZHEIMER'S DISEASE

All caregivers of people with Alzheimer's – both women and men – face a devastating toll. Due to the physical and emotional burden of caregiving, Alzheimer's and dementia caregivers had $9.3 billion in additional health care costs of their own in 2013. Nearly 60 percent of Alzheimer's and dementia caregivers rate the emotional stress of caregiving as high or very high, and more than one-third report symptoms of depression.

Mortality[1]

More than 500,000 seniors die each year because they have Alzheimer's. If Alzheimer's was eliminated, half a million lives would be saved a year.

Alzheimer's is officially the 6th leading cause of death in the United States and the 5th leading cause of death for those aged 65 and older. However, it may cause even more deaths than official sources recognize. It kills more than prostate cancer and breast cancer combined.

Deaths from Alzheimer's increased 68 percent between 2000 and 2010, while deaths from other major diseases decreased. Alzheimer's disease is the only cause of death among the top ten in America that cannot be prevented, cured or even slowed.

Researchers reported in 2014 that, "Since 2005, life expectancy at birth in the U.S. has increased by one year; however, the number of persons who died prematurely was relatively constant. The years of potential life lost declined for eight of the ten leading causes of death. Age-adjusted rates declined among all leading causes except deaths attributable to Alzheimer's disease and suicide, although the numbers of deaths increased for most causes. Heart disease, stroke, and deaths attributed to motor-vehicle injuries demonstrated notable declines since 2005. Numbers and rates increased for both Alzheimer's disease and suicide."[5]

---

[1]According to the Alzheimer's Association (alz.org).

WHAT IS ALZHEIMER'S DISEASE?

According to a December 2014 report[6], *memory lapses in people with higher levels of education may be associated with increased stroke risk.* The research included more than 9,100 people in the Netherlands, aged 55 and older, taking part in a long-term study. During the study, more than 1,100 of the participants suffered a stroke. Overall, memory problems were independently associated with a higher risk of stroke. The researchers also found that people with memory problems had a 39 percent higher risk of stroke if they also had a higher level of education.

Neuropathology

Alzheimer's disease is characterized by loss of neurons (nerve cells) in many parts of the brain. This loss results in gross atrophy (shrinkage) of the affected regions. Studies using imaging techniques, such as magnetic resonance imaging (MRI) and positron emission tomography (PET) scans, have documented reductions in the size of specific brain regions in people with AD as they progressed from mild cognitive impairment (described below) to Alzheimer's disease, and in comparison with similar images from healthy older adults.

Both amyloid plaques and neurofibrillary tangles are clearly visible by microscopy in brains of those afflicted by AD. Plaques are dense, mostly insoluble deposits of beta-amyloid peptide and cellular material outside and around neurons. Tangles (neurofibrillary tangles) are aggregates of the microtubule-associated protein tau which has become hyperphosphorylated and accumulate inside the cells themselves. Although many older individuals develop some plaques and tangles as a consequence of aging, the brains of people with AD have a greater number of them in specific brain regions such as the temporal lobe.

Residential Care

People living in residential care, including assisted living, are individuals that cannot live independently, but generally do not require the skilled level of care provided by nursing homes. On any given day in 2012, there were 713,300 residents in residential care communities. Using data from the first wave of the National Study of Long-Term Care Providers (NSLTCP), researchers described the characteristics of residents in residential care and compared selected characteristics to residential bed number. In 2012, 16 percent of residents living in residential care communities with 4-25 beds were under age 65 compared with 5 percent of residents living in communities with more than 50 beds. A higher percentage of residents in communities with 4-25 beds were male, minority, and receiving Medicaid, compared with residents in communities with 26-50 beds and more than 50 beds. The prevalence of Alzheimer's disease and other dementias was higher in communities with 4-25 beds (49 percent) than in communities with 26-50 beds (41 percent) and more than 50 beds (38 percent). The percentages of residents needing assistance with bathing, dressing, toileting, transferring in or out of a bed, and eating were highest in communities with 4-25 beds.[7]

Women and Alzheimer's[1]

Women are at the epicenter of the Alzheimer's crisis. A woman's estimated lifetime risk of developing Alzheimer's at age 65 is 1 in 6, compared with nearly 1 in 11 for a man. As real a concern as breast cancer is to women's health, women in their 60s are about twice as likely to develop Alzheimer's during the rest of their lives as they are to develop breast cancer.

Not only are women more likely to have Alzheimer's, they are also more likely to be caregivers of those with Alzheimer's. More than three of five unpaid Alzheimer's caregivers are women – and there are 2.5 more women than men who provide 24-hour care for someone with Alzheimer's.

Because of caregiving duties, women are likely to experience adverse consequences in the workplace. Nearly 19 percent of women Alzheimer's caregivers had to quit work either to become a caregiver or because their caregiving duties became too burdensome.

---

[1]According to the Alzheimer's Association (alz.org).

WHAT IS ALZHEIMER'S DISEASE?

The growing burden of Alzheimer's disease underscores the importance of enhancing current public health efforts to address dementia. Public health organizations and entities have substantial opportunities to contribute to efforts underway and to add innovations to the field. The Alzheimer's Association and the Centers for Disease Control and Prevention (CDC) worked with a 15-member leadership committee and hundreds of stakeholders to create The Healthy Brain Initiative: The Public Health Road Map for State and National Partnerships, 2013-2018 (Road Map). The actions in the Road Map provide a foundation for the public health community to anticipate and respond to emerging innovations and developments.[8]

Ten warning signs of Alzheimer's disease[1]

1. Memory loss that disrupts daily life

   One of the most common signs of Alzheimer's is memory loss, especially forgetting recently learned information. Others include forgetting important dates or events; asking for the same information over and over; increasingly needing to rely on memory aids (e.g., reminder notes or electronic devices) or family members for things they used to handle on their own.

   What's a typical age-related change?
   Sometimes forgetting names or appointments, but remembering them later.

2. Challenges in planning or solving problems

   Some people may experience changes in their ability to develop and follow a plan or work with numbers. They may have trouble following a familiar recipe or keeping track of monthly bills. They may have difficulty concentrating and take much longer to do things than they did before.

---
[1] From the Alzheimer's Association (alz.org).

ALZHEIMER'S DISEASE

What's a typical age-related change?

Making occasional errors when balancing a checkbook.

3. Difficulty completing familiar tasks at home, at work or at leisure

    People with Alzheimer's often find it hard to complete daily tasks. Sometimes, people may have trouble driving to a familiar location, managing a budget at work or remembering the rules of a favorite game.

    What's a typical age-related change?

    Occasionally needing help to use the settings on a microwave or to record a television show.

4. Confusion with time or place

    People with Alzheimer's can lose track of dates, seasons and the passage of time. They may have trouble understanding something if it is not happening immediately. Sometimes they may forget where they are or how they got there.

    What's a typical age-related change?

    Getting confused about the day of the week but figuring it out later.

5. Trouble understanding visual images and spatial relationships

    For some people, having vision problems is a sign of Alzheimer's. They may have difficulty reading, judging distance and determining color or contrast, which may cause problems with driving.

    What's a typical age-related change?

    Vision changes related to cataracts.

WHAT IS ALZHEIMER'S DISEASE?

6. New problems with words in speaking or writing

    People with Alzheimer's may have trouble following or joining a conversation. They may stop in the middle of a conversation and have no idea how to continue or they may repeat themselves. They may struggle with vocabulary, have problems finding the right word or call things by the wrong name (e.g., calling a "watch" a "hand-clock").

    What's a typical age-related change?
    Sometimes having trouble finding the right word.

7. Misplacing things and losing the ability to retrace steps

    A person with Alzheimer's disease may put things in unusual places. They may lose things and be unable to go back over their steps to find them again. Sometimes, they may accuse others of stealing. This may occur more frequently over time.

    What's a typical age-related change?
    Misplacing things from time to time and retracing steps to find them.

8. Decreased or poor judgment

    People with Alzheimer's may experience changes in judgment or decision-making. For example, they may use poor judgment when dealing with money, giving large amounts to telemarketers. They may pay less attention to grooming or keeping themselves clean.

    What's a typical age-related change?
    Making a bad decision once in a while.

9. Withdrawal from work or social activities

    A person with Alzheimer's may start to remove themselves from hobbies, social activities, work projects or sports. They may have trouble keeping up with a favorite sports team or remembering how to complete a favorite hobby. They may also avoid being social because of the changes they have experienced.

What's a typical age-related change?

Sometimes feeling weary of work, family and social obligations.

10. Changes in mood and personality

    The mood and personalities of people with Alzheimer's can change. They can become confused, suspicious, depressed, fearful or anxious. They may be easily upset at home, at work, with friends or in places where they are out of their comfort zone.

    What's a typical age-related change?

    Developing very specific ways of doing things and becoming irritable when a routine is disrupted.

CHAPTER THREE:
STAGES AND PROGRESSION OF ALZHEIMER'S DISEASE

The disease course can be divided into stages, with a progressive pattern of cognitive and functional impairment.

Subjective Memory Impairment (SMI)

Subjective memory impairment (SMI) is receiving increasing attention as a pre-mild cognitive impairment (MCI) condition in the course of the clinical manifestation of Alzheimer disease (AD). Elderly individuals with subjective memory impairment (SMI) report memory decline, but perform within the age-, gender-, and education-adjusted normal range on neuropsychological tests. Longitudinal studies indicate SMI as a risk factor or early sign of AD.

In one clinical study of SMI, a total of 2415 subjects without cognitive impairment 75 years or older were followed by researchers for three years. They found that, "SMI with worry at baseline was associated with greatest risk for conversion to dementia...The prediction of dementia in AD by SMI with subsequent amnestic MCI supports the model of a consecutive 3-stage clinical manifestation of AD from SMI via MCI to dementia."[9]

There is increasing evidence from neuroimaging that at the group level, subjects with SMI display evidence of AD-related brain pathology. In 2014, a group of researchers conducted a study aimed to determine differences in cortical (brain) thickness between individuals with SMI and healthy control subjects. One hundred and ten participants underwent brain imaging to determine cortical thickness in specific brain regions. Cortical thickness reduction was observed in the SMI group compared to controls, and the researchers concluded that, "We interpret our findings as evidence of early AD-related brain changes in persons with SMI."[10]

It is recognized that individuals with mild cognitive impairment (MCI) already demonstrate difficulty in aspects of daily functioning (also known as activities of daily living, or ADLs), which predicts disease progression. In 2014, researchers examined the relationship between self- versus informant-report of functional ability, and how those reports relate to objective disease measures across the disease spectrum (i.e. cognitively normal, MCI, Alzheimer's disease). A total of 1,080 subjects with self- and/or informant-rated Everyday Cognition questionnaires were included. Objective measures included cognitive functioning, structural brain atrophy, cerebrospinal fluid abnormalities, and a marker of amyloid deposition using positron emission tomography (PET) scans. The researchers concluded that, "Overall, informant-report was consistently more associated with objective markers of disease than self-report although self-reported functional status may still have some utility in early disease."[11]

Still other researchers reported in the October 2014 issue of *Neurology* the results of their research. They assessed subjective memory impairment (SMI) by older individuals as a predictor of subsequent cognitive impairment. Subjects (n = 531) enrolled while cognitively intact at the University of Kentucky were asked annually if they perceived changes in memory since their last visit. The association between SMI and Alzheimer-type neuropathology was assessed from autopsies (n = 243). They found that SMI was reported by more than half (55.7 percent) of the subjects, and were associated with increased risk of impairment. Mild cognitive impairment (MCI) occurred on average 9.2 years after SMI. They also found that SMI smokers took less time to transition to mild cognitive impairment, while SMI hormone-replaced women took longer to transition directly to dementia. The authors concluded that, "SMI reporters are at a higher risk of future cognitive impairment and have higher levels of Alzheimer-type brain pathology even when impairment does not occur. As potential harbingers of future cognitive decline, physicians should query and monitor SMI from their older patients."[12]

Mild Cognitive Impairment, MCI

The first symptoms are often mistakenly attributed to aging or stress. Detailed neuropsychological testing can reveal mild cognitive difficulties up to eight years before a person fulfills the clinical criteria for diagnosis of AD. These early symptoms can affect the most complex daily living activities. The most noticeable deficit is short term memory loss, which shows up as difficulty in remembering recently learned facts and inability to acquire new information.

Subtle problems with the executive functions of attentiveness, planning, flexibility, and abstract thinking, or impairments in semantic memory (memory of meanings, and concept relationships) can also be symptomatic of the early stages of AD. Apathy can be observed at this stage, and remains the most persistent neuropsychiatric symptom throughout the course of the disease. Depressive symptoms, irritability and reduced awareness of subtle memory difficulties are also common. The preclinical stage of the disease has also been termed mild cognitive impairment (MCI). This is often found to be a transitional stage between normal aging and dementia. MCI can present with a variety of symptoms, and when memory loss is the predominant symptom it is termed "amnestic MCI" and is frequently seen as a prodromal stage of Alzheimer's disease.

Mild cognitive impairment (MCI) is a brain function syndrome involving the onset and evolution of cognitive impairments beyond those expected based on the age and education of the individual, but which are not significant enough to interfere with their daily activities. It is often found to be a transitional stage between normal aging and dementia. Although MCI can present with a variety of symptoms, when memory loss is the predominant symptom it is termed "amnestic MCI" and is frequently seen as a prodromal stage of Alzheimer's disease. Studies suggest that these individuals tend to progress to probable AD at a rate of approximately 10 percent to 15 percent per year. Another group of researchers reports that, "At three years after diagnosis, the risk of AD for patients with MCI is estimated to be 18 percent to 30 percent."[13]

A group of researchers assessed how self-complaint of memory impairment relates to cognitive and neuro-imaging measures in older adults with MCI. They studied two groups based on the presence of self-reported memory complaint (no complaint n = 191, 77 ± 7 years; complaint n = 206, 73 ± 8 years). Cognitive outcomes included episodic memory, executive functioning, information processing speed, and language. They also used imaging to study brain thickness in specific areas of the brain. They concluded that, "Self-reported memory concern was unrelated to structural neuro-imaging markers of atrophy and measures of information processing speed, executive functioning, or language. In contrast, memory self-complaint related to objective verbal episodic learning performance."[14]

Subjective cognitive complaints are a criterion for the diagnosis of mild cognitive impairment (MCI), despite their uncertain relationship to objective memory performance in MCI. Researchers examined self-reported cognitive complaints in subgroups of the Alzheimer's disease Neuroimaging Initiative (ADNI) MCI group to determine whether they are a valuable inclusion in the diagnosis of MCI or, alternatively, if they contribute to misdiagnosis. They studied 448 individuals, and found that, "Overall, there was no relationship between self-reported cognitive complaints and objective cognitive functioning, but significant correlations were observed with depressive symptoms. The inclusion of self-reported complaints in MCI diagnostic criteria may cloud rather than clarify diagnosis and result in high rates of misclassification of MCI. Discrepancies between self- and informant-report demonstrate that overestimation of cognitive problems is characteristic of normal aging while underestimation may reflect greater risk for cognitive decline."[15]

Because of this difficulty of diagnosing Alzheimer's disease before typical symptoms arise, clinicians are developing other methods to detect pre-clinical AD. For example, researchers reported in the October 2014 issue of the journal *Neurology* the incidence and risk factors for motoric cognitive risk syndrome (MCR), a newly described pre-dementia syndrome characterized by slow gait and cognitive complaints. They studied 3,128 adults aged sixty years and older, MCR- and dementia-free at baseline over a median follow-up time of 3.2 years. MCR incidence was higher with older age but there were no sex differences. They found that strokes, Parkinson's disease, depressive symptoms, sedentariness, and obesity [in that order] predicted risk of incident MCR. The researchers concluded that, "The incidence of MCR is high in older adults. Identification of modifiable risk factors for MCR will improve identification of high-risk individuals and help develop interventions to prevent cognitive decline in aging."[16]

From the Division of Geriatrics and Nutritional Science, Department of Internal Medicine, Washington University School of Medicine, St. Louis, Missouri, researchers studied 435 cognitively normal adults aged sixty and older for an average of five years. They wanted to determine whether mildly impaired physical function, scored on the 9-item Physical Performance Test (PPT) is associated with development of Alzheimer's disease in cognitively normal older adults. During the follow-up period, 81 participants developed AD. Participants diagnosed with AD were older (81.0 vs 74) and had worse performance on the PPT than those who remained cognitively normal. Time to AD diagnosis was associated with PPT total score such that time to AD diagnosis was longer for participants with higher physical performance scores. PPT score significantly predicted time to AD diagnosis. The researchers noted, "*Mild physical impairment in cognitively normal older adults is associated with subsequent development of AD.* Although the physical impairment may be sufficiently mild that it is recognized only using performance-based assessments, its presence may predate clinically detectable cognitive decline."[17]

Loss of muscle strength is common and is associated with various adverse health outcomes in old age. To assess the possible relationship to

MCI and AD, another group of researchers studied more than 900 community-based older persons in retirement communities across the Chicago, Illinois metropolitan area. During a mean follow-up of 3.6 years, 138 persons developed AD. They found that for each one unit increase in muscle strength at baseline was associated with about a 43 percent decrease in the risk of AD. The researchers concluded that, *"Muscle strength was associated with a decreased risk of MCI."*[18]

Decline in cognitive performance is associated with gait deterioration. To study this relationship, researchers recruited 934 older community-dwellers without diagnosed dementia with an average age of 70 years. "A total of 294 (31.5 percent) participants presented with decline in cognitive performance. *Gait abnormalities and slower gait speed were associated with decline in episodic memory and executive performances."*[19]

Researchers designed a study to determine whether decline in cognitive function was greater among older individuals who experienced acute care or critical illness hospitalizations relative to those not hospitalized. They analyzed data from a study from 1994 through 2007 comprising 2,929 individuals 65 years old and older without dementia at baseline residing in the community in the Seattle area. During a mean follow-up of 6.1 years, 1,601 participants had no hospitalization, 1,287 had one or more noncritical illness hospitalizations, and 41 had one or more critical illness hospitalizations. There were 146 cases of dementia among those not hospitalized, 228 cases of dementia among those with one or more noncritical illness hospitalizations, and five cases of dementia among those with one or more critical illness hospitalizations. The researchers concluded that, *"Among a group of older adults without dementia at baseline, those who experienced acute care hospitalization and critical illness hospitalization had a greater likelihood of cognitive decline compared with those who had no hospitalization. Noncritical illness hospitalization was significantly associated with the development of dementia."*[20]

In order to understand the progression to cognitive decline in elderly persons, researchers studied ninety-five elders (mean age 84 years) who at entry into the study had no cognitive impairment. They were followed for up to thirteen years. Whereas 49 percent remained cognitively intact, 51 percent developed cognitive decline. Mean follow-up to the first sign of dementia was 3.8 years and age at conversion was 90.0 years. *Those who remained cognitively intact had better memory at entry than those who developed cognitive decline.*[21]

Moderate AD

Progressive deterioration eventually hinders independence, with subjects being unable to perform most common activities of daily living (ADLs). Speech difficulties become evident due to an inability to recall vocabulary, which leads to frequent incorrect word substitutions (paraphasias). Reading and writing skills are also progressively lost. Complex motor sequences become less coordinated as time passes and AD progresses, so the risk of falling increases. During this phase, memory problems worsen, and the person may fail to recognize close relatives. Long-term memory, which was previously intact, becomes impaired.

Behavioral and neuropsychiatric changes become more prevalent. Common manifestations are wandering, irritability and labile affect, leading to crying, outbursts of unpremeditated aggression, or resistance to caregiving. Sundowning (see below) can also appear. *Approximately 30 percent of people with AD develop illusionary misidentifications and other delusional symptoms.* Urinary incontinence can develop. These symptoms create stress for relatives and caregivers, which can be reduced by moving the person from home care to other long-term care facilities.

Advanced AD

During the final stages, the patient is completely dependent upon caregivers. Language is reduced to simple phrases or even single words, eventually leading to complete loss of speech. Despite the loss of verbal language abilities, people can often understand and return emotional signals. Although aggressiveness can still be present, extreme apathy and exhaustion are much more common symptoms. People with Alzheimer's disease will ultimately not be able to perform even the simplest tasks independently; muscle mass and mobility deteriorate to the point in which they are bedridden and unable to feed themselves. The cause of death is usually an external factor, such as infection of pressure ulcers or pneumonia, not the disease itself.

"Sundowning"

Sundowning is a phenomenon of increased confusion and restlessness in patients with some form of dementia. The term "sundowning" was coined due to the timing of the patient's confusion. For patients with sundowning syndrome, a multitude of behavioral problems begin to occur in the evening or while the sun is setting. Sundowning seems to occur more frequently during the middle stages of Alzheimer's disease and mixed dementia. Sundowning seems to subside with the progression of a patient's dementia. Research shows that 20–45 percent of Alzheimer's patients will experience some sort of sundowning confusion.

Symptoms are not limited to but may include:

- Increased general confusion as natural light begins to fade and increased shadows appear.
- Agitation and mood swings. Patients may become fairly frustrated with their own confusion as well as aggravated by noise. Patients found yelling and becoming increasingly upset with their caregiver is not uncommon.
- Mental and physical fatigue increase with the setting of the sun. This fatigue can play a role in the patient's irritability.
- A patient may experience an increase in their restlessness while trying to sleep. Restlessness can often lead to pacing and/or wandering which can be potentially harmful for a patient in a confused state.

Other researchers note the following about sundowning, "'Sundowning' in demented individuals, as distinct clinical phenomena, is still open to debate in terms of clear definition, etiology, operationalized parameters, validity of clinical construct, and interventions. In general, sundown syndrome is characterized by the emergence or increment of neuropsychiatric symptoms such as agitation, confusion, anxiety, and aggressiveness in late afternoon, in the evening, or at night. Sundowning is highly prevalent among individuals with dementia. It is thought to be associated with impaired circadian rhythmicity, environmental and social factors, and impaired cognition. *It appears to be mediated by decreased production of melatonin.* A variety of treatment options have been found to be helpful to ameliorate the neuropsychiatric symptoms associated with this phenomenon: bright light therapy, melatonin, acetylcholinesterase inhibitors [such as Aricept and Exelon], N-methyl-d-aspartate receptor antagonists [such as Namenda], antipsychotics [such as Abilify, Risperdal, and Seroquel], and behavioral modifications."[22]

Researchers from the Gertrude H Sergievsky Center, Columbia University Medical Center, New York, NY, determined that *disruptive behavior (wandering, verbal outbursts, physical threats/violence, agitation/restlessness, and sundowning) in people with Alzheimer's disease worsens prognosis.*[1] They studied 497 patients with early-stage AD for an average of 4.4 years. At least one disruptive behavioral symptom was noted in 48 percent of patients at baseline and in 83 percent at any evaluation. Their presence was associated with increased risks of cognitive decline, functional decline, and institutionalization. Sundowning was associated with faster cognitive decline, wandering with faster functional decline and institutionalization, and agitation/restlessness with faster cognitive and functional decline. There was no association between disruptive behavior and mortality. The authors concluded, "*Disruptive behavior is very common in AD and predicts*

---

[1]**Prognosis** is a medical term for predicting the likely outcome of one's current standing. A complete prognosis includes the expected duration, the function, and a description of the course of the disease, such as progressive decline, intermittent crisis, or sudden, unpredictable crisis.

cognitive decline, functional decline, and institutionalization but not mortality."[23]

In a separate analysis, researchers from the same institution, the Gertrude H Sergievsky Center, Columbia University Medical Center, New York, NY, studied the effect hallucinations and delusions had on the outcome of people with AD. They studied a total of 456 patients with AD at early stages. They were followed up semiannually for up to fourteen years (average, 4.5 years) in five university-based AD centers in the United States and Europe. The presence of delusions and hallucinations noted and compared with various outcome measures. During the course of follow-up, delusions were noted for 34 percent of patients at baseline and 70 percent at any evaluation. Their presence was associated with increased risk for cognitive and functional decline. Hallucinations were present in 7 percent of patients at initial visit and in 33 percent at any visit. Their presence was associated with increased risk for cognitive decline, functional decline, institutionalization, and death. The researchers concluded that, *"Delusions and hallucinations are very common in AD and predict cognitive and functional decline. Presence of hallucinations is also associated with institutionalization and mortality [death]."*[24]

Lifespan with Alzheimer's Disease

Family members of patients with Alzheimer's disease often wonder about the progression of the illness in their relative. This is a difficult question to answer in any particular individual. However, in 2014, researchers shed some light on this subject by reviewing the natural history of dementia with a focus on Alzheimer's disease and vascular dementia. They found that, "From the available published data, the life expectancy of elderly people with dementia is shorter than that of nondemented elderly. *Reports on survival after a diagnosis of dementia vary from three to twelve years.* The wide variation is partly due to the diagnostic criteria used in the studies and the sites where they were conducted (i.e., hospitals, clinics, or homes). There is an apparent difference in survival between AD patients with onset of illness before 75 years and those after 75 years: the younger patients have a longer life expectancy. However, there are conflicting data on survival (in years) comparing male and female patients and comparing patients of different ethnicities. For vascular dementia, published papers on life expectancy vary between three to five years. Vascular dementia appears to have a poorer prognosis than Alzheimer's disease. *The stages of severity of dementia were compared in a follow-up of a sample of Alzheimer's disease patients in Singapore, and the mean duration of the mild phase was 5.6 years, the moderate phase was 3.5 years, and the severe phase was 3.2 years.*"[25]

Predicting Alzheimer's Disease

Researchers studied 108 optimally healthy, elderly, cognitively intact individuals for an average follow-up of six years, to determine the ability of memory, memory area of the brain (hippocampal)[1] volume, and a gait speed (time to walk 30 ft) to independently predict cognitive decline in healthy elderly persons. They found that, "Questionable dementia occurred in 48 participants in a mean of 3.7 years. This progressed to persistent cognitive impairment in 38 of these participants in a mean of 4.4 years. Memory performance and hippocampal volume each predicted onset of questionable dementia, independent of age and sex. Time to walk thirty feet additionally contributed independently to the prediction of time to onset of persistent cognitive impairment."[26]

Researchers wanted to estimate the rates of dementia developing in initially non-demented subjects with and without mild memory impairment. To do so, they followed 264 initially non-demented, elderly community volunteers with examinations every 12 to 18 months for up

---

[1]The hippocampus is a major component of the brains of humans and other vertebrates. Humans and other mammals have two hippocampi, one in each side of the brain. It belongs to the limbic system and plays important roles in the consolidation of information from short-term memory to long-term memory and spatial navigation. The hippocampus is located under the cerebral cortex.

to ten years. Thirty-two cases of dementia developed during follow-up. The researchers found that *subjects with impaired recall (e.g., recent memory) at baseline had dementia develop over five years of follow-up at dramatically higher rates than subjects with intact recall.* The researchers concluded that, "These findings support the existence of a preclinical phase of dementia characterized by memory impairment, which is present for at least five years before diagnosis[27] In other words, elderly people with mild memory impairment are at much greater risk of developing dementia than those without any memory impairment.

A different group of researchers conducted a similar study to the one discussed above. They followed 532 individuals for up to six years. Among those, 459 remained non-demented and 73 developed AD during the follow-up period. They concluded that, *"The diagnosis of AD is preceded by a long preclinical phase in which deficits in memory performance are most common.* These deficits remain relatively stable up until the time that a dementia diagnosis can be rendered."[28]

In the September 2014 issue of the *Archives of Clinical Neuropsychology*, Dr. Triebel and colleagues reported the results of their research investigating financial skills in preclinical Alzheimer's disease using a new short form measure of financial capacity. In collaboration with the Mayo Clinic Study of Aging, they recruited 94 cognitively normal, community dwelling older adults age 70+ in Olmsted County, Minnesota. All participants brain PET scan imaging, and a short-form version of the Financial Capacity Instrument (FCI-SF). The FCI-SF measures performance accuracy on a series of everyday financial tasks, and also measures time to completion (in seconds) of four specific tasks: a medical deductible calculation, a simple income tax calculation, completion of a single-item checkbook/register task, and completion of a three-item checkbook/register task. They compared amyloid positive and negative cognitively normal subjects on their FCI-SF total performance score, and on the four timing variables.

Amyloid imaging resulted in a subdivision of the sample into groups of amyloid positive (n = 26) and amyloid negative cognitively normal subjects (n = 68). FCI-SF total score performance did not differ across groups. However, the amyloid positive group was slower completing the two checkbook tasks, and the four financial tasks as a whole. The authors concluded that, "Older cognitively normal subjects with a biomarker for preclinical AD [positive PET scans] performed equivalently with amyloid negative older subjects in accurately conducting different everyday financial tasks, but showed significantly slower time completing the tasks. These findings suggest that *diminished processing speed [but not inability to do calculations] is an initial preclinical change signaling future financial declines in patients with AD.*"[29]

Financial capacity (FC) clinically shows early impairment in patients with prodromal and clinical Alzheimer's disease (AD). Researchers used MRI imaging to investigate brain atrophy and FC in cognitively normal elderly (CN; N=44), patients with MCI due to AD (MCI; N=23), and patients with mild dementia due to AD (N=24). They found, as expected, that brain volume decreased with worsening signs of dementia. They also found that executive function (EF)[1] was the most significant cognitive predictor of the brain volume loss, with loss in arithmetic skills emerging later.[30]

Another group of researchers also studied the relationship between financial skill decline longitudinally in patients with mild cognitive impairment (MCI) due to an etiology of Alzheimer's disease. Study participants were cognitively normal older adults (n = 82) and patients with MCI (n = 91). Participants completed up to seven annual assessments using a standardized measure of financial skills (FCI). At baseline, and as expected, controls performed better than MCI patients across all FCI measures. The researchers found that, "Annualized decline in MCI global scores, calculated in relation to control performance, was 11-13 percent over the initial three-year time span, and 23 percent over six years. Annualized decline on the domains ranged from -6 percent (Knowledge of Assets/Estate) to -22 percent (Investment

---

[1]Executive functions is an umbrella term for the management (regulation, control) of cognitive processes, including working memory, reasoning, task flexibility, and problem solving as well as planning and execution.

Decision-Making) at three-year follow-up, and from -14 percent (Basic Monetary Skills) to -37 percent (Financial Judgment) over six years...Over a six-year period MCI patients demonstrated significant declines in multiple financial skills-in particular financial judgment.[31]

Researchers reported in December 2014 the results of an extensive literature review of the predictors of Alzheimer's disease progression. In doing so, they extracted information from fifteen clinical trials in mild-to-moderate AD patients (4,495 patients). Their analysis of the data, "...suggests that faster AD progression is associated with younger age and higher number of apolipoprotein E type 4 alleles (APOE*4)[1], after accounting for baseline disease severity. APOE*4, in particular, seems to be implicated in the AD pathogenesis. In addition, patients who are already on stable background AD medications [such as Aricept and Namenda] appear to have a faster progression relative to those who are not receiving AD medication [possibly implying that those on medications have more severe dementia to begin with]."[32]

A recent study investigated whether or not the rate of change of physical frailty and cognitive function in older adults are correlated. Researchers followed 2,167 older adults for six years. They found that, "Most individuals showed worsening frailty and cognition (82.8 percent); 17 percent showed progressive frailty alone and less than one percent showed only cognitive decline. The rates of change of frailty and cognition were strongly correlated."[33]

Early Onset Alzheimer Disease (EOAD)

Early Onset Alzheimer Disease (EOAD) is a rare condition, frequently associated with genetic causes. The dissemination of genetic testing along with biomarker[2] determinations have prompted a wider recogni-

---

[1]APOE*4, found in the genetic variant of AD, modulates LDL (low-density lipoproteins) metabolism, increases free radical formation and reduces plasma antioxidant concentrations.

[2]A biomarker, or biological marker, generally refers to a measurable indicator of some biological state or condition.

tion of EOAD in experienced clinical settings. However, despite the great efforts in establishing the contribution of causative genes to EOAD, atypical disease presentation and clinical features still makes its diagnosis and treatment a challenge for clinicians.[34]

In people with AD the increasing impairment of learning and memory eventually leads to a definitive diagnosis. In a small percentage, difficulties with language, executive functions, perception (agnosia), or execution of movements (apraxia) are more prominent than memory problems. AD does not affect all memory capacities equally. Older memories of the person's life (episodic memory), facts learned (semantic memory), and implicit memory (the memory of the body on how to do things, such as using a fork to eat) are affected to a lesser degree than new facts or memories.

Language problems are mainly characterized by a shrinking vocabulary and decreased word fluency, which lead to a general impoverishment of oral and written language. In this stage, the person with Alzheimer's is usually capable of communicating basic ideas adequately. While performing fine motor tasks such as writing, drawing or dressing, certain movement coordination and planning difficulties (apraxia) may be present but they are commonly unnoticed. As the disease progresses, people with AD can often continue to perform many tasks independently, but may need assistance or supervision with the most cognitively demanding activities.

CHAPTER FOUR: POSSIBLE RISK FACTORS FOR ALZHEIMER'S

Alcohol Consumption

Epidemiological studies have reported a reduction in the prevalence of Alzheimer's disease in individuals that ingest low amounts of alcohol. Also, it has been found that moderate consumption of alcohol might protect against β-amyloid (Aβ) toxicity. Researchers used an animal model to study this relationship, reporting their findings in the October 17, 2014 issue of *Neurobiology of Aging*. To summarize, they found a strong protective effect of a low concentration of alcohol (equivalent to moderate ethanol consumption). They concluded that, "These results may also provide an explanation for the *decrease in the risk of Alzheimer's disease in people who consume moderate doses of alcohol*."[35]

Anabolic Steroids

"Both genetic and environmental factors contribute to neurodegenerative disorders. In a large number of neurodegenerative diseases [for example, Alzheimer's disease], patients do not carry the mutant genes. Other risk factors, for example the environmental factors, should be evaluated. 17β-trenbolone is a kind of environmental hormone as well as an anabolic-androgenic steroid. 17β-trenbolone is used as a growth promoter for livestock in the USA. Also, a large portion of recreational exercisers inject 17β-trenbolone in large doses and for very long time to increase muscle and strength. 17β-trenbolone is stable in the environment after being excreted. In the present study, 17β-trenbolone was administered to adult and pregnant rats and the primary hippocampal

POSSIBLE RISK FACTORS FOR ALZHEIMER'S

[memory] neurons. 17β-trenbolone's distribution and its effects on serum hormone levels and Aβ42 accumulation in vivo and its effects on AD related parameters were assessed. 17β-trenbolone accumulated in adult rat brain, especially in the hippocampus, and in the fetus brain. It altered Aβ42 accumulation...*17β-trenbolone played critical roles in neurodegeneration*. Exercisers who inject large doses of trenbolone and common people who are exposed to 17β-trenbolone by various ways are all influenced chronically and continually."[36]

Antihistamines (and anticholinergics)

Many medications, including some antihistamines, have anticholinergic[1] effects. In general, anticholinergic-induced cognitive impairment is considered reversible on discontinuation of anticholinergic therapy. However, a few studies suggest that anticholinergics may be associated with an increased risk for dementia.

In order to examine whether cumulative anticholinergic use is associated with a higher risk for dementia, researchers followed 3,434 individuals 65 years or older with no dementia at study entry. All participants were followed up every two years. Computerized pharmacy dispensing data were used to ascertain cumulative anticholinergic exposure. The researchers reported that, "The most common anticholinergic classes used were tricyclic antidepressants [such as Elavil (amitriptyline) or Sinequan (doxepin)], first-generation antihistamines [such as Benadryl (diphenhydramine)], and bladder anti-muscarinics [such a Ditropan (oxybutynin) or Detrol (tolerodine)]. During a mean follow-up of 7.3 years, 797 participants (23.2 percent) developed dementia (637 of these

---

[1]An anticholinergic agent is a substance that blocks the neurotransmitter acetylcholine in the central and the peripheral nervous system. Anticholinergics inhibit parasympathetic nerve impulses by selectively blocking the binding of the neurotransmitter acetylcholine to its receptor in nerve cells. The nerve fibers of the parasympathetic system are responsible for the involuntary movement of smooth muscles present in the gastrointestinal tract, urinary tract, lungs, etc. Anticholinergic side effects from a medication might include dry mouth, constipation, blurry vision, confusion, difficulty urinating, memory impairment, and fast heart rate.

[79.9 percent] developed Alzheimer disease)...Higher cumulative [total] anticholinergic use is associated with an increased risk for dementia. Efforts to increase awareness among health care professionals and older adults about this potential medication-related risk are important to minimize anticholinergic use over time."[37]

The above findings, published in the January 26, 2015 issue of *JAMA Internal Medicine,* showed *people were at higher risk if they took at least 10mg a day of antidepressant doxepin, 4mg a day of antihistamine diphenhydramine, or 5mg a day of oxybutynin for more than three years.* Note that a typical dose of doxepin, when used for depression, is up to 300 mg per day, and a typical dose of diphenhydramine is 25 mg per day (or up to 100 mg per day)!

Examples of common anticholinergics:

- Amytriptyline (Elavil)
- Benztropine (Cogentin)
- Chlorpheniramine (Chlor-Trimeton)
- Dicyclomine (Dicycloverine)
- Dimenhydrinate (Dramamine)
- Diphenhydramine (Benadryl, Sominex, Advil PM, etc.)
- Doxylamine (Unisom)
- Doxepin (Sinequan)
- Glycopyrrolate (Robinul)
- Hydroxyzine (Atarax, Vistaril)
- Ipratropium (Atrovent)
- Oxitropium (Oxivent)
- Oxybutynin (Ditropan, Driptane, Lyrinel XL)
- Tolterodine (Detrol, Detrusitol)
- Tiotropium (Spiriva)

Adult Asthma

In 2015, Dr. Peng and colleagues reported their findings on the risk of dementia in patients diagnosed with adult asthma compared with that of people without asthma. Using data from the National Health Insurance Research Database, a total of 12,771 patients with newly diagnosed asthma between 2001 and 2003 were evaluated and 51,084 people without asthma were used as the comparison group. They found that, *"This nationwide study suggests that the risk of dementia development is significantly increased in patients with asthma compared with that of the general population. In addition, dementia risk increases substantially with asthma exacerbation and hospitalization frequency increases."*[38]

Benzodiazepine Use

Benzodiazepines (often colloquially called "benzos") are a class of psychoactive drugs. Benzodiazepines enhance the effect of the neurotransmitter gamma-aminobutyric acid (GABA) at the $GABA_A$ receptor, resulting in sedative, hypnotic (sleep-inducing), anxiolytic (anti-anxiety), anticonvulsant, and muscle relaxant properties. High doses of many shorter-acting benzodiazepines may also cause anterograde amnesia and dissociation. These properties make benzodiazepines useful in treating anxiety, insomnia, agitation, seizures, muscle spasms, alcohol withdrawal and as a premedication for medical or dental procedures. Benzodiazepines are categorized as either short-, intermediate-, or long-acting. Short- and intermediate-acting benzodiazepines are preferred for the treatment of insomnia; longer-acting benzodiazepines are recommended for the treatment of anxiety.

While the acute effects of benzodiazepines on memory and cognition are well documented, the possibility that they increased risk of dementia is still debated. To answer this question, researchers matched 1,796 people with a diagnosis of Alzheimer's with 7,184 people over the age of 66 who did not have the condition. The researchers examined benzodiazepine use begun at least five years before the start of the study. They reported, *"Findings showed an association with increased risk of Alzheimer's disease."* Increased exposure resulted in higher risk, and the use of long-acting benzodiazepines (such as Valium or diazepam, and Klonopin or clonazepam) increased the risk, compared to short-

acting agents (such as Xanax or alprazolam, and Ativan or lorazepam).[39]

Cancer

Epidemiological studies show an inverse association between cancer and Alzheimer's disease. In order to shed light on this relationship, researchers studied 1,609 people with information on baseline cancer history and AD diagnosis, age of AD onset, and baseline MRI scans. Participants were CA positive (N = 503) and CA negative (N = 1,106) diagnosed with AD, mild cognitive impairment (MCI), significant memory concerns (SMC), and cognitively normal older adults. The researchers note that, "As in previous studies, being CA positive was inversely associated with AD at baseline; interestingly, this effect appears to be driven by non-melanoma skin cancer (NMSC), the largest cancer category in this study. Being CA positive was also associated with later age of AD onset, independent of apolipoprotein E (APOE) ε4 allele status, and individuals with two prior cancers had later mean age of AD onset than those with one or no prior cancer, suggesting an additive effect. Thus, *cancer history is associated with a measurable delay in AD onset independent of APOE ε4.*"[40]

Diabetes

Dr.Mayeda and colleagues, from the Department of Epidemiology and Biostatistics, University of California, San Francisco published a scientific paper titled Diabetes and Cognition in the February 2015 issue of the journal *Clinical Geriatric Medicine*. They stated, "Dementia is a major cause of disability and death among older adults. *Those with type 2 diabetes (T2D) are 50-100 percent more likely to develop dementia than those without T2D*...Proposed mechanisms through which T2D could cause dementia include the effects of insulin dysregulation and chronic hyperglycemia [elevated blood sugar] on features of Alzheimer's disease and macrovascular [large blood vessels] and microvascular [small blood vessels] disorders in the brain."[41]

POSSIBLE RISK FACTORS FOR ALZHEIMER'S

The relationship between diabetes and Alzheimer's disease is discussed in much more detail in the section *Diabetes*, which is under Causes and Pathology, below.

Educational Level

Several epidemiological studies have found a lower incidence of Alzheimer's disease in highly educated populations. In order to study this phenomenon, researchers performed positron emission tomography (PET) scans and conducted neuropsychological testing in thirty cognitively normal older participants. Of the participants, sixteen had a period of education less than twelve years (low-education group) and fourteen had more than thirteen years (high-education group). Amyloid-β deposition was quantified and compared between the groups with different education levels. The researchers concluded that, "Our findings indicated a reduced amyloid pathology in highly educated, cognitively normal, participants. Our findings lead to the proposal that early-life education has a negative association with Alzheimer's disease pathology...People with more education might be prone to a greater inhibitory effect against amyloid-β deposition before the preclinical stage. At the same time, they have a greater reserve capacity, and greater pathological changes are required for dementia to manifest."[42]

Electromagnetic Fields

In late 2014, researchers reported on the relationship between electromagnetic fields and Alzheimer's disease. "The extensive use of an ever increasing worldwide demand for electricity has stimulated societal and scientific interest on the environmental exposure to low frequency electromagnetic fields (EMFs) on human health. Epidemiological studies suggest a positive association between 50/60-Hz power transmission fields and leukemia or lymphoma development. Consequent to the association between EMFs and induction of oxidative stress, concerns relating to development of neurodegenerative diseases, such as Alzheimer disease (AD), have been voiced as the brain consumes the greatest fraction of oxygen and is particularly vulnerable to oxidative stress. Exposure to extremely low frequency (ELF)-EMFs are reported to alter animal behavior and modulate biological variables, including gene expression, regulation of cell survival, promotion of cellular differentiation, and changes in cerebral blood flow in aged AD transgenic mice. Alterations in inflammatory responses have also been reported, but how these actions impact human health remains unknown." Using human brain cells, the researchers evaluated the effects of an electromagnetic wave, and found clearly detrimental effects and recommended further research.[43]

However, also in late 2014, a separate group of researchers found no detrimental effects in a study of 73,051 electricity generation and transmission workers for the period 1973-2010. Detailed assessments were made of exposures to magnetic fields. The researchers concluded that, *'There is no convincing evidence that electricity generation and transmission workers have suffered elevated risks from neurodegenerative diseases as a consequence of exposure to magnetic fields.*"[44]

Still other researchers reported on the possible association between exposures to magnetic fields and Alzheimer's disease. They said, "With the development and widespread use of electromagnetic field (EMF) technology, recent studies are focusing on the effects of EMF on human health. Recently, extremely low frequency electromagnetic fields (ELF-EMF) have been studied with great interest due to their possible effects on Alzheimer's disease (AD). The objective of the present study was to investigate the interaction between ELF-EMF exposure and memory impairment in rats...*The present study indicated that short-term exposure of 100 µT/50 Hz ELF-EMF had no effects on cognition and memory of rats, and did not alter the expression of Aβ and the neuron morphology.* However, more comprehensive studies are still required to elucidate the possible effects and underlying mechanisms of ELF-EMF exposure on living organisms."[45]

POSSIBLE RISK FACTORS FOR ALZHEIMER'S

Female Gender

The Alzheimer's Association recently reported that a woman's estimated lifetime risk of developing Alzheimer's at age 65 is 1 in 6, compared to nearly 1 in 11 for a man (i.e., female to male ratio 1.8).

Glaucoma

Glaucoma[1] is the leading cause of irreversible blindness worldwide and primary open-angle glaucoma (POAG) is the most common type of glaucoma. An association between POAG and the subsequent risk of Alzheimer's disease (AD) and Parkinson's disease (PD) was investigated by researchers. They studied a group of patients with and without POAG aged 60 years and older. They concluded that, "In elderly patients, *POAG is a significant predictor of AD*, but POAG is not a predictor of PD."[46]

SATNAV or GPS

A satellite navigation (SATNAV) or global positioning system (GPS) is a system of satellites that provide autonomous geo-spatial positioning with global coverage. It allows small electronic receivers to determine their location (longitude, latitude, and altitude) to high precision (within a few meters) using time signals transmitted along a line of sight by radio from satellites. The signals also allow the electronic receivers to calculate the current local time to high precision, which allows time synchronization. A satellite navigation system with global coverage may be termed a global navigation satellite system (GNSS). As of April 2013, only the United States NAVSTAR Global Position-

---

[1]Glaucoma is a term describing a group of ocular (eye) disorders resulting in optic nerve damage or loss to the field of vision, in many patients caused by a clinically characterized pressure buildup in regards to the fluid of the eye. In a large number of glaucoma patients, however, the intraocular pressure (IOP) is normal, i.e. below 20 mm Hg. These patients display the same signs of glaucomatous damage as those with an elevated IOP; their condition is thus called normal tension glaucoma.

ing System (GPS) and the Russian GLONASS are global operational GNSSs.

According to several research studies, over-reliance on these systems can be detrimental to one's memory:[47]

> "Can't recall a friend's phone number? Press the speed dial on your mobile. Don't know the way to their house? Use a satnav. Modern technology has taken the strain off our brains with the answers to so many problems available at the click of a button. But is there a dark side to all this convenience? Growing scientific evidence suggests a future where our brains may prematurely fail in later life through under-use, thanks to Mother Nature's rule that we 'use it or lose it.'
>
> You might describe this new threat to our mental health as 'e-mentia' - memory-related problems, and even depression, linked to our overuse of new technology.
>
> Some of the most worrying evidence regarding the problems we may be storing up for later relate to navigation aids. Research published in April 2011 shows our growing use of satnavs relieves us of using the brain's sophisticated capacity for mapping surroundings as we pass them and building those impressions into a mental picture.
>
> Dr. Rosamund Langston, a lecturer in neuroscience at the University of Dundee who conducted the study, said that by using satnavs, we wither away our 'caveman' ability to familiarize ourselves with new surroundings by memorizing snapshots of them.
>
> The disturbing thing is what happens--or more pertinently what doesn't happen--in our brain when we rely on an electronic arrow to lead us through the world. Last June,

POSSIBLE RISK FACTORS FOR ALZHEIMER'S

Dr Hugo Spiers, a senior lecturer in experimental psychology at University College London, scanned volunteers' brains as they navigated the maze of streets in Soho, Central London. Dr Spiers's scans revealed how we use two distinct areas of our brain to achieve this highly complex feat of mental calculation.

At the beginning of a journey, a region of the brain called the entorhinal cortex mentally constructs an as-the-crow-flies line to the destination. Once we are underway, however, a different area of the brain computes the precise distance along the path to get there. This region is the posterior hippocampus, which is also known for its role in forming memory. Disturbingly, the study, published in the journal *Current Biology*, found that neither of these brain regions was active when the volunteers used satnavs. In fact, the volunteers' brains were much less active in general.

Previous studies have shown how London taxi drivers who have done 'the knowledge' show an increase in the size of their hippocampus as a consequence of rote-learning the city's streetscape. Dr. Spiers, a member of the Memory Disorders Research Society, says his results may explain why London taxi drivers' brains grow: 'They indicate that it is the daily demand on processing paths in their posterior hippocampus that leads to the impressive expansion in their grey matter.'

Dr. Spiers told Good Health how this part of the brain, so vital to memory, may also shrink with disuse--such as relying on satnavs. 'My research with taxi drivers found indications which suggest there is some shrinkage of their hippocampus after they retire,' he explained.

Gout

It has been suggested that oxidative stress has a role in the pathogenesis or cause of Alzheimer's disease. Gout is caused by high levels of uric acid (UA). Uric acid has a positive effect on cognitive function and several lines of evidence suggest that UA may modulate outcome in neurological diseases. To study this relationship, researchers measured blood levels of UA in 41 AD patients and forty healthy controls. The researchers found that, "Demographic variables indicate that *individuals that are illiterate demonstrate a 7.5 fold increase in risk of developing AD*. The AD group shows 12.6 percent lower serum UA level than control subjects and the difference between groups is statistically significant...The results suggest that serum UA levels are significantly lower in AD patients in comparison to control subjects. *UA may have a protective role against AD*; however this role needs further investigations."[48]

Heavy Metal Exposure

A heavy metal is any metal of environmental concern. The term originated with reference to the harmful effects of cadmium, mercury and lead, all of which are denser than iron. It has since been applied to any other similarly toxic metal, such as arsenic, regardless of density. *Commonly encountered heavy metals are chromium, cobalt, nickel, copper, zinc, arsenic, selenium, silver, cadmium, antimony, mercury, thallium and lead.*

Environmental pollutants act as risk factors for Alzheimer's disease. In an animal model, researchers investigated early manifestations of AD-like pathology by a mixture of arsenic (As), cadmium (Cd), and lead (Pb), reported to impair neurodevelopment. They found that exposure to these heavy metals caused a dose-dependent[1] increase in amyloid-

---

[1]The dose–response relationship describes the change in effect on an organism caused by differing levels of exposure (or doses) to a stressor (usually a chemical) after a certain exposure time. This often means that a higher dose results in a greater effect. However, this relationship is frequently nonlinear (variable).

beta (Aβ) in specific parts of the brain, including the area were memories are formed (hippocampus). "The effect was strongly significant during early-adulthood...Investigating the mechanism of Aβ-induction revealed an augmentation in oxidative stress-dependent neuroinflammation...We then examined the effects of individual metals and mixture. Among individual metals, Pb [lead] triggered maximum induction of Aβ, whereas individual As [arsenic] or Cd [cadmium] had a relatively non-significant effect. Interestingly, when combined, the metals demonstrated synergism, with a major contribution by As. Eventually, increase in Aβ culminated in cognitive impairments in the young rats. Together, our data demonstrate that exposure to As+Cd+Pb induces premature manifestation of AD-like pathology that is synergistic, and oxidative stress and inflammation dependent."[49]

Researchers evaluated the levels of some of the most investigated metals (copper or Cu, selenium or Se, zinc or Zn, lead or Pb, and mercury or Hg) in the blood of patients affected by the most common chronic neurodegenerative diseases like Alzheimer's disease and multiple sclerosis (MS), in order to better clarify their involvement. "For the first time, we investigated a Sicilian population living in an area exposed to a potentially contaminated environment from dust and fumes of volcano Etna and consumer of a considerable quantity of fish in their diet, so that this represents a good cohort to demonstrate a possible link between metals levels and development of neurodegenerative disorders." They studied fifteen patients affected by AD, forty-one patients affected by MS, twenty-three healthy controls, and ten healthy elderly controls. The results of the study showed that higher levels of heavy metals were found in patients with AD, more than in other neurodegenerative pathologies, such as MS. They also determined that, in this particular study location, blood concentrations of these heavy metals were independent from the diet, but related to possible exposure to contaminated environment due both to occupation and place of residence.[50]

Arsenic toxicity is a worldwide health concern as several millions of people are exposed to this toxicant via drinking water, and exposure affects almost every organ system in the body including the brain. Recent studies have shown that even low concentrations of arsenic impair neurological function, particularly in children. Researchers from the Department of Neuroscience, University of New Mexico School of Medicine, Albuquerque, NM reviewed the scientific literature relevant to arsenic toxicity and documented a wide variety of pathologic processes caused by arsenic. Interestingly, they also discussed therapeutic strategies to combat arsenic toxicity, including the use of selenium and zinc."[51]

Dr. Mutter and colleagues reviewed the scientific literature related to the toxic effects of mercury and published their finding in the *Journal of Alzheimer's Disease*. They stated, "*Mercury is one of the most toxic substances known to humans*. It has been introduced into the human environment and has also been widely used in medicine. Circumstantial evidence exists that the pathology of Alzheimer's disease might be in part caused or exacerbated by mercury…Thirty-two studies, out of forty testing memory in individuals exposed to mercury, found significant memory deficits. Some autopsy studies found increased mercury levels in brain tissues of AD patients. Measurements of mercury levels in blood, urine, hair, nails, and cerebrospinal fluid were inconsistent. In vitro models showed that mercury reproduces all pathological changes seen in AD, and in animal models mercury produced changes that are similar to those seen in AD. Mercury may play a role as a co-factor in the development of AD. It may also increase the pathological influence of other metals. As the single most effective public health primary preventive measure, industrial, and medical usage of mercury should be eliminated as soon as possible."[52]

Other researchers note, "The homeostasis of *essential metals such as copper, iron, selenium and zinc* may be altered in the brain of subjects with Alzheimer's disease." In order to study the effects of various metals, they measured the concentrations of metals (magnesium, calcium, vanadium, manganese, iron, cobalt, nickel, copper, zinc, selenium, rubidium, strontium, molybdenum, cadmium, tin, antimony, cesium, mercury and lead) in blood and cerebrospinal fluid (CSF) in 173 patients with AD and in 87 patients with the combination of AD and minor vascular components (AD + vascular). Comparison was made with

POSSIBLE RISK FACTORS FOR ALZHEIMER'S

54 healthy controls. The major finding of the study was that patients with Alzheimer's disease had elevated blood mercury concentrations.[53]

Results of research by Dr. Drevnick and colleagues from the University of Michigan, reported February 2, 2015, found that levels of mercury in Hawaiian yellowfin tuna are increasing. Mercury is a potent toxin that can accumulate to high concentrations in fish, posing a health risk to people who eat large, predatory marine fish such as swordfish and tuna. In the open ocean, the principal source of mercury is atmospheric deposition from human activities, especially emissions from coal-fired power plants and gold mining. The researchers found that the concentration of mercury in yellowfin tuna increased at least 3.8 percent per year from 1998 to 2008 (the last year of the study). According to Dr. Drevick, "Mercury levels are increasing globally in ocean water, and our study is the first to show a consequent increase in mercury in an open-water fish. More stringent policies are needed to reduce releases of mercury into the atmosphere. If current deposition rates are maintained, North Pacific waters will double in mercury by 2050."[54]

Aluminum (Al) is a ubiquitous substance encountered both naturally (as the third most abundant element) and intentionally (used in water, foods, pharmaceuticals, and vaccines); it is also present in ambient and occupational airborne particulates. Researchers reviewed the scientific literature on the health effects of aluminum and reported their findings in 2014. They stated that, "Wide variations in diet can result in Al intakes that are often higher than the World Health Organization provisional tolerable weekly intake (PTWI)... Aluminum has been held responsible for human morbidity and mortality, but there is no consistent and convincing evidence to associate the Al found in food and drinking water at the doses and chemical forms presently consumed by people living in North America and Western Europe with increased risk for Alzheimer's disease. Neither is there clear evidence to show use of Al-containing underarm antiperspirants or cosmetics increases the risk of AD or breast cancer. Aluminum exposures during neonatal and pediatric parenteral nutrition (PN) can impair bone mineralization and delay neurological development. Adverse effects to vaccines with Al adjuvants have occurred; however, recent controlled trials found that the immunologic response to certain vaccines with Al adjuvants was no greater, and in some cases less than that after identical vaccination without Al adjuvants. The scientific literature on the adverse health effects of Al is extensive. Health risk assessments for Al must take into account individual co-factors (e.g., age, renal function, diet, gastric pH). Conclusions from the current review point to the need for refinement of the PTWI, reduction of Al contamination in PN solutions, justification for routine addition of Al to vaccines, and harmonization of OELs for Al substances."[55]

Herpes Simplex Virus (HSV)

Herpes simplex virus 1 (HSV-1)[1] has long been suspected to play a role in the cause of AD because of its effect on nerve cells, high rate of infection in the general population, and life-long persistence in nerve cells, particularly in the same brain regions that are usually altered in AD. It is proposed that virus is normally latent in many elderly brains but reactivates periodically (as in the peripheral nervous system) under certain conditions, for example stress, immuno-suppression, and peripheral infection, causing cumulative damage and eventually development of AD. Diverse approaches have provided data that explicitly support, directly or indirectly, these concepts.[57]

In order to study this relationship, researchers compared blood samples from 360 AD cases (75.3 percent women, mean age 61.2 years) and 360 age- and sex-matched dementia-free controls, taken on average 9.6 years before AD diagnosis. They concluded that, "Among persons with a follow-up time of 6.6 years or more, *HSV infection was significantly associated with AD.*"[58]

---

[1]Herpes simplex virus 1 and 2 (HSV-1 and HSV-2 are two members of the herpesvirus family, Herpesviridae, that infect humans. Both HSV-1 (which produces most cold sores) and HSV-2 (which produces most genital herpes) are very common and contagious.

POSSIBLE RISK FACTORS FOR ALZHEIMER'S

Height

That risk factors measured in middle age may not fully explain future dementia risk implicates exposures acting earlier in life. Height may capture early-life illness, adversity, nutrition and psychosocial stress. In order to investigate the little-explored association between height and dementia death further, researchers conducted a literature review of this topic. They reviewed eighteen general population studies (1994-2008; n = 181,800). Over an average follow-up of 9.8 years, there were 426 and 667 dementia deaths in men and women respectively. The mean heights were 174.4 cm for men and 161.0 cm for women. *Analysis revealed that increasing height was related to lower rates of death from dementia. They also found that the association observed in men was markedly stronger than that apparent in women. The researchers concluded that, "Early-life circumstances, indexed by adult height, may influence later dementia risk."*[59]

High Fat Diet

Mid-life hypercholesterolemia[1] is a risk factor for the development of Alzheimer's disease. Maternal obesity is associated with the development of obesity, hypertension and hypercholesterolemia in adulthood, suggesting that the risk for AD may also be influenced by early life environment. Researchers used an animal model to see if early life exposure to a high fat diet results in failure of Aβ amyloid (characteristic of AD) clearance from the brain. They also assessed if Aβ deposition is greater in the brains of aged humans with a history of hyperlipidemia, compared to age-matched controls with normal lipidemia. They stated, "Using a mouse model of maternal obesity, we found that exposure to a high fat diet during gestation and lactation induced changes in multiple components of the neurovascular [nerve-blood vessel] unit…Sustained high fat diet over the entire lifespan resulted in additional clearance of Aβ from the brain. In humans, vascular Aβ load was significantly in-

---

[1]Hypercholesterolemia (also called dyslipidemia) is the presence of high levels of cholesterol in the blood. It is a form of "hyperlipidemia" (elevated levels of lipids in the blood).

creased in the brains of aged individuals with a history of hypercholesterolemia. These results support a critical role for early dietary influence on the brain vasculature across the lifespan, with consequences for the development of age-related cerebrovascular and neurodegenerative diseases."[60] Translation: *a high fat diet contributes to the development of Alzheimer's disease, and this detrimental effect may begin in infancy.*

Inbreeding

Dr. Vardarajan and colleagues from the Taub Institute for Research on Alzheimer's disease and the Aging Brain, Columbia University, New York, New York, reported in the November 13, 2014 issue of *Genetic Medicine* on the relationship between inbreeding and Alzheimer's disease. They reported that, "We estimated the inbreeding coefficient in Caribbean Hispanics and examined its effects on risk of late-onset Alzheimer's disease. The inbreeding coefficient was calculated in 3,392 subjects (1,451 late-onset Alzheimer's disease patients and 1,941 age-matched healthy controls) of Caribbean Hispanic ancestry...the average inbreeding coefficient was found to close to third-cousin mating. Inbreeding coefficient was a significant predictor of Alzheimer's disease."[61]

Infections

The development of Alzheimer's disease is a multi-factorial process that may also involve infection with different bacteria. Recent studies suggest that bacteria have the potential to initiate a cascade of events, leading to inflammatory condition of the central nervous system. Infection with these organisms may be considered a risk factor for development of AD or to cognitive changes. Recent studies have revealed that exposure to these microorganisms induces Aβ accumulation and tau protein phosphorylation, and chronic infections with these pathogenic bacteria can possibly contribute to progression of AD. Controlling these chronic infections with antibacterial or anti-inflammatory drugs will allow preventing inflammation, a risk factor for AD.[62]

POSSIBLE RISK FACTORS FOR ALZHEIMER'S

Neurodegenerative diseases may be caused by chronic viral infections and may result in a loss of brain cells in the central nervous system that increases with age. To date, there is evidence of systemic viral infections that occur with some neurodegenerative conditions such as Alzheimer's disease, Parkinson's disease, amyotrophic lateral sclerosis, multiple sclerosis, autism spectrum disorders, and HIV-associated neuro-cognitive disorders. With increasing lifespan, the incidence of neurodegenerative diseases increases consistently. In addition to established non-viral-induced reasons for neurodegenerative diseases, viruses associated with neurodegenerative diseases have been proposed. Neuronal degeneration can be either directly or indirectly affected by viral infection. Viruses that attack the human immune system can also affect the nervous system and interfere with classical pathways of neurodegenerative diseases.[63]

Researchers reported in the August 8, 2014 issue of the *Journal of Infectious Disease* that, "Human cytomegalovirus (CMV)[1] is prevalent in older adults and has been implicated in many chronic diseases of aging. This study investigated the relation between CMV and the risk of Alzheimer's disease. Data come from three studies that included 849 participants (mean age 78.6 years). Of 849 participants, 73.4 percent had serologic evidence of exposure to CMV. During an average of five years of follow-up, 93 persons developed AD. CMV seropositivity was associated with an increased risk of AD. These results suggest that CMV infection is associated with an increased risk of AD and a faster rate of cognitive decline in older populations."[64]

---

[1]*Human cytomegalovirus* (HCMV or CMV) is a member of the viral family known as herpes viruses. HCMV infection is typically unnoticed in healthy people, but can be life-threatening for the immuno-compromised, such as HIV-infected persons, organ transplant recipients, or newborn infants. After infection, HCMV remains latent within the body throughout life and can be reactivated at any time. Congenital HCMV is the leading infectious cause of deafness, learning disabilities, and mental retardation in children. CMV also seems to have a large impact on immune parameters in later life and may contribute to increased morbidity and eventual mortality.

Another group of researchers reported in the July 30, 2014 issue of the *Journal of Alzheimer's disease* that, "Abnormal hyperphosphorylation of microtubule-associated protein tau is involved in the pathogenesis of several neurodegenerative disorders including Alzheimer's disease. Helicobacter pylori (H. pylori) infection [the bacteria that causes "stomach" ulcers] has been reported to be related with a high risk of AD...Our data provide evidence supporting the role of H. pylori infection in AD-like tau pathology, suggesting that H. pylori eradication may be beneficial in the prevention of tauopathy [and AD]."[65]

Other researchers reviewed the literature concerning the relationship between Helicobacter pylori (H. pylori) and Alzheimer's disease. They noted that, "...the infection was significantly associated with higher risk of developing dementia...Moreover, in another study evaluating the effect of H. pylori eradication on the progression of dementia in Alzheimer's disease, in patients with peptic ulcer, the cure of the bacterium was associated with a decreased risk of dementia progression compared to persistent infection."[66]

Lack of Purpose in Life

During up to seven years of follow-up (average, 4.0 years), 155 of 951 persons (16.3 percent) developed AD. Greater purpose in life was associated with a substantially reduced risk of AD. They found that, "A person with a high score on the purpose in life measure (score = 4.2, 90th percentile) was approximately 2.4 times more likely to remain free of AD than was a person with a low score (score = 3.0, 10th percentile). This association did not vary along demographic lines and persisted after the addition of terms for depressive symptoms, neuroticism, social network size, and number of chronic medical conditions...Greater purpose in life is associated with a reduced risk of AD and MCI in community-dwelling older persons."[67]

POSSIBLE RISK FACTORS FOR ALZHEIMER'S

Loneliness

The authors reviewed the relationship between loneliness and mental health. They reported that, "Human beings are social species which require safe and secure social surroundings to survive. Satisfying social relationships are essential for mental and physical well being. Impaired social relationship can lead to loneliness. Since the dawn of time, loneliness is perceived as a global human phenomenon. *Loneliness can lead to various psychiatric disorders like depression, alcohol abuse, child abuse, sleep problems, personality disorders and Alzheimer's disease.* It also leads to various physical disorders like diabetes, autoimmune disorders like rheumatoid arthritis, lupus and cardiovascular diseases like coronary heart disease, hypertension (HTN), obesity, physiological aging, cancer, poor hearing and poor health. Left untended, loneliness can have serious consequences for mental and physical health of people. Therefore it is important to intervene at the right time to prevent loneliness, so that physical and mental health of patients is maintained."[68]

Low Testosterone

Dr. Jayaraman and colleagues reported in the September 16, 2014 issue of the *Journal of Neuroinflammation* that, "Low testosterone and obesity are independent risk factors for dysfunction of the nervous system including neurodegenerative disorders such as Alzheimer's disease. In this study, we investigate the independent and cooperative interactions of testosterone and diet-induced obesity on metabolic, inflammatory, and neural health indices in the central and peripheral nervous systems." They used an animal model to study these relationships. They noted that, "Our results demonstrate that detrimental effects on both metabolic (blood glucose, insulin sensitivity) and pro-inflammatory responses caused by diet-induced obesity are exacerbated by testosterone depletion. In addition, low testosterone and diet-induced obesity combine to increase inflammation and evidence of nerve damage in the peripheral nervous system...Testosterone and diet-induced obesity independently and cooperatively regulate neuro-inflammation in central and peripheral nervous systems, which may contribute to observed impairments in neural health. Together, our findings suggest *that low testosterone and obesity are interactive regulators of neuro-inflammation that increase the risk of disorders including type 2 diabetes and Alzheimer's disease.*"[69]

Mental Issues

Researchers reported in the October 21, 2014 issue of *Neurology* the results of their study of the association between midlife neuroticism and extraversion and development of late-life dementia and long-standing distress in a sample of women followed for thirty-eight years. "A population-based sample of 800 women, aged thirty-eight to fifty-four years, was examined in 1968, with subsequent examinations in 1974, 1980, 1992, 2000, and 2005. During the 38-year follow-up, 153 women developed dementia; Alzheimer disease dementia was diagnosed in 104 of these. A higher degree of neuroticism in midlife was associated with increased risk of AD dementia and long-standing distress over thirty-eight years. The association between neuroticism and AD dementia diminished after adjusting for long-standing distress. Extraversion was associated with a lower degree of long-standing distress, but had no impact on AD dementia. When the two personality dimensions were combined, high neuroticism/low extraversion showed the highest risk of AD dementia. Our study suggests that *midlife neuroticism is associated with increased risk of AD dementia, and that distress mediates this association.*"[70]

Mild cognitive impairment (MCI) can be a prodromal stage of Alzheimer's disease. It is particularly relevant to focus on prodromal stages of AD such as MCI, because patho-physiological abnormalities of AD start years before the dementia stage. Researchers used magnetic resonance imaging (MRI) to study the brains of persons with MCI while also studying personality changes, because an increase in neuroticism and a decrease in conscientiousness have been reported in persons with MCI. This suggests that higher and lower scores, respectively, in neuroticism and conscientiousness are associated with an increased risk of developing AD. The researchers found a strong association between *"...specific abnormalities (white matter lesions[1], but not atrophy) on MRI scans and lower levels of conscientiousness and higher levels of neuroticism."*[71]

In order to examine the association of mid-life psychiatric disorders with the development of late-life dementia, researchers reviewed recorders, "...using Western Australian state-wide hospital inpatient, outpatient mental health and emergency records linked to death records. Incident dementia cases (2000-2009) aged sixty-five to eighty-four years were sex- and age-matched to an electoral roll control. Records as far back as 1970 were used to assess exposure to medical risk factors before age sixty-five years. Candidate psychiatric risk factors were required to be present at least ten years before dementia onset. A total of 13,568 dementia cases (median age 78.7 years, 43.4 percent male) were matched to a control. Depression, bipolar disorder, schizophrenia, anxiety disorder and alcohol dependence were found to be significant and independent risk factors for late-life dementia after adjusting for diabetes, heart disease, cerebrovascular disease and smoking risk factors. "The effect of a history of depression, schizophrenia and alcohol dependency on dementia risk varied with age, being strongest for earlier onset late-life dementia and waning at older ages. *Severe depression, anxiety disorder, bipolar disorder, schizophrenia and alcoholic dependency disorder treated by specialists in psychiatric facilities in mid-life are important risk factors for late-life dementia."*[72]

Obesity

Obesity is a medical condition in which excess body fat has accumulated to the extent that it may have a negative effect on health, leading to reduced life expectancy and/or increased health problems. In Western

---

[1]Leukoaraiosis or white matter hyperintensities (WMHs) describes the nonspecific changes in the cerebral white matter frequently seen on CT and MRI in aged individuals and even young adults sometimes. It is a condition routinely found in elderly people.

countries, people are considered obese when their body mass index (BMI), a measurement obtained by dividing a person's weight by the square of the person's height, exceeds 30 kg/m^2, with the range 25-30 kg/m^2 defined as overweight.

The association between body mass index (BMI) and cognition is complex: in younger adults, higher BMIs are associated with impaired cognition. Overweight and obesity in middle age are linked to increased future dementia risk in old age. However, when examined in old age, higher BMIs are associated with better cognition and decreased mortality. Little is known about the optimal BMI for well-being and survival in populations already suffering from dementia. Researchers note, *"Lifetime trends in weight, rather than single measures, might predict prognosis better and help untangle these apparent contradictions."*[73]

According to a review of the association between obesity and Alzheimer's disease, published in the September 13, 2014 issue of *Lancet Neurology*, "Being overweight or obese, as measured with body-mass index (BMI) or central adiposity (waist circumference), and the trajectory of body-mass index over the life course have been associated with brain atrophy, white matter changes, disturbances of blood-brain barrier integrity, and risk of all-cause late-onset dementia and Alzheimer's disease."[74]

Increasing evidence supports the idea that chronic low blood flow (hypo-perfusion) in the brain is associated with the pathology underling Alzheimer's disease. Obesity at midlife is associated with the risk of cognitive loss and AD at later life. Obesity decreases brain blood flow, which is in turn related to specific metabolic abnormalities related to AD. Researchers report that, "Obesity-induced endothelial [blood vessel] dysfunction and cerebral [brain] hypo-perfusion [low blood flow] enhance the production of β-amyloid that in turn impairs endothelial [blood vessel] function; this vicious cycle promotes the pathogenic changes leading to AD. Interrupting this cycle…is expected to promote prophylaxis against AD pathogenesis… therapeutic measures, including physical exercise, nutritionally adequate dietary intake, pharmacological treatments such as acetylcholinesterase inhibitors [such at

POSSIBLE RISK FACTORS FOR ALZHEIMER'S

Aricept and Namenda], antioxidants, and bariatric[1] surgery that are efficient in protecting and retarding the progress of cognitive failure and neuro-degeneration [are possible treatment strategies]."[75]

Obesity rates have been increasing dramatically and obesity is an independent risk factor for AD. Researchers studied an animal model of AD and the effects of a high calorie diet (HCD). They found that a HCD induced changes in the brain associated with AD as well as obesity. The researchers summarized their findings by noting that obesity caused elevated inflammation in the brain, consequently accelerating tau pathology, which is one of the characteristic pathological changes in Alzheimer's disease.[76]

Mild cognitive impairment (MCI), often considered an early stage of dementia, is heterogeneous, and not all subjects with MCI progress into clinically diagnosed dementia. *Low body weight* (and body mass index, BMI) as well as losing weight while having MCI have been proposed as possible risk factors of MCI-to-dementia conversion. In order to study this relationship, researchers conducted a two-year study of 102 MCI subjects. Data on 83 out of the originally included 102 subjects were available after two years; twenty-seven of those (32.5 percent) progressed to dementia. Analysis revealed that, among other things, lower baseline BMI (and losing weight on 2-year follow-up) were associated with conversion to dementia. Apathetic subjects had lower BMI and higher weight loss. The authors concluded that, "MCI subjects presenting with apathy, low initial BMI and losing weight on follow-up have a significantly greater risk of developing dementia."[77]

Osteoporosis

---

[1]Bariatric surgery (weight loss surgery) includes a variety of procedures performed on people who have obesity. Weight loss is achieved by reducing the size of the stomach with a gastric band or through removal of a portion of the stomach (sleeve gastrectomy or biliopancreatic diversion with duodenal switch) or by resecting and rerouting the small intestine to a small stomach pouch (gastric bypass surgery).

Osteoporosis is a progressive bone disease that is characterized by a decrease in bone mass and density which can lead to an increased risk of fracture. Researchers studied the relationship between low bone mineral density (BMD) and conversion from mild cognitive impairment (MCI) to Alzheimer's disease in a group of men and women (n=946), aged 60-75, who were followed annually for five years. *They found that there was a positive relationship between osteoporosis and a decline in cognition and function* (measured by activities of daily living or ADLs). The subjects with BMD values in the lowest quartile[1] had a 2-fold increased risk of AD conversion compared with the controls. The authors concluded that, *"Osteoporosis was associated with an increased risk of AD dementia. Additionally, low BMD at baseline was associated with an increased risk of AD in both women and men."*[78]

Periodontitis

Periodontitis is a set of inflammatory diseases affecting the periodontium (i.e., the tissues that surround and support the teeth). Periodontitis involves progressive loss of the bone around the teeth, and if left untreated, can lead to the loosening and subsequent loss of teeth. Periodontitis is caused by microorganisms that adhere to and grow on the tooth's surfaces, along with an over-aggressive immune response against these microorganisms.

Neuro-inflammation--inflammation of the brain, is strongly implicated in Alzheimer's disease, which can be enhanced by systemic inflammation. Therefore, the initiation and progression of AD are affected by systemic diseases such as cardiovascular disease and diabetes. This concept suggests a possible link between periodontitis and AD because periodontitis is a peripheral, chronic infection that elicits a significant systemic inflammatory response. There is now growing clinical evidence that chronic periodontitis is closely linked to the initiation and progression of AD. It is estimated that a high percentage of adults are suffering from periodontitis, and the prevalence of periodontitis in-

---

[1]The lowest (or fourth) quarter of the data.

creases with age. Therefore, chronic periodontitis can be a significant source of covert systemic inflammation within the general population.[79]

To compare periodontal health status in individuals with and without Alzheimer's disease, researchers studied fifty-eight individuals with AD and sixty cognitively normal (ND) adult individuals, ranging in age from fifty to eighty years, who were assessed for periodontal health status. Individuals with AD were further divided as mild, moderate, and severe. In 2014, they reported that, "All the evaluated periodontal parameters were higher in individuals with AD than that in ND individuals, and the periodontal status deteriorated with the progression of AD. *The periodontal health status of individuals with AD deteriorates with disease progression and was closely related to their cognitive function.*"[80]

Dr. Kamer and sixteen colleagues reported in the November 5, 2014 issue of *Neurobiology of Aging* on research of the relationship between periodontal disease and Alzheimer's disease. They noted that, "The accumulation of amyloid-β (Aβ) plaques is a central feature of Alzheimer's disease (AD). First reported in animal models, it remains uncertain if peripheral inflammatory and/or infectious conditions in humans can promote Aβ brain accumulation. Periodontal disease, a common chronic infection, has been previously reported to be associated with AD." The researchers studied thirty-eight cognitively normal, healthy, and community-residing elderly (mean age, 61 and 68 percent female) to test the hypothesis that periodontal disease, assessed by clinical attachment loss, was associated with brain Aβ load, using positron emission tomography (PET) imaging. The found that, "clinical attachment loss (≥3 mm), representing a history of periodontal inflammatory/infectious burden, was associated with increased PIB uptake in Aβ vulnerable brain regions. *We show for the first time in humans an association between periodontal disease and brain Aβ load. These data are consistent with the previous animal studies showing that peripheral inflammation/infections are sufficient to produce brain Aβ accumulations.*"[81]

Pesticides

Researchers from the Environmental Chemistry and Toxicology Laboratory, Department of Environmental Science, Policy, and Management, University of California, Berkeley, California reviewed the potential risk of developing Alzheimer's disease or Parkinson's disease due to exposure to pesticides. They concluded in 2013 that, *"Possible associations between pesticides and Parkinson's and Alzheimer's diseases are proposed but not established* based on epidemiological observations and mechanistic considerations."[82]

However, in 2014, Dr. Richardson, from the Department of Environmental and Occupational Medicine, Rutgers Robert Wood Johnson Medical School, Piscataway, New Jersey, and colleagues, reported the following in the journal *JAMA Neurology*:[83]

> "Alzheimer's disease is the most common neurodegenerative disease worldwide and cases are expected to increase 3-fold over the next 40 years. The most common form of AD is the late-onset form, which typically develops after 60 years of age. The etiological factors of late-onset AD are not yet completely understood but include genetic, environmental, and lifestyle factors that influence a person's risk for developing the disease. Although there is a growing list of AD susceptibility genes, only having an apolipoprotein E4 (*APOE4*) allele has a relatively strong effect (relative risk approximately 2-3), and, cumulatively, the more than ten genes identified thus far account for only less than half of AD cases. To our knowledge, few studies have explored the potential of environmental exposures to contribute to AD, but occupational exposure to metals, solvents, and pesticide is reported to be a potential environmental contributor. Previously, we reported that serum levels of p,p'-dichlorodiphenyldichloroethylene (DDE), a metabolite of the organochlorine pesticide dichlorodiphenyltrichloroethane (DDT), were significantly higher in a small co-

hort (n = 20) of patients with AD compared with control participants, and that there was a significant association between DDE levels and a diagnosis of AD.

In the present study, we evaluated the associations between serum DDE levels, AD, and Mini-Mental State Examination (MMSE) scores in a larger number of cases and control participants from two geographical sites, and we explored differential susceptibility by *APOE4* genotype status. We also examined the relationship between brain and serum levels of DDE and whether DDT or DDE alters the expression of the amyloid precursor protein (APP) in cultured neuronal cells.

[The research was] A case-control study consisting of existing samples from patients with AD and control participants from the Emory University Alzheimer's Disease Research Center and the University of Texas Southwestern Medical School's Alzheimer's Disease Center. Serum levels of DDE were measured in 79 control and 86 AD cases.

Levels of DDE were 3.8-fold higher in the serum of those with AD when compared with control participants. The highest tertile of DDE levels was associated with an odds ratio of 4.18 for increased risk for AD and lower Mini-Mental State Examination scores. The Mini-Mental State Examination scores in the highest tertile of DDE were −1.753 points lower in the subpopulation carrying an *APOE* ε4 allele compared with those carrying an *APOE* ε3 allele. Serum levels of DDE were highly correlated with brain levels of DDE. Exposure of human neuro-blastoma cells to DDT or DDE increased levels of amyloid precursor protein.

[In conclusion] *Elevated serum DDE levels are associated with an increased risk for AD and carriers of an*

APOE4 ε4 allele may be more susceptible to the effects of DDE. Both DDT and DDE increase amyloid precursor protein levels, providing mechanistic plausibility for the association of DDE exposure with AD. Identifying people who have elevated levels of DDE and carry an APOE ε4 allele may lead to early identification of some cases of AD."

Pollution

Several studies with animal research associate air pollution in Alzheimer's disease (AD) neuropathology. Researchers investigated the relationship between long-term exposure to ozone (O3) and particulate matter (PM) and newly diagnosed AD. They studied 95,690 individuals age 65 or older during 2001-2010. They discovered a clear and more severe detrimental effect with increasing levels of pollution. They concluded that, *"These findings suggest long-term exposure to O3 and PM above the current US EPA standards are associated with increased risk of AD.*[84] The people in Beijing, the capital of China, should be really worried, as there air pollution is extreme!

In late 2014, researchers from Mexico, the United States, and Canada summarized the concerns about air pollution as follows:[85]

> "Research links air pollution mostly to respiratory and cardiovascular disease. The effects of air pollution on the central nervous system (CNS) are not broadly recognized. Urban outdoor pollution is a global public health problem particularly severe in megacities and in underdeveloped countries, but large and small cities in the United States and the United Kingdom are not spared. *Fine and ultrafine particulate matter pose a special interest for the brain effects given the capability of very small particles to reach the brain. In adults, ambient pollution is associated to stroke and depression, whereas the emerging picture in children show significant sys-*

POSSIBLE RISK FACTORS FOR ALZHEIMER'S

temic inflammation, immunodysregulation at systemic, intratechal and brain levels, neuro-inflammation and brain oxidative stress, along with the main hallmarks of Alzheimer and Parkinson's diseases: hyperphosphorilated tau, amyloid plaques and misfolded α-synuclein. Animal models exposed to particulate matter components show markers of both neuro-inflammation and neuro-degeneration. Epidemiological, cognitive, behavioral and mechanistic studies into the association between air pollution exposures and the development of CNS damage particularly in children are of pressing importance for public health and quality of life. Primary health providers have to include a complete prenatal and postnatal environmental and occupational history to indoor and outdoor toxic hazards and measures should be taken to prevent or reduce further exposures."

Relatives With Alzheimer's Disease

A positive family history (FH) raises the risk for late-onset Alzheimer's disease though, other than the known risk conferred by apolipoprotein ε4 (ApoE4), much of the genetic variance remains unexplained. In order to study this relationship, researchers examined the effect of family history on brain atrophy (shrinkage) rates in 184 subjects (mean age 79.9; FH+ in 42 percent) with mild cognitive impairment (MCI), over a period of four years. The researchers stated, "We conclude that a positive family history of AD may influence cortical and temporal lobe [brain] atrophy in subjects with mild cognitive impairment, *but it does not have a significant additional effect beyond the known effect of the E4 genotype.*[86]

Sleep Apnea

In late 2014, researchers reviewed the scientific literature on the potential relationship between obstructive sleep apnea (OSA)[1] and Alzheimer's disease. They concluded that, "Although a causal relationship between OSA and AD is not yet established, OSA induces neurodegenerative changes as a result of two major contributing processes: sleep fragmentation and intermittent hypoxia. As such, inflammation and cellular stress are sufficient to impair cell-cell interactions, synaptic function, and neural circuitry, leading to a decline of cognitive behavior. *Sustained OSA could promote cognitive dysfunction, overlapping with that in AD and other neurodegenerative diseases.* Early treatment by positive airway pressure and other current standards of care should have a positive impact to alleviate structural and functional deterioration."[87] Bottom line, if you have obstructive sleep apnea, use your Continuous Positive Airway Pressure (CPAP) machine!

Sleep Issues

Trouble falling or staying asleep, poor sleep quality, and short or long sleep duration are gaining attention as potential risk factors for cognitive decline and dementia, including Alzheimer's disease. Sleep-disordered breathing has also been linked to these outcomes. In late 2014, researchers reviewed recent observational and experimental studies investigating the effect of poor sleep on cognitive outcomes and Alzheimer's disease. They concluded that, *"Findings indicate that poor sleep is a risk factor for cognitive decline and Alzheimer's disease.* Although mechanisms underlying these associations are not yet clear,

---

[1]Obstructive sleep apnea (OSA) is the most common type of sleep apnea and is caused by obstruction of the upper airway. It is characterized by repetitive pauses in breathing during sleep, despite the effort to breathe, and is usually associated with a reduction in blood oxygen saturation. These pauses in breathing, called "apneas," typically last 20 to 40 seconds. The individual with OSA is rarely aware of having difficulty breathing, even upon awakening. It is recognized as a problem by others witnessing the individual during episodes or is suspected because of its effects on the body, such as fatigue or feeling tired. OSA is commonly accompanied with snoring.

POSSIBLE RISK FACTORS FOR ALZHEIMER'S

healthy sleep appears to play an important role in maintaining brain health with age, and may play a key role in Alzheimer's disease prevention."[88]

To study the association between self-reported sleep disturbances and dementia risk, in 2014 researchers studied men at ages 50 (n = 1,574) and 70 (n = 1,029) years. Dementia incidence was determined by reviewing their patient history between ages 50 and 90 years. In addition, plasma levels of β-amyloid (Aβ) peptides 1-40 and 1-42 were measured at ages 70, 77, and 82 years. They found that, *"Men with self-reported sleep disturbances had a higher risk of developing dementia (+33 percent) and Alzheimer's disease (+51 percent) than men without self-reported sleep disturbances."* The researchers noted that the increased risk for Alzheimer's disease was highest when sleep disturbance was reported at age 70 years. No group differences were found in Aβ levels. They concluded that, *"Improving sleep quality may help reduce the neurodegenerative risk in older men."*[89]

A different group of researchers, reporting in the October 21, 2014 issue of *Neurology*, found that *long sleep duration was associated with increased risk of dementia mortality.* For the study, the authors studied 3,857 people without dementia aged 65 years and. The average daily total sleep duration was grouped into three categories: ≤5 hours (short sleepers), 6-8 hours (reference category), and ≥9 hours (long sleepers). Community-dwelling elders were followed for a median of 12.5 years, after which the death certificates of those who died were examined.

During the above study, a total of 1,822 (47.2 percent) of 3,857 participants died, including 201 (11.0 percent) deaths among short sleepers, 832 (45.7 percent) among long sleepers, and 789 (43.3 percent) among those participants in the reference category. Of 1,822 deceased participants, 92 (5.1 percent) had a dementia condition reported on the death certificate (49 [53.3 percent] were long sleepers, 36 [39.1 percent] reported sleeping between six and eight hours, and 7 [7.6 percent] were short sleepers). The researchers concluded that, *"Self-reported long sleep duration was associated with 58 percent increased risk of demen-*

tia-specific mortality in this cohort [group] of elders without dementia."[90]

How does a good night's sleep decrease the risk of Alzheimer's disease? Recently, researchers have discovered how *the brain removes potentially toxic molecules that accumulate with normal brain function. A molecular clearance system that removes toxic metabolites in the brain has been described. This so-called "glymphatic system" is strongly stimulated by sleep.* Moreover, anesthesia can activate the glymphatic system to clear potentially toxic proteins known to contribute to the pathology of Alzheimer's disease such as beta-amyloid (Abeta). Clearance during sleep is as much as two-fold faster than during waking hours. The researchers conclude stating, "These results support a new hypothesis to answer the age-old question of why sleep is necessary. Glymphatic dysfunction may pay a hitherto unsuspected role in the pathogenesis of neurodegenerative diseases as well as maintenance of cognition. *Furthermore, clinical studies suggest that quality and duration of sleep may be predictive of the onset of AD, and that quality sleep may significantly reduce the risk of AD for apolipoprotein E (ApoE) ε4 carriers, who have significantly greater chances of developing AD.* Further characterization of the glymphatic system in humans may lead to new therapies and methods of prevention of neurodegenerative diseases. *A public health initiative to ensure adequate sleep among middle-aged and older people may prove useful in preventing AD, especially in apolipoprotein E (ApoE) ε4 carriers.*"[91]

Smoking

Researchers studied whether or not smoking and drinking alcohol were associated with the risk of dementia, including Alzheimer's disease and vascular dementia (VaD) after seven years of follow-up. They studied 3,170 elderly men, according to their smoking and alcohol drinking status. They concluded that, "*Current smoking and daily drinking were found to be significantly associated with dementia in elderly men.*"[92] They also found the risk was highest when both smoking and drinking were done together, as opposed to just drinking or just smoking.

POSSIBLE RISK FACTORS FOR ALZHEIMER'S

Stress

An important factor that may affect the severity and time of onset of Alzheimer's disease is chronic stress. Epidemiological studies report that chronically stressed individuals are at an increased risk for developing AD. In 2014, *researchers reviewed the scientific literature on this topic and documented the wide range of pathologic processes associated with AD that are negatively affected by stress, such as inflammation, glucose metabolism, accumulation of β-amyloid, TAU hyperphosphorylation, oxidative stress and impairment of mitochondrial function.* They conclude by stating that, *"All these data support the idea that chronic stress could be considered a risk factor for AD."*[93]

Cardiovascular disease contributes to Alzheimer's disease (see below), and stress clearly exacerbates cardiovascular disease. The relationship between psychological distress and vascular disease (peripheral vascular disease, abdominal aortic aneurysm, and heart failure) was examined by a group of researchers, with the results reported in 2014. They reviewed the data from numerous studies, which included 166,631 male and female participants. During a mean follow-up 9.5 years there were 17,368 deaths of which 8,625 were cardiovascular disease-related. Relative to the asymptomatic group, the highly distressed group experienced a greatly elevated risk of peripheral vascular disease and heart failure. The researchers concluded, *"As anticipated, distress was associated with cardiovascular disease, coronary heart disease, and all strokes combined."*[94]

Using an animal model, researchers reported in the August 12, 2014 issue of *Molecular Neurobiology* the results of their research on how chronic stress affects the severity and time of onset of Alzheimer's disease. Without discussing the complicated details of the experiment, the researchers concluded that, chronic stress resulted in impaired learning and memory. The authors concluded that, *"chronic stress may accelerate the emergence of AD in susceptible individuals."*[95]

Tooth Loss

Similar to periodontal disease (previously discussed), tooth loss may be a modifiable risk factor for memory disorders. In order to better understand this relationship, researchers conducted a 5-year study investigating the effect of tooth loss on the development of mild memory impairment (MMI) among the elderly. They studied 2,335 community residents who were cognitively intact at baseline. The number of remaining teeth at baseline was classified as zero, 1-8, 9-16, 17-24, and 25-32. The main outcome for the analysis was the development of MMI at follow-up. They concluded that, *"Tooth loss predicts the development of MMI among the elderly."*[96]

Traumatic Brain Injury (TBI)

Traumatic brain injury (TBI) occurs when an external force traumatically injures the brain. TBI can be classified based on severity, mechanism (closed or penetrating head injury), or other features. TBI has been identified as a risk factor for Alzheimer's disease, but the relationship to Mild Cognitive Impairment (MCI), a prodromal stage of AD, is unknown. Researchers wanted to examine whether a history of TBI without chronic deficits leads to an earlier age of MCI diagnosis. To do so, they enlisted subjects with and without MCI. Subjects were categorized based on lifetime reported TBI with less than five minutes loss of consciousness (n = 214) or greater than five minutes loss of consciousness (n = 104) and compared to MCI subjects without TBI (n = 3,090). The researchers found that "Subjects with a history of self-reported TBI of less than five minutes as well as those with greater than five minutes loss of consciousness were diagnosed with MCI an average of 2.5 years earlier than those without TBI. This parallels findings in AD and *supports emerging literature of TBI as a risk factor for cognitive decline later in life.*"[97]

POSSIBLE RISK FACTORS FOR ALZHEIMER'S

Use of Proton Pump Inhibitors

In late 2014, Dr. Haenisch and nineteen colleagues studied the association between proton pump inhibitors (PPIs)[1] and the risk of dementia in elderly people. Data were derived from a longitudinal, multicenter study in elderly primary care patients, and included 3,327 community-dwelling persons aged 75 years or older. They were followed for eighteen months, and during that time, a total of 431 patients developed some type of dementia, including 260 patients with Alzheimer's disease. The researchers found that, *"Patients receiving PPI medication had a significantly increased risk of any dementia and Alzheimer's disease compared with nonusers."*[98] Uh oh. Lots of people have to take these, and there is no good alternative.

Vascular and Cholesterol Risk

Cardiovascular disease (CVD)[2] and related risk factors are associated with Alzheimer's disease. This association is less well-defined in normal cognition (NC) or prodromal AD (mild cognitive impairment, MCI). Researchers wanted to understand this relationship better. In order to do so, they studied 3,117 individuals with MCI (74 ± 8 years, 56 percent female) and 6,603 normal cognition or NC participants (72 ± 8 years, 68 percent female). A composite measure of *vascular risk was defined using the Framingham Stroke Risk Profile (FSRP) score (i.e., age, systolic blood pressure, anti-hypertensive medication, diabetes, cigarette smoking, CVD history, atrial fibrillation)*. The researchers found that, "In NC participants, increasing FSRP was related to worse baseline global cognition, information processing speed, sequencing

---

[1] Proton-pump inhibitors (PPIs) are a group of drugs whose main action is a pronounced and long-lasting reduction of gastric acid production. They are the most potent inhibitors of acid secretion available, and include drugs such as omeprazole (Gasec, Omepral, Prilosec, Zegerid, etc.), lansoprazole (such as Prevacid), esomeprazole (Nexium, Esotrex, esso), and pantoprazole (Protonix, Somac, etc.).

[2] Cardiovascular disease (CVD) is a class of diseases that involve the heart, the blood vessels (arteries, capillaries, and veins) or both. The causes of cardiovascular disease are diverse but atherosclerosis ("hardening of the arteries") and hypertension are the most common.

abilities and a worse longitudinal trajectory on all cognitive measures. In MCI individuals, increasing FSRP correlated with worse longitudinal delayed memory...*Conclusions: An adverse vascular risk profile is associated with worse cognitive trajectory*, especially global cognition, naming, and information processing speed, among NC elders."[99]

In 2014, using an animal model of Alzheimer's disease, researchers were able to show that *high blood pressure (hypertension)* "*leads to age-dependent Aβ accumulation similar to that observed in AD.*"[100]

Also in 2014, a different group of researchers noted that, "The cerebrovasculature [brain blood vessels] plays an important role in the elimination of Aβ from the brain and hypertension is a well-known risk factor for AD...Cerebrovascular impairment is frequent in patients with Alzheimer disease and is believed to influence clinical manifestation and severity of the disease. Cardiovascular risk factors, especially hypertension, have been associated with higher risk of developing Alzheimer's disease." They used an animal to study this relationship, and concluded that, "*Our results indicate that hypertension accelerates the development of Alzheimer's disease-related structural and functional alterations...*"[101]

Dr. Son and colleagues reported in 2015 the results of their research on thirty-seven Alzheimer's disease patients (eighteen patients with hypertension and nineteen patients without hypertension), who underwent functional magnetic resonance imaging (fMRI). *Most notably, they found decreased nerve connections in specific parts of the brain in the hypertensive group*, and concluded that, "This finding may account for an additional contribution of hypertension to the pathophysiology [abnormal function and structure] of AD."[102]

Coronary heart disease (CHD)[1] has been linked with cognitive decline and dementia in several studies. CHD is strongly associated with blood

---

[1]Coronary artery disease (CAD) also known as atherosclerotic heart disease (ASHD), coronary heart disease (CHD), or ischemic heart disease (IHD), is the most common type of heart disease and cause of heart attacks. The disease is caused by plaque

POSSIBLE RISK FACTORS FOR ALZHEIMER'S

pressure, but it is not clear how blood pressure levels or changes in blood pressure over time affect the relation between CHD and dementia-related pathology. To study this relationship, researchers evaluated "69 elderly at risk of dementia who participated in the Cardiovascular Risk Factors[1], Aging and Dementia (CAIDE) study. CAIDE participants were examined in midlife, re-examined twenty-one years later, and then after additionally seven years (in total up to thirty years follow-up)." MRIs from the second re-examination were used to compare various aspects of brain structure. The researchers found that CHD was associated with specific brain abnormalities, particularly in people with longer disease duration (>10 years). Associations between CHD and several abnormalities were strongest in people with CHD and hypertension in midlife, and those with CHD and declining blood pressure after midlife. The researchers concluded by noting that, *"Based on these results, long-term CHD seems to have detrimental effects on brain tissue, and these effects are influenced by blood pressure levels and their changes over time."*[103]

Between 2003-2006, 2,364 non-demented persons underwent computed tomography (CT scans) of the arteries of the heart (coronaries), aortic arch, extracranial (e.g., outside the skull), and intracranial (e.g., inside the skull) carotid arteries to quantify atherosclerotic calcification (e.g., deposition of calcium in the artery wall, which is abnormal). Participants were followed for the development of dementia (n = 90) until April 2012. Researchers conducting the study found that, *"Atherosclerosis, in particular in the extracranial carotid arteries, is related to a higher risk of dementia and cognitive decline."*[104]

---

building up along the inner walls of the arteries of the heart, which narrows the lumen (opening) of arteries and reduces blood flow to the heart.

[1] Cardiovascular Risk Factors: Traditional risk factors include such things as high blood pressure (hypertension), smoking, obesity, age, lack of physical activity, high cholesterol (hyperlipidemia). However, there are now many other risk factors that also have to be considered. For a full discussion, see:
http://emedicine.medscape.com/article/164163-overview

Cholesterol[1] is an organic molecule. It is a sterol (or modified steroid), a lipid molecule and is biosynthesized by all animal cells because it is an essential structural component of animal cell membranes. In addition to its importance within cells, cholesterol also serves as a precursor for the biosynthesis of steroid hormones, bile acids, and vitamin D. Cholesterol is the principal sterol synthesized by animals. All kinds of cells in animals can produce it. In vertebrates the hepatic (liver) cells typically produce greater amounts than other cells.

Cholesterol is only slightly soluble in water; it dissolves into the (water-based) bloodstream only at exceedingly small concentrations. Instead, cholesterol is transported inside lipoproteins, complex particles There are several types of lipoproteins in the blood. In order of increasing density, they are very-low-density lipoprotein (VLDL), low-density lipoprotein (LDL; "bad cholesterol"), intermediate-density lipoprotein (IDL), and high-density lipoprotein (HDL; "good cholesterol"). Cholesterol within different lipoproteins is identical, although some is carried as "free" alcohol, while others as fatty acyl esters, known also as cholesterol esters.

According to one group of researchers, "High-density lipoproteins (HDLs) are a heterogeneous group of lipoproteins composed of various lipids and proteins. HDL is formed both in the systemic circulation and in the brain. In addition to being a crucial player in the reverse cholesterol transport pathway, HDL possesses a wide range of other functions including anti-oxidation, anti-inflammation, pro-endothelial [blood vessel] function, anti-thrombosis [anti-blood clot], and modulation of immune function. It has been firmly established that high plasma levels of HDL protect against cardiovascular disease. Accumulating evidence indicates that the beneficial role of HDL extends to many other systems including the central nervous system. Cognition is a complex brain function that includes all aspects of perception, thought, and memory. Cognitive function often declines during aging and this decline mani-

---

[1] For a nice chart of cholesterol values, go to:
http://www.newhealthguide.org/Cholesterol-Levels-Chart.html

POSSIBLE RISK FACTORS FOR ALZHEIMER'S

fests as cognitive impairment/dementia in age-related and progressive neurodegenerative disorders such as Alzheimer's disease, Parkinson's disease, Huntington's disease, and amyotrophic lateral sclerosis. A growing concern is that no effective therapy is currently available to prevent or treat these devastating diseases. *Emerging evidence suggests that HDL may play a pivotal role in preserving cognitive function under normal and pathological conditions."*[105] *Keep in mind that exercise increases blood levels of HDL!*

A wide range of vascular burden factors has been found to increase the risk of Alzheimer's disease. In 2014, researchers reported the results of their research evaluating various vascular risk factors, clustered in a vascular burden index (VBI), and their relationship to Alzheimer's disease. They investigated 1,102 elderly patients at risk for dementia, and the impact of the VBI on cognitive performance. They included age and gender in the risk analysis. Results showed that, "*...in order of impact, the following factors had a negative effect: age (0.26), obesity (0.18), hypertension (0.14), sex (0.09), smoking (0.08), diabetes (0.07), and atherosclerosis (0.05), whereas other cardiovascular diseases or hypercholesterolemia were not significant in this study."*[106]

Another group of researchers examined the relationships among elevated vascular risk burden, age, cerebral blood flow (CBF; the blood supply to the brain), and cognition in seventy-one non-demented older adults. They found that, ..."among older adults with elevated vascular risk burden (i.e., multiple vascular risk factors), advancing age was significantly associated with reduced CBF, whereas there was no such relationship for those with low vascular risk burden. Furthermore, among those with elevated vascular risk, reduced CBF was associated with poorer cognitive performance. *Such findings suggest that older adults with elevated vascular risk burden may be particularly vulnerable to cognitive change as a function of CBF reductions.*[107]

CHAPTER FIVE:
CAUSE(S) AND PATHOLOGY

The cause for most Alzheimer's cases is still mostly unknown (or unproven) except for one percent to five percent of cases where genetic differences have been identified. Several competing hypotheses exist trying to explain the cause of the disease.

Introduction

In late 2014, a group of researchers outlined the overall underlying mechanisms in Alzheimer's disease. These are complicated, but they help explain why some experimental treatments haven't worked as hoped, and help establish a descriptive model of the disease process which can be used for the development of therapeutic agents. The authors propose seven key elements of importance to the pathogenesis (biologic cause) of AD as follows:[108]

1. amyloid beta [amyloid-β; amyloid-beta peptide; abeta; Aβ]
2. tau
3. beta-secretase
4. glutamate
5. cyclin-dependent kinase 5
6. phosphoinositide 3-kinase
7. hypoxia-induced factor 1 alpha

In total, they describe thirty-nine biologic mechanisms in the development of AD, discuss interconnections between pathways, and identified combinations for potential treatments of AD. Some of these mechanisms are discussed in more detail below.

CAUSE(S) AND PATHOLOGY

Arginine

A very interesting theory of the cause of Alzheimer's disease (not included in the list above) was published in the April 15, 2015 issue of the *Journal of Neuroscience* by Dr. Kan and colleagues. This is a new, and contrary, theory, and so we have included the entire summary of the authors' explanation of their new theory:[109]

> The pathogenesis [cause] of Alzheimer's disease is a critical unsolved question; and although recent studies have demonstrated a strong association between altered brain immune responses and disease progression, the mechanistic cause of neuronal dysfunction and death is unknown. We have previously described the unique CVN-AD mouse model of AD, in which immune-mediated nitric oxide is lowered to mimic human levels, resulting in *a mouse model that demonstrates the cardinal features of AD [see the following paragraphs for more details], including amyloid deposition, hyperphosphorylated and aggregated tau, behavioral changes, and age-dependent hippocampal neuronal loss*. Using this mouse model, we studied longitudinal changes in brain immunity in relation to neuronal loss and, *contrary to the predominant view that AD pathology is driven by proinflammatory factors, we find that the pathology in CVN-AD mice is driven by local immune suppression*. Areas of hippocampal neuronal death are associated with the presence of immunosuppressive CD11c(+) microglia and extracellular arginase [an enzyme], *resulting in arginine catabolism [destruction] and reduced levels of total brain arginine*. Pharmacologic disruption of the arginine utilization pathway by an inhibitor of arginase and ornithine decarboxylase protected the mice from AD-like pathology and significantly decreased CD11c expression. *Our findings strongly implicate local immune-mediated amino acid catabolism [destruction] as a novel and potentially critical mecha-*

nism mediating the age-dependent and regional loss of neurons in humans with AD.

Genetics

The genetic heritability of Alzheimer's disease, based on reviews of twin and family studies, range from 49 percent to 79 percent. However, only 0.1 percent of the cases are familial forms of autosomal (not sex-linked) dominant inheritance, which have an onset before age 65. This form of the disease is known as early onset familial Alzheimer's disease (EOAD).

Most cases of Alzheimer's disease do not exhibit autosomal-dominant inheritance and are termed *sporadic Alzheimer's disease,* in which environmental and genetic differences may act as risk factors. The best known genetic risk factor is the inheritance of the ε4 allele[1] of the apolipoprotein E (APOE)[2]. Between 40 and 80 percent of people with AD possess at least one APOEε4 allele. *Those who possess two APOEε4 alleles are at much higher risk of contracting AD.* Like many human diseases, environmental effects and genetic modifiers result in variable effects.

Cholinergic Hypothesis

The oldest hypothesis of AD, on which most currently available drug therapies are based, is the *cholinergic hypothesis,* which proposes that AD is caused by reduced synthesis of the neurotransmitter acetylcholine. Other cholinergic effects have also been proposed, for example, initiation of large-scale aggregation of amyloid, leading to generalized neuroinflammation.

---

[1] An allele, or allel, is one of a number of alternative forms of the same gene.
[2] A specific isoform of apolipoprotein, APOE4, is a major genetic risk factor for AD. Whilst apolipoproteins enhance the breakdown of beta amyloid, some isoforms are not very effective at this task (such as APOE4), leading to excess amyloid buildup in the brain.

CAUSE(S) AND PATHOLOGY

Amyloid Hypothesis

In 1991, the *amyloid hypothesis* postulated that amyloid beta (A$_\beta$) deposits are the fundamental cause of Alzheimer's disease. One of the hallmarks of AD is the formation of *senile plaques* in the brain, which contain Aβ (amyloid β-peptide).[110] Support for this postulate comes from the location of the gene for the amyloid precursor protein (APP) on chromosome 21, together with the fact that people with trisomy 21 (Down Syndrome) who have an extra gene copy almost universally exhibit AD by 40 years of age. Also, as mentioned above, a specific form of apolipoprotein, APOE4, is a major genetic risk factor for AD. *Whilst apolipoproteins enhance the breakdown of beta amyloid, some isoforms are not very effective at this task (such as APOE4), leading to excess amyloid buildup in the brain.*

In late 2014, *researchers used an animal model of AD to show that impairment in beta-amyloid clearance from the brain into cerebrospinal fluid (CSF) plays a significant role in senile plaque formation.*[111]

Also in 2014, a different group of researchers were able to show for the first time, in an animal model of AD, the propagation or transfer of AD pathology via cell-to-cell transfer of amyloid beta (Aβ) residues. The researchers concluded, "Furthermore, cell-to-cell transfer is shown to be an early event that is seemingly independent of later appearances of cellular toxicity. This phenomenon could explain how seeds for the AD pathology could pass on to new brain areas and gradually induce AD pathology, even before the first cell starts to deteriorate, and how cell-to-cell transfer can act together with the factors that influence cellular clearance and/or degradation in the development of AD."[112]

The amyloid hypothesis has driven drug development strategies for Alzheimer's disease for over 20 years. *Recently, however, researchers have called into question the amyloid hypothesis with new data and interpretations. They note several unresolved issues in the field including the presence of Aβ deposition in cognitively normal individuals, the weak correlation between plaque load and cognition, questions regarding the biochemical nature, the bias of pre-clinical AD models toward the amyloid hypothesis and the poorly explained pathological heterogeneity and comorbidities associated with AD, and suggest several future directions for AD research.*[113]

While the amyloid hypothesis of AD is compelling, therapeutic trials targeting this pathology have not been successful to date. High-profile clinical trials of of two agents (bapineuzumab and solanezumab), antibodies targeted at amyloid-beta (Aβ) removal, have failed to meet their primary endpoints. Neither drug improves clinical outcomes in patients with late onset AD, joining a long list of unsuccessful attempts to treat AD with anti-amyloid therapies.[114]

Tau Hypothesis

In Alzheimer's disease, changes in tau protein lead to the disintegration of microtubules in brain cells. The *tau hypothesis* proposes that tau protein abnormalities initiate the disease cascade. In this model, *hyperphosphorylated tau* begins to pair with other threads of tau. Eventually, they form neurofibrillary tangles inside nerve cell bodies. When this occurs, the microtubules disintegrate, collapsing the neuron's transport system. This may result first in malfunctions in biochemical communication between neurons and later in the death of the cells.

Recent studies have demonstrated an important interaction between tau and cholesterol. The researchers note that, "This argues for an impact of tau pathology on cellular cholesterol homeostasis. We suggest that there is a bidirectional mode of action: Disturbances in cellular cholesterol metabolism may promote tau pathology, but tau pathology may also alter neuronal cholesterol homeostasis; once it is established, a vicious cycle may promote neurofibrillary tangle formation."[115]

In an animal model of AD, researchers found a link between tau and inflammation. They concluded that, "*...the pathogenesis of Alzheimer's disease may be driven by tau dysfunction, in addition to the direct effects of beta-amyloid.*"[116]

CAUSE(S) AND PATHOLOGY

TDP-43 (A Protein)

In 2014, researchers reported in the *Journal of Alzheimer's disease*, a new abnormality associated with Alzheimer's disease. They reviewed the brain pathology (abnormalities) of 228 individuals, whose age of death ranged from 78 to 106 years. They looked for a particular protein, called TDP-43. They found that, "TDP-43 neuronal [nerve cell] inclusions were present in 27 percent of the sample, 36 percent of those with clinical dementia and 18 percent without dementia. Individuals who died later (>90 years) or with clinical dementia were more likely to show TDP-43 inclusions. Hippocampal and entorhinal [memory areas] TDP-43 inclusions were significantly associated with dementia severity and increasing age…TDP-43 neuronal inclusions appeared to be co-localize with severe neuronal loss…Findings indicate that hippocampal and entorhinal TDP-43 inclusions are important abnormalities of late onset dementia which appear to co-localize with severe neuronal loss, but not with Alzheimer's disease markers of amyloid and tau. This broadens the accepted view of TDP-43 pathology in dementias."[117]

Homocysteine

Homocysteine is a non-protein α-amino acid. It is a homologue[1] of the amino acid cysteine. It is biosynthesized from methionine. Homocysteine can be recycled into methionine or converted into cysteine with the aid of certain B-vitamins.

A high level of homocysteine in the blood (hyperhomocysteinemia) makes a person more prone to endothelial (blood vessel) cell injury, which leads to inflammation in the blood vessels, which in turn may lead to atherogenesis, which can result in ischemic injury. Hyperhomocysteinemia is therefore a possible risk factor for coronary artery disease. Coronary artery disease occurs when an atherosclerotic plaque blocks blood flow to the coronary arteries, which supply the heart with oxygenated blood.

---

[1]Homologous: having similar characteristics or function; derived from a common origin.

Hyperhomocysteinemia has been correlated with the occurrence of blood clots, heart attacks, strokes, and possibly AD, though it is unclear whether hyperhomocysteinemia is an independent risk factor for these conditions.

A recent study, reported in the *Journal of Alzheimer's disease*, noted that, "*High levels of homocysteine is a risk factor for developing Alzheimer's disease, and the effect that this amino acid has on amyloid-β (Aβ) protein precursor metabolism is considered one of the potential mechanism(s) involved in this effect.*"[118]

B vitamins can decrease homocysteine levels, and their use in preventing AD is discussed in detail below.

Inflammation

Inflammation is part of the complex biological response of cells to harmful stimuli, such as pathogens (bacteria, viruses, fungi, and so forth), damaged cells, or irritants (such as trauma or chemicals). Inflammation is a protective response involving cells, blood vessels, and proteins and other mediators that is intended to eliminate the initial cause of cell injury, as well as the dead or damaged cells and tissues resulting from the original insult, and to initiate the process of repair.

The classical signs of acute inflammation are pain, heat, redness, swelling, and loss of function. Inflammation is a protective attempt by the organism to remove the injurious stimuli and to initiate the healing process.

Inflammation can be classified as either *acute* or *chronic*. *Acute inflammation* is the initial response of the body to harmful stimuli and is achieved by the increased movement of plasma and leukocytes (especially granulocytes) from the blood into the injured tissues. A cascade of biochemical events propagates and matures the inflammatory response, involving the local vascular system, the immune system, and various cells within the injured tissue. Prolonged inflammation, known as *chronic inflammation*, leads to a progressive shift in the type of cells present at the site of inflammation and is characterized by simultaneous destruction and healing of the tissue from the inflammatory process.

Inflammation is now known to cause or to be related to many diseases. Recently, for example, inflammation has been found to be associated with depression and psychosis.

Numerous lines of evidence indicate that chronic inflammation plays a major role in the development of various neurodegenerative diseases, including Alzheimer's disease, Parkinson's disease, multiple sclerosis, brain tumor, and meningitis. Why these diseases are more common among people from some countries than others is not fully understood, but lifestyle factors have been linked to the development of neurodegenerative diseases. For example, the incidence of certain neurodegenerative diseases among people living in the Asian subcontinent, where people regularly consume spices, is much lower than in countries of the western world. *Extensive research over the last ten years has indicated that nutraceuticals derived from such spices as turmeric, red pepper, black pepper, licorice, clove, ginger, garlic, coriander, and cinnamon target inflammatory pathways, thereby may prevent neurodegenerative diseases.*[119]

According to a recent scientific article, "*Neuroinflammation has long been known as an accompanying pathology of Alzheimer's disease.* Microglia [inflammatory nerve cells] surrounding amyloid plaques in the brain of Auguste D [the first patient diagnosed with Alzheimer's disease] were described in the original publication of Alois Alzheimer [the German physician who first described the condition]."[120]

Another group of researchers also report that, "Increased production of amyloid β-peptide (Aβ) and altered processing of tau in Alzheimer's disease are associated with synaptic dysfunction, neuronal death and cognitive and behavioral deficits. *Neuroinflammation is also a prominent feature of AD brain and considerable evidence indicates that inflammatory events play a significant role in modulating the progression of AD.* The role of microglia [inflammatory nerve cells] in AD inflammation has long been acknowledged. Substantial evidence now demonstrates that astrocyte[1]-mediated inflammatory responses also influence pathology development, synapse health and neurodegeneration in AD. Several anti-inflammatory therapies targeting astrocytes show significant benefit in models of disease, particularly with respect to tau-associated neurodegeneration."[121]

Other researchers report a more complicated relationship between astrocytes and nerve cells. They state, "A growing body of research suggests that astrocytes play roles as contributors to the pathophysiology of Alzheimer's disease. Several lines of evidence propose that activated astrocytes produce and release proinflammatory molecules that may be critical for the generation of amyloid-β peptide (Aβ). However, accumulating evidence indicates that Aβ may activate astrocytes, which leads to an increase in cytokines[2] that has been suggested to be a causative factor in the cognitive dysfunction of AD; thus, a vicious circle may be created. Intrinsic inflammatory mechanisms may provide a regulatory system that is capable of influencing the neuronal microenvironment that affects neuronal survival."[122]

A recent scientific article in the *Frontiers of Aging Neuroscience* stated that, "Alzheimer disease is the most common form of dementia and is characterized by progressive cognitive impairment. In addition to classical neuropathological features such as amyloid plaques and neurofibrillary tangles (NFT), accumulation of activated immune cells has been documented in the AD brain, suggesting a contribution of neuroinflammation in the pathogenesis of AD. Besides cognitive dete-

---

[1] Astrocytes also known collectively as astroglia, are characteristic star-shaped glial cells in the brain and spinal cord. They are the most abundant cells of the human brain. They perform many functions, including biochemical support of endothelial cells that form the blood–brain barrier, provision of nutrients to the nervous tissue, maintenance of extracellular ion balance, and a role in the repair and scarring process of the brain and spinal cord following traumatic injuries.

[2] Cytokines are a broad and loose category of small proteins that are important in cell signaling. They are released by cells and affect the behavior of other cells. Cytokines include chemokines, interferons, interleukins, lymphokines, and tumor necrosis factor. They act through receptors, and are especially important in the immune system. They are important in health and disease, specifically in host responses to infection, immune responses, inflammation, trauma, sepsis, cancer, and reproduction.

rioration, non-cognitive symptoms, such as agitation, aggression, depression and psychosis, are often observed in demented patients, including those with AD, and these neuropsychological symptoms place a heavy burden on caregivers. These symptoms often exhibit sudden onset and tend to fluctuate over time, and in many cases, they are triggered by an infection in peripheral organs, suggesting that inflammation plays an important role in the pathogenesis of these non-cognitive symptoms...Observations from experimental mouse models indicate that alteration of brain blood vessels, especially blood-brain barrier (BBB) dysfunction, may contribute to the relationship."[123]

In 2014, researchers reported the results of study where they followed 247 patients with Alzheimer's disease for approximately thirteen years. At follow-up, 89 percent of the patients had died. The mean survival time was 6.4 ± 3.0 years. The noted that, *"The AD pathology that independently predicted an early death caused by dementia was cerebral inflammation...This is the first study to link neuroinflammation independently to early death in AD and, hence, a rapidly progressing disease...Our results suggest that inflammation, and not amyloid or tau pathology, is an independent underlying mechanism in the malignancy[1] of AD."*[124]

Dr. Popp and seventeen colleagues reported a study of the relationship between cortisol (a stress hormone) and cognitive decline in the October 2014 issue of *Neurobiology of Aging*. They found that, *"higher baseline cerebrospinal fluid (CSF) cortisol levels ['stress hormone'] were associated with faster clinical worsening and cognitive decline in mild cognitive impairment of AD type (MCI-AD)."*[125]

Reporting in the *Journal of Neuroinflammation*, researchers reported that, "Recently, a rapid form of AD has been described." They compared the inflammatory response in the rapid form and the standard form of Alzheimer's disease, and found that, *"In conclusion, we found a characteristic proinflammatory response in the serum [blood] of rap-*

---

[1]Malignancy is the tendency of a medical condition to become progressively worse. Also used to refer to cancer.

id AD patients. It might explain the more rapid course of the rapid AD subform and can be helpful in distinguishing between classical AD and rapid AD."[126]

Mitochondrial Dysfunction

The mitochondrion (plural mitochondria) is a membrane bound organelle[1] found in most eukaryotic cells (the cells that make up plants, animals, fungi, and many other forms of life). These structures are sometimes described as "the powerhouse of the cell" because they generate most of the cell's supply of adenosine triphosphate (ATP), used as a source of chemical energy. In addition to supplying cellular energy, mitochondria are involved in other tasks such as signaling, cellular differentiation, cell death, as well as maintaining the control of the cell cycle and cell growth. Mitochondria have been implicated in several human diseases, including mitochondrial disorders, cardiac dysfunction, autism, Alzheimer's disease, and play a role in the aging process.

Mitochondrial functions can be negatively affected by amyloid β peptide (Aβ), an important component in Alzheimer's disease pathogenesis, and Aβ can interact with mitochondria and cause mitochondrial dysfunction. *One of the most accepted hypotheses for AD onset implicates mitochondrial dysfunction and oxidative stress as primary events triggering AD.*[127]

Cells from patients with mild cognitive impairment, early AD, late AD, and age-matched normal controls were used to study mitochondrial functions. Researchers found a variety of dysfunctions, and concluded that, "Comparison of protein changes throughout the progression of AD suggests *the most pronounced changes occur in early AD mitochondria.*"[128]

The relationship between diabetes mellitus (DM) and Alzheimer's disease is discussed in detail below (see Diabetes). According to one group of re-

---

[1] In cell biology, an organelle is a specialized subunit within a cell that has a specific function.

searchers, "Hyperglycemia [elevated blood sugar] in DM is associated with damage of hippocampal cells [where memories are formed], reflected by changes in mitochondrial functionality. Similar mitochondrial damage has been observed when amyloid beta (Aβ) accumulates in the brain of AD patients...*we suggest that hyperglycemia in the diabetic patient could change the structure and functionality of mitochondria in hippocampal cells, accelerating neuronal damage, and favoring the start of AD.*"[129]

Diabetes

Type 2 diabetes (T2D)[1] and Alzheimer disease are two major health issues nowadays. T2D is an ever increasing epidemic, affecting millions of elderly people worldwide, with major repercussions in the patients' daily life. This is mostly due to its chronic complications that may affect brain and constitutes a risk factor for AD. T2D principal hallmark is insulin resistance[2] which also occurs in AD, rendering both pathologies more than mere unrelated diseases. This hypothesis has been reinforced in the recent years, with a high number of studies high-

---

[1]Diabetes mellitus (DM), commonly referred to as diabetes, is a group of metabolic diseases in which there are high blood sugar levels over a prolonged period. Symptoms of high blood sugar include frequent urination, increased thirst, and increased hunger. Serious long-term complications include cardiovascular disease, stroke, kidney failure, foot ulcers, damage to the eyes, damage to peripheral nerves, and neurodegenerative diseases, such as Alzheimer's disease. Diabetes is due to either the pancreas not producing enough insulin or the cells of the body not responding properly to the insulin produced. There are two main types of diabetes mellitus: Type 1 DM results from the body's failure to produce enough insulin. This form was previously referred to as "insulin-dependent diabetes mellitus" (IDDM) or "juvenile diabetes." The cause is unknown. Type 2 DM begins with insulin resistance, a condition in which cells fail to respond to insulin properly. As the disease progresses a lack of insulin may also develop. This form was previously referred to as "noninsulin-dependent diabetes mellitus" (NIDDM) or "adult-onset diabetes." This type may be caused by excessive body weight and not enough exercise.

[2]Insulin resistance is a condition in which cells fail to respond to the normal actions of the hormone insulin. The body (pancreas) produces insulin, but the cells in the body become resistant to insulin and are unable to use it as effectively, leading to elevated blood sugar (hyperglycemia). Beta cells in the pancreas subsequently increase their production of insulin, further contributing to elevated insulin levels (hyperinsulinemia).

lighting the existence of several common molecular links. As such, it is not surprising that AD has been considered as the "type 3 diabetes" or a "brain-specific T2D," supporting the idea that a beneficial therapeutic strategy against T2D might be also beneficial against AD.[130]

Along the same lines, another group of researchers state, *"The emerging data suggest that type 2 diabetes mellitus (T2DM) can contribute significantly to the onset or progression of Alzheimer's disease either directly or as a cofactor*. Various animal and human clinical studies have provided evidence that T2DM is a major risk factor in the pathology of AD and the two diseases share common biological mechanisms at the molecular level. The biological mechanisms that are common in the pathology of both T2DM and AD include insulin resistance, impaired glucose metabolism, β-amyloid formation, oxidative stress, and the presence of advanced glycation end products. With better understanding of the degree of association between AD and T2DM and the underlying molecular mechanisms explaining this relationship, it is hoped that researchers will be able to develop effective therapeutic interventions to treat or control T2DM and, as a consequence, delay the onset or progression of AD."[131]

A group of researchers investigated whether higher blood sugar levels in cognitively normal, nondiabetic adults were associated with lower brain metabolism. They studied 124 cognitively normal persons aged 64 ± 6 years with a first-degree family history of AD. They reported that, *"As predicted, higher fasting serum glucose levels were significantly correlated with lower brain blood flow, and these decreases were confined to the vicinity of brain regions preferentially affected by AD*.[132]

Vascular risk factors[1] are associated with a higher incidence of dementia. In fact, diabetes mellitus is considered a main risk factor for Alz-

---

[1]Cardiovascular Risk Factors: Traditional risk factors include such things as high blood pressure (hypertension), smoking, obesity, age, lack of physical activity, high cholesterol (hyperlipidemia). However, there are now many other risk factors that also have to be considered. For a full discussion, see:
http://emedicine.medscape.com/article/164163-overview

heimer's disease and both diseases are characterized by vascular (blood vessel) dysfunction. Researchers recently studied this relationship in an animal model and concluded that, *"In conclusion, AD and T2D promote similar vascular dysfunction of the aorta [the main blood vessel from the heart], this effect being associated with elevated oxidative and nitrosative stress and inflammation. Also, AD-associated vascular alterations are potentiated by T2D. These findings support the idea that metabolic alterations predispose to the onset and progression of dementia."*[133]

In late 2014, another group of researchers reviewed the scientific literature on the relationship between diabetes and Alzheimer's disease, and the common blood vessel abnormalities found in both diseases. They stated that, *"Accordingly, evidence-based epidemiological factors support a compelling hypothesis stating that metabolic rundown encountered in Type 2 diabetes causes severe cerebral vascular [brain blood vessel] insufficiencies that are causally linked to long term neural degenerative processes in AD."*[134]

A different group of researchers, also in late 2014, note the following, *"Emerging evidence suggests that diabetes affects cognitive function and increases the incidence of dementia.* Clinically, diabetic patients show decreased executive function, information processing, planning, visuospatial construction[1], and visual memory. Therefore, in comparison with the characteristics of AD brain structure and cognition, diabetes seems to affect cognitive function through not only simple AD pathological feature-dependent mechanisms but also independent mechanisms. Diabetes compromises cerebrovascular function, and might alter the blood-brain barrier. Diabetes also affects glucose metabolism, insulin signaling, and mitochondrial function in the brain. Diabetes also modifies metabolism of Aβ and tau and causes Aβ/tau-dependent pathological changes. Moreover, there is evidence that suggests an interaction between Aβ/tau-dependent and independent mechanisms. *Therefore, diabetes modifies cognitive function through Aβ/tau-*

---

[1]Visual-spatial construction is the ability to mentally manipulate 2-dimensional and 3-dimensional figures. It is typically measured with simple cognitive tests.

dependent and independent mechanisms. Interaction between these two mechanisms forms a vicious cycle."[135]

Insulin is a key hormone regulating metabolism. Insulin binding to cell surface insulin receptors engages many signaling intermediates to control glucose, energy, and lipids as well as a variety of other cell functions. Abnormalities in the function of any of these intermediates, which occur in a variety of diseases, including Alzheimer's disease, cause reduced sensitivity to insulin and insulin resistance[1] with consequent metabolic dysfunction. Chronic inflammation ensues which exacerbates compromised metabolic homeostasis. Insulin resistance is a big topic in Alzheimer's research as of late, as the following points out.

Dr. McGregor and colleagues, reporting in the December 3, 2014 issue of *Molecular Endocrinology*, "The hippocampus [the area in the brain where memories are formed], in particular expresses high levels of both insulin and leptin[2] receptors as well as key components of their associated signaling cascades. Moreover, recent studies indicate that both hormones are potential cognitive enhancers. Indeed, it has been demonstrated that both leptin and insulin markedly influence key cellular events that underlie hippocampal learning and memory. The hippocampal formation is also a prime site for the neurodegenerative processes that occur during Alzheimer's disease, and *impairments in either leptin or insulin function have been linked to CNS-driven diseases like AD.* Thus the capacity of the metabolic hormones, leptin and insulin to

---

[1]Insulin resistance is a condition in which cells fail to respond to the normal actions of the hormone insulin. The body (pancreas) produces insulin, but the cells in the body become resistant to insulin and are unable to use it as effectively, leading to elevated blood sugar (hyperglycemia). Beta cells in the pancreas subsequently increase their production of insulin, further contributing to elevated insulin levels (hyperinsulinemia).

[2]Leptin the "satiety hormone," is a hormone made by fat cells, which regulates the amount of fat stored in the body. It does this by adjusting both the sensation of hunger, and adjusting energy expenditures. Hunger is inhibited (satiety) when the amount of fat stored reaches a certain level. Leptin is then secreted and circulates through the body, eventually activating leptin receptors in the hypothalamus.

CAUSE(S) AND PATHOLOGY

regulate hippocampal synaptic function has significant implications for normal brain function and also CNS-driven disease."[136]

One group of researchers note, *"Insulin resistance has been identified as a major risk factor for the onset of AD.* Animal models of AD or insulin resistance or both demonstrate that AD pathology and impaired insulin signaling form a reciprocal relationship...Exploiting the connection between insulin resistance and AD provides powerful opportunities to delineate therapeutic interventions that slow or block the pathogenesis of AD."[137]

"A critical role of insulin resistance (IR) in Alzheimer's disease (AD) includes beta-amyloid (Aβ) production and accumulation, the formation of neurofibrillary tangles (NFTs), failure of synaptic transmission and neuronal degeneration...IR induces oxidative stress and inflammation in the brain which contributes to Aβ and tau pathology. Aβ accumulation can enhance IR through Aβ-mediated inflammation and oxidative stress. IR is a possible linking between amyloid plaques and NFTs pathology via oxidative stress and neuroinflammation. Additionally, IR could disrupt acetylcholine activity and lead to cognitive impairment in AD. *Preclinical and clinical studies have supported that insulin could be useful in the treatment of AD.* Thus, an effective measure to inhibit IR may be a novel drug target in AD."[138]

In clinical research reported in late 2014, researchers studied the level of impairment in executive functioning in a group of elderly individuals with both Alzheimer's disease and Diabetes Mellitus (DM) as compared to three control groups. Individuals who received neuropsychological testing were identified through a search of electronic medical records at a memory disorder clinic in Florida. Those who had both diagnoses of AD and DM (n = 44) were compared to individuals with AD without DM (n = 44), no AD with DM (n = 52), and no AD without DM (n = 35). Mean age was 79.4 (SD = 5.69. Levels of executive functioning of the four groups were compared. The researchers stated, "Results indicate the AD with DM group was more likely to have impaired functioning. Additionally, the no-AD no-DM group was more likely to have average functioning. There were no differences for the

AD without DM and DM without AD groups...*Individuals diagnosed with both AD and DM are more likely to exhibit impaired executive functioning. These findings support previous studies that reported an increased risk of executive dysfunction in comorbid AD and DM.*"[139]

In the August 26, 2014 issue of *Journal of Alzheimer's disease*, Dr. Ma and colleagues reported their findings on the association between type 2 diabetes mellitus (T2DM), mild cognitive impairment (MCI), and dementia. Their study group included 634 participants with T2DM-MCI, 261 T2DM participants who were cognitively intact, and 585 MCI participants without diabetes. All participants received detailed annual evaluations to detect dementia onset during the five years of follow-up. During follow-up, 152 and 49 subjects developed dementia in the MCI and cognitively-intact groups respectively. In their analysis of the groups, MCI accelerated the median progression to dementia by 2.74 years. *Major risk factors for dementia were age >75 years and longer durations of diabetes, while significantly reduced risks of dementia were associated with oral hypoglycemic agents and lipid lowering agents (HMG-CoA reductase inhibitors, such as Lipitor, Crestor, and others).* Insulin was not associated with significantly changed risk. The researchers concluded that, *"To minimize progression to dementia, it may be worthwhile to target several modifiable diabetes-specific features, such as the duration of disease, glycemic [blood sugar] control, and antidiabetic agents."*[140]

Other Hypotheses

The cellular homeostasis[1] of copper, iron, and zinc is disrupted in AD, though it remains unclear whether this is produced by or causes the changes in proteins. These metals affect and are affected by tau, amy-

---

[1] Homeostasis is the property of a system in which variables are regulated so that internal conditions remain stable and relatively constant. Examples of homeostasis include the regulation of temperature and the balance between acidity and alkalinity (pH). It is a process that maintains the stability of the human body's internal environment in response to changes in external conditions.

loid precursor protein (APP)[1], and APOE. Some studies have shown an increased risk of developing AD with environmental factors such as the intake of metals, particularly aluminum. The quality of some of these studies has been criticized, and other studies have concluded that there is no relationship between these environmental factors and the development of AD.

Some have hypothesized that dietary copper may play a causal role. For example, in 2014, researchers postulated that, "Since low brain copper levels have been described in...various brain regions in Alzheimer's disease [and several other neurodegenerative disorders], a mechanism has been proposed that may underlie the neurodegenerative processes that occur when copper protection against free radicals is impaired."[141]

Also in 2014, a researcher stated, "A myriad of complex factors contribute to AD, promoting the deposition in plaques of amyloid-beta (Aβ), which is the main constituent of this pathognomonic sign of AD at autopsy brain inspection. Aβ toxicity is related to oxidative stress, which results in synaptic loss in specific brain areas, eventually leading to cognitive decline. Metal, and especially copper, is a key factor in these processes."[142]

---

[1] Amyloid precursor protein (APP) is an integral membrane protein expressed in many tissues and concentrated in the synapses of neurons. Its primary function is not known, though it has been implicated as a regulator of synapse formation, neural plasticity and iron export. APP is best known as the precursor molecule whose proteolysis generates beta amyloid (Aβ), a 37 to 49 amino acid peptide whose amyloid fibrillar form is the primary component of amyloid plaques found in the brains of Alzheimer's disease patients.

CHAPTER SIX:
DIFFERENTIAL DIAGNOSIS OF ALZHEIMER'S DISEASE

Other illnesses or conditions may have signs or symptoms in common with Alzheimer's disease. These must be excluded before a diagnosis of AD can be made. Some of these other conditions are briefly discussed below.

Other Types of Dementia (DSM-V)

Alzheimer's dementia is the most common form of dementia, but other types exist as well. It is vital to determine the type of dementia a person has, as treatment, if it exists, is specific. According to the American Psychiatric Association's *Diagnostic and Statistical Manual of Mental Disorders, 5th Edition: DSM-5*, these are the most common types besides Alzheimer's:

- Frontotemporal Lobar Degeneration

    Behavioral variant (three or more of the following):

    Behavioral disinhibition.

    Apathy or inertia.

    Loss of sympathy or empathy.

    Perseverative, stereotyped, or compulsive/ritualistic behavior.

    Hyperorality and dietary changes.

DIFFERENTIAL DIAGNOSIS OF ALZHEIMER'S DISEASE

Language variant:

> Prominent decline in language ability, speech production, word finding, object naming, grammar, or word comprehension.
>
> Relative sparing of learning and memory and perceptual-motor function.
>
> Insidious onset and gradual progression.

- Lewy Body Disease

    Core diagnostic features:

    > Fluctuating cognition and pronounced variations in attention and alertness.
    >
    > Recurrent visual hallucinations that are well-formed and detailed.

    Spontaneous features of Parkinsonism, with onset subsequent to the development of cognitive decline.

    Suggestive diagnostic features:

    > Meets criteria for rapid eye movement sleep behavior disorder.
    >
    > Severe neuroleptic sensitivity.

- Vascular Disease

    Clinical features are consistent with a vascular etiology:

    > Onset of the cognitive deficits is temporally related to one or more cerebrovascular events.
    >
    > Evidence for decline is prominent in complex attention (including processing speed) and frontal-executive function.

    There is evidence of the presence of cerebrovascular disease from history, physical examination, and/or neuro-imaging considered sufficient to account for the neuro-cognitive deficits.

- Traumatic Brain Injury
- Substance/medication Use
- Parkinson's Disease

    The disturbance occurs in the setting of established Parkinson's disease:

    Tremor at rest.

    Stiffness.

    Slowing of movement.

    Postural instability.

    There is insidious onset and gradual progression of impairment.

- Huntington's Disease
- Another medical condition
- Multiple etiologies
- Unspecified

Depression

Depression is one of the most common conditions affecting humanity. Elderly people can develop clinical depression, referred to as "major depressive disorder," but sometimes this can present as having dementia or Alzheimer's dementia. This is referred to as "pseudodementia," because the person doesn't really have dementia, they just appear to have it--but they really have depression. Because of this, any person who appears to have AD should be screened for depression.

Delirium

Delirium, or acute confusional state, is an organically-caused decline from a previously attained baseline level of cognitive function. It is typ-

DIFFERENTIAL DIAGNOSIS OF ALZHEIMER'S DISEASE

ified by fluctuating course, attentional deficits and generalized severe disorganization of behavior. It typically involves other cognitive deficits, changes in arousal (hyperactive, hypoactive, or mixed), perceptual deficits, altered sleep-wake cycle, and psychotic features such as hallucinations and delusions.

It is important to be able to recognize this condition, because it is pretty common in those with dementia, and the incidence increases dramatically with age. In other words, all too often, dementia and delirium are found together.

Delirium itself is not a disease, but rather a clinical syndrome (a set of symptoms), which results from an underlying disease, from medications administered during treatment of that disease in a critical phase, from a new problem with mentation or from varying combinations of two or more of these factors.

Delirium may present in hyperactive, hypoactive, or mixed forms. In its hyperactive form, it is manifested as severe confusion and disorientation, developing with relatively rapid onset and fluctuating in intensity. In its hypoactive form, it is manifested by an equally sudden withdrawal from interaction with the outside world. Delirium may occur in a mixed type where someone may fluctuate between both hyper- and hypoactive periods. Delirium as a syndrome is one which occurs more frequently in people in their later years.

Delirium may be caused by a disease process outside the brain that nonetheless affects the brain, such as infection (urinary tract infection, pneumonia) or drug effects, particularly anticholinergics or other CNS depressants (benzodiazepines and opioids). Although hallucinations and delusions are sometimes present in delirium, these are not required for the diagnosis. Delirium must by definition be caused by an organic process, i.e., a physically identifiable structural, functional, or chemical problem in the brain.

Delirium requires both a sudden change in mentation, and an organic cause for this. Thus, without careful assessment and history, delirium can easily be confused with a number of psychiatric disorders or long term organic brain syndromes, because many of the signs and symptoms of delirium are conditions also present in dementia, depression, and psychosis. Delirium may newly appear on a background of mental illness, baseline intellectual disability, or dementia, without being due to any of these problems.

Treatment of delirium requires treatment of the underlying organic cause(s). In some cases, temporary or symptomatic treatments are used to comfort patients or to allow better patient management (for example, a patient who, without understanding, is trying to pull out a ventilation tube that is required for survival). Delirium is probably the single most common acute disorder affecting adults in general hospitals. It affects 10-20 percent of all hospitalized adults, and 30-40 percent of elderly hospitalized patients and up to 80 percent of ICU patients. In ICU patients or in other patients requiring critical care, delirium is not simply an acute brain disorder but in fact is a harbinger of much greater likelihood of death within the twelve months which follow the ICU patient's hospital discharge.

In the April 2014 issue of the journal *JAMA Psychiatry*, Dr. Hatta and colleagues reported on a study to examine whether ramelteon (Rozerem), a melatonin agonist, is effective for the prevention of delirium. Sixty-seven patients were randomly assigned to receive ramelteon (8 mg/d; 33 patients) or placebo (34 patients) every night for seven days. The researchers concluded that, *"Ramelteon administered nightly to elderly patients admitted for acute care may provide protection against delirium. This finding supports a possible pathogenic role of melatonin neurotransmission in delirium."*[143]

It should be noted, however, that no treatment has shown a robust effect in clinical studies in preventing delirium (much less treating it).

Primary Progressive Aphasia

Primary progressive aphasia (PPA) is a group of disorders characterized by progressive language and speech difficulties. Primary Progressive Aphasias have a clinical and pathological overlap with the Frontotemporal Lobar Degeneration spectrum of disorders and Alzheimer's disease. Studies have shown that verbal communication of people affected by AD at early to moderate stages is abnormal in quality and reduced in quantity compared to those without AD.[144]

Logopenic progressive aphasia is a form of primary progressive aphasia characterized by slow speech and impaired syntactic comprehension and naming. It is defined clinically by impairments in naming and sentence repetition. *It is suspected that an atypical form of Alzheimer's disease is the most common cause of logopenic progressive aphasia.*

Although patients with the logopenic variant of PPA are still able to produce speech, their speech rate may be significantly slowed down due to word retrieval difficulty; composed clinically of speech paucity (scarcity) and dysfluency (impairment of the ability to produce smooth, fluent speech). Over time, they may experience the inability to retain lengthy information, causing problems with understanding complex verbal information. Some additional behavioral features include irritability, anxiety and agitation.

Compared to those people with primary progressive aphasia, patients with the logopenic variant of primary progressive aphasia have been found to be associated with cognitive and behavioral characteristics. Studies have shown that patients with the logopenic variant perform significantly worse on tests of calculation than other primary progressive aphasia patients. Several logopenic variant patients, especially those with Alzheimer's disease pathology, have also been found to perform poorly on memory tasks.

ALZHEIMER'S DISEASE

CADASIL (Cerebral Autosomal-Dominant Arteriopathy with Subcortical Infarcts and Leukoencephalopathy)

CADASIL is the most common form of hereditary stroke disorder, and is thought to be caused by mutations of the *Notch 3* gene on chromosome 19. The disease belongs to a family of disorders called the leukodystrophies. The most common clinical manifestations are migraine headaches and transient ischemic attacks (TIAs)[1] or strokes, which usually occur between forty and fifty years of age, although MRI is able to detect signs of the disease years prior to clinical manifestation of disease.

CADASIL may start with attacks of migraine with aura or subcortical transient ischemic attacks or strokes, or mood disorders between 35 to 55 years of age. The disease progresses to subcortical dementia associated with pseudobulbar palsy and urinary incontinence.

Ischemic strokes are the most frequent presentation of CADASIL, with approximately 85 percent of symptomatic individuals developing transient ischemic attacks or stroke (s). The mean age of onset of ischemic episodes is approximately 46 years (range 30–70). A classic lacunar syndrome occurs in at least two-thirds of affected patients while hemispheric strokes are much less common. It is worthy of note that ischemic strokes typically occur in the absence of traditional cardiovascular risk factors. Recurrent silent strokes, with or without clinical strokes, often lead to cognitive decline and overt subcortical dementia.

MRIs show hypointensities on T1-weighted images and hyperintensities on T2-weighted images, usually multiple confluent white matter lesions of various sizes, are characteristic. These lesions are concentrated around the basal ganglia, periventricular white matter, and the pons, and are similar to those seen in Binswanger disease (see be-

---

[1] A transient ischemic attack (TIA) is a transient episode of neurologic dysfunction caused by ischemia (loss of blood flow) – either focal brain, spinal cord, or retinal – without acute infarction (tissue death). TIAs have the same underlying cause as strokes: a disruption of cerebral blood flow (CBF), and are often referred to as mini-strokes.

low). These white matter lesions are also seen in asymptomatic individuals with the mutated gene. While MRI is not used to diagnose CADASIL, it can show the progression of white matter changes even decades before onset of symptoms.

The definitive test is sequencing the whole Notch 3 gene, which can be done from a sample of blood. However, as this is quite expensive and CADASIL is a systemic arteriopathy, evidence of the mutation can be found in small and medium-size arteries. Therefore, skin biopsies are often used for the diagnosis.

Binswanger's Disease

Binswanger's disease, also known as subcortical leukoencephalopathy, is a form of small vessel vascular dementia caused by damage to the white brain matter. White matter atrophy can be caused by many circumstances including chronic hypertension as well as old age. This disease is characterized by loss of memory and intellectual function and by changes in mood. These changes encompass what are known as executive functions of the brain. It usually presents between fifty-four and sixty-six years of age, and the first symptoms are usually mental deterioration or stroke.

Binswanger's disease can usually be diagnosed with a CT scan, MRI, and a proton MR spectrography in addition to clinical examination. Indications include infarctions, lesions, or loss of intensity of central white matter and enlargement of ventricles, and leukoaraiosis. Leukoaraiosis (LA) refers to the imaging finding of white matter changes that are common in Binswanger disease. However, LA can be found in many different diseases and even in normal patients, especially in people older than sixty-five years of age.

There is controversy regarding whether LA and mental deterioration actually have a cause and effect relationship. Recent research is showing that different types of LA can affect the brain differently, and that proton MR spectroscopy would be able to distinguish the different types more effectively and enable better diagnosis to treat the issue. Because of this information, white matter changes indicated by an MRI or CT cannot alone diagnose Binswanger disease, but can aid to a broader picture in the diagnosis process. *There are many diseases similar to Binswanger's disease including CADASIL syndrome and Alzheimer's disease, which makes this specific type of white matter damage hard to diagnose.*

Progressive Supranuclear Palsy (PSP)

Progressive supranuclear palsy (PSP) is a form of dementia that is characterized by problems with eye movements. Generally the problems begin with difficulty moving the eyes up and/or down (vertical gaze palsy). Since difficulty moving the eyes upward can sometimes happen in normal aging, problems with downward eye movements are the key in PSP. Other key symptoms of PSP include falling backwards, balance problems, slow movements, rigid muscles, irritability, apathy, social withdrawal and depression. The person may also have certain "frontal lobe signs" such as perseveration, a grasp reflex and utilization behavior (the need to use an object once you see it). People with PSP often have progressive difficulty eating and swallowing, and eventually with talking as well. Because of the rigidity and slow movements, PSP is sometimes misdiagnosed as Parkinson's disease.

On scans of the brain, the midbrain of people with PSP is generally shrunken (atrophied), but there are no other common brain abnormalities visible on images of the person's brain.

Less common causes of dementia include normal pressure hydrocephalus (NPH), Creutzfeldt–Jakob disease, and other causes.

Why Early and Accurate Diagnosis is Important

In November 2014, a large group of researchers reported that, "Several lines of evidence from Alzheimer's disease research continue to support the notion that the biological changes associated with AD are occurring possibly *several decades* [emphasis added] before an individual will experience the cognitive and functional changes associated with the disease. The National Institute on Aging-Alzheimer's Association revised criteria for AD provided a framework for this new thinking. As a result of this growing understanding, several research efforts have launched or will be launching large secondary prevention[1] trials in AD."[145]

In late 2014, researchers studied patients with mild cognitive impairment and mild Alzheimer's disease using electroencephalography (EEG)[2]. They found that, "Our results indicate a declined functional network organization even during the prodromal phase. *Degeneration is evident even in the preclinical phase* and coexists with transient network reorganization due to compensation."[146]

Lifestyle modification offers a promising way of preventing or delaying Alzheimer's disease. In particular, nutritional interventions can contribute to decrease the risk of dementia. The efficacy of such interventions should be assessed in individuals thought to be prone to AD. It is therefore necessary to identify markers that may help detecting AD as early as possible. Episodic memory decline appears consistently as the earliest sign of incipient typical AD. An episodic memory test that ensures deep encoding of information and assesses retrieval with free as well as cued recall appears as a useful tool to detect patients at an early stage of AD. Beyond the memory domain, category verbal fluency has been shown to decline early and to predict progression to AD. Moreover, in line with current diagnosis criteria for prodromal AD, combining neuropsychological scores and neuroimaging data allows a better discrimination of future AD patients than neuroimaging or neuropsychological data alone. *Altogether, the detection of cognitive changes*

---

[1]Secondary prevention: Methods to detect and address an existing disease prior to the appearance of symptoms.
[2]Electroencephalography (EEG) is the recording of electrical activity along the scalp. EEG measures voltage fluctuations resulting from electrical current flows within the neurons of the brain. In clinical contexts, EEG refers to the recording of the brain's spontaneous electrical activity over a short period of time, usually 20–40 minutes, as recorded from multiple electrodes placed on the scalp.

that are predictive of the typical form of probable AD already in the pre-dementia stage points to at risk people who are the best target for therapeutic interventions, such as nutrition or physical exercise counseling or dietary interventions.[147]

However, *many cases of Alzheimer's disease remain undiagnosed.* In 2014, researchers stated that, "Overall, we estimate over 100,000 undiagnosed dementia patients in Medicare."[148]

CHAPTER SEVEN:
DIAGNOSIS

Introduction

Even though, as noted above, more than 100,000 people remain undiagnosed with Alzheimer's disease, the U.S. Preventive Services Task Force (USPSTF) concluded in 2013 that, "The USPSTF concludes that the current evidence is insufficient to assess the balance of benefits and harms of screening for cognitive impairment. This recommendation applies to universal screening with formal screening instruments in community-dwelling adults in the general primary care population who are older than 65 years and have no signs or symptoms of cognitive impairment."[149]

Elaborating on the views of the Alzheimer's Association on this topic, Maria Carrillo, PhD, vice president of medical and scientific relations, explained to *Medscape Medical News* that "inadequate evidence of benefit" means there is not enough evidence to make an informed recommendation one way or the other about screening for cognitive decline. More well-designed, long-term research is needed to generate the evidence.

She noted that the Alzheimer's Association is not in favor of "one-time" screening — in which a brief test is conducted on one occasion — which it believes is associated with a high rate of false-positive and false-negative results. Rather, *it advocates cognitive evaluation and regular follow-up assessments in a medical setting to establish a baseline and track change over time, such as through the Medicare Annual Wellness Visit.* "Routine cognitive assessments are not screening, but are a way to detect change over time that could indicate underlying pathology," Dr. Carrillo notes.

She points out that as many *as 50 percent of people with Alzheimer's disease or another form of dementia do not receive a formal diagnosis. In addition, when a diagnosis is received, it is often after the dementia has progressed significantly.*[150]

So who gets a "cognitive assessment" in the United States? Reporting in the January 6, 2015 issue of *Neurology*, Dr. Kotagal and his group answered this question. In order to determine which factors were associated with clinical evaluations for cognitive impairment among older residents of the United States, they studied 297 individuals from the Aging, Demographics, and Memory Study (ADAMS), a nationally representative community-based group, who met criteria for dementia. Informants for these subjects reported whether or not they had ever received a clinical cognitive evaluation. The researchers then evaluated demographic, socioeconomic, and clinical factors associated with an informant-reported clinical cognitive evaluation.

Of the 297 participants with dementia in ADAMS, 55.2 percent (representing about 1.8 million elderly Americans in 2002) reported no history of a clinical cognitive evaluation by a physician. They found that marital status was the only significant independent predictor of receiving a clinical cognitive evaluation, and concluded that, *"Many elderly individuals with dementia do not receive clinical cognitive evaluations. The likelihood of receiving a clinical cognitive evaluation in elderly individuals with dementia associates with certain patient-specific factors, particularly severity of cognitive impairment and current marital status."*[151]

Studies suggest that most people support screening for and disclosure of dementia, but it is not clear whether respondents have reflected on the benefits and risks of diagnosis. Do people actually want more information about Alzheimer's disease and their risk of acquiring it? In order to understand this question better, researchers conducted a survey. The Alzheimer's Prevention Registry is an online community of people at least eighteen years of age who are interested in AD prevention research for purely informational purposes or to be considered for possible research participation in future studies.

DIAGNOSIS

To explore the self-expressed desire for, envisioned reaction to, and basic understanding of pre-symptomatic Alzheimer disease-related genetic and biomarker tests, information about pre-symptomatic testing and an online multiple choice format survey were posted from November 1, 2012, through June 20, 2013, on the registry website. Of 4,036 respondents, 80.8 percent (3195/3952) wanted genetic testing if paid by insurance and 58.7 percent (2261/3851) if it would cost them at least $100. A total of 80.2 percent (3112/3879) wanted biomarker testing. If at high risk for AD, 90.5 percent (3478/3841) endorsed that they would "pursue a healthier lifestyle," but 11.6 percent (427/3706) endorsed "seriously consider suicide."

The implication of a positive genetic test result was incorrectly understood by 13.1 percent (500/3812) and 32.6 percent (1255/3848) failed to view a positive biomarker test result as evidence of increased risk for or the presence of AD. The researchers concluded that, "Despite efforts to increase public awareness of AD, our survey results suggest that greater education of the public is needed. Interested patients should probably undergo psychological screening to identify those at high risk of adverse psychological outcomes, and disclosure of pre-symptomatic test results should be anchored to tangible constructive action plans, such as healthy lifestyle changes, long-term care planning, and, when available and appropriate, participation in research trials."[152]

In order to shed light on this topic, another group of researchers studied 132 individuals' preferences for diagnosis, disclosure and screening for AD before and after discussion of the potential benefits and hazards of diagnosis. At baseline the percentages with a positive attitude were 79.6 percent for diagnosis, 85.7 percent for disclosure and 59.3 percent for screening. The authors concluded that, "although most people want to 'know' if they have AD, there is a diminishing degree of support from disclosure to diagnostic assessment to screening. Preferences for diagnosis and screening decline when respondents have the opportunity to consider the consequences of their decision.[153]

Currently, Alzheimer's disease can be diagnosed with a fair degree of accuracy, using a combination of clinical history, paper-and-pencil tests, and brain imaging. Very soon, we will be able to diagnose it with great accuracy, using a simple blood test.

Paper-and-Pencil Testing

There are too many "paper-and-pencil tests" to list that are designed to assist in the diagnosis of dementia. It seems like every country has their own test(s) used to screen for dementia. Only the most common tests used in the United States are listed below.

ADCS Preclinical Alzheimer Cognitive Composite (ADCS-PACC)

Alzheimer's disease Cooperative Study - Preclinical Alzheimer Cognitive Composite (ADCS-PACC) combines tests that assess episodic memory, timed executive function, and global cognition. The ADCS-PACC is the primary outcome measure for the first clinical trial in preclinical AD (ie, the Anti-Amyloid Treatment in Asymptomatic Alzheimer's study).[154]

Alzheimer Disease Assessment Scale-Cognitive Subscale (ADAS-Cog)

ADAS was designed to measure the severity of the most important symptoms of Alzheimer's disease. Its subscale ADAS-cog is the most popular cognitive testing instrument used in clinical trials of nootropics[1]. It consists of eleven tasks measuring the disturbances of memory, language, praxis[2], attention and other cognitive abilities which are often referred to as the core symptoms of AD.

---

[1]Nootropics, also referred to as *smart drugs, memory enhancers, neuro enhancers, cognitive enhancers*, and *intelligence enhancers*, are drugs, supplements, nutraceuticals, and functional foods that improve one or more aspects of mental function, such as working memory, motivation, and attention.
[2]Praxis: in neurology, the ability to carry out tasks.

DIAGNOSIS

Alzheimer's Disease 8 Screening Questionnaire (AD8)

The AD8 is an informant-based measure that validly and reliably differentiates non-demented from demented individuals. It is sensitive to the earliest signs of cognitive change as reported by an informant. The AD8 takes less than three minutes to complete, and it can be reliably administered either in person or over the phone. Researchers found that, in detecting early dementia, it was superior to the MMSE.

BIMS (Brief Interview for Mental Status)

This is similar to the MMSE, but is used primarily for elderly *patients in nursing homes* as part of the Minimum Data Set 3.0 (MDS 3.0), which is part of the Centers for Medicare and Medicaid Services (CMS) requirements. It is used as a performance-based cognitive screener that can be easily completed by nursing home staff. The range of scores is 0-15, with 15 being the best possible scores. The cutoff for normal is 12. Below this is considered abnormal, and indicates possible early dementia.

A word of caution with the BIMS: It is possible that in some instances, even with a score above 12 (even a score of "15"), some individuals can have dementia, which is apparent by clinical evaluation or by more sophisticated testing, such as neuropsych tests.

Blessed Dementia Rating Scale (BDRS)

The BDRS is a clinical rating scale with twenty-two items that measure changes in performance of everyday activities (eight items), self-care habits (three items), and changes in personality, interests, and drives (eleven items). Ratings are based on information from relatives or friends and concern behavior over the preceding six months. The content of each rating is indicated, but precise question phrasing is not indicated.

A group of researchers compared the Blessed Dementia Rating Scale (BDRS), the Mini Mental State Examination (MMSE), and the Clinical Dementia Rating Scale (CDR). They studied 3,027 individuals for two years, and reported that, "BDRS might be considered as a better tool than MMSE to screen for MCI and dementia."[155]

CFI (Cognitive Function Instrument)

According to an article published February 26, 2015:[156]

> "Researchers with the Alzheimer's Disease Cooperative Study (ADCS) have developed a simple tool to track early changes in cognitive function in older adults without cognitive impairment at the outset. In a longitudinal study, they found that subjective self and partner report of change in cognitive function on the Cognitive Function Instrument (CFI) was associated with traditional measures of cognitive decline; *greater subjective report of memory concerns was associated with worse memory performance over time.*
>
> The CFI asks the participant and partner (usually a family member) fourteen questions that cover the "full realm" of early functional change, the researchers note. Among the "yes-no-maybe" questions: Compared to one year ago, do you feel that your memory (or the subject's memory) has declined substantially? Do others tell you that you tend to repeat questions over and over? (Does the subject tend to do this?) Have you been misplacing things more often, or has the subject?"

Clinical Dementia Rating (CDR)

The Clinical Dementia Rating (CDR) is a numeric scale used to quantify the severity of symptoms of dementia or stage. Using a structured-interview protocol, a qualified health professional assesses a patient's cognitive and functional performance in six areas: memory, orientation, judgment and problem solving, community affairs, home and hobbies, and personal care. Scores in each of these are combined to obtain a composite score ranging from 0 through 3, with 3 being the worst, while a score of zero indicating no impairment.

Clock Drawing Test (CDT)

The Clock drawing test (CDT) is a brief cognitive task that can be used by clinicians who suspect neurological dysfunction based on history. The procedure of the CDT begins with the instruction to the participant to draw a clock reading a specific time. After the task is complete, the test administrator draws a clock with the hands set at the same specific time. Then the patient is asked to copy the image. Errors in clock drawing are classified according to the following categories: omissions, perseverations, rotations, misplacements, distortions, substitutions and additions. Memory, concentration, initiation, energy, mental clarity and indecision are all measures that are scored during this activity. *Those with deficits in executive functioning will often make errors on the first clock but not the second. In other words, they will be unable to generate their own example, but will show proficiency in the copying task.*

A group of researchers found that writing skills deteriorate sooner than the ability to draw in a group of patients with minimal-moderate Alzheimer's disease. They concluded that, *"The findings suggest that the deterioration of writing skills observed in the spontaneous writings of AD patients shows a pattern of impairment..., which is later joined by a disruption of visuospatial and graphomotor processing (e.g., clock drawing).*[157]

A word of caution when administering the CDT (or any paper-and-pencil test): A group of researchers compared the cognitive profile from screening tests of older adults with bipolar disorder (BD) with and without dementia. To do so, they studied 209 older adults. They concluded that, *"Elderly subjects with BD showed greater impairment in*

CDT in both groups (bipolar patients with normal cognition and bipolar patients with AD).[158]

Dementia Severity Rating Scale (DSRS)

The Dementia Severity Rating Scale (DSRS) is a brief, informant-rated questionnaire to quantify functional impairment in Alzheimer's disease. Items are comparable to the Clinical Dementia Rating scale (CDR), but incorporate a broader range of scores to detect finer increments of change across time.

Instrumental Activities of Daily Living (IADL)

Instrumental activities of daily living (IADLs) are not necessary for fundamental functioning, but they let an individual live independently in a community:

- Housework
- Taking medications as prescribed
- Managing money
- Shopping for groceries or clothing
- Use of telephone or other form of communication
- Using technology (as applicable)
- Transportation within the community

A useful mnemonic is SHAFT: shopping, housekeeping, accounting, food preparation/meds, and telephone/transportation.

Impairment in instrumental activities of daily living (IADL) starts as individuals with amnestic mild cognitive impairment (MCI) transition to Alzheimer's disease. However, most IADL scales have not shown IADL alterations in clinically normal (CN) elderly. Researchers conducted a study to determine which of the IADL-related Everyday Cognition (ECog) scale items are most sensitive for detection of early functional changes. To do so, they assessed 290 CN and 495 MCI participants from the Alzheimer's disease Neuroimaging Initiative. *They* found, "...worse performance on 'remembering a few shopping items,' 'remembering appointments,' 'developing a schedule in advance of anticipated events,' 'balancing checkbook,' and 'keeping mail and papers organized' best discriminated MCI from CN. Our results indicate that a few simple questions targeting early functional changes, addressed either to the individual or informant, can effectively distinguish between CN elderly and individuals with MCI."[159]

Another group of researchers, using a different questionnaire, also examined which activities of daily living impairments could identify individuals with mild cognitive impairment (MCI). To do so, they assessed 447 subjects, 289 of whom were cognitively normal (CN) and 158 of whom had MCI. They found that, "...four items best discriminated between CN and MCI subjects (MCI performing worse than CN): 'participating in games that involve retrieving words,' 'navigating to unfamiliar areas,' 'performing mental tasks involved in a former primary job,' and 'fixing things or finishing projects.' Our results point to the earliest functional changes seen in elderly at risk for AD, which could be captured by a few simple questions."[160]

MMSE (Mini-Mental State Exam)

The mini–mental state examination (MMSE) is a sensitive, valid and reliable questionnaire that is *used extensively* to measure cognitive impairment. It is commonly used to screen for dementia. It is also used to estimate the severity and progression of cognitive impairment and to follow the course of cognitive changes in an individual over time; thus making it an effective way to document an individual's response to treatment. Administration of the test takes between 5–10 minutes and examines functions including registration, attention and calculation, recall, language, ability to follow simple commands and orientation. The range of scores is 1-30, with 30 being the best possible score.

Neuropsychological Testing

Neuropsychological tests are specifically designed tasks used to measure a psychological function known to be linked to a particular brain structure or pathway. Tests are used for research into brain function and in a clinical setting for the diagnosis of deficits, including dementia. They usually involve the systematic administration of clearly defined procedures in a formal environment. Neuropsychological tests are typically administered to a single person working with an examiner in a quiet office environment, free from distractions. As such, it can be argued that neuropsychological tests at times offer an estimate of a person's peak level of cognitive performance. Neuropsychological tests are a core component of the process of conducting neuropsychological assessment, along with personal, interpersonal and contextual factors.

Neuropsychological testing is considered the gold standard of paper-and-pencil testing for mental functioning. It can only be administered by Ph.D.-level psychologists. (Neurologists and psychiatrists, who are medical doctors, are generally not trained to administer this type of testing.) It is time-consuming and expensive, but can reveal a great deal about actual brain function. Lack of availability in some areas, cost, and time constraints, limit its general use, however.

Researchers used several neuropsychological tests to identify those best suited to distinguishing Mild Cognitive Impairment (MCI) and early AD from normal aging. Impairments in long-term memory were found in older adults and these were even greater in MCI and AD. Notably, "older adults outperformed young controls on category fluency and produced later acquired and less familiar words. Older adults also outperformed both patient groups on this task, producing more words which were significantly later acquired, less familiar and less typical. *Decline in long-term memory appears nonspecific and in the early stage of AD cannot help the differentiation between normal and pathological brain aging. Normal aging has no negative effects on verbal fluency, and impairment on this task signals not only established AD, but also its prodromal MCI stage.*"[161]

Researchers conducted a study using neuropsychological tests to distinguish between persons with mild Alzheimer's disease who will progress slowly from persons who will progress at an average or faster rate. Participants were classified as Faster (n = 45) or Slower (n = 51) progressors and followed for two years. No disease-specific, health, or demographic variable predicted rate of progression; however, history of heart disease showed a trend. Among the neuropsychological variables, *Trail Making Test - A best distinguished Faster from Slower Progressors.*[162]

Clinical Evaluation

Current state-of-the-art diagnostic measures of Alzheimer's disease are invasive (cerebrospinal fluid (CSF) analysis, which requires a spinal tap), expensive (neuroimaging, such as CAT scans, PET scans, or MRIs), and time-consuming (neuropsychological assessment) and thus have limited accessibility as frontline screening and diagnostic tools for AD.[163]

At the present time, therefore, this leaves clinical evaluation as the centerpiece in the diagnosis of Alzheimer's disease. It involves obtaining a history of the person's ability to function mentally, from birth to the present. Obtaining this information from the patient can be difficult, for self evident reasons. Impaired awareness of memory deficits has been recognized as a common phenomenon in Alzheimer's disease. In order to better understand awareness in groups at risk for future dementia, in 2014, researchers reported findings of their research aimed at determining whether levels of awareness differ among healthy elderly people and patients with subjective cognitive decline (SCD), amnestic and non-amnestic subtypes of mild cognitive impairment (aMCI, naMCI), Alzheimer's disease (AD) and Parkinson's disease (PD). To do so, they studied 756 outpatients of a memory clinic and 211 healthy controls, who underwent thorough neuropsychological testing. They reported that, "At group level, awareness significantly decreased along the naMCI→aMCI→AD continuum, with naMCI patients showing a tendency toward overestimation of memory dysfunction. PD patients showed accurate self-appraisals as long as memory function was largely unaffected. However, there was a considerable between-group overlap in awareness scores…In general, unawareness seems to be associated with decreased cognitive performance in various domains (especially memory)."[164]

Given the above, clinical history is best obtained from family members or other knowledgeable informants, as the patient may not be able to give an accurate history due to a decline in cognitive ability and memory. *Researchers recently confirmed the usefulness of informants in detecting individuals with early dementia.*[165]

And, a different group of researchers found that in their research, *"Informant-based assessments may be superior to performance-based screening measures such as the Mini Mental State Examination in corresponding to underlying Alzheimer's disease pathology, particularly at the earliest stages of decline."*[166]

Depression Screening

In elderly people, sometimes those with depression can appear to have dementia but not be demented. This is sometimes referred to as "pseudodementia." The presence of depression must, therefore, be considered in each person evaluated for dementia. Individuals with dementia may also have concomitant depression, as discussed below. There are numerous paper-and-pencil tests used to detect depression, and some are highlighted below.

The American Psychiatric Association's *Diagnostic and Statistical Manual, Fifth Edition (DSM-V)* criteria for diagnosis of major depressive disorder: At least five of the following symptoms have been present during the same 2-week period, represent a change from previous functioning, and include either depressed mood or loss of interest or pleasure:

- Depressed mood
- Marked diminished interest or pleasure

DIAGNOSIS

- Significant weight loss or weight gain
- Insomnia or hypersomnia
- Psychomotor agitation or retardation
- Fatigue or loss of energy
- Feelings of worthlessness or excessive guilt
- Diminished ability to concentrate
- Recurrent thoughts of death or suicidal ideation

In order to determine the level of depression in individuals with dementia, Dr. Snowden and colleagues studied 27,776 individuals with dementia, mild cognitive impairment (MCI), or normal cognition from 34 Alzheimer's Disease research centers. Reporting their findings in the September 21, 2014 issue of the *American Journal of Geriatric Psychiatry*, they found that, *"MCI and dementia were associated with significantly higher rates of depression*. These findings suggest that efforts to effectively engage and treat older adults with dementia will need also to address co-occurring depression.[167]

A group of researchers in Canada recently came to a similar conclusion. They studied 216 rural individuals who attended a memory clinic between March 2004 and July 2012, where 51 patients were diagnosed with mild cognitive impairment (MCI) and 165 with either dementia due to Alzheimer's disease (AD) or non-AD dementia. They found that, *"The prevalence of elevated depressive symptoms was 51.0 percent in the MCI patients and 30.9 percent in the dementia patients.* Depressive symptoms were more severe in the MCI patients than in the dementia patients. Elevated depressive symptoms were statistically associated with younger age for the MCI group, with lower self-rated memory for the dementia group, and with increased alcohol use and lower quality of life ratings for all patients.[168]

Researchers studied the effects of depression on cognition, while also studying the level of education and reading ability to modify those effects. In order to do so, they included non-demented participants (n = 3,484); a subsample of these participants without dementia (n = 703), who had brain imaging data, was also selected for a separate analysis. Depressive symptomatology was assessed, as well as reading level and years of education. Four distinct cognitive composite scores were calculated: executive function, memory, visual-spatial, and language. Results "revealed interaction effects between reading level and years of education and depressive symptoms on all the cognitive outcome measures except for visual-spatial ability...Our findings indicate that the association between late-life depressive symptoms and core aspects of cognition varies depending on one's reading level and years of education. *Those that had greater levels of education and/or reading ability showed a greater decrease in memory, executive, and language performances as depressive symptoms increased than those with lower years of education and reading ability.*"[169]

Another group of researchers found that race was an important determinant in how depression affects cognition or thinking. They examined 292 non-Hispanic Whites and 37 African Americans over age 54 and found that, "...associations between depressive symptoms and cognition differed by race, independent of age, education, reading level, income, health, and recruitment site. Depressive symptoms were associated with slowed processing speed among Whites and worse task-switching, inhibition, and episodic memory among African Americans. African Americans may be more vulnerable to negative effects of depression on cognition than non-Hispanic Whites."[170]

Dr. Khundakar and colleagues published a very interesting article in the September 10, 2014 issue of the *Journal of Alzheimer's disease* on the treatment of depression in people with Alzheimer's disease. They report that, "Depression is among the most common behavioral and psychological symptoms of dementia, and leads to more rapid decline and higher mortality. Treatment for depression in dementia has centered on conventional antidepressant drug treatment. However, recent major studies have suggested that conventional antidepressant treatments are not effective for depression in dementia. Postmortem studies have also suggested that depression in dementia does not arise from serotonergic or noradrenergic abnormalities, or indeed from the degenerative pathology associated with Alzheimer's disease. In contrast, considerable recent evidence has suggested that alterations in glutamatergic[1] transmission may contribute to the pathophysiology of depression. *This supports the view that treatment-resistant depressed patients, such as many dementia patients, may benefit from agents affecting glutamate transmission.*"[171]

Hamilton Depression Rating Scale (abbreviated HAM-D)

The Hamilton Rating Scale for Depression (HRSD), also called the Hamilton Depression Rating Scale (HDRS), abbreviated HAM-D, is a multiple item questionnaire used to provide an indication of depression, and as a guide to evaluate recovery. The questionnaire is designed for adults and is used to rate the severity of their depression by probing mood, feelings of guilt, suicide ideation, insomnia, agitation or retardation, anxiety, weight loss, and somatic symptoms.

Initially considered the "Gold Standard" for rating depression in clinical research, it is criticized as a test instrument for clinical practice in part because it places more emphasis on insomnia than on suicide ideas and gestures. An antidepressant may show statistical efficacy even when thoughts of suicide increase but sleep is improved, or for that matter, an antidepressant that as a side effect increase sexual and gastrointestinal symptom ratings may register as being less effective in treating the depression itself than it actually is. Hamilton maintained that his scale should not be used as a diagnostic instrument.

The original 1960 version contains seventeen items to be rated (HRSD-17), but four other questions are not added to the total score and are used to provide additional clinical information. Each item on the questionnaire is scored on a 3- or 5-point scale, depending on the item, and the total score is compared to the corresponding descriptor. Assessment time is estimated at twenty minutes.

---

[1]Glutamate is an important neurotransmitter that plays the principal role in neural activation. Glutamate is involved in cognitive functions like learning and memory in the brain.

The Geriatric Depression Scale (GDS)

The GDS questions are answered "yes" or "no" instead of a five-category response set. This simplicity enables the scale to be used with ill or moderately cognitively impaired individuals. The scale is commonly used as a routine part of a comprehensive geriatric assessment. One point is assigned to each answer and the cumulative score is rated on a scoring grid. The grid sets a range of 0-9 as "normal," 10-19 as "mildly depressed," and 20-30 as "severely depressed."

A diagnosis of clinical depression should not be based on GDS results alone. Although the test has well-established reliability and validity evaluated against other diagnostic criteria, responses should be considered along with results from a comprehensive diagnostic work-up. A short version of the GDS (GDS-SF) containing fifteen questions has been developed, and the scale is available in languages other than English. The conducted research found the GDS-SF to be an adequate substitute for the original 30-item scale.

The GDS was validated against Hamilton Rating Scale for Depression (HRS-D) and the Zung Self-Rating Depression Scale (SDS). It was found to have a 92 percent sensitivity and a 89 percent specificity when evaluated against diagnostic criteria.

Cornell Scale for Depression in Dementia (CSDD)

The Cornell Scale for Depression in Dementia (CSDD) is *designed for use in elderly patients with underlying cognitive deficits.* Because this patient population may give unreliable answers, the CSDD additionally uses information from a patient informant, someone who knows and has frequent contact with the patient, and can include family members or care staff.

The CSDD takes approximately twenty minutes to administer. The CSDD is a 19-item scale, with scores of 0 for absent, 1 for mild or intermittent, and 2 for severe symptoms. A total score of 10 indicate probable major depression and greater than 18 indicate definite major depression. However, a recent study found a score of 6 or more has a sensitivity of 93 percent and specificity of 97 percent. The same questions are asked of both the patient and the informant and include mood-related signs of anxiety, sadness, lack of reactivity to pleasant events, and irritability; behavioral disturbance including psychomotor agitation and retardation, physical complaints, acute loss of interest; physical signs such as appetite loss, weight loss, and lack of energy; cyclic functions including diurnal variations and sleep difficulties; and ideation disturbance including suicide, self-deprecation, pessimism, and mood congruent delusions.

Researchers compared the effectiveness or validity of the Geriatric Depression Scale (GDS) and the Cornell Scale for Depression in Dementia (CSDD). They concluded that, "The CSDD retained its validity and specificity as a screening tool for depression in a population of demented, while the GDS versions all diminished in validity. The GDS and the CSDD are both valid screening tools for depression in the elderly; however, *the CSDD alone seems to be equally valid in populations of demented and non-demented.*"[172]

Patient Health Questionnaire (PHQ-9)

The Patient Health Questionnaire can be self-administered or administered by someone other than the patient; it is a tool of 2 (PHQ2) or 9 (PHQ9) items. A meta-analysis found sensitivity to be 80 percent and specificity of 92 percent. The PHQ2 is a screening tool for depression. The PHQ 9 establishes the clinical diagnosis of depression and can additionally be used over a period of time to track the severity of symptoms. PHQ-9 scores of 5, 10, 15, and 20 are representative of mild, moderate, moderately severe, and severe depression, respectively.

Basic Blood Tests

These tests are routinely done in order to provide an overview of a patient's general health status.

Complete Metabolic Panel (CMP)

A comprehensive metabolic panel is a panel of blood tests that measure your sugar (glucose) level, electrolyte (such as sodium and potassium) and fluid balance, kidney function, and liver function. (A BMP or basic metabolic panel is similar to a CMP, but includes fewer tests, excluding liver functions, for example.)

Without noting cause or effect, researchers found an association between decreasing kidney (renal) function and declining cognition. They noted that, "Decline in cognitive functioning in association with declining renal functioning was observed despite statistical adjustment for demographic variables [such as age] and [cardiovascular disease] CVD risk factors and the exclusion of persons with dementia or a history of acute stroke."[173]

Complete Blood Count (CBC)

A complete blood count (CBC) is a blood panel that gives information about the cells in a patient's blood. The cells that circulate in the bloodstream are generally divided into three types: white blood cells (leukocytes), red blood cells (erythrocytes), and platelets (thrombocytes). Abnormally high or low counts may indicate the presence of many forms of disease, and hence blood counts are among the most commonly performed blood tests in medicine.

Without going into details of the study, researchers reported in the *Journal of Neurology* that, "In older persons without dementia, *both lower and higher hemoglobin[1] levels are associated with an increased hazard for developing AD and more rapid cognitive decline.*"[174] The RDW (red blood cell distribution width; discussed in the Longevity setion) is also associated with longevity. The lower the number, the greater the probability of longer life.

---

[1]Hemoglobin, found in red blood cells, carries oxygen from the lungs to the rest of the body.

Lipid Profile or Panel (Cholesterol)

Lipid profile or lipid panel is a group of blood tests that typically includes: total cholesterol, triglycerides, low-density lipoprotein (LDL; "bad" cholesterol), and high-density lipoprotein (HDL; "good" cholesterol). Very-low-density lipoprotein (VLDL) is a type of lipoprotein made by the liver. VLDL is one of the five major groups of lipoproteins that enable fats and cholesterol to move within the water-based solution of the bloodstream. VLDL is assembled in the liver from triglycerides, cholesterol, and apolipoproteins. VLDL is converted in the bloodstream to low-density lipoprotein (LDL).

In a sophisticated research study in healthy older and amnestic mild cognitive impairment (aMCI) individuals, researchers reported, among other things, that *"Interestingly, levels of high-density lipoprotein (HDL) [so called 'good cholesterol'] cholesterol were positively correlated with brain connectivity in aMCI subjects, and increased triglycerides accompanied brain atrophy in specific areas of aMCI subjects..."*[175]

Vitamin D

Vitamin D deficiency is very common, and testing for vitamin D levels in the blood has become routine. Vitamin D is discussed in more detail in the Prevention Section, below.

Hemoglobin A_1C (HgbA_1C)

Hemoglobin A_1C is a form of hemoglobin that is measured to identify the average plasma glucose (sugar) concentration over prolonged periods of time. As the average amount of plasma glucose increases, the fraction of Hemoglobin A_1C increases in a predictable way. *This serves as a marker for average blood glucose levels over the previous three months prior to the measurement.* In diabetes mellitus, higher levels of Hemoglobin A_1C, indicating poorer control of blood glucose levels, have been associated with cardiovascular disease, and other medical complications. Monitoring HgbA₁C in diabetic patients may improve outcomes. Because diabetes is a risk factor for Alzheimer's disease, and a portion of people with AD also have diabetes, ordering this test is not uncommon in people with Alzheimer's disease.

More Specialized Blood Tests

There are many specialized blood tests, and only those more commonly done in people who have, or may have, dementia are mentioned below.

B12

B12 is discussed in more detail in the Prevention Section, below. Inexpensive blood tests for B12 levels are obtained for a variety of reasons, one of which is to rule out a B12 deficiency that can present as cognitive dysfunction, including dementia.

NOTE: Some healthcare providers may look at specific elements of a complete blood count (CBC), namely the mean corpuscular volume (MCV) and mean corpuscular hemoglobin (MCH), and infer that one's B12 level is normal, if the MCV and MCH are normal. However, serum B12 levels can be low, even if the MCV and/or the MCH are normal. Therefore, in order to determine the correct level of B12 in the blood, a specific blood test for B12 must be done.

In addition, even "normal" B12 levels might not be good enough. Quest Diagnostics, one of the largest laboratories in the country, provides laboratory services across the United States. Recently, they have been printing this warning about test results for B12 levels on their lab slips:

> "Please note: Although the reference range for vitamin B12 is 200-1100 pg/mL [picograms per milliliter], *it has been reported that between 5 and 10 percent of patients with values between 200 and 400 pg/mL may experience neuropsychiatric [mental] and hematologic [blood] abnormalities due to occult B12 deficiency*; less than 1

percent of patients with values above 400 pg/mL will have symptoms."

This means that low "normal" B12 levels can be associated with clinically meaningful abnormalities.

C-reactive Protein (CRP)

C-reactive protein (CRP) is manufactured by the liver in response to factors released by white blood cells. Levels in the blood rise in response to inflammation, due to many causes. Because of this, levels are sometimes measured in people with Alzheimer's disease, because it is now known that inflammation is associated with mild cognitive impairment (MCI) and Alzheimer's dementia. (There are many other, less common, more expensive blood tests for immune function or inflammation which are rarely done in people with AD.)

Human immunodeficiency virus (HIV)

The human immunodeficiency virus (HIV) is a virus that causes the acquired immunodeficiency syndrome (AIDS). People infected with this virus, especially if not diagnosed and treated, can present with dementia. Because of this, and in appropriate at-risk populations, patients can be tested for the HIV virus (hopefully in order to exclude its presence). Because so few elderly people are felt to be at risk for infection with this virus, this test is not done very often.

Homocysteine

Epidemiological studies show a positive, dose-dependent relationship between mild-to-moderate increases in plasma total homocysteine concentrations (Hcy) and the risk of neurodegenerative diseases, such as Alzheimer's disease, vascular dementia, cognitive impairment or stroke. The concept of improving patients' clinical outcomes by lowering of Hcy with B vitamins seems to be attractive. Recent B vitamin supplementation trials demonstrated a slowing of brain atrophy and improvement in some domains of cognitive function. Other studies showed that B vitamins supplementation caused a decrease in plasma Hcy and a trend for lowering the risk of stroke. Elevated homocysteine levels are common in elderly people. Therefore, it seems prudent to identify B vitamin deficient subjects and to ensure sufficient vitamin intake. Recent evidence supports the role of Hcy as a potential biomarker in age-related neurodegenerative diseases[176]

A simple blood test can measure the level of homocysteine. The role of B vitamins in preventing Alzheimer's disease is discussed in more detail below, in the Prevention Section.

In late 2014, researchers reported the results of their study of the relationship between serum cholesterol and homocysteine levels, and cognitive function. In order conduct the research, they enlisted 1,889 individuals, measuring total cholesterol, high-density lipoprotein, triglycerides, and homocysteine blood levels. The researchers discovered that, "There was a significant interaction between the homocysteine and cholesterol levels on cognitive scores. In participants with normal homocysteine levels, an inverse U-shaped relationship between total cholesterol level and cognitive score was found, *indicating that both low and high cholesterol levels were associated with lower cognitive scores. In participants with high homocysteine levels, no significant association between cholesterol and cognition was found*...The relationship between cholesterol levels and cognitive function depends upon homocysteine levels, suggesting an interactive role between cholesterol and homocysteine on cognitive function in the elderly population."[177]

Homocysteine is discussed in more detail below, with regard to blood levels of folate, in the Prevention section.

Methylmalonic Acid

Increased methylmalonic acid levels may indicate a vitamin B_{12} deficiency. However, it is sensitive (those with the disease almost always test positive) but not specific (those that test positive do not always have the disease). MMA is elevated in 90-98 percent of patients with B_{12} deficiency. It has lower specificity as 20-25 percent of patients over the age of seventy have elevated levels of MMA, but 25-33 percent of them do not have B_{12} deficiency. For this reason, MMA test is not routinely recommended in the elderly.

Thyroid Tests

The thyroid hormones, triiodothyronine (T_3) and thyroxine (T_4), which are produced by the thyroid gland, which is located in the front of the neck, are primarily responsible for regulation of metabolism. Thyroid-stimulating hormone (TSH) is secreted from the pituitary gland, which is located in the brain. It stimulates the thyroid gland to produce thyroxine (T_4), and triiodothyronine (T_3). Because symptoms of thyroid dysfunction can overlap with depression and poor cognitive function, a TSH is often ordered to exclude thyroid dysfunction.

Venereal Disease Research Laboratory test (VDRL)

The Venereal Disease Research Laboratory test (VDRL) is a blood test for syphilis, which if untreated, can present with dementia. This is rare. Because of this, and in appropriate at-risk populations, patients can be tested for the syphilis (hopefully in order to exclude its presence). Because so few elderly people are felt to be at risk for infection with this bacterium, this test is not done very often.

Brain-derived neurotrophic factor (BDNF)

BDNF acts on certain neurons of the central nervous system and the peripheral nervous system, helping to support the survival of existing neurons, and encourage the growth and differentiation of new neurons and synapses. In the brain, it is active in specific areas vital to learning, memory, and higher thinking. BDNF itself is important for long-term memory.

Dr. Weinstein and colleagues reported the results of their study to examine whether or not higher serum BDNF levels in cognitively healthy adults protect against the future risk for dementia and Alzheimer's disease in the January 2014 issue of *JAMA Neurology*. The authors note that, "In animal studies, brain-derived neurotrophic factor (BDNF) has been shown to improve nerve cell survival and function and improve long-term memory. *Circulating BDNF levels increase with physical activity and caloric restriction, thus BDNF may mediate some of the observed associations between lifestyle and the risk for dementia.* Some prior studies showed lower circulating BDNF in persons with AD compared with control participants."

In order to conduct their study, they followed 2,131 dementia-free participants aged 60 years and older (mean age, 72 years; 56 percent women). "During follow-up, 140 participants developed dementia, 117 of whom had AD...Higher serum BDNF levels may protect against future occurrence of dementia and AD. *Our findings suggest a role for BDNF in the biology and possibly in the prevention of dementia and AD, especially in select subgroups of women and older and more highly educated persons.*"[178]

This test is not typically done in clinical practice as of yet. It is expensive and more of a research tool. One can assume, however, that the more you exercise, the higher your BDNF!

Below we briefly discuss more sophisticated (and unusual) diagnostic tests for Alzheimer's disease, including genetic tests, imaging studies, and so forth.

Dr. Wurtman summarized the current state of affairs in diagnosing Alzheimer's disease at the earliest stage (or even diagnosing it before clinical symptoms develop) in the October 30, 2014 issue of *Metabo-*

lism. The following is the summary of his article. It is technical, and therefore may only be of interest to some readers.

Biomarkers in the diagnosis and management of Alzheimer's disease:[179]

> "Traditionally Alzheimer's disease has been diagnosed and its course followed based on clinical observations and cognitive testing, and confirmed postmortem by demonstrating amyloid plaques and neurofibrillary tangles in the brain. But *the growing recognition that the disease process is ongoing, damaging the brain long before clinical findings appear* [emphasis added], has intensified a search for biomarkers that might allow its very early diagnosis and the objective assessment of its responses to putative [generally considered or reputed to be] treatments. At present at least eight biochemical measurements or scanning procedures are used as biomarkers, usually in panels, by neurologists and others.
>
> "The biochemical measurements are principally of amyloid proteins and their A-beta precursors, or of tau proteins; the scanning procedures identify brain atrophy (MRI), decreased blood flow and metabolism (fMRI), energy utilization and synaptic number (FDG-PET), impaired connectivity between brain regions (DTI), and metabolic markers of diminished cell number (MRS). Additional proposed biomarkers utilize EEG or MEG for quantifying impairments in connectivity, or genetic analyses to illustrate the heterogeneity of disease processes that can cause MCI syndromes. *Recent observations awaiting confirmation suggest that levels of some plasma [blood] phospholipids can also be biomarkers of AD and that reductions in these levels can enable the accurate prediction that a cognitively normal individual will go on to develop MCI or AD within two years.* [This is clearly one of the most exciting developments in the

diagnosis of Alzheimer's disease that has ever occurred.]"

Does the above sound farfetched? It isn't. Some of these tests for Alzheimer's disease are discussed below. The following is just one example of how rapidly scientific advances are coming, in many medical areas!

FDA Approves Blood Test That Gauges Heart Attack Risk

The U.S. Food and Drug Administration (FDA) approved a new blood test, in December 2014, that can help determine a person's future odds for heart attack and other heart troubles. The test is designed for people with no history of heart disease, and it appears to be especially useful for women, and black women in particular, the agency said. "A cardiac test that helps better predict future coronary heart disease risk in women, and especially black women, may help health care professionals identify these patients before they experience a serious [heart disease] event, like a heart attack," Alberto Gutierrez, director of the Office of In Vitro Diagnostics and Radiological Health in the FDA's Center for Devices and Radiological Health, said in an agency news release.[180]

The test tracks the activity of a *specific biological signal of vascular inflammation, called Lp-PLA2*. Vascular inflammation is strongly associated with the buildup of artery-clogging plaques in blood vessels, the FDA explained. As plaque accumulates, arteries narrow and the chances of a serious cardiovascular event increase. The test seems especially sensitive for black women, because they experienced a "higher jump" in the rate of heart attack and other heart disease events when their blood levels of Lp-PLA2 exceeded a certain level. "As a result, the test's labeling contains separate performance data for black women, black men, white women and white men," the FDA said.

Specific Blood Tests for Alzheimer's Disease

NOTE: Most of the specific blood tests or genetic tests (discussed below) are not available in routine clinical practice currently. However, some of them will be. It's just a question of time.

According to Drs. Khan and Alkon, as published in the November 5, 2014 issue of the *Journal of Alzheimer's disease*, *"Although commonly viewed as an abnormality of the brain, Alzheimer's disease is a systemic disease with associated dysfunction in metabolic, oxidative, inflammatory, and biochemical pathways in peripheral tissues, such as the skin and blood cells.* This has led researchers to investigate and develop assays of peripheral AD biomarkers[1] that require minimally invasive skin or blood samples."[181]

To develop preventive therapy for Alzheimer's disease, it is essential to develop AD-related biomarkers that identify at-risk individuals in the same way that cholesterol levels identify persons at risk for heart disease. An early diagnosis is necessary to intervene and slow down the progression of Alzheimer's disease. Unfortunately, the disease typically isn't spotted until symptoms have already appeared and amyloid plaques have begun to accumulate and cause damage to the brain. A variety of tests attempt to predict the development of AD, with new tests now being developed quite often. Some of these tests are discussed below. Many are quite technical and, no doubt, only of interest to some readers.

Insulin Receptor Substrate-1 (IRS-1)

According to a recent article, *a protein, insulin receptor substrate-1 (IRS-1), may be able to predict Alzheimer's disease up to ten years before clinical symptoms appear.* Brain insulin resistance occurs in AD even in the absence of peripheral insulin resistance, but until now, no brain biomarker of brain insulin resistance has been discovered. Re-

---

[1]A biomarker, or biological marker, generally refers to a measurable indicator of some biological state or condition.

search by Dimitrios Kapogiannis, PhD, from the National Institute on Aging in Baltimore, Maryland reported that *the blood test, "near-perfectly discriminates patients with AD from cognitively normal elderly adults, adults with diabetes, and those with frontotemporal dementia."* However, this test is still in the research stage according to Dr. Kapogiannis, who emphasized that a blood test for AD is not around the corner.[182]

Platelet Proteins

Studies have identified Alzheimer's disease-specific cerebrospinal fluid (CSF) biomarkers but sample collection requires invasive lumbar puncture. To identify AD-modulated proteins in easily accessible blood platelets, which share biochemical signatures with neurons (nerve cells), researchers compared platelets from 62 AD, twenty-four amnestic mild cognitive impairment (aMCI), thirteen vascular dementia (VaD), and twelve Parkinson's disease (PD) patients with those of 112 matched controls. They found four proteins that, "…yielded a sensitivity of 94 percent and a specificity of 89 percent to differentiate AD patients from healthy controls. To bridge the gap between bench and bedside, we developed a high-throughput multiplex protein biochip with great potential for routine AD screening…Based on minimally invasive blood drawing, *this innovative protein biochip enables identification of AD patients with an accuracy of 92 percent in a single analytical step in less than 4h.*[183]

CoQ10 Blood Levels

Mitochondrial impairment and increased oxidative stress are considered to be involved in the pathogenesis of neurodegenerative diseases, such as Alzheimer's disease. Coenzyme Q10 (CoQ10) is a component of the electron transport chain localized on the inner membrane of the mitochondria. In addition to its activity in energy production, CoQ10 also has antioxidant activity in mitochondrial and cell membranes, which protects against the reactive oxidative species generated during oxidative stress. Several previous studies have reported no significant differences in serum CoQ10 levels between patients with and without dementia, such as Alzheimer's disease. However, in late 2014, Yamagishi and his colleagues demonstrated for the first time that a lower serum CoQ10 level is associated with a greater risk of dementia. These findings suggest that *assessing blood CoQ10 levels could be useful for predicting the development of dementia*, rather than as a biomarker for the presence of dementia.[184]

N-terminal pro-brain natriuretic peptide (NT-proBNP)

Researchers studied 7,158 subjects without previous memory disorders in a study with a median follow-up of 13.8 years. They tested whether elevated N-terminal pro-brain natriuretic peptide (NT-proBNP) levels would predict any dementia or Alzheimer's disease. The researchers found that, "A total of 220 new dementia cases occurred, of which 149 were AD. Baseline NT-proBNP levels were associated significantly with the risk of dementia in the entire study population...*NT-proBNP is an independent risk marker for dementia, and patient discrimination regarding dementia risk could be improved by using it.*"[185]

Tests Related to Abeta Amyloid and Tau Proteins

Researchers studied individuals with PET scans (described in more detail below) positive for brain abnormalities (i.e., amyloid plaques) found in people who may develop Alzheimer's disease, or already show clinical signs of the disease. Forty PET+ individuals, including cognitively healthy controls (HC), and mild cognitive impairment and AD individuals, and 22 PET- healthy cognitive individuals participated. They noted, "We evaluated the performance of the ratio of APP669-711 to Aβ1-42 (APP669-711/Aβ1-42) as a biomarker. APP669-711/Aβ1-42 significantly increased in the PET+ groups. The sensitivity and specificity to discriminate PiB+ individuals from PiB- individuals were 0.925 and 0.955, respectively. Our plasma biomarker precisely surrogates cerebral [brain] amyloid deposition."[186]

Blood amyloid-β (Aβ) peptide levels have been examined as a low-cost accessible marker for risk of incident Alzheimer's disease and dementia, but results have varied between studies. In order to shed light on this discrepancy, researchers reassessed these associations in one of the largest, prospective, community-based studies to date, the Framingham Study. They studied a total of 2,189 dementia-free participants, aged 60 years or older (mean age, 72; 56 percent women), who had blood amyloid-β (Aβ) peptide levels ($A\beta_{1-42}$ and $A\beta_{1-40}$) measured and were followed prospectively for an average of 7.6 years for the development of dementia, including AD. They concluded that, *"Our results suggest that lower plasma Aβ levels are associated with [higher] risk of AD and dementia."*[187]

Another group of researchers studied proteins pathogenic in Alzheimer's disease by extracting them from blood samples, and then quantifying them to develop biomarkers for the staging of AD. In order to do so, they obtained blood at one time-point from patients with AD (n = 57) or frontotemporal dementia (FTD) (n = 16), and at two time-points from others (n = 24) when cognitively normal and 1 to 10 years later when diagnosed with AD. The researchers concluded that, *"Levels of P-S396-tau, P-T181-tau, and Aβ1-42 in blood predict the development of AD up to 10 years before clinical onset."*[188]

Henrikesen and colleagues studied the Tau-A/Tau-C ratio, which has been linked to nerve cell death and may serve a blood biomarker of cognitive loss. They reported their findings in the August 28, 2014 issue of the *Journal of Alzheimer's disease*, stating that, "These data indicate that *measuring the balance between tau fragments in blood may provide a marker of the rate of progression of AD.*"[189]

Immune Function and Oxidative Stress

A growing awareness exists that pro-oxidative state and neuro-inflammation are both involved in AD. However, the extent of this relationship is still a matter of debate. Artificial neural networks (ANNs) are computational models inspired by central nervous system networks, capable of machine learning and pattern recognition. Researchers used ANNs to better understand the relationship between immunological and oxidative stress markers in AD and MCI. They reported that, "Through a machine learning approach, we were able to construct an algorithm to classify MCI and AD with high accuracy. Such an instrument, requiring a small amount of immunological and oxidative-stress parameters, would be useful in the clinical practice. Moreover, applying an innovative non-linear mathematical technique, *a global immune deficit was shown to be associated with cognitive impairment. Surprisingly, both adaptive and innate immunity were peripherally defective in AD and MCI patients.*"[190]

Blood Test Panels

There have been other tests for Alzheimer's disease announced in 2014 that use different biomarkers to predict the disease. Based on *ten proteins* found in the blood, a team from Oxford predicted onset of AD within *a year* for over 1,100 participants, with 87 percent accuracy. A team from Georgetown University screened for *10 lipids* in 525 participants, and was 90 percent accurate in predicting disease in *three years*.

Dr. Olazaran and colleagues published the results of their research on blood tests for Alzheimer's disease in the February 3, 2015 issue of *Journal of Alzheimer's disease*. Without going into the details of the research, they found that, "Metabolite alterations common to both aMCI [amnestic mild cognitive impairment] and AD patients were used to generate a model that accurately distinguished AD from NC [normal cognition] patients. *The final panel consisted of seven metabolites: three amino acids (glutamic acid, alanine, and aspartic acid), one non-esterified fatty acid (22:6n-3, DHA), one bile acid (deoxycholic acid), one phosphatidylethanolamine [PE(36:4)], and one sphingomyelin [SM(39:1)]*...The final model accurately distinguished AD from NC patients. Importantly, *the model also distinguished aMCI from NC patients, indicating its potential diagnostic utility in early disease stages. These findings describe a sensitive biomarker panel that may facilitate the specific detection of early-stage AD through the analysis of plasma samples.*"[191]

Another group of researchers compared serum metabolites of demented patients (Alzheimer's disease and vascular dementia) and controls, and explored serum metabolite profiles of nondemented individuals five years preceding the diagnosis. In the study, cognitively healthy participants were followed up for 5-20 years. Cognitive assessment, serum sampling, and diagnosis were completed every five years. Of the metabolites studied, *3,4-dihydroxybutanoic acid, docosapentaenoic acid, and uric acid (associated with gout) were found to be predictive of dementia.* The researchers found that, *"Serum metabolite profiles are altered in demented patients, and detectable up to five years preceding the diagnosis. Blood sampling can make an important contribution to the early prediction of conversion to dementia.*"[192]

Genetic Testing

According to one author, *"In should be kept in mind that pre-test counseling and the identification of genetic defects are important in both patients and asymptomatic at risk family members."*[193]

Alzheimer's disease has a strong genetic component and, because of this, much research in AD has focused on identifying genetic causes and risk factors. Much of this research, however, is too complex for the average reader, and therefore will not be discussed in detail. Suffice it to say that researchers are making great strides in this area. According to one group of researchers, "The identification of these recently identified genes has implicated previously unsuspected biological pathways in the pathophysiology of AD."[194]

Fortunately for those with a burning desire to understand more of the details of the genetics associated with Alzheimer's disease, Dr. Bai and colleagues, reported on their database in the November 29, 2014 issue of *Molecular Neurobiology*:[195]

DIAGNOSIS

"To facilitate novel discoveries in this field, here, we have integrated information from multiple sources for the better understanding of gene functions in AD pathogenesis. Several categories of information have been collected, including (1) gene dysregulation in AD and closely related processes/diseases such as aging and neurological disorders, (2) correlation of gene dysregulation with AD severity, (3) a wealth of annotations on the functional and regulatory information, and (4) network connections for gene-gene relationship. In addition, we have also provided a comprehensive summary for the top ranked genes in AlzBase. By evaluating the information curated in AlzBase, researchers can prioritize genes from their own research and generate novel hypotheses regarding the molecular mechanism of AD. To demonstrate the utility of AlzBase, we examined the genes from the genetic studies of AD. It revealed links between the upstream genetic variations and downstream endo-phenotype and suggested several genes with higher priority. This integrative database is freely available on the web at http://alz.big.ac.cn/alzBase."

The apolipoprotein E (APOE) ε4 allele (variant or type) is a major genetic risk factor for Alzheimer's disease. It remains unclear, however, whether blood levels of apoE confer additional risk of developing AD. In order to test this, researchers, reporting in the December 3, 2014 issue of the *Annals of Neurology*, studied 75,708 individuals from the general population. They tested whether low plasma levels of apoE at study enrollment were associated with increased risk of future Alzheimer's disease, and whether this association was independent of ε2/ε3/ε4 APOE genotype. They found that, "*Low plasma levels of apoE are associated with increased risk of future Alzheimer's disease in the general population, independent of ε2/ε3/ε4 APOE genotype. This is clinically relevant, because no plasma biomarkers currently are implemented. Hence, plasma levels of apoE may be a new, easily accessible preclinical biomarker.*"[196]

In late 2014, researchers reported on their extensive literature analysis of the association of the apolipoprotein E (ApoE) gene and exceptional longevity (EL, i.e. reaching 100+years), by identifying possible unequal distribution of alleles/genotypes in the common variants ε2, ε3 and ε4 among centenarians and younger population. The association of ApoE with EL was analyzed in a total of 2,776 centenarians (cases; those living to or beyond 100 years) and 11,941 younger controls (from 13 case-control studies). The researchers found that, "The main result for all ethnic groups combined was that *the likelihood of reaching EL was negatively associated with ε4-allele type* and *the ε3-allele was...positively associated with EL*. The present analysis confirms that, besides its previously documented influence on Alzheimer's and cardiovascular disease risk, *the ApoE gene is associated with the likelihood of reaching EL.*"[197]

Dr. Begum and colleagues reported the results of their very interesting research on specific immune cells found in blood and their relationship to Alzheimer's disease, in the July 29, 2014 issue of *Translational Psychiatry*. Due to its complexity and difficulty translating their work into everyday English, the summary of their findings is included in its entirety below:[198]

> "Adaptive immunity to self-antigens causes autoimmune disorders, such as multiple sclerosis, psoriasis and type 1 diabetes; paradoxically, T- and B-cell [immune cells] responses to amyloid-β (Aβ) reduce Alzheimer's disease (AD)-associated pathology and cognitive impairment in mouse models of the disease. The manipulation of adaptive immunity has been a promising therapeutic approach for the treatment of AD, although vaccine and anti-Aβ antibody approaches have proven difficult in patients, thus far. CD4(+) T cells have a central role in regulating adaptive immune responses to antigens, and Aβ-specific CD4(+) T cells have been shown to reduce AD pathology in mouse models. As these cells may facilitate endogenous mechanisms that counter AD, an evaluation of their abundance before and during AD

could provide important insights. Aβ-CD4see is a new assay developed to quantify Aβ-specific CD4(+) T cells in human blood, using dendritic cells derived from human pluripotent stem cells. In tests of >50 human subjects Aβ-CD4see showed an age-dependent decline of Aβ-specific CD4(+) T cells, which occurs earlier in women than men. In aggregate, men showed a 50 percent decline in these cells by the age of seventy years, but women reached the same level before the age of sixty years.

Notably, women who carried the AD risk marker apolipoproteinE-ε4 (ApoE4) showed the earliest decline, with a precipitous drop between forty-five and fifty-two years, when menopause typically begins. Aβ-CD4see requires a standard blood draw and provides a minimally invasive approach for assessing changes in Aβ biology that may reveal AD-related changes in physiology by a decade. Furthermore, CD4see probes can be modified to target any peptide, providing a powerful new tool to isolate antigen-specific CD4(+) T cells from human subjects."

Exciting new research by Dr. Lill and and more than fifty colleagues, reported in the April 30, 2015 issue of the journal *Alzheimer's & Dementia* that:[199]

"A rare variant in TREM2[1] (p.R47H, rs75932628) [a protein] was recently reported to increase the risk of Alzheimer's disease (AD) and, subsequently, other neurodegenerative diseases, i.e. frontotemporal lobar degeneration (FTLD), amyotrophic lateral sclerosis (ALS), and Parkinson's disease (PD). Here we comprehensively assessed TREM2 rs75932628 for association with these

---

[1]TREM2: "Receptor expressed on myeloid cells 2" also known as TREM-2 is a protein that in humans is encoded by the TREM2 gene.

diseases in a total of 19,940 previously untyped subjects of European descent. These data were combined with those from twenty-eight published data sets by meta-analysis. Furthermore, we tested whether rs75932628 shows association with amyloid beta ($A\beta_{42}$) and total-tau protein levels in the cerebrospinal fluid (CSF) of 828 individuals with AD or mild cognitive impairment.

Our data show that rs75932628 [a varient of TREM2] is highly significantly associated with the risk of AD across 24,086 AD cases and 148,993 controls of European descent (odds ratio or OR = 2.71). No consistent evidence for association was found between this marker and the risk of FTLD, PD, and ALS. Furthermore, carriers of the rs75932628 risk allele showed significantly increased levels of CSF-total-tau (P = .0110) but not $A\beta_{42}$ suggesting that TREM2's role in AD may involve tau dysfunction."

Cerebral Spinal Fluid (CSF)

Cerebrospinal fluid (CSF) is a clear, colorless bodily fluid found around the brain and spine. It is produced in the brain. It acts as a cushion or buffer for the brain and spinal cord, providing basic mechanical and immunological protection to the brain inside the skull, and it serves a vital function in regulation of cerebral or brain blood flow.

CSF can be tested for the diagnosis of a variety of neurological diseases, usually obtained by a procedure called lumbar puncture. This is carried out under sterile conditions by inserting a needle into the space around the spinal cord (subarachnoid space), usually between the third and fourth lumbar vertebrae. CSF is extracted through the needle, and tested. Cells in the fluid are counted, as are the levels of protein and glucose. These parameters alone may be extremely beneficial in the diagnosis of subarachnoid hemorrhage and central nervous system infections (such as meningitis).

For some, but not all, people with Alzheimer's disease there can be abnormalities found in CSF. Unfortunately, this is "invasive," somewhat traumatic, relatively expensive, and is generally only performed by certain types of physicians, such as neurologists, interventional radiologists, hospitalists (hospital specialists), and ER physicians. Examining CSF in order to diagnose Alzheimer's disease is not standard practice, and is mostly limited to specific research studies. However, obtaining CSF can be helpful in making a diagnosis of AD.[200]

CSF Amyloid Beta (Aß) and Tau

Abnormal levels of amyloid-beta, t-tau, and p-tau CSF biomarkers and decreased brain uptake of glucose have recently been used in the early diagnosis of AD in experimental studies. Although presently, there are no Food and Drug Administration (FDA)-approved diagnostics for early detection of AD, a panel of promising AD biomarkers in CSF may be a likely candidate for the clinical diagnosis of AD.[201]

Dr. Ritchie and colleagues, from the Imperial College London, London, UK, conducted an extensive literature review on the value of blood and CSF amyloid beta for the diagnosis of Alzheimer's disease dementia and other dementias in people with mild cognitive impairment (MCI). Publishing their finding in June 2014, they concluded that, "The proposed diagnostic criteria for prodromal dementia and MCI due to Alzheimer's disease, although still being debated, would be fulfilled where there is both core clinical and cognitive criteria and a single biomarker abnormality. From our review, the measure of abnormally low CSF Aß[42] levels has very little diagnostic benefit with likelihood ratios suggesting only marginal clinical utility. The quality of reports was also poor, and thresholds and length of follow-up were inconsistent. *We conclude that when applied to a population of patients with MCI, CSF Aß[42] levels cannot be recommended as an accurate test for Alzheimer's disease.*"[202]

However, Dr. Palmqvist and colleagues, reporting in the October 7, 2014 issue of *JAMA Neurology*, came to a different conclusion from the authors above. They conducted research to study whether CSF biomarkers, analyzed consecutively in routine clinical practice during two years, can predict brain Aβ deposition and to establish a threshold for Aβ42 abnormality. They compared amyloid positron emission tomography (brain PET scan) imaging with CSF levels of amyloid beta (Aβ) in patients with mild cognitive impairment (MCI). The found that, *"Cerebrospinal fluid Aβ42 levels can be used with high accuracy to determine whether a patient has normal or increased cortical [brain] Aβ deposition and so can be valuable for the early diagnosis of Alzheimer disease."*[203]

Other researchers came to a similar conclusion as the group above. Without going into the details, they stated, *"Our results confirm the key role of CSF biomarkers [Aβ1-42, p-tau181] in predicting patient conversion from [mild cognitive impairment] MCI to dementia. The study suggests that CSF biomarkers may also be reliable in a real world clinical setting."*[204]

Dr. Seeburger and fifteen colleagues, reporting in the November 12, 2014 issue of the *Journal of Alzheimer's disease*, studied the relationship between numerous CSF biomarkers and Alzheimer's disease compared to normal "controls." This study is technical but important, because it is one of the few studies to compare results with actual brain pathology, examined after death. The researchers noted, "Cerebrospinal fluid (CSF) amyloid-β (Aβ) and tau [another protein associated with AD] have been studied as markers of Alzheimer's disease. Combined Aβ42 and t-tau distinguishes AD from healthy controls with a sensitivity and specificity (sens/spec) near 89 percent across studies. This study examined these markers using extensive longitudinal follow up and postmortem evaluation to confirm clinicopathological status. Baseline CSF was analyzed from 227 participants with AD (97 percent autopsy-confirmed), mild cognitive impairment (MCI; 73 percent confirmed), other dementia syndrome (ODS; 100 percent confirmed), and controls (CTL; 27 percent confirmed, follow up 9-13 years). Biomarker concentrations were analyzed. AD patients had lower CSF Aβ42 and higher t-tau, p-tau, t-tau/Aβ42, and t-tau/Aβ40 compared to CTLs, with MCI intermediate. CTL and MCI participants who progressed to

AD demonstrated more AD-like profiles...In a well-characterized, homogeneous population, *a single cutoff for baseline CSF Aβ and tau markers can distinguish AD with a high level of sens/spec compared to other studies.*"[205]

Researchers conducted an extensive literature review to evaluate the clinical importance of cerebrospinal fluid (CSF) β-amyloid 42 (Aβ42) in mild cognitive impairment (MCI), Alzheimer's disease and other dementias, more specifically: frontotemporal dementia (FTD), dementia with Lewy bodies (DLB), Parkinson's disease (PD) with dementia (PDD) and vascular dementia (VaD). Fifty eligible articles were identified. The researchers stated, *"We found that CSF Aβ42 concentrations were significantly lower in AD compared to MCI, FTD, PDD, and VaD... Results from this meta-analysis hinted that CSF Aβ42 is a good biomarker for discriminating Alzheimer's disease from other dementias and MCI."*[206]

In a scientific paper from late 2014, entitled "The Clinical Use Of Cerebrospinal Fluid Biomarker Testing For Alzheimer's Disease Diagnosis: A Consensus Paper From The Alzheimer's Biomarkers Standardization Initiative [European]," the authors, concluded that, *"Consensus was reached that lumbar puncture for AD CSF biomarker analysis be considered as a routine clinical test in patients with early-onset dementia, at the prodromal stage or with atypical AD. Moreover, consensus was reached on which biomarkers to use, how results should be interpreted, and potential confounding factors. Changes in Aβ$_{1-42}$, T-tau, and P-tau$_{181P}$ allow diagnosis of AD in its prodromal stage. Conversely, having all three biomarkers in the normal range rules out AD. Intermediate conditions require further patient follow-up."*[207]

CSF Apolipoprotein E (ApoE)

Apolipoprotein E (ApoE) is a type of protein. In the central nervous system (CNS), ApoE is mainly produced by brain cells (astrocytes), and transports cholesterol to nerve cells (neurons).

Apolipoprotein E plays a role in the cause or pathogenesis of Alzheimer's disease. Cerebrospinal fluid (CSF) and blood (plasma) level alterations have been reported in AD patients. In search of a potential biomarker, which would be predictive of cognitive, functional, or motor decline, researchers analyzed CSF apolipoprotein E (ApoE) levels of AD patients. Without going into details, the researchers found "No association of CSF ApoE levels and speed of decline on the various scales could be established...Herein, *CSF ApoE at time of AD diagnosis could not be shown to be a viable biomarker for future cognitive, functional, or motor decline.*"[208]

Dr. Lautner and seventeen colleagues, reporting in the October 2014 issue of *JAMA Psychiatry*, noted that, "Several studies suggest that the apolipoprotein E (APOE) ε4 allele [type] modulates cerebrospinal fluid (CSF) levels of β-amyloid 42 (Aβ42)." They conducted a study "To evaluate whether the APOE genotype affects the diagnostic accuracy of CSF biomarkers for Alzheimer disease (AD), in particular Aβ42 levels, and whether the association of APOE ε4 with CSF biomarkers depends on cortical [brain] Aβ status." Without going into details of the study, they concluded that, "*Cerebrospinal fluid levels of Aβ42 are strongly associated with the diagnosis of AD* and cortical Aβ accumulation *independent of APOE genotype*. The clinical cutoff for CSF levels of Aβ42 should be the same for all APOE genotypes."[209]

CSF Endostatin

Endostatin, a fragment of collagen that accumulates in the brain of patients with Alzheimer's disease, in the cerebrospinal fluids (CSF) of patients with neurodegenerative diseases. Researchers measured the level of total protein, endostatin, amyloid-β1-42 peptide, tau, and hyperphosphorylated tau proteins in CSF of patients with AD (n = 57), behavioral frontotemporal dementia (bvFTD, n = 22), non-AD and non FTD dementia (nAD/nFTD, n = 84), and 45 subjects without neurodegenerative diseases. They found that, "The concentration of endostatin in CSF was higher than the levels of the three markers of AD both in control subjects and in patients with neurodegenerative diseases. The endostatin/amyloid-β1-42 ratio was significantly increased in patients with AD and nAD/nFTD compared to controls. The endostatin/tau protein ratio was significantly decreased in patients with AD but was increased in bvFTD patients compared to controls. In the same way, the endostatin/hyperphosphorylated tau protein ratio was decreased in patients with AD but increased in patients with bvFTD compared to controls. *The measurement of endostatin in CSF and the calculation of its ratio relative to well-established AD markers improve the diagnosis of bvFTD patients and the discrimination of patients with AD from those with bvFTD and nAD/nFTD.*"[210]

In summary, endostatin helps clarify the diagnosis of Alzheimer's disease by excluding other potential causes of dementia.

So what is the real-world impact of the use of cerebrospinal fluid (CSF) biomarkers for Alzheimer's disease on decision making and patient management. In order to answer this question, researchers studied patients attending a high-level or "tertiary" memory clinic. They included all patients, for one year, visiting the clinic for cognitive screening. Neurologists completed questionnaires before and after CSF results were known. They assessed the change of diagnosis, diagnostic confidence, and impact on patient management. A total of 438 patients (age 63 ± 8 years, 39 percent women) were included, of whom 351 (80 percent) underwent lumbar puncture. After the disclosure of CSF results, 23/351 (7 percent) diagnoses were changed. Diagnostic confidence increased from 84 percent to 89 percent. There were consequences for management in 44/351 (13 percent) patients with CSF, and 13/87 (15 percent) patients because of unavailable CSF. There was no effect of age on these results. The researchers concluded that, *"CSF biomarkers aid clinicians with decision making during diagnostic work-up of cognitive disorders. This study may be useful for developing guidelines for the implementation of CSF biomarkers in daily practice."*[211]

Neuroimaging (Brain Scans)

NOTE: A variety of scans and other procedures can aid in the diagnosis of Alzheimer's disease but when used alone, cannot be relied upon to make the diagnosis of AD. To date, there is no single blood test or other test that is 100 percent accurate. Many of the following article summaries are quite technical, but are included for those interested in such details.

As one author notes, "In clinical practice, neuroimaging examinations such as X-ray CT and MRI of the brain are useful to exclude cerebrovascular disorders [such as strokes and aneurysms], brain tumors, subdural hematomas, and normal pressure hydrocephalus from neurodegenerative disorders [such as Alzheimer's disease)] After differentiating those disorders, the regional distribution patterns of atrophy [brain shrinkage], neuronal [nerve] injury, or functional impairment detected by morphological MRI, perfusion SPECT, or 18F-FDG PET are useful for the differential diagnosis of neurodegenerative diseases [such as Alzheimer's disease]…Those structural, functional, and pathology specific neuroimaging tools can be used not only for the early diagnosis, but also for tracing disease progression in understanding the relationship between lifestyle diseases and dementia, and developing disease modifying therapies."[212]

In a review article published in 2014, titled, *The Appropriate Use Of Neuroimaging In The Diagnostic Work-Up Of Dementia: An Evidence-Based Analysis*, researchers sought to determine the appropriate use of neuroimaging during the diagnostic work-up of dementia, including indications for neuroimaging and comparative accuracy of alternative technologies. After an extensive review of the relevant scientific literature, they found that, "Approximately ten percent of dementia cases are potentially treatable, though less than one percent reverse partially or fully. *Neither prediction rules nor clinical indications reliably select the subset of patients who will likely benefit from neuroimaging. Clinical utility is highest in ambiguous cases or where dementia may be mixed, and lowest for clinically diagnosed Alzheimer disease or clinically excluded vascular dementia. There is a lack of evidence that MRI is superior to CT in detecting a vascular component to dementia. Accuracy of structural imaging is moderate to high for discriminating different types of dementia."*[213]

"Computed tomography and magnetic resonance imaging are considered first-line imaging modalities for the routine evaluation of Alzheimer's disease."[214]

CT (Computed Tomography) Scan

X-ray computed tomography (X-ray CT) is a technology that uses computer-processed X-rays to produce tomographic images (virtual 'slices') of specific areas of the scanned object, allowing the user to see inside without cutting. Digital geometry processing is used to generate a three-dimensional image of the inside of an object from a large series of two-dimensional radiographic images taken around a single axis of rotation. Medical imaging is the most common application of X-ray CT. Its cross-sectional images are used for diagnostic and therapeutic purposes in various medical disciplines.

As X-ray CT is the most common form of CT in medicine and various other contexts, the term computed tomography alone (or CT) is often used to refer to X-ray CT, although other types exist (such as positron emission tomography [PET] and single-photon emission computed tomography [SPECT]). Older and less preferred terms that also refer to X-ray CT are computed axial tomography (CAT scan) and computer-aided/assisted tomography.

Use of CT has increased dramatically over the last three decades in many countries. An estimated 72 million scans were performed in the United States in 2007. CT scans can be performed with and without contrast dye. Risks associated with CT scans include possible allergy to the dye and radiation exposure.

In contrast to the article above, where the use of CT and MRI scans were found to be equally sensitive in the differential diagnosis of Alzheimer's disease, a special type of CT scan has been found to be more sensitive to a particular type of brain atrophy or shrinkage in AD. The article reporting this research is quite technical. In summary, "The voxel-based morphometry (VBM) technique using brain magnetic resonance imaging (MRI) objectively maps gray matter [brain nerve cell] loss. *This newly developed CT-based VBM technique can detect significant atrophy in the entorhinal cortex [a specific area of the brain] in probable AD patients as previously reported using MRI-based VBM. However, CT-VBM was more sensitive and revealed larger areas of significant atrophy than MR-VBM.*"[215]

MRI (Magnetic Resonance Imaging)

Magnetic resonance imaging (MRI) is a medical imaging technique used in radiology to investigate the anatomy and physiology of the body. MRI scanners use strong magnetic fields and radio waves to form images of the body. The technique is widely used in hospitals for medical diagnosis, staging of disease and for follow-up without exposure to radiation.

MRI has a wide range of applications in medical diagnosis and there are estimated to be over 25,000 scanners in use worldwide. Since MRI does not use any ionizing radiation, its use is recommended in preference to CT when either modality could yield the same information. Contraindications to MRI include most cochlear implants and cardiac pacemakers, shrapnel and metallic foreign bodies in the orbits.

There are many studies of the use of MRI in the diagnosis of Alzheimer's disease, and only a few are highlighted below.

According to one research group, "Structural MRI measures of the hippocampus [primary memory area of the brain] and medial temporal lobe are still the most clinically validated biomarkers for AD, but newer techniques such as functional MRI and diffusion tensor imaging offer great scope in tracking changes in the brain, particularly in functional and structural connectivity, which may precede gray matter atrophy [brain shrinkage]."[216]

Another detailed study noted that, "Even though the role of hippocampal atrophy is well known in the later stages of decline, the ability of fornix-hippocampal markers to predict the earliest clinical deterioration is less clear." To examine the involvement of the hippocampus-fornix circuit in the very earliest stages of cognitive impairment and to determine whether the volumes of fornix white matter and hippocampal gray matter would be useful markers for understanding the onset of dementia and for clinical intervention, researchers studied a group of individuals for four years. They found that, "Fornix body volume and axial diffusivity were highly significant predictors of cognitive decline from normal cognition. Hippocampal volume was not significant as a predictor of decline but was significantly associated with fornix volume and diffusivity. This could be among the first studies establishing fornix degeneration as a predictor of incipient cognitive decline among healthy elderly individuals. Predictive fornix volume reductions might be explained at least in part by clinically silent hippocampus degeneration. The importance of this finding is that white matter tract measures may become promising candidate biomarkers for identifying incipient cognitive decline in a clinical setting, possibly more so than traditional gray matter measures."[217]

According to one group of researchers, reporting the results of their study in late 2014, "Normal aging is associated with a decline in cognitive abilities, particularly in the domains of psychomotor speed and executive functioning. However, 'aging,' per se, is not a cause of cognitive decline but rather a variable that likely captures multiple accumulating biological changes over time that collectively affect mental abilities. Recent work has focused on the role of cerebrovascular disease as one of the biological changes. In the current study, we examined whether lobar [frontal, temporal, parietal, occipital lobe regions] microbleeds [small hemorrhages] - magnetic resonance imaging (MRI) signal voids due to hemosiderin [iron] deposits secondary to cerebral amyloid angiopathy - are associated with cognitive decline in normal aging...Here, we used a longitudinal design to examine whether the presence of lobar microbleeds is associated with the rate of cognitive decline among non-demented older adults. Participants came from an ongoing longitudinal community-based aging study, in which subjects were evaluated at 18-24 months intervals and received a full medical, neurological, and neuropsychological examination at each of the follow-up visits. A total of 197 non-demented participants (mean age: 84.15) were studied...We compared cognition between individuals with two or more (n = 11) and fewer than 2 (n = 186) lobar microbleeds and examined longitudinal cognitive change beginning 9.47 years before the MRI scan. Subjects with two or more lobar microbleeds had worse executive functioning at the visit closest to the MRI scan and had a faster decline in executive function over time than subjects with fewer than 2 lobar microbleeds...Conclusion: *Lobar microbleeds, a marker of cerebral amyloid angiopathy, are associated with an accelerated rate of executive function decline.* The presence of cerebral amyloid angiopathy may be an important source of cognitive decline in aging. Future work should examine how cerebral amyloid angiopathy interacts with neurodegenerative processes, such as Alzheimer's disease."[218]

There is growing evidence that vascular health plays a significant role in the cause of Alzheimer's disease. Understanding the timing of vascular changes in relation to progression from cognitive impairment to AD has become of increasing importance, being both possible pre-clinical markers and potentially modifiable risk factors. White matter hyperintensities (WMH) detected with magnetic resonance imaging (MRI), are commonly used to assess cerebrovascular burden in cognitive impairment and appear to be associated with an increased risk of cognitive decline due to many causes. One group of researchers reported in 2014 that, "*Overall, current findings across the literature suggest that WMH may predict AD at least a decade before the clinical stage of the disease*, independently of biomarkers of AD pathology, thus indicating that vascular factors may constitute important targets for pre-clinical detection and intervention."[219]

Cross-sectional volumetric measures of WMH, particularly in the parietal lobes, are associated with increased risk of AD. Researchers sought to determine whether the longitudinal regional progression of WMH predicts the development of AD above-and-beyond traditional radiological markers of neurodegeneration (i.e., hippocampal atrophy and cortical thickness). "Three hundred three nondemented older adults (mean age = 79.24) received high-resolution magnetic resonance imaging (MRI) at baseline and then again 4.6 years later. Over the follow-up interval 26 participants progressed to AD...Smaller baseline hippocampus volume, change in hippocampus volume (i.e., atrophy), higher baseline parietal lobe WMH, and increasing parietal lobe WMH volume but not WMH in other regions or measures of cortical thickness, independently predicted progression to AD. *The findings provide strong evidence that regionally accumulating WMH [in the parietal lobe] predict AD onset in addition to hallmark neurodegenerative changes typically associated with AD."*[220]

Hippocampal (one of the main areas where memories are formed) atrophy is frequently observed on magnetic resonance images (MRIs) from patients with Alzheimer's disease and persons with mild cognitive impairment. Even in asymptomatic elderly, a small hippocampal volume on magnetic resonance imaging is a risk factor for developing Alzheimer's disease. However, not everyone with a small hippocampus develops dementia. With the increased interest in the use of sequential magnetic resonance images as potential surrogate biomarkers of the disease process, it has also been shown that the rate of hippocampal atrophy is higher in persons with Alzheimer's disease compared to those with mild cognitive impairment and the healthy elderly. Whether a higher rate of hippocampal atrophy also predicts Alzheimer's disease or subtle cognitive decline in non-demented elderly is unknown.

In order to study this relationship, researchers followed a group of 518 elderly (age 60-90 years, 50 percent female) for an average of ten years. Without going into the details of the study, the researchers concluded that, "We found an increased risk to develop dementia per faster rate of decline in hippocampal volume. Furthermore, decline in hippocampal volume predicted onset of clinical dementia when corrected for baseline hippocampal volume. In people who remained free of dementia during the whole follow-up period, we found that decline in hippocampal volume paralleled, and preceded, specific decline in delayed word recall. No associations were found in this sample between rate of hippocampal atrophy, Mini Mental State Examination and tests of executive function. *Our results suggest that rate of hippocampal atrophy is an early marker of memory decline and dementia*, and could be of additional value when compared with a single hippocampal volume measurement as a surrogate biomarker of dementia."[221]

There is growing recognition that poor brain blood flow (cerebral hypoperfusion) is related to the pathogenesis of Alzheimer's disease, implicating the measurement of cerebral blood flow (CBF) as a possible biomarker of AD. The ability to identify the earliest and most reliable markers of incipient cognitive decline and clinical symptoms is critical to developing effective preventive strategies and interventions for AD. In 2014, researchers noted that, "Arterial spin labeling (ASL) magnetic resonance imaging (MRI) measures CBF. *Studies using ASL MRI in humans indicate that CBF changes are present several years before the development of the clinical symptoms of AD.* Moreover, ASL-measured CBF has been shown to distinguish between cognitively normal individuals, adults at risk for AD, and persons diagnosed with AD. Some studies indicate that CBF may even be sensitive for predicting cognitive decline and conversion to mild cognitive impairment and AD over time. Taken together, evidence suggests that the current staging models of AD biomarker pathology should incorporate early changes in CBF as a useful biomarker, possibly present even earlier than amyloid-β accumulation. Though still a research tool, ASL imaging is a promising non-invasive and reliable method with the potential to serve as a future clinical tool for the measurement of CBF in preclinical AD."[222]

Positron Emission Tomography (PET) Scan

NOTE: Expense and availability limit the use of PET scans in the diagnosis of AD.

Positron emission tomography (PET) is a nuclear medicine, functional imaging technique that produces a three-dimensional image of functional processes in the body. The system detects pairs of gamma rays emitted indirectly by a positron-emitting radionuclide (tracer), which is injected into the body on a biologically active molecule. Three-dimensional images of tracer concentration within the body are then constructed by computer analysis. In modern PET-CT scanners, three dimensional imaging is often accomplished with the aid of a CT X-ray scan performed on the patient during the same session, in the same machine.

If the biologically active molecule chosen for PET is fluorodeoxyglucose (FDG), an analogue of glucose, the concentrations of tracer imaged will indicate tissue metabolic activity by virtue of the regional glucose uptake. Use of this tracer to explore the possibility of cancer metastasis (i.e., spreading to other sites) is the most common type of PET scan in standard medical care (90 percent of current scans). However, on a minority basis, many other radioactive tracers are used in PET to image the tissue concentration of many other types of molecules of interest.

To conduct the scan, a short-lived radioactive tracer isotope is injected into the living subject (usually into blood circulation). The tracer is chemically incorporated into a biologically active molecule. There is a waiting period while the active molecule becomes concentrated in tissues of interest; then the subject is placed in the imaging scanner. The molecule most commonly used for this purpose is fluorodeoxyglucose (FDG), a sugar, for which the waiting period is typically an hour. During the scan, a record of tissue concentration is made as the tracer decays.

PET scans are increasingly read alongside CT or magnetic resonance imaging (MRI) scans, with the combination (called "co-registration") giving both anatomic and metabolic information (i.e., what the structure is, and what it is doing biochemically). Because PET imaging is most useful in combination with anatomical imaging, such as CT, modern PET scanners are now available with integrated high-end multi-detector-row CT scanners (so-called "PET-CT"). Because the two scans can be performed in immediate sequence during the same session, with the patient not changing position between the two types of scans, the two sets of images are more-precisely registered, so that areas of abnormality on the PET imaging can be more perfectly correlated with anatomy on the CT images. This is very useful in showing detailed views of moving organs or structures with higher anatomical variation, which is more common outside the brain.

At present, by far the most commonly used radiotracer in clinical PET scanning is fluorodeoxyglucose (also called FDG or fludeoxyglucose), an analogue of glucose that is labeled with fluorine-18. This radiotracer is used in essentially all scans for oncology and most scans in neurology, and thus makes up the large majority of all of the radiotracer (> 95 percent) used in PET and PET-CT scanning.

While some imaging scans such as CT and MRI isolate organic anatomic changes in the body, PET and SPECT are capable of detecting areas of molecular biology detail (even prior to anatomic change). Changing of regional blood flow in various anatomic structures (as a measure of the injected positron emitter) can be visualized and relatively quantified with a PET scan.

In practice, since the brain is normally a rapid user of glucose, and since brain pathologies such as Alzheimer's disease greatly decrease brain metabolism of both glucose and oxygen in tandem, standard FDG-PET of the brain, which measures regional glucose use, may also be successfully used to differentiate Alzheimer's disease from other dementing processes, and also to make early diagnosis of Alzheimer's disease.

Therapies targeting amyloid-β peptide currently represent approximately 50 percent of drugs now being developed for Alzheimer's disease. Some, including active and passive anti-Aβ immunotherapy, directly target the amyloid plaques. The new PET scan amyloid tracers are increasingly being included in the proposed updated diagnostic criteria, and may allow earlier diagnosis. Those targeting amyloid-β peptide allow identification of amyloid plaques in live patients. Florbetapir (Amyvid™) and flutemetamol (Vizamyl™) have received marketing authorization for this purpose.[223]

Pittsburgh compound B (PiB) is a radioactive agent which can be used in positron emission tomography scans to image beta-amyloid plaques in nerve tissue. Due to this property, Pittsburgh compound B was the original compound used to identify amyloid plaques in Alzheimer's disease.

Magnetoencephalographic Imaging (MEGI)

Magnetoencephalography (MEG) is a functional neuroimaging technique for mapping brain activity by recording magnetic fields produced by electrical currents occurring naturally in the brain, using very sensitive magnetometers. Applications of MEG include basic research into perceptual and cognitive brain processes, localizing regions affected by pathology before surgical removal, determining the function of various parts of the brain, and neurofeedback. This can be applied in a clinical setting to find locations of abnormalities as well as in an experimental setting to simply measure brain activity.

Recent studies have reported successful classification of patients with multiple sclerosis, Alzheimer's disease, schizophrenia, Sjögren's syndrome, chronic alcoholism, and facial pain. MEG can be used to distinguish these patients from healthy control subjects, suggesting a future role of MEG in diagnostics.

Understanding neural (nerve) network dysfunction in neurodegenerative disease is imperative to effectively develop network-modulating therapies. Researchers report that, *"In Alzheimer's disease (AD), cognitive decline associates with deficits in resting-state functional connectivity of diffuse brain networks.* The goal of the current study was to test whether specific cognitive impairments in AD spectrum correlate with reduced functional connectivity of distinct brain regions. We recorded resting-state functional connectivity of alpha-band activity in twenty-seven patients with AD spectrum—twenty-two patients with probable AD (5 logopenic variant primary progressive aphasia, seven posterior cortical atrophy, and ten early-onset amnestic/dysexecutive AD) and five patients with mild cognitive impairment due to AD. We used magnetoencephalographic imaging (MEGI) to perform a search for regions where patterns of functional connectivity correlated with disease severity and cognitive performance. Functional connectivity measured the strength of coherence between a given region and the rest of the brain...Our findings indicate that reductions in region-specific alpha-band resting-state functional connectivity are strongly correlated with, and might contribute to, specific cognitive deficits in AD spectrum. In the future, MEGI functional connectivity could be an important biomarker to map and follow defective networks in the early stages of AD."[224]

EEG (Electroencephalogram)

Electroencephalography (EEG) is the recording of electrical activity along the scalp. EEG measures voltage fluctuations resulting from ionic current flows within the neurons of the brain. In clinical contexts, EEG refers to the recording of the brain's spontaneous electrical activity over a short period of time, usually 20–40 minutes, as recorded from multiple electrodes placed on the scalp.

EEG is most often used to diagnose epilepsy, which causes obvious abnormalities in EEG readings. It is also used to diagnose sleep disorders, coma, encephalopathies, and brain death. EEG used to be a first-line method of diagnosis for tumors, stroke and other focal brain disorders, but this use has decreased with the advent of high-resolution anatomical imaging techniques such as MRI and CT. Despite limited spatial resolution, EEG continues to be a valuable tool for research and diagnosis, especially when millisecond-range temporal resolution (not possible with CT or MRI) is required.

This is a brain wave test, measuring the very small electric currents generated by the brain. No radiation or IV contrast dyes are used when performing this test. It is a poor test for diagnosing various types of dementias, but is very helpful in diagnosing delirium, which is very common in the elderly. Symptoms of delirium can sometimes be confused with dementia. Obtaining an EEG is helpful in ruling in or out delirium in the face of dementia.

Slowing of the electroencephalogram (EEG) is frequent in Parkinson's (PD) and Alzheimer's disease (AD) and correlates with cognitive decline. As overlap pathology plays a role in the pathogenesis of dementia, it is likely that demented patients in PD show similar physiological alterations as in AD. To analyze distinctive quantitative EEG characteristics in early cognitive dysfunction in PD and AD, researchers studied forty patients (20 PD- and twenty AD patients with early cognitive impairment) and twenty normal controls (NC). Resting state EEG was recorded from 256 electrodes. The researchers found that, "*Relative theta power in left temporal region and median frequency separated the three groups significantly. Relative theta power was increased and median frequency reduced in patients with both diseases compared to NC. Median frequency was higher in AD than in PD and classified groups significantly.* Increase of theta power in the left temporal region and a reduction of median frequency were associated with presence of AD or PD. *PD patients are characterized by a pronounced slowing as compared to AD patients.*"[225]

The cholinergic hypothesis (see Causes and Pathology, Cholinergic Hypothesis, above) is well established and has led to the development of pharmacological treatments for Alzheimer's disease. However, there has previously been no physiological means of monitoring cholinergic activity in live subjects. In order to accomplish this, researchers developed an electroencephalography (EEG)-based acetylcholine (Ach) index reflecting the cholinergic activity in the brain was developed using data from a scopolamine challenge study. The applicability of the Ach index was examined in an elderly population of healthy controls and patients suffering from various causes of cognitive decline. The researchers concluded that, "The Ach index showed a strong reduction in the severe stages of AD dementia. A high correlation was demonstrated between the Ach index and cognitive function. The index was reduced in patients with mild cognitive impairment and prodromal AD, indicating a decreased cholinergic activity. When considering the distribution of the Ach index in a population of healthy elderly subjects, an age-related threshold was revealed, beyond which there is a general decline in cholinergic activity. *The EEG-based Ach index provides, for the first time, a physiological means of monitoring the cholinergic activity in the human brain in vivo [in living people]. This has great potential for aiding diagnosis and patient stratification as well as for monitoring disease progression and treatment response.*"[226]

Other Tests

Smell Test

Olfactory[1] dysfunction is a recognized risk factor for the pathogenesis of Alzheimer's disease, while the mechanisms are still not clear.[227]

In order to determine whether odor identification impairment contributes to the prediction of cognitive decline, Dr. Schubert and colleagues followed 1,920 participants in the Epidemiology of Hearing Loss Study (mean age 66.9) for five years. Study participants had normal cognition at the beginning of the study. The researchers found that, "There was a significant association between olfactory impairment at baseline and 5-year incidence of cognitive impairment...*Olfactory impairment at baseline was strongly associated with 5-year incidence of cognitive impairment*...Odor identification testing may be useful in high-risk settings, but not in the general population, to identify patients at risk for cognitive decline."[228]

Another study to determine the predictive utility of baseline odor identification deficits for future cognitive decline and the diagnosis of Alzheimer's disease was conducted by Dr. Devanand and colleagues, who reported their findings in the December 3, 2014 issue of *Neurology*. They followed 1,037 participants without dementia; in 757 participants, follow-up occurred at two years and four years. They discovered that, "*Impairment in odor identification was superior to deficits in verbal episodic memory in predicting cognitive decline in cognitively intact*

---

[1]Olfaction is the sense of smell.

participants. The findings support the cross-cultural use of a relatively inexpensive odor identification test as an early biomarker of cognitive decline and AD dementia."[229]

Researchers conducted a study to explore the relationship between olfactory impairment, cognitive measures, and brain structure volumes in healthy elderly individuals, compared to patients with amnestic mild cognitive impairment (aMCI) or early Alzheimer's disease. They found that, "The aMCI/AD group with reduced olfactory ability had significantly smaller hippocampal volume [the area of the brain where memories are formed]...Similar changes with tests of executive function and memory were not found...*The results from this pilot study suggest that the reduction in the size of hippocampus in connection with early AD is associated more with loss of olfactory ability rather than loss of memory*, thus demonstrating that impaired olfaction is an early marker of medial temporal lobe [where the hippocampus is located] degeneration."[230]

Another study examined whether conversion to dementia can be predicted by self-reported olfactory impairment and/or by an inability to identify odors. Researchers followed a sample of 1529 participants, who were within a normal range of overall cognitive function at baseline, over a 10-year period during which 159 were classified as having a dementia disorder. Dementia conversion was predicted from demographic[1] variables, Mini-Mental State Examination (MMSE) score, and olfactory assessments. The researchers found that, "*Self-reported olfactory impairment emerged as an independent predictor of dementia.* After adjusting for effects of other predictors, individuals who rated their olfactory sensitivity as "worse than normal" were more likely to convert to dementia than those who reported normal olfactory sensitivity. Additionally, low scores on an odor identification test also predicted conversion to dementia, but these two effects were additive. We sug-

---

[1]Demography involves the statistical study of human populations. Demographic analysis can cover whole societies, or groups defined by criteria such as education, nationality, religion, birth rate, death rate, and ethnicity.

gest that assessing subjective olfactory complaints might supplement other assessments when evaluating the risk of conversion to dementia."[231]

Dr. Growdon and colleagues, from Harvard Medical School and affiliated institutions in Boston, MA, reported the results of their research on smell and dementia in the May 1, 2015 issue of the journal of *Neurology*. (Details of their study are included for healthcare providers and scientists.) They noted the following:[232]

> "Our objective was to investigate cross-sectional associations between odor identification ability and imaging biomarkers of neurodegeneration and amyloid deposition in clinically normal (CN) elderly individuals, specifically testing the hypothesis that there may be an interaction between amyloid deposition and neurodegeneration in predicting odor identification dysfunction.
>
> Data were collected on 215 CN participants from the Harvard Aging Brain Study. Measurements included the 40-item University of Pennsylvania Smell Identification Test and neuropsychological testing, hippocampal volume (HV) and entorhinal cortex (EC) thickness from MRI, and amyloid burden using Pittsburgh compound B (PiB) PET. A linear regression model evaluated the cross-sectional association between the University of Pennsylvania Smell Identification Test and amyloid burden, HV, and EC thickness, assessing for effect modification by PiB status. Covariates included age, sex, premorbid intelligence, APOE ε4 carrier status, and Boston Naming Test.
>
> In unadjusted univariate analyses, worse olfaction was associated with decreased HV, thinner EC, worse episodic memory, and marginally associated with greater amyloid burden (binary PiB status). In the multivariate

model, thinner EC in PiB-positive individuals (interaction term) was associated with worse olfaction.

In CN elderly, worse odor identification was associated with markers of neurodegeneration. Furthermore, individuals with elevated cortical amyloid and thinner EC exhibited worse odor identification, elucidating the potential contribution of olfactory testing to detect preclinical AD in CN individuals."

Sleep Study

For some individuals, severely impaired sleep, either in quantity or quality, can impair brain function. A sleep study is the only way to accurately determine if someone has significantly impaired sleep. Sleep studies can be useful in some patients who may have sleep apnea or other abnormalities of sleep, but they are not often used in the clinical evaluation of individuals who may have Alzheimer's disease. Incidentally, sleep quality, severe insomnia or sleeping too much has been found to be associated with a shortened life span. Some research shows that sleeping about 6-8 hours per night is healthiest. (See Sleep in the Longevity section below for more details.)

Virtual Reality

Recent research supports the potential of virtual reality (VR)[1] applications in assessing cognitive functions, highlighting the possibility of using a VR application for mild cognitive impairment (MCI) screening. Reporting in the November 25, 2014 issue of the *Journal of Alzheimer's Disease,* Dr. Zygouris and colleagues reported the results of their study to investigate whether a VR cognitive training application, the virtual supermarket (VSM), could be used as a screening tool for

---

[1] Virtual Reality (VR), is a computer-simulated environment that can simulate physical presence in places in the real world or imagined worlds. Virtual reality can recreate sensory experiences, which include virtual taste, sight, smell, sound, and touch.

MCI. They studied two groups, one of healthy older adults (n = 21) and one of MCI patients (n = 34), who were recruited from day centers for cognitive disorders and administered the VSM and a neuropsychological test battery. The performance of the two groups in the VSM was compared and correlated with performance in established neuropsychological tests. At the same time, the effectiveness of a combination of traditional neuropsychological tests and the VSM was examined. The researchers found that, "VSM displayed a correct classification rate (CCR) of 87.30 percent when differentiating between MCI patients and healthy older adults...At the same time, the VSM correlates with various established neuropsychological tests...*VSM appears to be a valid method of screening for MCI in an older adult population* though it cannot be used for MCI subtype assessment. VSM's concurrent validity is supported by the large number of correlations between the VSM and established tests. *It is considered a robust test on its own* as the inclusion of other tests failed to improve its CCR significantly."[233]

Memory complaints of patients sometimes are not verified via standard cognitive testing. Acquisition of information in everyday life requires memorization in complex three-dimensional environments. Researchers mimicked this with a virtual environment (VE) experiment. Memory for verbal material and spatial scenery was tested in healthy controls (HC) and patients with mild Alzheimer's disease (mini-mental state evaluation or MMSE on average of 25.7). The researchers found that, "The number of memorized items increased to 90 percent in both classical list learning and for items memorized in VE in HC. In contrast, only 40 percent of items were recalled in list learning and 20 percent in VE in AD patients. Unlike the gender difference favoring female HC on list learning, performance was alike for both genders in VE. We conclude that verbal learning abilities in healthy elderly subjects are alike in standard settings and under virtual reality conditions. *In AD patients memory deficits that are relevant to everyday life, yet not detectable with list learning, are unmasked in virtual reality.*"[234]

Gait & Balance Assessment

Dr. Hsu and colleagues, reporting in the *Journal of Biomedical Health Information* in November 2014, noted that many patients with Alzheimer's disease have gait and balance problems. They further studied this phenomenon in twenty-one AD patients and fifty healthy controls (HCs). The researchers found that, *"Experimental results show that the wearable instrument with the designed gait and balance analyzing system is a promising tool for automatically analyzing gait information and balance ability, serving as assistant indicators for early diagnosis of AD."*[235]

Life Space

As an indicator of physical and cognitive functioning in community-dwelling older adults, there is increasing interest in measuring life space, defined as the geographical area a person covers in daily life. Typically measured through questionnaires, life space can be challenging to assess in amnestic dementia associated with Alzheimer's disease. Global positioning system (GPS) technology has been suggested as a potential solution. In order to shed light on this, researchers studied nineteen community-dwelling older adults with mild-to-moderate AD (Mini-Mental State Examination score 14-28, age 70.7) and thirty-three controls (CTL; age 74.0) who wore a GPS-enabled mobile phone during the day for three days. Measures of geographical territory (area, perimeter, mean distance from home, and time away from home) were calculated from the GPS log. Construct validity of the GPS measures was tested by examining the correlation between the GPS measures and indicators of physical function [steps/day, gait velocity, and Disability Assessment for Dementia (DAD)] and affective state (Apathy Evaluation Scale and Geriatric Depression Scale).

Researchers found that, *"GPS-derived area, perimeter, and mean distance from home were smaller in the AD group compared to CTL. The correlation analysis found significant associations of the GPS measures area and perimeter with all measures of physical function (steps/day, DAD, and gait velocity), symptoms of apathy), and depression. Gait velocity and dependence were the strongest variables associated with GPS measures. This study demonstrated that GPS-derived area and perimeter: (1) distinguished mild-to-moderate AD patients from CTL and (2) were strongly correlated with physical function and affective state. These findings confirm the ability of GPS technology to assess life space behavior and may be particularly valuable to continuously monitor functional decline associated with neurodegenerative disease, such as AD.*"[236]

Primitive Reflexes

Knowing where pathology is located in the brain associated with various types of dementia helps make a correct diagnosis. This is where primitive reflexes[1] become important. When present, they indicate frontal lobe dysfunction, which can be associated with different types of dementia. The strongest relationship is found with frontotemporal lobar dementia followed by Alzheimer's dementia, as the following study shows.

Dr. Matias-Guin and colleagues, from the Department of Neurology, Hospital Clínico San Carlos, San Carlos Health Research Institute (IdISSC) Universidad Complutense de Madrid, Madrid, Spain, reported the results of their research in the April 29, 2015 issue of the *European Journal of Neurology* and noted the following:[237]

> "Although primitive reflexes (PRs) are inhibited during the first years of childhood, they may reappear with

---

[1]Primitive reflexes are reflex actions originating in the central nervous system that are exhibited by normal infants, but not neurologically intact adults, in response to particular stimuli. These reflexes are absent due to the development of the frontal lobes as a child transitions normally into child development. These primitive reflexes are also called infantile, infant or newborn reflexes, and sometimes frontal release signs. For example, the palmar grasp reflex appears at birth and persists until five or six months of age. When an object is placed in the infant's hand and strokes their palm, the fingers will close and they will grasp it with a palmar grasp, In dementia that affects the frontal lobes, these reflexes may return. See wikipedia.org "primitive reflexes" for a full discussion.

brain injury. PRs have been linked to frontal lobe dysfunction, but their precise topography has not yet been defined. The purpose of this study was to map which regions of the brain display a reduced glucose metabolism in patients with cognitive impairment and PRs.

A prospective study was conducted to evaluate PRs in a group of patients assessed due to suspected cognitive decline. Neurological and neuropsychological examinations and ^{18}F-fluorodeoxyglucose positron emission tomography [PET] fused with computerized tomography were performed.

The study included 99 patients (33 diagnosed with Alzheimer's disease, 33 on the frontotemporal dementia spectrum and 33 with other diagnoses). Mean age was 71 ± 9.7 years; time since symptom onset was 3.6 ± 2.9 years. *At least one PR was observed in 43 cases (43.4 percent of the whole sample; 48.5 percent in the Alzheimer's disease group, 63.6 percent in frontotemporal [lobar] dementia and 18.2 percent in the group with other diagnoses).* The group of patients with PRs exhibited a decreased cerebral metabolism in the bilateral superior frontal gyri (Brodmann area 6), bilateral putamina and thalami.

The presence of PRs was associated with hypometabolism at the superior frontal gyrus and putamen. This suggests that dysfunction in the corticostriatal motor circuit (supplementary motor area-putamen-thalamus) may constitute the anatomical basis of the recurrence of PRs."

ALZHEIMER'S DISEASE

Pulse Wave Velocity (PWV)

Drs. Scuteri and Wang, reporting in the January 1, 2014 issue of the *Journal of Alzheimer's Disease*, note that, "Carotid-femoral pulse wave velocity (PWV), an index of large artery stiffness, is a good proxy of arterial aging and also an independent marker of cardiovascular disease. *A consistently growing number of studies has shown a significant inverse association of arterial aging and cognitive function: the greater the PWV, the lower the cognitive performance (and the greater its decline over time)*-regardless of heterogeneity in study populations, sample size, and measure of cognitive functions adopted in each study. Therefore the epidemiological evidence and the biological plausibility require adoption of strategies to foster the routine measurement of PWV and cognitive function measurements in each and every older subject, particularly those at higher cardiovascular risk. *Consistently, limited available healthcare resources should be progressively shifted from a sterile differential diagnosis between Alzheimer-type and vascular dementia to interventions aimed to reduce PWV and, thus, to prevent dementia before its onset or to decrease its rate of progression.*"[238]

Dr. Fabiani and colleagues, reporting in the November 2014 issue of the journal *Psychophysiology,* note that, "*Cerebrovascular support is crucial for healthy cognitive and brain aging. Arterial stiffening is a cause of reduced brain blood flow, a predictor of cognitive decline, and a risk factor for cerebrovascular accidents and Alzheimer's disease.* Arterial health is influenced by lifestyle factors, such as cardiorespiratory fitness (CRF). We investigated new noninvasive optical measures of cerebrovascular health, which provide estimates of arterial pulse parameters (pulse pressure, transit time, and compliance/elasticity) within specific cerebral arteries and cortical regions, and low-resolution maps of large superficial cerebral arteries. *We studied naturally occurring variability in these parameters in adults (aged 55-87), and found that these indices of cerebrovascular health are negatively correlated with age and positively with CRF and gray and white matter volumes. Further, regional pulse transit time predicts specific neuropsychological performance.*"[239]

Retinal Assessment

Although cerebral small vessel disease has been implicated in the development of Alzheimer's disease, the cerebral microcirculation is difficult to visualize directly. As the retina and the brain share similar embryological origin, anatomical features and physiological properties with the cerebral small vessels, the retinal vessels thus offer a unique and easily accessible "window" to study the consequences of cerebral small vessel diseases. Retinal microvasculature can now be visualized, quantified and monitored non-invasively using state-of-the-art retinal imaging technology. According to researchers, *"Recent clinic- and population-based studies have demonstrated a link between retinal vascular changes and dementia, in particular AD, and cerebral small vessel disease."*[240]

Eye Movements

A growing body of literature has investigated changes in eye movements as a result of Alzheimer's disease. Researchers note that, *"When compared to healthy, age-matched controls, patients display a number of remarkable alterations to oculomotor[1] function and viewing behavior. AD-related changes to fundamental eye movements, include such things as saccades[2] and smooth pursuit motion, in addition to changes to eye movement patterns during more complex tasks like visual search and scene exploration."*[241]

Volatile Organic Compounds (VOCs)

Alzheimer's disease is a profoundly life changing condition and once diagnosis occurs, this is typically at a relatively late stage into the disease process. Therefore, a shift to earlier diagnosis, which means several decades before the onset of the typical manifestation of the disease,

---

[1]Oculomotor: of or pertaining to movement of the eyeball.
[2]Saccades: a rapid jerky movement of the eye (voluntary or involuntary) from one focus to another.

will be an important step forward for the patient. According to researchers, "A promising diagnostic and screening tool to answer this purpose is represented by breath and exhaled volatile organic compounds (VOCs) analysis. In fact, human exhaled breath contains several thousand of VOCs that vary in abundance and number in correlation with the physiological status. The exhaled VOCs reflect the metabolism, including the neuronal ones, in healthy and pathological conditions. A growing number of studies clearly demonstrate the effectiveness of VOCs analysis in identifying pathologies, including neurodegenerative diseases. In the present study we recorded, in real time, breath parameters and exhaled VOCs. *We were able to demonstrate a significant alteration in breath parameters induced by the pathology of AD. Further, we provide the putative VOCs fingerprint of AD. These vital findings are an important step toward the early diagnosis of AD.*"[242]

Transcranial Ultrasound

One of the pathologic processes that underlie Alzheimer's disease is impairment of brain microvasculature or small blood vessels. According to researchers, "Transcranial ultrasound is a non-invasive[1] examination of cerebral blood flow that can be employed as a simple and useful screening tool for assessing the vascular status of brain circulation in preclinical and clinical stages of AD. With transcranial ultrasound, the most frequently studied parameters are cerebral blood flow velocities and pulsatility indices, cerebrovascular reserve capacity, and cerebral microembolization. On the basis of current knowledge, we recommend using as a transcranial Doppler sonography screening method of choice the assessment of cerebrovascular reserve capacity with breath-holding test."[243]

---

[1]Non-invasive procedure: one that does not penetrates or breaks the skin or enters a body cavity. (Examples of invasive procedures include those that involve perforation, an incision, a catheterization, or other entry into the body. Surgery is a typical medical invasive procedure.)

Event Related Potential P3

An event-related potential (ERP) is the measured brain response that is the direct result of a specific sensory, cognitive, or motor event. More formally, it is any stereotyped electrophysiological response to a stimulus. The study of the brain in this way provides a non-invasive means of evaluating brain function in patients with cognitive diseases.

ERPs are measured by means of electroencephalography (EEG). The magnetoencephalography (MEG) equivalent of ERP is the ERF, or event-related field.

Subjective cognitive decline (SCD) has recently been proposed as the earliest stage of pathologic cognitive decline in older adults. Longitudinal research suggests that many individuals with SCD go on to develop mild cognitive impairment or Alzheimer's disease. However, those with SCD typically appear normal on standardized neuropsychological testing, and as of yet there are no reliable objective measures discriminating those with SCD from healthy peers. To shed light on this problem, researchers studied two groups of healthy older adults (ages 65-80), who self-identified as being with (n=17) or without SCD (n=23), completed self-report measures and objective measures of cognition. "Groups did not differ on demographic variables, estimated cognitive reserve, or clinical neuropsychological testing. However, self-identifying as having SCD predicted clear differences in the P3 [P300] event-related potential in response to an attention control task, over and above any contributions from mood, anxiety, or neuroticism. *Results suggest that using direct neural measures of information processing might be useful where standardized clinical tools are insensitive in those with SCD.*"[244]

CHAPTER EIGHT:
TREATMENT

Introduction

Current treatments for Alzheimer's disease are not very satisfactory. The best they can do is slow the progression of the disease, not stop or reverse it. As previously noted, currently there is no cure for AD. The anticipated increase of AD patients in next few decades makes development of better therapies an urgent issue.[245]

Keep in mind, every medication is absolutely unique. No matter how similar, no two medications are the same. In addition, getting some medications into the brain can be challenging, depending upon a variety of factors, including but not limited to, the blood-brain barrier[1] and blood-cerebrospinal fluid barrier, which can limit the delivery of medications to the brain. One possible solution is nanotechnology[2]. Advancement in nanotechnology-based drug delivery systems over the last decade exemplifies the effective drug delivery and targeting to the brain with controlled rate in various diseases including AD.[246]

Delivering certain medications transdermally (e.g., across the skin) or intranasally (e.g., through the nose) is already being done. The delivery of some medications intranasally is currently being explored for Alz-

---

[1]The blood–brain barrier (BBB) is a highly selective permeability barrier that separates the circulating blood from brain fluid in the central nervous system (CNS). The blood–brain barrier is formed by capillary endothelial cells, which are connected by tight junctions. The blood–brain barrier allows the passage of water, some gases, and lipid (fat) soluble molecules by passive diffusion, as well as the selective transport of molecules such as glucose (sugar) and amino acids that are crucial to neural function.
[2]Nanotechnology is the manipulation of matter with at least one dimension sized from 1 to 100 nanometers.

heimer's disease. Recently, direct intranasal delivery of medications to the central nervous system (CNS) has emerged as a therapeutically viable alternative to oral and parenteral[1] routes. Intranasal delivery bypasses the blood-brain barrier by delivering drugs directly to the CNS.[247]

In December 2014, Hayward and colleagues developed a model of pre-symptomatic treatment of Alzheimer's disease after a screening diagnostic evaluation and explored the circumstances required for an AD prevention treatment to produce aggregate net population benefit. Computer software (Monte Carlo) simulation methods were used to estimate outcomes in a simulated population derived from data on AD incidence and mortality. A wide variety of treatment parameters were explored. The researchers found that, *"In the base-case scenario, treatment effects were uniformly positive, and net benefits increased with increasing age at screening...Highly efficacious pre-symptomatic screen and treat strategies for AD are likely to produce substantial aggregate population benefits that are likely greater than the benefits of aspirin in primary prevention of moderate risk cardiovascular disease, even in the context of an imperfect treatment delivery environment."*[248]

FDA-approved Medications

All of the medications discussed below may be helpful in slowing the decline in a variety of areas, not just memory. For example, they may help improve behaviors, gait, and stabilize mood or activities of daily living (ADLs).[2]

---

[1]Parenteral dosage forms are intended for administration as an injection or infusion. Common injection types are intravenous (IV; into a vein), subcutaneous (SC; under the skin), and intramuscular (IM; into muscle).
[2]Activities of daily living (ADLs) is a term used in healthcare to refer to daily self care activities. ADLs are defined as "the things we normally do...such as feeding ourselves, bathing, dressing, grooming, work, homemaking, and leisure."

Cholinergic Medications

The oldest hypothesis of Alzheimer's disease, on which most currently available drug therapies are based, is the *cholinergic hypothesis*, which proposes that AD is caused by reduced synthesis of the neurotransmitter acetylcholine. This led to the development of cholinesterase inhibitors (ChEIs), which are at present the main therapy used for mild-to-moderate AD. ChEIs prevent the degradation of acetylcholine (ACh) by the acetylcholinesterase enzyme, resulting in higher levels of ACh available in the synaptic cleft for receptor absorption. The treatment enhances the cholinergic transmission, thus improving the communication between neurons.

Until an effective and especially disease-modifying treatment for Alzheimer's disease is available, the currently available pharmacological therapeutic arsenal aims at merely improving symptomatology. Both for cholinesterase inhibitors and, to a lesser extent, for memantine it can be claimed that the direct cost of the drug itself is eclipsed by the cost savings associated with delaying institutionalization or delaying the time of progression into a more severe disease state.[249]

Dr. Wattmo and colleagues reported the findings from their very interesting research into the relationship between cholinesterase inhibitor (ChEI) treatment (Aricept or donepezil, Exelon or rivastigmine, and Reminyl or galantamine) and longevity, in the September 10, 2014 issue of *BioMed Central Neurology*. They studied the relationship between the 6-month response to ChEI and lifespan. Six hundred and eighty-one deceased patients with a clinical AD diagnosis and a Mini-Mental State Examination (MMSE) score of 10-26 at the start of ChEI therapy (baseline) were included. The individuals' socio-demographic characteristics, ChEI dose, and date of death were recorded. Responses to ChEI and the association of possible risk factors with survival were analyzed. Among other findings, the researchers discovered that, *"The patients who received a higher ChEI dose during the first six months had a mean lifespan after baseline that was fifteen months longer than that of those who received a lower dose…In individuals who received and tolerated higher ChEI doses, a longer lifespan can be expected."*[250]

TREATMENT

In order to shed light on the typical duration of acetylcholinesterase inhibitor (AChEI) therapy for mild-to-moderate Alzheimer's disease patients, researchers reviewed the relevant literature, ultimately including five of forty possible studies in their analysis. Reporting their findings in 2014, they concluded that, *"There were no studies identified that suggested an optimal duration of AChEI therapy for AD patients."*[251]

In a 2015 review of how long acetylcholinesterase inhibitors (AchEIs) should be used in patients with advanced Alzheimer's disease, Dr. Tan, Associate Professor, Department of Medicine, Division of Geriatrics, University of California, Los Angeles; Medical Director, UCLA Alzheimer's and Dementia Care Program, Ronald Reagan UCLA Medical Center, Los Angeles, California, in association with the UCLA Alzheimer's and Dementia Care Program, had the following to say:[252]

> "Three cholinesterase inhibitors are currently available in the United States: donepezil (Aricept®), rivastigmine (Exelon® and Exelon® patch), and galantamine (Razadyne®). All are comparable in efficacy and adverse effects…The decision of whether and when to stop treatment with AChEIs in persons in the advanced stages of the disease can be challenging. Unlike in mild to moderate AD, the evidence of benefit of this class of medication in persons with severe disease is less clear. In a study of 295 community-dwelling patients with moderate to severe AD (MMSE score 5-13), those who were randomly assigned to continue donepezil therapy for a year had higher MMSE scores and scores on an activities of daily living scale, indicating less impairment compared with those who stopped it. Other trials report similar results.
>
> *Thus, AChEIs may be beneficial in some persons with advanced AD. However, this potential benefit will need to be weighed against the risk for adverse effects, pill burden, and goals of care in determining when it is time*

to discontinue the medication. Discontinuation should be considered if after 6-8 weeks, no benefit is observed, adverse effects are intolerable, or a severe disease stage is reached. If a decision is made to discontinue an AChEI, it can be tapered over 2-3 weeks, and the patient should be observed for any changes in cognition, function, or behavior."

As an interesting aside, Drs. Rossignol and Frye, reporting in the August 22, 2014 issue of *Frontiers of Pediatrics*, note that:[253]

"Autism spectrum disorder[1] (ASD) is a neurodevelopmental disorder that affects 1 in 68 children in the United States. Even though it is a common disorder, only two medications (Risperidol or risperidone and Abilify or aripiprazole) are approved by the U.S. Food and Drug Administration (FDA) to treat symptoms associated with ASD. However, these medications are approved to treat irritability, which is not a core symptom of ASD. A number of novel medications, which have not been approved by the FDA to treat ASD have been used off-label in some studies to treat ASD symptoms, including medications approved for Alzheimer's disease. Interestingly, some of these studies are high-quality, double-blind, placebo-controlled (DBPC) studies. This article systematically reviews studies published through April, 2014, which examined the use of Alzheimer's medications in ASD, including donepezil [Aricept] (seven stud-

---

[1] Autism spectrum disorder describes a range of conditions classified as neurodevelopmental disorders in the fifth revision of the American Psychiatric Association's *Diagnostic and Statistical Manual of Mental Disorders 5th edition* (DSM-5). The DSM-5, published in 2013, redefined the autism spectrum to encompass the previous (DSM-IV-TR) diagnoses of autism, Asperger syndrome, pervasive developmental disorder not otherwise specified (PDD-NOS), and childhood disintegrative disorder. These disorders are characterized by social deficits and communication difficulties, stereotyped or repetitive behaviors and interests, sensory issues, and in some cases, cognitive delays.

ies, two were DBPC, five out of seven reported improvements), galantamine [Reminyl] (four studies, two were DBPC, all reported improvements), rivastigmine [Exelon] (one study reporting improvements), tacrine [Cognex] (one study reporting improvements), and memantine [Namenda] (nine studies, one was DBPC, eight reported improvements). An evidence-based scale was used to rank each medication.

Collectively, these studies reported improvements in expressive language and communication, receptive language, social interaction, irritability, hyperactivity, attention, eye contact, emotional lability, repetitive or self-stimulatory behaviors, motor planning, disruptive behaviors, obsessive-compulsive symptoms, lethargy, overall ASD behaviors, and increased REM sleep. Reported side effects are reviewed and include irritability, gastrointestinal problems, verbal or behavioral regression, headaches, irritability, rash, tremor, sedation, vomiting, and speech problems. Both galantamine [Exelon] and memantine [Namenda] had sufficient evidence ranking for improving both core and associated symptoms of ASD. Given the lack of medications approved to treat ASD, further studies on novel medications, including Alzheimer's disease medications, are needed."

Cognex (tacrine)

Tacrine was the first centrally acting cholinesterase inhibitor approved for the treatment of Alzheimer's disease, and was marketed under the trade name Cognex in 1993. Tacrine acts by inhibiting the metabolism of acetylcholine and thus prolonging its activity and raising levels in the brain. Because of continuing concerns over safety and availability of other acetylcholinesterase inhibitors, tacrine was withdrawn from use in 2013.

Although tacrine is no longer in clinical use, researchers are trying to develop effective and safer sister drugs.[254] One such candidate not only had 2-fold higher potency against human AchE but, according to researchers reporting in late 2014, "showed simultaneous inhibitory effects against both Aβ aggregation and β-secretase. *We therefore conclude that tacrine-coumarin hybrid is an interesting multifunctional lead for the AD drug discovery.*"[255]

Aricept (donepezil)

Approved by the Food and Drug Administration (FDA) in 1996 for the treatment of mild to moderate Alzheimer's disease, and in 2006 for treatment of severe AD. As of 2011, Aricept was the world's best-selling Alzheimer's disease treatment. The first generic donepezil became available in November 2010. Common side effects include bradycardia, nausea, diarrhea, anorexia, abdominal pain, and vivid dreams. It has an oral bioavailability of 100 percent and easily crosses the blood–brain barrier. Currently, no definitive proof shows the use of donepezil or other similar agents alters the course or progression of Alzheimer's disease. However, 6 to 12-month controlled studies have shown modest benefits in cognition and/or behavior.

Gait deficits are prevalent in people with dementia and increase their fall risk and future disability. Few treatments exist for gait impairment in Alzheimer's disease but preliminary studies have shown that cognitive enhancers may improve gait in this population. To determine the efficacy of donepezil, a cognitive enhancer that improves cholinergic activity, on gait in older adults newly diagnosed with Alzheimer's disease, researchers studied forty-three seniors with mild AD who received donepezil (Aricept). Participants had not previously received treatment with cognitive enhancers. The researchers reported that, "primary outcome variables were gait velocity (GV) and stride time variability (STV)…Secondary outcomes included attention and executive function…*Donepezil improved gait in participants with mild AD.* The enhancement of dual-task gait suggests that the positive changes achieved in executive function as a possible causal mechanism."[256]

On January 14, 2015, Dr. Dubois and twenty-five colleagues, published the results of their research studying the effects of 10 mg per day of donepezil (Aricept) on the rate of hippocampal atrophy (shrinkage of the main area of the brain where memory is formed) in individuals with early or prodromal Alzheimer's disease. They followed 92 patients on placebo and 82 patients on Aricept for twelve months. They found that *"A 45 percent reduction of rate of hippocampal atrophy was observed in prodromal AD following one year of treatment with donepezil compared with placebo."*[257] Their results mean that taking Aricept early on in the dementing process of Alzheimer's disease helps prevent the damage to memory that would otherwise take place.

Exelon (rivastigmine)

Rivastigmine is a cholinergic agent approved by the FDA for the treatment of mild to moderate dementia of the Alzheimer's type and dementia due to Parkinson's disease. The drug can be administered orally or via a transdermal patch; the latter form reduces the prevalence of side effects, which typically include nausea and vomiting. It has been available in capsule and liquid formulations since 1997. In 2006, it became the first product approved globally for the treatment of mild to moderate dementia associated with Parkinson's disease, and in 2007 the rivastigmine transdermal patch became the first patch treatment for dementia.

Rivastigmine, an acetylcholinesterase inhibitor, inhibits both butyrylcholinesterase and acetylcholinesterase (unlike Aricept), which selectively inhibits acetylcholinesterase). It is thought to work by inhibiting these cholinesterase enzymes, which would otherwise break down the brain neurotransmitter acetylcholine. It has been used in more than 6 million patients worldwide. It has demonstrated significant treatment effects on the cognitive (thinking and memory), functional (activities of daily living) and behavioral problems commonly associated with Alzheimer's and Parkinson's disease dementias.

In patients with either type of dementia, rivastigmine has been shown to provide meaningful symptomatic effects that may allow patients to remain independent and 'be themselves' for longer. In particular, it appears to show marked treatment effects in patients showing a more aggressive course of disease, such as those with younger onset ages, poor nutritional status, or those experiencing symptoms such as delusions or hallucinations. For example, the presence of hallucinations appears to be a predictor of especially strong responses to rivastigmine, both in Alzheimer's and Parkinson's patients. These effects might reflect the additional inhibition of butyrylcholinesterase, which is implicated in symptom progression and might provide added benefits over acetylcholinesterase-selective drugs in some patients. Side effects may include nausea and vomiting, decreased appetite and weight loss.

Reminyl (galantamine)

Galantamine (Nivalin, Razadyne, Razadyne ER, Reminyl, Lycoremine) *is approved by the FDA for the treatment of mild to moderate Alzheimer's disease.* It is a potent cholinesterase inhibitor (like Aricept and Exelon) and increases the concentration of acetylcholine in certain parts of the brain. As with Aricept and Exelon, there is no evidence that galantamine alters the course of the underlying dementing process.

Absorption of galantamine is rapid and complete with absolute oral bioavailability between 80 and 100 percent. The U.S. Food and Drug Administration (FDA) and international health authorities published an alert about galantamine based on data from two studies during the treatment for mild cognitive impairment (MCI); higher mortality rates were seen in drug-treated patients. On April 27, 2006, FDA approved labeling changes concerning all forms of galantamine preparations (liquid, regular tablets, and extended release tablets) warning of the risk of bradycardia (slow resting heart rate), and sometimes atrioventricular block, especially in predisposed persons. At the same time, the risk of syncope (fainting) seems to be increased relative to placebo. "In randomized controlled trials, bradycardia was reported more frequently in galantamine-treated patients than in placebo-treated patients, but was rarely severe and rarely led to treatment discontinuation." These side effects have not been reported in Alzheimer's disease related studies.

In 2014, researchers reported their results of their investigation assessing the effect of galantamine on brain atrophy in individuals with mild cognitive impairment (MCI). Data from 364 MCI patients with 24-month MRI data (galantamine, n = 176; placebo, n = 188) were included in the analysis. They found that, "Patients with MCI who were treated with galantamine demonstrated a lower rate of whole brain atrophy, but not of hippocampal [memory area] atrophy, over a 24-month treatment period, compared to those treated with placebo. *This protective effect of galantamine on whole brain atrophy rate in MCI was only present in APOE ϵ4 carriers.*"[258]

Reporting in the February 26, 2015 issue of the *Journal of Alzheimer's disease*, Dr. Bhattacharya and colleagues reported the results of their use of Memogain (a precursor to galantamine, which is formed in the brain from enzymatic action on Memogain) in an animal experiment. They administered the drug intranasally, noting that, "The possibility to deliver Memogain intranasally may further circumvent side effects, allowing higher dosing compared to galantamine…Eight weeks of chronic treatment resulted in improved performance in behavioral tests, such as open field and light-dark avoidance, and in fear conditioning already at mildly affected stages at the age of eighteen weeks compared to untreated controls. Furthermore, after treatment a significantly lower plaque density in the brain, i.e., in the entorhinal cortex (reduction 20 percent females, 40 percent males) and the hippocampus (19 percent females, 31 percent males) at the age of 18 weeks was observed. *These results show that nasal application of Memogain effectively delivers the drug to the brain with the potential to retard plaque deposition and improve behavioral symptoms in AD similar to the approved galantamine.*"[259]

NMDA (*N*-Methyl-D-aspartate) Medication

Namenda XR (memantine)

Memantine is the first in a novel class of Alzheimer's disease medications acting on the glutamatergic system by blocking NMDA receptors. Memantine is approved by the U.S. F.D.A and the European Medicines Agency for treatment of moderate-to-severe Alzheimer's disease.

Memantine has been associated with a moderate decrease in clinical deterioration with only a small positive effect on cognition, mood, behavior, and the ability to perform daily activities in moderate to severe Alzheimer's disease.

Memantine is, in general, well-tolerated. Common adverse drug reactions (≥ 1 percent of patients) include confusion, dizziness, drowsiness, headache, insomnia, agitation, and/or hallucinations. Less common adverse effects include vomiting, anxiety, hypertonia, cystitis, and increased libido.

Sales of the drug reached $1.8 billion for 2014. The cost of Namenda is $269 to $489 a month.

Namenda XR is approved by the FDA for the treatment of moderate to severe Alzheimer's disease. Some experts recommend that it be prescribed at the first sign of Alzheimer's disease, although doing so is considered "off-label" use (i.e., not approved by the FDA for use in mild Alzheimer's disease). A special word of caution with this medication: one research study had to be stopped due to excessive agitation caused by Namenda. This is a good reminder that no medication is perfect, works for everyone, or is absolutely free of potential problems.

Namenda is frequently used in combination with Aricept, as research has shown that the combination may provide the best results. In fact, a pill combining these medications may soon be available.

TREATMENT

Genetics is helping healthcare providers select the right medications for the right patients, at the right doses. This is sometimes referred to as 'genomic' medicine.[1] The following summary of research reported in late 2014 is included for readers who are also providers:[260]

> "The K variant of butyrylcholinesterase (BCHE-K) exhibits a reduced acetylcholine-hydrolyzing capacity; so the clinical response to rivastigmine may differ in Alzheimer's disease (AD) patients with the BCHE-K gene. Objective: To investigate the clinical response to rivastigmine transdermal patch monotherapy or memantine plus rivastigmine transdermal patch therapy in AD patients based on the BCHE-K gene. Methods: A total of 146 probable AD patients consented to genetic testing for butyrylcholinesterase and underwent the final efficacy evaluations. Responders were defined as patients with an equal or better score on the Alzheimer's disease Assessment Scale-cognitive subscale (ADAS-cog) at 16 weeks compared to their baseline score. Results: BCHE-K carriers showed a lower responder rate on the ADAS-cog than non-carriers (38.2 vs. 61.7 percent, p = 0.02), and this trend was evident in AD patients with apolipoprotein E ε 4 (35 vs. 60.7 percent, p = 0.001). The presence of the BCHE-K allele predicted a worse response on the ADAS-cog (odds ratio 0.35, 95 percent confidence interval 0.14-0.87), after adjusting for demographic and baseline cognitive and functional variables. Conclusion: *The BCHE-K genotype may be related to a poor cognitive response to rivastigmine patch or memantine add-on therapy, especially in the presence of apolipoprotein E ε 4.*"

Behavioral symptoms (such as agitation, aggression, mood lability, irritability) are common in moderate to severe Alzheimer's disease and are

---

[1]Genomic medicine: health care which utilizes advances made by the science of genomics, a branch of molecular biology; also called genomic health care.

improved by Namenda with the most pronounced effect on agitation/aggression. Nuedexta (dextromethorphan in combination with quinidine) is the only drug approved by U.S. Food and Drug Administration for the treatment of pseudobulbar affect (PBA)[1] on the basis of efficacy in patients with multiple sclerosis (MS) or amyotrophic lateral sclerosis (ALS).

Researchers reported the findings of their study, in late 2013, of the effect of Namenda on patients with Alzheimer's disease who also had PBA. Alzheimer's patients with pathological laughter and crying were administered memantine (final dose of 20 mg daily) or citalopram (20 mg once daily), each for ten weeks. The researchers found that, "Although memantine had beneficial effects on PBA, *it also had a crucial impact on behavioral symptoms, especially aggression and agitation (to an average of 3.5 times higher [than patients not taking Namenda]... Therefore, the study was prematurely stopped.* In addition, we had evidenced a drop of platelet 5-HT [serotonin] concentration (to an average of 73 percent of initial value). Surprisingly, our research showed the opposite action of memantine on neuropsychiatric symptoms as expected. *In a limited number of AD patients with PBA, memantine had a beneficial effect on involuntary emotional expression, but it potentiated agitation/aggression, irritability and caused a crucial drop of the platelet 5-HT concentration."*[261]

The results of this study once again underscore the fact that every medication has potential risks as well as benefits, and that treatment has to be individualized for every person.

---

[1]Pseudobulbar affect (PBA) refers to a neurologic disorder characterized by involuntary crying or uncontrollable episodes of crying and/or laughing, or other emotional displays. PBA occurs secondary to a neurologic disease or brain injury.

TREATMENT

Combination Treatments

Namzaric (donepezil + memantine)

Scheduled to be approved by the FDA, possibly in 2015, to treat moderate-to-severe Alzheimer's dementia, by combining in a single capsule Namenda XR (memantine) and Aricept (donepezil) — the ingredients in two drugs that are often prescribed together.

Medications Used for Agitation in Alzheimer's Patients

Apart from the medications described above, which are used to slow the progression of the disease, other medications are commonly used to treat behavioral and psychological symptoms of dementia (BPSD; such as agitation, aggression, assaultiveness, or psychosis) that can be associated with Alzheimer's disease. The prevalence of the behavioral and psychological symptoms of dementia (BPSD) in late stage Alzheimer's disease varies between 20-90 percent, depending on the care settings and severity of the dementia syndrome. BPSD is the major reason for referrals to secondary care.

In order to quantify the efficacy and safety of pharmacological treatments on neuropsychiatric symptoms in patients with Alzheimer's disease, Wang and colleagues conducted a comprehensive review (meta-analysis) comparing pharmacological agents with placebo. Reporting in the January 2015 issue of the Journal of Neurology Neurosurgery, and Psychiatry, they found that, "Cholinesterase inhibitors (ChEIs, such as Aricept and Exelon) and atypical antipsychotics [see below] *improved total score on the Neuropsychiatric Inventory (NPI)*, but antidepressants and memantine (Namenda) *did not. However, ChEIs and atypical antipsychotics increased the risk of dropouts due to adverse events and the incidence of adverse events.* For typical antipsychotics [such as Haldol and Prolixin], no study was included." [262]

"Mood Stabilizers"

The term "mood stabilizer" does not describe a mechanism, but rather an effect. Drugs commonly classified as mood stabilizers include: Tegretol (carbamazepine), Depakote (valproic acid), Neurontin (gabapentin), Topamax (topiramate), Lamictal (lamotrigine), Trileptal (oxcarbazepine) and lithium.

Researchers reviewed the scientific literature available on the effectiveness of mood stabilizers in the treatment of behavioral and psychological symptoms of dementia (BPSD). The researchers reported in 2012 that, "We found one meta-analysis and three randomized controlled trials (RCTs) supporting the efficacy of carbamazepine in managing global BPSD, particularly aggression and hostility. With regard to valproate, current evidence from one meta-analysis and five RCTs did not strongly support its efficacy for global BPSD, including agitation and aggression. Only open trials or case series showed some efficacy of gabapentin, topiramate and lamotrigine in controlling BPSD. The single RCT investigating the effect of oxcarbazepine on agitation and aggression showed negative results. Case series reports on lithium tended to show it to be ineffective. *Thus far, among mood stabilizers, carbamazepine [Tegretol] has the most robust evidence of efficacy on BPSD.* More RCTs are needed to strengthen evidence regarding the efficacy of gabapentin, topiramate and lamotrigine. Valproate, oxcarbazepine and lithium showed low or no evidence of efficacy."[263]

Second-generation or "Atypical" Antipsychotic Medications

- Abilify (aripiprazole)
- Geodon (ziprazadone)
- Invega (palperidone)
- Latuda (lurasidone)
- Risperdal (risperidone)
- Saphris (asenapine)

TREATMENT

- Seroquel (quetiapine)
- Zyprexa (olanzapine)

These agents are approved by the FDA for the treatment of schizophrenia and bipolar disorder. They are not approved by the FDA for the treatment of agitation associated with Alzheimer's disease. In fact, some research has shown that these agents are associated with an increased risk of stroke and death in the elderly. For this reason, the FDA issued a very strong warning against the use of these medications in the elderly. This warning is called a "black box warning" (and the warning actually has a black box around it). Nevertheless, these medications, most commonly Risperdal, Abilify, and Seroquel, are frequently used for agitation, aggression, assaultiveness or for psychosis (delusions and hallucinations) in the elderly. While there is a national trend against the use of these medications in the elderly, they are still widely used due to the need to control agitated, sometimes assaultive, or psychotic patients. It should also be noted that some research has found little or no increase in stroke or death with the use of some these medications.

According to one group of researchers, "Recent findings of neuropathological, neurochemical and neuroimaging studies yielded unequivocal evidence that the behavioral and psychological symptoms of dementia (BPSD) symptoms are not a consequence of a single neurotransmitter imbalance, but rather of disproportionate level changes in biogenic amines, excitatory and inhibitory transmitters in the central nervous system. Consequently, the available pharmacotherapy should target the balancing of the dopaminergic, serotoninergic, noradrenergic, excitatory and GABAergic neurotransmission by using antipsychotics, antidepressants, phase-prophylactic agents, and benzodiazepines. *Several clinical studies have proven the efficacy of atypical antipsychotics that target multiple neurotransmitter systems in treating BPSD. The first results of the CATIE-AD[1] study also confirm these findings and*

---

[1]The National Institutes of Mental Health (NIMH)-funded Clinical Antipsychotic Trials of Intervention Effectiveness (CATIE) Study was a multimillion-dollar nationwide public health-focused clinical trial that compared the effectiveness of older ("typical;" first available in the 1950s) and newer ("atypical;" available since the 1990s) antipsychotic medications used to treat schizophrenia.

indicate that the atypical antipsychotics are effective in controlling anger, aggression and delusions in Alzheimer's disease, while cognitive symptoms, quality of life and care needs are not improved."[264]

In 2011, another group of researchers reviewed the literature pertaining to the efficacy and safety of atypicals in people with Alzheimer's disease. They found that, *"Atypical antipsychotics confer modest benefits for short-term (up to twelve weeks) treatment of aggression and psychosis in AD. These benefits have to be balanced against the risk of serious adverse events including 1.5 - 1.8-fold increased mortality. The benefits are less clear-cut with longer term prescribing, but the mortality risk remains significantly elevated.*[265]

Researchers reviewed the scientific literature in 2013 on the use of aripiprazole (Abilify) in patients with Alzheimer's disease, noting that, "In randomized placebo-controlled clinical trials, *aripiprazole shows modest efficacy in the treatment of AD-related psychosis*. Neuropsychiatric symptoms alleviated were predominantly psychotic features and agitation. In individual trials, aripiprazole was generally well-tolerated, serious side effects were seldom reported and included accidental injury and somnolence. Meta-analyses, however, demonstrated increased mortality as a class effect for atypical, but also for typical antipsychotics. No increased cardiovascular outcomes, cerebrovascular accidents, increased appetite or weight gain were demonstrated in meta-analyses for aripiprazole-treated patients with psychosis of dementia. Aripiprazole was found to induce sedation. Aripiprazole should only be used in selected patient populations resistant to non-pharmacological treatment with persisting or severe psychotic symptoms and/or agitation, and in which symptoms lead to significant morbidity, patient suffering and potential self-harm. The indication for continuing treatment should be revised regularly."[266]

On the plus side, several research studies in animal models of Alzheimer's disease have shown that Seroquel (quetiapine) can not only prevent, but can even treat and alleviate the neuropathology of AD, and thus indicate that *quetiapine may actually have therapeutic effects in the treatment of AD.*[267] Seroquel can also be administered by gel, so it can be rubbed on the skin of patients who are refusing oral medications.

"Antidepressants"

(Discussed here for possible treatment of agitation, and discussed in the "Prevention" section, which is below, as well.) Selective Serotonin Reuptake Inhibitors (SSRIs; FDA-approved for the treatment of depression and various anxiety disorders, such as generalized anxiety disorder, panic disorder, agoraphobia, and OCD):

- Celexa (citalopram): This has recently been shown in some studies to be helpful for agitation that can be associated with AD. Its usefulness in preventing AD is discussed in the Prevention section.

    Drs. Gallagher and Herrmann, reported in the February 2015 issue of *Neurodegenerative Disease Management* that, "There has been a growth in the evidence base for psychosocial interventions, and non-pharmacological approaches to care should ordinarily be the first option. *Antipsychotics remain the pharmacological agents with most evidence to support their use while there is more limited evidence for other agents such as carbamazepine [Tegretol] and selective serotonin reuptake inhibitors [SSRIs] such as citalopram.*"[268]

    In 2014, researchers reported that, "Neuropsychiatric symptoms (NPS) are common among individuals with Alzheimer's disease, associated with excess morbidity and mortality, greater healthcare use, earlier institutionalization, and caregiver burden. Agitation presents as emotional distress, excessive psychomotor activity, aggressive behaviors, disruptive irritability and disinhibition. There is an unmet need to find pharmacologic treatment for agitation in patients with AD that can be safely and effectively used as a concurrent treatment alongside psychosocial interventions. A recent, multicenter, randomized, placebo-controlled trial explored the efficacy of a 30-mg daily dose of citalopram for agitation in patients with AD and showed a significant decrease in agitation for citalopram compared with placebo. Both QTc prolongation and cognitive worsening, as measured by the Mini Mental State Examination, were observed in the citalopram group and present a concern to clinicians. *Citalopram at a 20-mg daily dose should be considered as a possible first-line treatment in addition to psychosocial intervention.*[269] (Twenty milligrams or mg is the maximum FDA-approved dose in people 60 or older; 40 mg in is the maximum in adults up to age 60.)

- Zoloft (sertraline): less research has been done on this medication vis-à-vis agitation in AD, but it has a similar mechanism of action to Celexa (as all SSRIs do). It may help prevent AD as well, as is discussed below, in the Prevention section.

CAUTION: *In 2015, researchers discovered an unexpected neurotoxic interaction between sertraline and carbamazepine (Tegretol), and these two medications should not be used together.*[270]

- Paxil (paroxetine): used by millions of people worldwide, and is approved for use in the U.S. for the treatment of major depressive disorder, obsessive-compulsive disorder, panic disorder, social anxiety disorder, generalized anxiety disorder, posttraumatic stress disorder, and premenstrual dysphoric disorder. However, its use has significant drawbacks. Although not relevant for adults concerned about dementia, paroxetine can cause birth defects (FDA Pregnancy Category D[1]). It can cause weight

---

[1] The Food and Drug Administration (FDA) has developed a rating system to provide therapeutic guidance based on potential benefits and fetal risks. Drugs have been classified into categories A, B, C, D and X based on this system of classification. Drugs, and some multivitamins, that have demonstrated no fetal risks after controlled studies in humans are classified as Category A, while drugs like thalidomide with proven fetal risks that outweigh all benefits are classified as Category X. Most medications fall into category B (Animal reproduction studies have failed to demonstrate a risk to

gain. It has a property referred to as "anticholinergic," which can cause blurry vision, constipation, urinary hesitancy, dry mouth, rapid heart rate, and most importantly in the elderly, confusion.

Its use is contraindicated in breast cancer patients taking the anti-cancer drug tamoxifen, because it increases its metabolism, which results in lower levels of tamoxifen. This is clearly associated with an increased death rate when these two medications are used together. [271, 272, 273, 274] Given all of these potential problems, and the availability of several more suitable agents, why use it?

- Lexapro (escitalopram): a derivative of Celexa, a suitable alternative to Celexa or Zoloft.

In 2011, researchers compared escitalopram and risperidone (Risperdal) for psychotic symptoms and agitation associated with AD. Inpatients with AD, who had been hospitalized because of behavioral symptoms, were recruited to a six-week randomized, double-blind, controlled trial. Participants (n = 40) were randomized to once daily risperidone 1 mg or escitalopram 10 mg. The researchers reported that, "Onset was earlier in the risperidone-treated group, but improvement did not significantly differ between groups by study end. Completion rates differed for escitalopram (75 percent) and risperidone (55 percent), mainly due to adverse events. There were no adverse events in the escitalopram group, while in the risperidone group two patients suffered severe extrapyramidal symptoms and four patients suffered acute physical illness necessitating transfer to

---

the fetus and there are no adequate and well-controlled studies in pregnant women) or category C (Animal reproduction studies have shown an adverse effect on the fetus and there are no adequate and well-controlled studies in humans, but potential benefits may warrant use of the drug in pregnant women despite potential risks). Category D: There is positive evidence of human fetal risk based on adverse reaction data from investigational or marketing experience or studies in humans, but potential benefits may warrant use of the drug in pregnant women despite potential risks.

general hospital. *Escitalopram and risperidone did not differ in efficacy in reducing psychotic symptoms and agitation in patients with AD. Completion rates were higher for escitalopram-treated patients.*[275]

- Prozac (fluoxetine): although this was the first SSRI, it is still widely used. One problem is that it has an extremely long half-life, meaning that even after it is discontinued, it is still present in tissues for a long period of time (weeks). It also has more potential drug-drug interactions than the other SSRIs. It shares the potential harmful drug-drug interaction with tamoxifen that paroxetine does, and so should not be used in those taking tamoxifen.

Benzodiazepines (Minor Tranquilizers)

Benzodiazepines: FDA-approved for the treatment of anxiety, including panic attacks or agoraphobia, these are often used "off-label" to treat agitation associated with AD. *These medications also carry risks, such as sedation, impaired balance and coordination, confusion, and memory impairment.* Nevertheless, due to severe agitation or anxiety, they are often used, even in the elderly.

- Xanax (alprazolam): short-acting (half-life of 11.2 hours [16.3 in elderly]; can be given up to four times per day).
- Ativan (lorazepam): intermediated acting (half-life of 14 hours; can be given up to four times per day). Ativan can be given by injection (or gel, which can be rubbed on the skin) and, because of this, it often used for agitated patients of all ages.
- Klonopin (clonazepam): long-acting (half-life of 20-50 hours; usually given only 1-2 times per day)"

A further concern with the use of benzodiazepines was highlighted in the September 9, 2014 issue of the *British Medical Journal* by Dr. Billiote de Gage and colleagues. In order to study the possible link between benzodiazepines and Alzheimer's dementia, the authors followed

1,796 people with a first diagnosis of Alzheimer's disease and 7,184 individuals who did not develop AD, for six years. Both groups were randomly sampled from older people (age >66) living in the community in 2000-09. They found that, *"Benzodiazepine use was associated with an increased risk of Alzheimer's disease. The strength of association increased with exposure density [e.g., greater use] and with the drug half-life [the greater the half-life, the greater the risk]...Unwarranted long term use of these drugs should be considered as a public health concern."*[276]

Other Medications for Agitation

Nuedexta (dextromethorphan hydrobromide and quinidine sulfate)

Nuedexta is a new drug on the (U.S.) market that has shown some benefit for agitation in people with Alzheimer's disease, although it is not approved (yet) by the FDA for this indication. The Nuedexta web site (nuedexta.com) notes the following:

> If you or someone you care for suddenly bursts out crying or laughing for no apparent reason, it may be due to a neurologic condition doctors call PseudoBulbar Affect (PBA). PBA is caused by neurologic conditions such as Alzheimer's disease or other dementias, stroke, traumatic brain injury (TBI), Parkinson's disease, multiple sclerosis (MS), or Lou Gehrig's disease (ALS). PBA results in episodes of crying or laughing that are often sudden and exaggerated or do not match what the person is feeling inside. Though frequently mistaken for depression, PBA is thought to be the result of a 'short circuit' in the areas of the brain that control emotional expression. Nearly two million people may have PBA. NUEDEXTA (dextromethorphan hydrobromide and quinidine sulfate)

20mg/10mg capsules is the first and only prescription medicine specifically approved to treat PBA.

We have found this medication to be helpful for some (but not all, or even most) patients with agitation associated with Alzheimer's disease. For example, we treated an elderly patient in a nursing home, a surgeon, who was very angry, irritable, and episodically agitated. On Nuedexta, he calmed down and became much more pleasant and less negative, and had no side effects.

Medications Used for Inappropriate Sexual Behaviors

Unfortunately, patients with different types of dementia, including Alzheimer's disease, can develop inappropriate sexual thoughts and/or actions. These can become very disturbing to the patients' families, fellow residents, and staff. Different medications have been tried to stop these thoughts and behaviors, mostly with limited success. However, there is one medication, Medroxyprogesterone acetate (Depo-Provera), that has been shown to be very effective, in both men and women, and it seems to be safe. It is not approved by the FDA for this indication, and so its use in this context would be considered "off label." If this medication is indicated for a patient, it is typically their primary care provider (PCP) who prescribes it, as PCPs are more familiar with hormones than psychiatrists are. The dose varies from 150 mg every three months, to up to 450 mg per week. Like almost all medications, it is recommended to start with the lowest dose, and then to increase if necessary. There are few scientific studies about this problem, but several are reviewed below.

Researchers from the University of Ottawa, Department of Psychiatry and Royal Ottawa Mental Health Centre, Ottawa, Canada, note the following:[277]

> "Inappropriate sexual behavior (ISB) is an important topic in geriatrics; etiologies remain unclear and evidence for the efficacy of treatment strategies is limited.

The aims of this study were to provide a description of the phenomenology of ISB in the geriatric population, to identify potential contributing factors, and to review the efficacy of interventions aimed at reducing ISB.

A retrospective chart review was conducted of ten patients admitted to an academic inpatient geriatric psychiatry ward because of their ISB (study group) and ten patients matched in age and gender (control group). A comprehensive chart review inventory was done to determine variables that may contribute to ISB. A significant finding was the association of a history of right frontal lobe stroke with ISB. Also significant was performance on cognitive testing and the presence of dementia in the study group. Citalopram [Celexa] was well tolerated but with minimal reduction of ISB. Atypical antipsychotics olanzapine [Zyprexa] and risperidone [Risperdal] were effective in some cases but also had adverse effects. Medroxyprogesterone acetate[1] [Depo-Provera; injectable, not oral] was well tolerated and effective in all cases in which it was utilized (n = 5)."

In 2008, Dr. Guay, from the Department of Experimental and Clinical Pharmacology, College of Pharmacy, University of Minnesota, Minneapolis, Minnesota published the results of his literature review in the *American Journal of Geriatric Pharmachotherapy*. Following is his report:[278]

"Agitated and aggressive behaviors are common in older patients with dementia (33 percent of the community-dwelling and 80 percent of the institutionalized populations). Although inappropriate verbal and physical sexual behaviors are among the least common of these

---

[1]Medroxyprogesterone acetate (Depo-Provera) is a steroidal progestin, a synthetic variant of the steroid hormone progesterone. It is used as a contraceptive, in hormone replacement therapy and for the treatment of endometriosis as well as several other indications.

actions, they can be profoundly disruptive to caregivers (spouse, institutional staff, or both) and other individuals in the immediate surroundings. Substantial mental and physical harm can occur secondary to these behaviors. The common perception is that such behavior cannot be treated.

This review summarizes the epidemiology, etiology, and biology of abnormal sexual behaviors in cognitively impaired older individuals and highlights potentially useful drug therapies. Use of pharmacotherapy in managing inappropriate sexual behaviors in cognitively impaired older individuals has been detailed in only twenty-three case reports and case series (N = 55 subjects). Additional supportive data from case reports and case series are available in nonsexual agitation/aggression in elderly patients with dementia (N = 16 subjects) and abnormal sexual behaviors in cognitively intact elderly (N = 2 subjects). One comparative trial in nonsexual agitation/aggression in elderly patients with dementia also exists (N = 27 subjects).

There are no practice guidelines available for the treatment of abnormal sexual behaviors in the cognitively impaired elderly population. Recommendations must be individualized on the basis of clinical exigency and pragmatism; they should also be predicated on medical clearance to use estrogen or anti-androgen (progestogen, luteinizing hormone-releasing hormone [LHRH] agonist) therapies, if necessary. Very few data exist regarding the treatment of females of any age exhibiting abnormal sexual behaviors. For males, reasonable data support the use of serotoninergics (eg, tricyclic antidepressants [TCAs], selective serotonin reuptake inhibitors [SSRIs]), estrogens (oral, transdermal), antiandrogens (cyproterone acetate, medroxyprogesterone acetate), and the LHRH agonists (eg, leuprolide, triptorelin). Com-

TREATMENT

parative trial data, both within and between these drug classes from the paraphilia literature, provide additional information that can be used to generate at least a provisional approach to drug treatment of abnormal sexual behaviors in older subjects with impaired cognition.

In general, unless the patient is engaging in or threatening dangerous acts involving physical contact, serotoninergics (first choice, SSRIs; second choice, TCAs) are first-line agents followed by antiandrogens (cyproterone acetate or medroxyprogesterone acetate) as second-line agents. LHRH agonists (first choice) and estrogens (second choice) are considered third-line agents. Combination therapy is reasonable if the patient fails to respond to monotherapy."

We have found in our extensive nursing home experience, that Depo-Provera works very well, and we have not seen any side effects. We do not agree with Dr. Guay with the use of tricyclic antidepressants (e.g., Elavil, which is amitriptyline, for example). They have many potential side effects in this population. We have not found SSRIs to be effect with these behaviors.

In the March 2006 issue of the *Journal of Psychiatry & Neuroscience*, Drs. Light and Holroyd from the Department of Psychiatric Medicine, University of Virginia, Charlottesville, VA, noted the following, "Sexually inappropriate behavior in a patient with dementia can be a problem for caregivers. Little research has been done concerning treatment for this behavioral disorder. The hormone medroxyprogesterone acetate [Depo-Provera] (MPA) is a known, but infrequently used, treatment option. We describe a series of five cases in which MPA was used successfully to control inappropriate sexual behaviors in men with dementia."[279]

Other Possible Treatments

Cognitive Training & Mindfulness

There is much interest in early intervention for the prevention or postponement of dementia in Alzheimer's disease. The results of drug trials in this regard have thus far been disappointing, and non-pharmacological interventions are receiving increased attention. Evidence from epidemiological studies suggests that participation in stimulating mental activities is associated with lowered dementia risk. The introduction of novel and complex cognitive interventions to healthy adults and those with cognitive impairment may represent an efficacious treatment option to improve cognition, lower dementia incidence, and slow rate of decline.

Cognitively based interventions (i.e., cognitive training, cognitive rehabilitation) hold particular promise for maximizing patients' functioning, are relatively inexpensive, and have virtually no side effects. Everyday life is complex and multifaceted, which means that a personalized approach is essential for maximizing and prolonging functioning in each patient. "While limited at this time, there is some evidence of the long-term benefits of cognitive intervention."[280]

Researchers examined the evidence for restorative cognitive training (CT) and addresses a number of clinically relevant issues regarding cognitive benefit and its transfer and persistence. They found that, "Although the number of randomized controlled trials is limited, *preliminary evidence suggests that CT may provide immediate and longer term cognitive benefits which generalize to non-trained domains and non-cognitive functions, with supervised small group multi-domain training providing greatest benefits.*"[281]

Researchers studied a rehabilitation program (RP) adapted for people diagnosed with various phases of Alzheimer's disease. The RP is a cognitive stimulation program that integrates the recommendations of the American College of Sports Medicine for aerobic, resistance, and balance exercises. In order to do so, they enrolled 64 participants with AD for an RP intervention lasting twelve months. They found that, "The RP has a positive effect on patients with mild- to moderate-phase AD. However, we identified no effect for the RP on cognitive ability. *These findings provide empirical evidence to support the use of RP as an effective complementary therapy. Improving the physical capacity and the quality of life may have important long-term benefits for the older adults and their caregivers.*"[282]

Unawareness of deficit (e.g., failure to appreciate that one has memory or thinking impairments) has been shown to affect the outcome of targeted cognitive intervention programs applied to patients with Alzheimer disease. In order to further explore this phenomenon, in 2014 researchers investigated the efficacy of the Multi-Intervention Program (MIP) approach on improving cognitive, functional, affective, and behavioral symptoms in people with mild AD. In addition, they examined whether the presence of unawareness influences the MIP outcomes. "Sixty-one mild stage AD patients were randomly assigned to either an experimental group which carried out an MIP individually (forty-eight sessions, sixteen weeks duration), combining diverse cognitive tasks, training in daily life and recreational activities, or a waiting list group which did not receive any treatment for the same time period. The results showed that patients overall benefited from the MIP in terms of both cognitive and non-cognitive symptoms. AD patients with awareness of deficits showed positive effects on all outcome measures in comparison with the waiting list group, while AD patients with unawareness showed improvements in non-cognitive symptoms only. *In conclusion, the presence of unawareness reduces the cognitive and functional effects of MIP in patients with mild AD.*"[283]

Although there is a vast body of literature linking education and later health outcomes, the mechanisms underlying these associations are relatively unknown. However, in 2014 researchers were able to show evidence that "the genetic effects of the "risky" APOE variant on old-age cognitive decline are absent in individuals who complete college (vs. high school graduates). Auxiliary analyses suggest that the likely mechanisms of education are most consistent through changing brain processes (i.e., "how we think") and potentially building cognitive reserves, rather than alleviating old age cognitive decline through the channels of higher socioeconomic status and resources over the life course."[284]

The following article, published November 21, 2014, is a good summary of the state of affairs vis-à-vis "brain training:[285]

> "Growing evidence suggests brain training may help maintain cognition and lower dementia risk, resulting in the rise of a billion dollar brain training industry. However, new research examining the efficacy of such programs suggests not all are created equal and that it may be a case of buyer beware.
>
> A meta-analysis[1] of fifty-one randomized clinical trials (RCTs) that included more than 4,800 older participants showed that *group-based brain training under the supervision of a trainer was significantly more effective for overall cognition, memory, and processing speed than self-directed, home-based training programs.*
>
> "Our results send a key message to the public. They show that brain training carried out in a center can improve cognition in older adults, but commercial products promoted for solo training use at home just don't work. There are better ways to spend your time and money," senior author Michael Valenzuala, PhD, associate professor and leader of the Regenerative Neuroscience Group at the Brain and Mind Research Institute (BMRI) at the University of Sydney, Australia, said in a release.

---

[1]Meta-analysis: In statistics, meta-analysis comprises statistical methods for contrasting and combining results from different studies in the hope of identifying patterns among study results, sources of disagreement among those results, or other interesting relationships that may come to light in the context of multiple studies. Meta-analysis can be thought of as "conducting research about previous research."

In addition, *training one to three times per week was effective, but more than that appeared to neutralize benefits.* "The brain's plastic mechanisms may saturate if training is too frequent. Like strenuous physical exercise, we recommend at least one rest day between training sessions," lead author Amit Lampit, postdoctoral research fellow at BMRI, said in the same release."

Neurosurgical Treatments

In September 2014, Dr. Pereira and colleagues from the Department of Neurosurgery, David Geffen School of Medicine, University of California Los Angeles, USA, report that, "After decades of investigation, Alzheimer's disease is now understood to be a complex disease that affects behavior and cognition through several mechanisms: Disrupted neuronal communication, abnormal regional tissue metabolism, and impaired cellular repair. Existing therapies have demonstrated limited efficacy, which has spurred the search for specific disease markers and predictors as well as innovative therapeutic options. Deep brain stimulation (DBS) of the memory circuits is one such option, with early studies suggesting that modulation of neural activity in these networks may improve cognitive function. Encapsulated cell biodelivery (ECB) is a device that delivers nerve growth factor (NGF) to the cholinergic basal forebrain to potentially improve cognitive decline in AD patients."[286]

In 2014, Dr. Laxton and colleagues reviewed the scientific literature on neurosurgical approaches that have been attempted or are currently being investigated for the treatment of Alzheimer's disease. They concluded that, "The following five categories of neurosurgical treatment were identified: cerebrospinal fluid shunting, intraventricular infusions, tissue grafting, gene therapy, and electrical neural stimulation. *While none of the neurosurgical approaches applied to the treatment of AD have proven effective to date, recent trials involving gene therapy and electrical neural stimulation are showing promising early results.* Larger trials investigating these treatments have been proposed or are currently under way."[287]

Social Interaction

To test the association between several social network variables with the risk of dementia and Alzheimer's disease, researchers followed 2,089 individuals for fifteen years. During the follow-up period, 461 people developed dementia and, of those, 373 developed Alzheimer's disease. The researchers found that, "Participants who felt satisfied with their relations had a 23 percent reduced dementia risk. Participants who reported that they received more support than they gave over their lifetime had a 55 percent and 53 percent reduced risk for dementia and Alzheimer's disease, respectively...*The only variables associated with subsequent dementia or Alzheimer's disease were those reflecting the quality of relationships [higher quality, less dementia]*."[288]

Dr. Hsiao and colleagues, reported their findings on the impact of social interactions in reversing the pathology of Alzheimer's disease in an animal model, in the December 3, 2014 issue of the *Journal of Neuroscience*. Without going into the complexities of their findings, suffice it to say that they were able to catalog the biochemical events underlying the improvement in memory in "Alzheimer's" mice after increased social interaction.[289]

Support Groups

Dr. Dal Belo-Hass and colleagues, reporting in the July-September 2014 issue of *Rural Remote Health,* noted that,[290]

> "Worldwide, countries are calling for a chronic disease management approach to people with dementia. In response, 'living well' with dementia and 'supported self-care' frameworks are being adopted by advocacy and volunteer organizations, and more attention is being directed toward health and wellness promotion as a critical component for 'living well.' This exploratory study examined the health and wellness self-management behaviors of patients attending a rural and remote memory clinic; and relationships between engaging in health and

wellness behaviors and psychological and neuropsychological function, independence in daily activities, and balance...The cross-sectional sample comprised 260 patients referred to the Rural and Remote Memory Clinic (RRMC), Saskatchewan, Canada. Patients were diagnosed with amnestic or non-amnestic mild cognitive impairment, Alzheimer's disease (AD), or non-AD dementia. Via questionnaire, patients were asked how many days a week they exercised for at least twenty minutes, if their diet met the Canada's Food Guide to Healthy Eating recommendations, and what they did to maintain their psychological health.

Patients completed a depression scale, a neuropsychological battery, and a balance scale. Caregivers completed the Functional Assessment Questionnaire... Participants were aged between forty-four and ninety-seven years, and had between 0 and 20 years of formal education. About half of those with Alzheimer's disease and more than half of the other diagnostic groups reported having five or more chronic conditions. Over a third of the total sample reported not exercising at all on a weekly basis. Less than half (42.7 percent) of the Alzheimer's disease group reported exercising for twenty minutes less than three times per week, while more than half of the other groups reported exercising for twenty minutes less than three times per week. Associations between exercise and tests of neuropsychological function and balance were statistically non-significant for the non-AD dementia group. In contrast, for the group with AD, engagement in exercise for twenty minutes for three or more times a week was moderately associated with better Stroop interference test scores and better balance...Patients referred to the RRMC reported good nutrition habits and participating in a variety of activities to maintain psychological health. *Engaging in exercise and good nutrition was found to have beneficial effects for the sub-sample of patients with AD."*

Tailored Lighting Intervention

Light therapy has shown great promise as a non-pharmacological method to improve symptoms associated with Alzheimer's disease and related dementias, with preliminary studies demonstrating that appropriately timed light exposure can improve nighttime sleep efficiency, reduce nocturnal wandering, and alleviate evening agitation. Since the human circadian[1] system is maximally sensitive to short-wavelength (blue) light, lower, more targeted lighting interventions for therapeutic purposes, can be used. To further evaluate this potential, researchers used a low-level "bluish-white" lighting designed to deliver high circadian stimulation during the daytime, which was installed in fourteen nursing home resident rooms for a period of four weeks. Without going into the specifics of the study, the researchers found that, *"A lighting intervention, tailored to increase daytime circadian stimulation, can be used to increase sleep quality and improve behavior in patients with dementia."*[291]

Transcranial LED Therapy (TCLT)

During the aging processes, there is a range of functional changes, including reduced cerebral (brain) blood flow. Researchers "investigated the effects of transcranial[2] light emitting diode (LED) on cerebral blood

---

[1]Circadian: A circadian rhythm is any biological process that displays an endogenous, entrainable oscillation of about 24 hours. These 24-hour rhythms are driven by a circadian clock, and they have been widely observed in plants, animals, fungi, and cyanobacteria. The term *circadian* comes from the Latin *circa*, meaning "around" (or "approximately"), and *diēs*, meaning "day." The formal study of biological temporal rhythms, such as daily, tidal, weekly, seasonal, and annual rhythms, is called chronobiology. Although circadian rhythms are endogenous ("built-in", self-sustained), they are adjusted (entrained) to the local environment by external cues called zeitgebers, commonly the most important of which is daylight.

[2]Transcranial: passing or performed through the skull.

flow in healthy elderly women analyzed by transcranial Doppler ultrasound (TCD) of the right and left middle cerebral artery and basilar artery. Twenty-five non-institutionalized elderly women (mean age seventy-two years old), with a cognitive status >24, were assessed using transcranial Doppler ultrasound on two separate occasions: pre-irradiation and post-transcranial LED therapy (TCLT)...results showed that there was a significant improvement after TCLT with increase in the systolic and diastolic velocity of the left middle cerebral artery (25 and 30 percent, respectively) and basilar artery (up to 17 and 25 percent), as well as a decrease in the pulsatility index and resistance index values of the three cerebral arteries analyzed. *TCD parameters showed improvement in the blood flow on the arteries analyzed.*[292]

Transcranial Stimulation

Repetitive transcranial magnetic stimulation (rTMS) is a noninvasive[1] tool for modulating cortical (brain) activity. In order to study the effects of rTMS on cognitive functions in patients with amnestic mild cognitive impairment (MCI) or incipient dementia due to Alzheimer's disease, researchers studied ten patients (six men; four women, mean age of 72. They found that *"High frequency rTMS induced significant improvement of attention and psychomotor speed in patients with MCI/mild dementia due to AD.* This pilot study is part of a more complex protocol and ongoing research."[293]

Reminiscence Therapy

Reminiscence therapy is defined by the American Psychological Association (APA) as "the use of life histories - written, oral, or both - to improve psychological well-being. The therapy is often used with older people." This form of therapeutic intervention respects the life and experiences of the individual with the aim to help the patient maintain good mental health.

---

[1]Noninvasive: not requiring the introduction of instruments into the body.

Autobiographical memory deficits are prominent from the early stages of Alzheimer's disease and result in a loss of personal identity. Nevertheless, standardized methods of autobiographical memory stimulation for the neuropsychological rehabilitation of patients with AD remain underdeveloped. In order to improve this situation, researchers conducted a study to evaluate the impact of a new cognitive training program for autobiographical memory (REMau) on autobiographical memory performance across lifetime periods, as well as on mood. "Pre/post evaluations were conducted on two groups of patients with early to moderate AD, assigned to one of two different training activities: either the REMau or a cognitive training program focused on collective semantic memory. *Statistical comparisons showed significant improvement of memory performance in the REMau group, as well as improved mood. By contrast, deleterious pre/post differences were observed in the other group. Most interestingly, this study showed that the REMau program boosted autobiographical memory from the reminiscence bump period, which is considered crucial for the construction and maintenance of personal identity.*"[294]

In order to study certain aspects of verbal reminiscence, in 2014 researchers assessed a simple computer-aided program for helping patients with moderate Alzheimer's disease engage in verbal reminiscence. The program was aimed at fostering the patient's verbal engagement on a number of life experiences/topics previously selected for him or her and introduced in the sessions through a friendly female, who appeared on the computer screen. "The female asked the patient about the aforementioned experiences/topics, and provided him or her with positive attention, and possibly verbal guidance (i.e., prompts/encouragements). *Eight patients were involved in the study, and seven of them showed clear improvement during the intervention phase* [i.e., with the program]."[295]

Experimental Treatments

Alzheimer's disease is one of the most complex diseases researchers have ever studied. There are many reasons Alzheimer's research is so challenging. To start, the brain is the most complex and inaccessible organ in the body and the disease is correspondingly complicated. However, as our understanding of the disease grows so does our ability to find new potential treatment approaches and, ultimately, effective new medicines.

America's biopharmaceutical research companies are investigating or developing 93 medicines to help the more than five million patients in the United States who are living with Alzheimer's. The medicines in development – all in either clinical trials or under review by the Food and Drug Administration – include eighty-one for Alzheimer's, eleven for cognition disorders and two for dementias, according to a new report released by the Pharmaceutical Research and Manufacturers of America (PhRMA). What follows is a review of just some of this research, in order to give one a sense of what is going on in the field of Alzheimer's research.

Antibodies and Immunotherapy

Recent advances in the understanding of Alzheimer's disease pathogenesis have led to the development of numerous compounds that might modify the disease process. Amyloid β peptide represents an important molecular target for intervention in Alzheimer's disease. Researchers recently conducted a literature search to review immunotherapy studies in relation to the Alzheimer's disease. They found that:[296]

> "Several types of amyloid β peptide immunotherapy for Alzheimer's disease are under investigation, active immunization and passive administration with monoclonal antibodies directed against amyloid β peptide. Although immunotherapy approaches resulted in clearance of amyloid plaques in patients with Alzheimer's disease, this clearance did not show significant cognitive effect for the moment. Currently, several amyloid β peptide im-

munotherapy approaches are under investigation but also against tau pathology.

Results from amyloid-based immunotherapy studies in clinical trials indicate that intervention appears to be more effective in early stages of amyloid accumulation, in particular solanezumab, with a potential impact at mild Alzheimer's disease, highlighting the importance of diagnosing Alzheimer's disease as early as possible and undertaking clinical trials at this stage. In both phase III solanezumab and bapineuzumab trials, PET imaging revealed that about a quarter of patients lacked fibrillar amyloid pathology at baseline, suggesting that they did not have Alzheimer's disease in the first place. So a new third phase 3 clinical trial for solanezumab, called Expedition 3, in patients with mild Alzheimer's disease and evidence of amyloid burden has been started. Thus, currently, amyloid intervention is realized at early stage of the Alzheimer's disease in clinical trials, at prodromal Alzheimer's disease, or at asymptomatic subjects or at risk to develop Alzheimer's disease and/or at asymptomatic subjects with autosomal dominant mutation."

The following summary, reported in late 2014, is included primarily for researchers in Alzheimer's disease, as it is too detailed for most of us mere mortals to comprehend. "Pathologically modified tau protein is the main feature of Alzheimer's disease and related tauopathies. Therefore, immunotherapies that target mis-disordered tau represent a promising avenue for the disease-modifying treatment of AD...We have discovered defined determinants on mis-disordered truncated tau protein which are responsible for tau oligomerization leading to neurofibrillary degeneration. Antibody DC8E8 reactive with these determinants is able to inhibit tau-tau interaction *in vitro* and *in vivo*. DC8E8 is able to discriminate between the healthy and diseased tau proteome, making its epitopes suitable targets, and DC8E8 a suitable candidate molecule, for AD immunotherapy."[297]

TREATMENT

Also reported in late 2014, and also too complicated for most readers to understand (or care about), "Among active and passive anti-β-amyloid (Aβ) immunotherapies for Alzheimer's disease, bapineuzumab and solanezumab, two humanized monoclonal antibodies, failed to show significant clinical benefits in mild-to-moderate AD patients in large Phase III clinical trials. Another ongoing Phase III trial of solanezumab aims to confirm positive findings in mild AD patients. Gantenerumab is the first fully human anti-Aβ monoclonal antibody directed to both N-terminal and central regions of Aβ. A 6-month PET study in sixteen AD patients showed that gantenerumab treatment dose-dependently reduced brain Aβ deposition, possibly stimulating microglial-mediated phagocytosis. Two ongoing Phase III trials of gantenerumab in patients with prodromal or mild dementia due to AD will determine if any reduction in brain Aβ levels will translate into clinical benefits. An ongoing secondary prevention trial of gantenerumab in presymptomatic subjects with genetic mutations for autosomal-dominant AD will verify the utility of anti-Aβ monoclonal antibodies as prevention therapy."[298]

Alzheimer's disease is a chronic neurodegenerative disease associated with intracerebral accumulation of aggregated amyloid-beta (Aβ) and tau proteins, as well as neuroinflammation. Researchers report that: [299]

> "Human intravenous immunoglobulin (IVIG) is a mixture of polyclonal IgG antibodies isolated and pooled from thousands of healthy human donors. The scientific rationale for testing IVIG as a potential AD treatment include its natural anti-Aβ antibody activity, its favorable safety profile and inherent anti-inflammatory/ immunomodulatory properties...Anti-amyloid antibodies in IVIG show significantly higher binding avidity for amyloid oligomers and fibrils than for Aβ monomers. In a double transgenic murine model of AD, intracerebral injection of IVIG causes suppression of Aβ fibril pathology whereas long term peripheral IVIG treatments causes elevation of total brain Aβ levels with no measurable impact on Aβ deposits or tendency for inducing cerebral microhemmorhage. Furthermore, chronic IVIG

treatment suppressed neuroinflammation and fostered adult hippocampal neurogenesis.

In clinical studies with AD patients, IVIG showed an acceptable safety profile and has not been reported to increase the incidence of amyloid-related imaging abnormalities. Preliminary studies on a small number of patients reported clinical benefits in mild to moderate stage AD patients. However, double blind, placebo controlled studies later did not replicate those initial findings. Interestingly though, in APOE4 carriers and in moderate disease stage subgroups, positive cognitive signals were reported. Nevertheless, both clinical and experimental (mouse) studies show that antibodies in IVIG can accumulate in CNS and its biological activities include neutralization of Aβ oligomers, suppression of neuroinflammation and immunomodulation. Identifying mediators of IVIG's effects at the cellular and molecular level is warranted. In light of its favorable safety profile and aforementioned biological properties, *IVIG is still an enigmatic experimental candidate with enormous potential for being an AD therapeutic.*"

According to another group of researchers, "Tau pathology is the main pathological characteristic of mild cognitive impairment (MCI) and Alzheimer disease (AD), and tau-based therapeutic strategies have great implications in the prevention of MCI and AD. The phosphorylation of threonine 231 preceding proline 232 (pThr231-Pro232) triggers tau hyperphosphorylation, tau aggregation, and tau pathology. Interestingly, the pThr231-Pro232 motif may be in a cis or trans configuration, but several recent studies have firstly indicated that cis, but not trans, pThr231-Pro232 tau is a striking therapeutic target for MCI and AD. Cis pThr231-Pro232 tau appears firstly in MCI and accumulates exclusively in the development of AD. Moreover, cis pThr231-Pro232 tau has low affinity to microtubules, high resistance to dephosphorylation and degradation, and a potent tendency to aggregate. On the contrary, trans pThr231-Pro232 tau has normal physiological activity in vivo.

Fortunately, Pin1 is the only known isomerase that catalyzes pThr231-Pro232 tau from the neurotoxic cis to nontoxic trans configuration, which prevents MCI and AD. Nonetheless, as we have mentioned before, Pin1 is frequently inactivated under abnormal physiological conditions in vivo. Therefore, it is necessary to clear cis pThr231-Pro232 tau by immunotherapy when Pin1 is insufficient, in order to avoid the occurrence of MCI and AD."[300] So, everything is clear then!

Diabetic Medications

Dr. Claxton and colleagues, reported the results of their research in the January 1, 2015 issue of the *Journal of Alzheimer's Disease*. They studied the effects of intranasal long-lasting insulin detemir) in adults with Alzheimer's disease dementia or amnestic mild cognitive impairment (MCI). "Sixty adults diagnosed with MCI or mild to moderate AD received placebo (n = 20), 20 IU of insulin detemir (n = 21), or 40 IU of insulin detemir (n = 19) for twenty-one days, administered with a nasal drug delivery device. Results revealed a treatment effect for the memory composite for the 40 IU group compared with placebo. *This effect was moderated by APOE status, reflecting improvement for APOE-ε4 carriers, and worsening for non-carriers.* Higher insulin resistance at baseline predicted greater improvement with the 40 IU dose. Significant treatment effects were also apparent for verbal working memory and visuospatial working memory, reflecting improvement for subjects who received the high dose of intranasal insulin detemir. No significant differences were found for daily functioning or executive functioning. In conclusion, *daily treatment with 40 IU insulin detemir modulated cognition for adults with AD or MCI, with APOE-related differences in treatment response for the primary memory composite.*"[301]

Epigenetic Therapies

Available treatments for neurodegenerative diseases such as Alzheimer's disease, Parkinson's disease, amyotrophic lateral sclerosis (ALS), and Huntington's disease, do not arrest disease progression but mainly help keeping patients from getting worse for a limited period of time. "Increasing evidence suggests that epigenetic[1] mechanisms such as DNA methylation and histone tail modifications are dynamically regulated in neurons and play a fundamental role in learning and memory processes. In addition, both global and gene-specific epigenetic changes and deregulated expression of the writer and eraser proteins of epigenetic marks are believed to contribute to the onset and progression of neurodegeneration. *Studies in animal models of neurodegenerative diseases have highlighted the potential role of epigenetic drugs, including inhibitors of histone deacetylases and methyl donor compounds, in ameliorating the cognitive symptoms and preventing or delaying the motor symptoms of the disease, thereby opening the way for a potential application in human pathology.*"[302]

Hyperketonemia

Results of a very interesting experimental treatment, conducted by Dr. Newport and colleagues, were reported in the October 7, 2014 issue of *Alzheimer's Dementia*. They noted that, "Providing ketone bodies[2] to the brain can bypass metabolic blocks to glucose utilization and improve function in energy-starved neurons. For this, plasma ketones must be elevated well above the ≤0.2 mM default concentrations normally prevalent. Limitations of dietary methods currently used to produce therapeutic hyperketonemia have stimulated the search for better approaches. Described herein is a new way to produce therapeutic hyperketonemia, entailing prolonged oral administration of a potent ketogenic agent-ketone monoester (KME)-to a patient with Alzheimer's disease dementia and a pretreatment Mini-Mental State Exam-

---

[1]Epigenetics is the study of cellular and physiological trait variations that are *not* caused by changes in the DNA sequence; epigenetics describes the study of dynamic alterations in the transcriptional potential of a cell. These alterations may or may not be heritable, although the use of the term epigenetic to describe processes that are not heritable is controversial.

[2]Ketone bodies are three water-soluble molecules that are produced by the liver from fatty acids during periods of low food intake (fasting) or carbohydrate restriction for cells of the body to use as energy instead of glucose.

ination score of 12 [MMSE; highest score is 30]. *The patient improved markedly in mood, affect, self-care, and cognitive and daily activity performance. The KME was well tolerated throughout the 20-month treatment period. Cognitive performance tracked plasma β-hydroxybutyrate concentrations, with noticeable improvements in conversation and interaction at the higher levels, compared with predose levels. KME-induced hyperketonemia is robust, convenient, and safe, and the ester can be taken as an oral supplement without changing the habitual diet.*"[303]

The most popular retail ketogenic agent is Raspberry Ketone Supplement, which is primarily marketed for weight loss. It seems that it would be more appropriate for use with individuals with neurodegenerative disorders, such as Alzheimer's disease. That is, those whose ability to utilize glucose is known to be compromised, and for whom an alternate source of energy (e.g., ketones) might be useful.

Nanosolution

"Neuritic plaques are mainly composed of aggregates of amyloid-β (Aβ) protein while neurofibrillary tangles are composed of the hyperphosphorylated tau protein. Despite intense investigations, no effective therapy is currently available to halt the progression of this disease. Here, we have undertaken a novel approach to attenuate apoptosis and tau phosphorylation in cultured neuronal [nerve] cells and in a transgenic animal model of AD. RNS60 is a 0.9 percent saline solution containing oxygenated nanobubbles...Furthermore, RNS60 also decreased Aβ(1-42)-induced tau phosphorylation via (PI-3 kinase-Akt)-mediated inhibition of GSK-3β. Similarly, RNS60 treatment suppressed neuronal apoptosis, attenuated Tau phosphorylation, inhibited glial activation, and reduced the burden of Aβ in the hippocampus and protected memory and learning in 5XFAD transgenic mouse model of AD. *Therefore, RNS60 may be a promising pharmaceutical candidate in halting or delaying the progression of AD.*"[304]

Nanotubes

Defective autophagy[1] in Alzheimer's disease promotes disease progression in diverse ways. In 2014, researchers studied the effect of nanotubes on this phenomenon. "Here, we demonstrate impaired autophagy flux in primary glial cells derived from CRND8 mice that over-express mutant amyloid precursor protein (APP). Functionalized single-walled carbon nanotubes (SWNT) restored normal autophagy by reversing abnormal activation of mTOR signaling and deficits in lysosomal proteolysis, thereby facilitating elimination of autophagic substrates. *These findings suggest SWNT as a novel neuroprotective approach to AD therapy.*"[305]

Stem Cells

Stem cells[2] have the remarkable potential to develop into many different cell types, essentially without limit to replenish other cells as long as the person or animal is still alive, offering immense hope of curing Alzheimer's disease, repairing damaged spinal cords, treating kidney, liver and lung diseases and making damaged hearts whole. Until recently, scientists primarily worked with two kinds of stem cells from animals and humans: embryonic stem cells and non-embryonic "somatic" or "adult" stem cells. Recent breakthrough make it possible to convert or "reprogram" specialized adult cells to assume a stem stem-like cells with different technologies.[306]

Currently, no effective therapies for Alzheimer's disease have been developed. However, recent advances in the fields of neural stem cells and human induced pluripotent stem cells now provide us with the first real hope for a cure. According to one researcher, reporting in 2014, "*The recent discovery by Blurton-Jones and colleagues that neural*

---

[1] Autophagy (or autophagocytosis) is the basic catabolic mechanism that involves cell degradation of unnecessary or dysfunctional cellular components.
[2] Stem cells are undifferentiated biological cells that can differentiate into specialized cells and can divide (through mitosis) to produce more stem cells. In mammals, there are two broad types of stem cells: embryonic stem cells, which are isolated from the inner cell mass of blastocysts, and adult stem cells, which are found in various tissues.

stem cells can effectively deliver disease-modifying therapeutic proteins throughout the brains of our best rodent models of Alzheimer's disease, combined with recent advances in human nuclear reprogramming, stem cell research, and highly customized genetic engineering, may represent a potentially revolutionary personalized cellular therapeutic approach capable of effectively curing, ameliorating, and/or slowing the progression of Alzheimer's disease."[307]

Using an animal model of Alzheimer's disease, researchers stated, "The purpose of this study was to evaluate the therapeutic potential of human induced pluripotent stem (iPS) cell-derived macrophage-like cells for Alzheimer's disease...We observed significant reduction in the level of Aβ in the brain interstitial fluid following administration of iPS-ML/NEP2. *These results suggested that iPS-ML/NEP2 may be a potential therapeutic agent in the treatment of AD.*"[308]

Ultrasound

As you are now well aware, amyloid-β (Aβ) peptide has been implicated in the pathogenesis of Alzheimer's disease. In March 2015, researchers studied a non-pharmacological approach for removing Aβ and restoring memory function in a mouse model of AD in which Aβ is deposited in the brain. "We used repeated scanning ultrasound (SUS) treatments of the mouse brain to remove Aβ, without the need for any additional therapeutic agent such as anti-Aβ antibody...Plaque burden was reduced in SUS-treated AD mice compared to sham-treated animals, and cleared plaques were observed in 75 percent of SUS-treated mice. Treated AD mice also displayed improved performance on three memory tasks: the Y-maze, the novel object recognition test, and the active place avoidance task. *Our findings suggest that repeated SUS is useful for removing Aβ in the mouse brain without causing overt damage, and should be explored further as a noninvasive method with therapeutic potential in AD.*"[309]

Vaccines

Dr. Kontsekova and colleagues, reporting their research using an animal of Alzheimer's disease in the August 1, 2014 issue of *Alzheimer's Research and Therapy*, note that, "We have identified structural determinants on tau protein that are essential for pathological tau-tau interaction in Alzheimer's disease. These regulatory domains, revealed by monoclonal antibody DC8E8, represent a novel target for tau-directed therapy. In order to validate this target, we have developed an active vaccine, AADvac1...Active immunization targeting crucial domains of Alzheimer tau eliminated tau aggregation and neurofibrillary pathology. Most importantly, the AD type of tau hyperphosphorylation was abolished by vaccination across a wide range of AD phospho-epitopes. *Our results demonstrate that active immunization led to elimination of all major hallmarks of neurofibrillary pathology, which was reflected by a profound improvement in the clinical presentation of transgenic rats. This makes the investigated tau peptide vaccine a highly promising candidate therapeutic for the disease-modifying treatment of AD. The tested vaccine displayed a highly favorable safety profile in preclinical toxicity studies, which opens up the possibility of using it for AD prophylaxis in the future.* The vaccine has already entered phase I clinical trial[1] under the name AADvac1."[310]

---

[1]Clinical trials are conducted in a series of steps, called phases - each phase is designed to answer a separate research question.
- Phase I: Researchers test a new drug or treatment in a small group of people for the first time to evaluate its safety, determine a safe dosage range, and identify side effects.
- Phase II: The drug or treatment is given to a larger group of people to see if it is effective and to further evaluate its safety.
- Phase III: The drug or treatment is given to large groups of people to confirm its effectiveness, monitor side effects, compare it to commonly used treatments, and collect information that will allow the drug or treatment to be used safely.
- Phase IV: Studies are done after the drug or treatment has been marketed to gather information on the drug's effect in various populations and any side effects associated with long-term use.

TREATMENT

Johnson & Johnson boosted its research efforts in Alzheimer's research in January 2015 by striking a deal potentially worth up to $509 million with unlisted Swiss biotech firm AC Immune to develop anti-tau vaccines. According to the news release, "Tau is a protein known for forming tangles inside brain cells and is linked to cell death. It is one of two abnormal proteins tied to Alzheimer's disease. The other is beta amyloid. The Swiss company already has another major tie-up with Roche for a beta amyloid-fighting drug called crenezumab. The hope is that therapeutic vaccines targeting tau will offer a way to treat Alzheimer's patients earlier in the disease…J&J will further develop AC Immune's lead therapeutic vaccine, ACI-35, which is currently in an early-stage Phase Ib clinical trial. ACI-35 is designed to stimulate the patient's immune system to produce a response against tau protein."[311]

Chapter Nine:
PREVENTION

Introduction

As with any medical illness, it is better to prevent a disease altogether, than to have to treat it. Think of heart disease. Would you rather have to have coronary bypass surgery or a stent, or even a heart attack (MI or myocardial infarction), or would you rather keep your cholesterol low, exercise, not smoke, and eat a healthy diet? The answer is obvious, at least to most people. It is the same with Alzheimer's disease. It is much better to prevent it than to treat it. Prevention is the key! The good news is that Alzheimer's disease can be prevented, or at a minimum the onset delayed, in most people.

As scientists have relentlessly chipped away for more than fifty years at the causes and potential treatments of most common diseases, impressive discoveries have slowly accumulated. With Alzheimer's disease, we are now on the verge of having a simple blood test that can diagnose this condition, and we are also on the verge of having the ability to prevent it, for most people.

Some of the same things that prevent Alzheimer's disease may also help prevent other neurodegenerative diseases (for example, Parkinson's disease), heart disease, and cancer, and may even promote longevity.

FDA-approved Medications (Used "Off-label")

The only approved medications for AD are symptomatic and there are no currently available disease modifying treatments. Hence, a disease modifying treatment is desperately needed for AD not only for proper

PREVENTION

care and management of affected patients, but also to reduce society's socioeconomic burden. Developing novel compounds for any indication is a time, effort, and money consuming endeavor and most treatments never make it to market. Other research and development strategies are needed, especially for the treatment of AD. *One viable strategy is the repurposing of medications currently used for non-AD indications.*

The use of FDA-approved medications for an illness, condition, or indication for which the medication is not approved is referred to as "off-label" use. Off-label use is very common. Generic drugs generally have no sponsor as their indications and use expands, and incentives are limited to initiate new clinical trials to generate additional data for approval agencies to expand indications of proprietary drugs. *Up to one-fifth of all drugs are prescribed off-label and amongst psychiatric drugs, off-label use rises to 31 percent.* In the United States, no law prohibits a physician or other healthcare practitioner from prescribing an approved medication for other uses than their specific FDA-approved indications. *The use of any of the medications discussed below for Alzheimer's disease would be off-label.*

Reflecting the widespread interest in this area, and for example, the Alzheimer's Drug Discovery Foundation (ADDF) and the Michael J. Fox Foundation for Parkinson's Research (MJFF) convened an advisory panel in October 2013 on repurposing FDA-approved drugs for neurodegenerative diseases."[312]

Although written in 2006, the following is a good overview of the issue of repurposing supplements and/or FDA-approved medications for the prevention or treatment of Alzheimer's disease:[313]

"This review examines key pharmacological strategies that have been clinically studied for the primary[1] or sec-

---

[1]Primary prevention: Methods to avoid occurrence of disease either through eliminating disease agents or increasing resistance to disease. Examples include immunization against disease, maintaining a healthy diet and exercise regimen, and avoiding smoking. Secondary prevention: Methods to detect and address an existing disease prior to

ondary prevention of Alzheimer's disease. Much information (neuropsychological, genetic and imaging) is already available to characterize an individual's risk for developing Alzheimer's disease. However, *regulatory pathways for obtaining a prevention indication are less well charted, and such trials tend to involve 3- to 7-year studies of 1000 - 5000 individuals, depending on baseline status.* Treatments developed for prevention will also need to have superior safety. *For these reasons, > 100 proprietary pharmacological products are currently being developed for an Alzheimer's disease treatment, but only a few are being studied for prevention.* Randomized trial data are available for antihypertensive agents (calcium channel blockers, angiotensin-converting enzyme inhibitors), pravastatin, simvastatin, conjugated estrogen, raloxifene, rofecoxib, CX516 (AMPA agonist) and cholinesterase inhibitors regarding efficacy for Alzheimer's disease prevention.

At least four large prevention trials of conjugated estrogen, selenium and vitamin E, Ginkgo biloba and statins are currently underway. Strategies using other agents have not yet been evaluated in Alzheimer's disease prevention clinical trials. These include anti-amyloid antibodies, active immunization, selective secretase inhibitors and modulators, microtubule stabilizers (e.g., paclitaxel), R-flurbiprofen, xaliproden, ONO-2506, FK962 (somatostatin releaser), SGS 742 (GABA(B) antagonist), TCH 346 (apoptosis inhibitor), Alzhemed®, phophodiesterase inhibitors, rosiglitazone, leuprolide, interferons, metal-protein attenuating compounds (e.g., PBT2), CX717, rasagaline, huperzine A, antioxidants and memantine. Studies combining lifestyle modifica-

---

the appearance of symptoms. Examples include treatment of hypertension (a risk factor for many cardiovascular diseases), cancer screenings

tion and drug therapy have not been conducted. Full validation of surrogate markers for disease progression (such as amyloid imaging) should further facilitate drug development. Reducing the complexity of prevention trials and gaining regulatory consensus of design is a high priority for the field."

Many different compounds from many different pharmacological classes have already been studied in an AD context. *According to one analysis, current data suggest compounds worthy of further study as treatments for AD include lithium, minocycline, exenatide, valproic acid, methylene blue, and nicotine.*[314] *Other studies have shown that lithium, Prozac (fluoxetine), and antipsychotics have the potential to modify AD.*[315] In fact, there are many studies, too numerous to list here, that indicate the potential of current FDA-approved mediations to prevent and/or treat Alzheimer's disease. However, more research is needed in order to determine their true benefits. Below, we review specific medications that have shown benefit in the prevention of Alzheimer's disease.

Antidepressants

FDA Warning: *Antidepressants increased the risk of suicidal thoughts and behavior in children, teenagers, and young adults.* In patients of all ages who are started on antidepressant therapy, watch closely for worsening depression and for suicidal thoughts and behaviors. Families and caregivers of patients on antidepressants should talk with the patient's doctor if depression becomes worse.

SSRIs (Selective Serotonin Reuptake Inhibitors such as Celexa or citalopram; Zoloft or sertraline; Prozac, or fluoxetine; Lexapro, or escitalopram):

NOTE: It is important to keep in mind that elderly people can develop clinical depression, referred to as "major depressive disorder," but sometimes they can present as having dementia or Alzheimer's dementia. This is referred to as "pseudodementia," because the person doesn't really have dementia, they just appear to have it, but they really have depression.

One of the most exciting types of currently FDA-approved medications with the potential to prevent Alzheimer's disease are antidepressants. Antidepressants are already used to treat depression, anxiety, and behavioral symptoms in AD. In fact, one study found that these medications are used in about 30 percent of patients with AD, compared to the general population, where they are used in approximately ten percent of people (primarily for anxiety and depression).[316] It has been known for more than ten years that antidepressants might be helpful in the prevention of AD.[317]

Celexa (citalopram; 5-20 mg in those 60 or older; up to 40 mg otherwise):

Citalopram is considered safe and well tolerated in the therapeutic dose range. Distinct from some other agents in its class, it exhibits linear pharmacokinetics[1] and minimal drug interaction potential, making it a better choice for the elderly patients.

Celexa is one of the most exciting compounds when it comes to the prevention of Alzheimer's disease. It has been shown in animal models of AD to have amazing therapeutic or beneficial effects on a variety of enzymes, proteins, and other cellular structures, some of which will be described below.

Social isolation is considered as a chronic stress and, in one experiment using animal models of AD, was shown to be quite damaging to a variety of brain proteins, and other cellular structures—even though it did

---

[1]Linear pharmacokinetics: the rate of change in drug concentration depends only on the current concentration; it is a direct or 1:1 relationship (for example, the higher the dose given, the higher the blood concentration, in direct propotion to the amount given). The half-life will remain constant, no matter how high the concentration.

not lead to depression or anxiety-like behaviors. In this experiment, memory deficits and other abnormalities could be almost completely reversed by citalopram. Interestingly, *melatonin levels were decreased in the social isolation group, and citalopram could partly restore the level of melatonin. Even more significantly, it was also shown that citalopram could increase melatonin (MT1 and MT2) receptors* in mRNA (messenger RNA) levels. All of this suggested to the researchers that social isolation might constitute a risk factor for Alzheimer's disease, and *"citalopram may represent a therapeutic strategy for the treatment of AD."*[318]

Aggregation of amyloid-β (Aβ) and amyloid plaques within the brain appears to be the main pathogenic event that initiates Alzheimer's disease lesions. One therapeutic strategy has been to reduce Aβ levels to limit its accumulation. In an exciting experiment in an animal model of AD, citalopram arrested the growth of preexisting amyloid plaques, which are characteristic of AD pathology, and reduced the appearance of new plaques by 78 percent. The same researchers reported that *in healthy human volunteers, acute (not even long-term) dosing of citalopram decreased Aβ concentrations in cerebrospinal fluid (CSF) by 38 percent in the citalopram group compared to placebo.* The researchers found, *"The ability to safely decrease Aβ concentrations is potentially important as a preventive strategy for AD."*[319]

In a very similar report, researchers assessed the ability of serotonin to alter brain Aβ levels and plaques in a mouse model of AD and in humans. In mice, brain fluid Aβ levels were decreased by 25 percent following administration of several selective serotonin reuptake inhibitor (SSRI) antidepressant drugs. Chronic treatment with citalopram caused a 50 percent reduction in brain plaque load in mice. To test whether antidepressants could impact Aβ plaques in humans, the researchers compared brain amyloid load in cognitively normal elderly participants who were exposed to antidepressant drugs within the past five years (of testing) to participants who were not. Antidepressant-treated participants had significantly less amyloid load as quantified by PET scans. *Cumulative time of antidepressant use within the five-year period preceding the scan correlated with less plaque load.* The researchers concluded that, *"These data suggest that serotonin signaling was associated with less Aβ accumulation in cognitively normal individuals."*[320]

One study found that the clinical benefit from combined use of galantamine (Nivalin, Razadyne, Razadyne ER, Reminyl, Lycoremine; approved by the FDA for mild to moderate AD) and citalopram may be related to a "synergistic" [i.e., more than additive] inhibition of butyrylcholinesterase, facilitating cholinergic neurotransmission."[321] In other words, *the addition of citalopram increased the effectiveness of galantamine.*

Researchers studied human brain (nerve) networks involved in depression and cognition, and discovered that, while there was some overlap in the networks, they were quite distinct from each other. The study evaluated the cerebral glucose metabolic effects of citalopram treatment. The researchers reported that, "Sixteen geriatric depressed patients (who didn't have AD) underwent positron emission tomography (PET) studies of cerebral glucose metabolism and assessment of affective symptoms (depression and anxiety) and cognitive function before and after eight weeks of treatment with citalopram. Functional connectivity analyses revealed two networks which were uniquely associated with improvement of affective symptoms and cognitive function during treatment. One network was associated with improvement in affect, while another network was associated with improvement in cognition (immediate verbal learning/memory and verbal fluency). Notably, the regions that comprise the cognitive network overlap with the regions that are affected in Alzheimer's dementia. *Thus, alterations in specific brain networks associated with improvement of affective symptoms and cognitive function are observed during citalopram treatment in geriatric depression.*"[322]

Prozac (fluoxetine; 5-80 mg)

Fluoxetine was approved by the U.S. Food and Drug Administration (FDA) for the treatment of major depressive disorder in December 1987. Fluoxetine is used for the treatment of major depressive disorder (including pediatric depression), obsessive–compulsive disorder (in both adults and children), bulimia nervosa, panic disorder, and premenstrual dysphoric disorder.

In 2010, over 24.4 million prescriptions for generic formulations of fluoxetine were filled in the United States, making it the third-most prescribed antidepressant after sertraline and citalopram.

Fluoxetine is one of the antidepressants used for the treatment of depression and anxiety associated with AD. *It was shown in a recent scientific study, in an animal model of AD, that fluoxetine improved spatial memory, learning and emotional behaviors. It was also shown to have profound effects on β-amyloid (Aβ) in brain tissue, cerebrospinal fluid (CSF) and blood, as well as one of the main proteins associated with AD, amyloid precursor protein (APP).*[323]

Another study found that fluoxetine can enhance nerve cell development, and that it has protective effects against cell death caused by proteins associated with AD. The researchers noted that *"taken together, these results clearly show that the use of fluoxetine…is applicable for cell therapy for various neurodegenerative diseases, such as Alzheimer's and Parkinson's diseases."*[324]

Zoloft (Sertraline; 12.5-200 mg)

In a very large study, at multiple locations in the United States, *researchers found that treatment with sertraline in patients with AD was not associated with greater improvement in cognition after 24 weeks of treatment than with placebo.*[325] So, once again, prevention is shown to be better than treatment.

The take home message is that once AD is present, no medication has been shown to be beneficial, to decrease symptoms or to improve thinking. This includes medications, vitamins, and natural supplements that may, in fact, help prevent AD if given long before AD develops.

Fetzima (levomilnacipran; 20-120 mg)

Fetzima is an antidepressant approved by the FDA in 2013 for the treatment of major depressive disorder in the United States. It acts as a serotonin-norepinephrine reuptake inhibitor (SNRI). For reference, other SNRIs include Cymbalta (duloxetine), Effexor XR (venlafaxine), and Pristiq (desvenlafaxine).

This is a new and novel antidepressant that, unlike SSRIs (such as citalopram and sertraline), affects serotonin transporters (SERT) as well as an enzyme associated with AD. This enzyme is called beta-site amyloid precursor protein cleaving enzyme-1 (BACE-1), and is responsible for amyloid β plaque formations. Researchers noted in 2014, *"Hence, Fetzima (levomilnacipran) might act as a potent dual inhibitor of SERT and BACE-1 and [is] expected to form the basis of a future dual therapy against depression and AD."*[326]

Norepinephrine (a neurotransmitter):

Antidepressants that increase norepinephrine:

- Cymbalta (duloxetine)
- Effexor XR (venlafaxine)
- Fetzima (levomilnacipran)
- Pristiq (desvenlafaxine)
- Tofranil (imipramine)
- Vivactil (protriptyline)
- Wellbutrin (bupropion)

Increasing norepinephrine decreases the neuropathology and cognitive deficits in animal models of AD. Researchers have found that increasing norepinephrine protects neurons (nerve cells) from cognitive deficits in animal models of the disease. They note, "These results indicate that *norepinephrine can protect against amyloid-β toxicity...and have implications for potential therapies for the disease* [AD]."[327]

PREVENTION

Protriptyline (a tricyclic antidepressant or TCA)

The discovery of drug molecules capable of targeting multiple factors involved in AD pathogenesis would greatly facilitate therapeutic strategies. The repositioning of existing non-toxic drugs could dramatically reduce the time and costs involved in developmental and clinical trial stages. *To this end, in 2014 researchers studied 140 FDA-approved nervous system drugs. They discovered the tricyclic group of antidepressants (the oldest class of antidepressants) was the most powerful against three major AD targets (e.g., Acetylcholinesterase (AChE), β-secretase (BACE-1), and amyloid β (Aβ) aggregation), with one member, protriptyline, showing the highest inhibitory activity.* The results of this study, conducted in 2014, led the authors to conclude that *protriptyline was "a promising candidate for AD treatment."*[328]

Keppra (levetiracetam)

In 2015, researchers noted that "studies of individuals with amnestic mild cognitive impairment (aMCI) have detected *hyperactivity in the hippocampus* [memory area of the brain] during task-related functional magnetic resonance imaging (fMRI)." Without going into the details of their research, the investigators "assessed the effects of levetiracetam in three groups of aMCI participants, each receiving a different dose of levetiracetam. Elevated activation in the DG/CA3 region [a specific area of the hippocampus], together with impaired task performance, was detected in each aMCI group relative to an aged control group. *We observed significant improvement in memory task performance under drug treatment relative to placebo in the aMCI cohorts at the 62.5 and 125 mg BID doses of levetiracetam*...Similar to findings in animal studies, higher dosing at 250 mg BID had no significant benefit on either task performance or fMRI activation.[329]

Lithium

Lithium carbonate is an inorganic compound, the lithium salt of carbonate with the formula Li_2CO_3. This white salt is widely used in the processing of metal oxides. For the treatment of bipolar disorder, it is on the World Health Organization's List of Essential Medicines, a list of the most important medication needed in a basic health system.

In 1843, lithium carbonate was used as a new solvent for stones in the bladder. In 1859, some doctors recommended a therapy with lithium salts for a number of ailments, including gout, urinary calculi, rheumatism, mania, depression, and headache. In 1949, John Cade discovered the antimanic effects of lithium ions. This finding led lithium, specifically lithium carbonate, to be used to treat mania associated with bipolar disorder.

Lithium carbonate is used to treat mania, the elevated phase of bipolar disorder. Lithium ions interfere with ion transport processes that relay and amplify messages carried to the cells of the brain. Mania is associated with irregular increases in protein kinase C (PKC) activity within the brain. Lithium carbonate and sodium valproate (Depakote), another drug used to treat the disorder, act in the brain by inhibiting PKC's activity and help to produce other compounds that also inhibit the PKC. Despite these findings, a great deal remains unknown regarding lithium's mood-controlling properties.

Use of lithium salts exhibit a number of risks and side effects, especially at higher doses. Lithium intoxication affects the central nervous and renal systems and is potentially lethal. It can also adversely affect thyroid functioning. If this occurs, it is a temporary problem and thyroid replacement is given, rather than lithium treatment being discontinued.

Researchers have noted that, "Clinical and epidemiological studies in bipolar disorder show that...*long-term treatment [with lithium] lowers the risk of dementia.*"[330]

Lithium is one of the most widely used mood-stabilizing agents for the treatment of bipolar disorder. Although the underlying mechanism(s) of this mood stabilizer remains controversial, evidence linking lithium to neurotrophic/neuroprotective effects suggests novel benefits of this drug in addition to mood stabilization. *More than ten years ago, re-*

PREVENTION

searchers used an animal model of Alzheimer's disease to demonstrate the ability of lithium (and Depakote) to inhibit beta-amyloid peptide (Abeta) production and reduce plaque burden.[331]

Also more than ten years ago, other researchers found that lithium exerts neuroprotective effects in vitro (in the laboratory) and stimulates nerve cell growth in the part of the brain where memories are stored (hippocampus).[332]

From the Molecular Neurobiology Section, Mood and Anxiety Disorders Program, National Institute of Mental Health, National Institutes of Health, Bethesda, Maryland, Dr. Chuang, in 2004, reported on a variety of cellular and animal experiments. He concluded, "The neuroprotective and neurotrophic actions of lithium have profound clinical implications. In addition to its present use in bipolar patients, *lithium could be used to treat acute brain injuries such as stroke and chronic progressive neurodegenerative diseases [such as Alzheimer's disease]*."[333]

Other experimental and clinical studies also have provided evidence that lithium may exert neuroprotective effects. In animal and cell culture models, lithium has been shown to increase nerve cell viability through a combination of mechanisms. In humans, lithium treatment has been associated with a multitude of evidence of neuroprotection, "such as increased expression of anti-apoptotic genes, inhibition of cellular oxidative stress, synthesis of brain-derived neurotrophic factor (BDNF), cortical thickening, increased grey matter density, and hippocampal enlargement...A recent placebo-controlled clinical trial in patients with amnestic mild cognitive impairment (MCI) showed that long-term lithium treatment may actually slow the progression of cognitive and functional deficits...Therefore, *lithium treatment may yield disease-modifying effects in AD*, both by the specific modification...and by the unspecific provision of neurotrophic and neuroprotective support. Although the clinical evidence available so far is promising, further experimentation and replication of the evidence in large scale clinical trials is still required to assess the benefit of lithium in the treatment or prevention of cognitive decline in the elderly."[334]

ALZHEIMER'S DISEASE

Lithium has been shown to have considerable neuroprotective effects, even in trace or low doses. In a recent review of the literature, authors summarize the current understanding of lithium benefits in trace or low doses in dementia prevention and for other behavioral or medical benefits. They noted that, "Five out of seven epidemiological studies found an association between standard-dose lithium and low dementia rates. Nine out of eleven epidemiological studies, usually of drinking water sources, found an association between trace-dose lithium and low suicide/homicide/mortality and crime rates. *All four small randomized clinical trials of lithium for Alzheimer's dementia have found at least some clinical or biological benefits versus placebo.*"[335]

A lower incidence of dementia in bipolar patients treated with lithium has been described. This metal inhibits some of the mechanisms related to degenerative neurologic conditions, including Alzheimer's disease. *Recently, researchers found that lithium has disease-modifying properties in amnestic mild cognitive impairment with potential clinical implications for the prevention of Alzheimer's disease, when a dose ranging from 150 to 600 mg is used.* More recently, a different group of researchers evaluated the effect of a *microdose of 300 μg (not mg, or milligrams but micrograms)*, administered once daily on AD patients for fifteen months. "The treated group showed no decreased performance in the mini-mental state examination test (MMSE), in opposition to the lower scores observed for the control group during the treatment, with significant differences starting three months after the beginning of the treatment, and increasing progressively. *This data suggests the efficacy of a microdose lithium treatment in preventing cognitive loss, reinforcing its therapeutic potential to treat AD using very low doses.*"[336]

Researchers studied the effects of chronic lithium treatment, using an animal model of AD. They published their results in the *Journal of Alzheimer's Disease*, and found that chronic lithium treatment, "...reduced...amyloid-β production and senile plaque formation, accompanied by the improvement in spatial learning and memory abilities...*Our results suggest that prolonged lithium treatment, even during the later stages of AD, could be an effective therapy.*"[337]

PREVENTION

To evaluate the effect of long-term lithium treatment on people with amnestic mild cognitive impairment (aMCI), researchers studied forty-five individuals, twenty-four of whom received lithium, over a twelve-month period. The researchers concluded that, "Overall tolerability of lithium was good and the adherence rate was 91 percent. *The present data support the notion that lithium has disease-modifying properties with potential clinical implications in the prevention of Alzheimer's disease.*"[338]

To investigate whether treatment with lithium in patients with mania or bipolar disorder is associated with a decreased rate of subsequent dementia, researchers studied a total of 4,856 patients with a diagnosis of bipolar disorder. Among these patients, 2,449 were exposed to lithium (50.4 percent), 1,781 to anticonvulsants (36.7 percent), 4,280 to antidepressants (88.1 percent), and 3,901 to antipsychotics (80.3 percent) during the study period. A total of 216 patients received a diagnosis of dementia during follow-up. The researchers concluded that, "*Continued treatment with lithium was associated with a reduced rate of dementia in patients with bipolar disorder in contrast to continued treatment with anticonvulsants, antidepressants, or antipsychotics.*"[339]

Results from a recent clinical trial suggest that long-term lithium treatment at subtherapeutic doses may have the potential to delay the progression of disease, and observational studies have shown that lithium reduces the prevalence of dementia in subjects with bipolar disorder on long-term lithium therapy. Dr. Wallace, as reported in the March 2014 edition of the journal *Cellular Calcium,* advanced the hypothesis that *lithium may protect against cognitive decline by stabilizing intracellular calcium.*[340]

In order to evaluate the effect of long-term lithium treatment at subtherapeutic doses on renal (kidney) function in older adults, as well as its effects on thyroid, immune, and glycemic functions, researchers conducted a four-year clinical study of sixty-one patients with mild cognitive impairment. These patients received either lithium or placebo. Results showed that no significant changes in renal function were detected after four years of lithium treatment. However, significant increases in the number of neutrophils (a type of white blood cell), serum TSH (thyroid stimulating hormone), and body weight were observed in the lithium group. The lithium group presented more overall adverse events, particularly interfering in daily activities. In addition, those patients had a higher incidence of diabetes mellitus and arrhythmia. The authors concluded, *"Chronic use of lithium at low doses did not affect renal function and was clinically safe.* However, some other potentially relevant adverse events were observed and others could not be ruled out due to limitations of the study design."[341]

Researchers used an animal model of Alzheimer's disease to study the protective effects of lithium. The scientists concluded, *"Our data suggest that progression of the pathology can be prevented by administration of lithium when the first signs of neuropathology appear. Further, it is possible to partially reverse this pathology in advanced stages of the disease, although the presence of already assembled neurofibrillary tangle-like structures cannot be reversed."*[342]

To assess the safety and feasibility of prescribing long term lithium to elderly people with mild to moderate Alzheimer's disease, researchers prescribed low dose lithium for up to one year to twenty-two people with AD. The conclusion, *"Lithium treatment in elderly people with AD has relatively few side effects and those that were apparently due to treatment were mild and reversible.* Nonetheless discontinuation rates are high. *The use of lithium as a potential disease modification therapy in AD should be explored further but is not without problems."*[343]

Researchers studied the short-term use of lithium in 71 patients with mild Alzheimer's disease. The 10-week treatment included a 6-week titration phase to reach the target serum level of lithium (0.5-0.8 mmol/L). The authors concluded that, "The current results do not support the notion that lithium treatment may lead to reduced biochemical signs associated with AD after a short 10-week treatment in the Alzheimer's disease target population.[344] (It would be shocking if the results were different, given that the researchers were trying to treat Alzheimer's disease, number one, and number two, that the treatment was so short. This, once again, underscores the need for long-term preventive measures, just the opposite of short-term treatment.)

As in all of medical research, it is good to keep in mind that nothing is 100 percent one way, and there are almost always conflicting scientific studies. This is also true with the effects of lithium and AD. There is at least one study, done in 2005 in the U.K., that found that the use of lithium was associated with a higher incidence of AD, for example.[345] Ultimately, one has to weigh all the evidence, for and against a particular treatment option, and make an informed decision to take the treatment or not.

Researchers, using a new animal model of Alzheimer's disease, reported in 2014 that *specific cognitive deficits and molecular pathology were reversed by lithium incubation.*[346]

Dr. Sofola-Adesakin and eleven colleagues also reported in 2014, using two different animal modes of AD. They concluded that, *"Our data highlight a role for lithium...for AD pathogenesis."* They found in one animal model that the use of lithium was also associated with an increased lifespan.[347]

Statins (HMG-CoA Reductase Inhibitors)

Most common statins:

- Crestor (rosuvastatin)
- Lescol (fluvastatin)
- Lipitor (atorvastatin)
- Livalo (pitavastatin)
- Mevacor; Altocor (lovastatin)
- Pravachol (pravastatin)
- Vytorin (simvastatin + ezetimibe)
- Zocor (simvastatin)

ALZHEIMER'S DISEASE

Note: *Consumer Reports* has an excellent discussion of these medications, including costs. It is a PDF file; just google "Consumer Reports 2014 statins."

The best-selling statin has been Lipitor (atorvastatin), which by 2003 became the best-selling pharmaceutical in history. The manufacturer Pfizer reported sales of $12.4 billion in 2008. Due to patent expirations (including Lipitor), several statins are now available as inexpensive generics.

Side effects of statins include muscle pain, increased risk of diabetes and abnormalities in liver enzyme tests. Additionally, they have rare but severe adverse effects, particularly muscle damage. They deplete mitochondrial CoQ10, and some experts recommend CoQ10 supplementation for those taking statins.

Statins are a class of drugs used to lower cholesterol levels by inhibiting the enzyme HMG-CoA reductase, which plays a central role in the production of cholesterol in the liver, which produces about 70 percent of total cholesterol in the body. High cholesterol levels have been associated with cardiovascular disease (CVD). Statins have been found to prevent cardiovascular disease and mortality in those who are at high risk. The evidence is strong that statins are effective for treating CVD in the early stages of a disease (secondary prevention) and in those at elevated risk but without CVD (primary prevention).

Blood cholesterol levels are not consistently elevated in subjects with age-related cognitive decline, although epidemiological studies suggest that Alzheimer's disease and cardiovascular diseases share common risk factors. There is now evidence that statins might help prevent AD. Alzheimer's disease shares many risk factors with atherosclerosis, and several observational studies have reported a lower risk of developing this condition in patients taking statins.

In light of the fact that several studies have shown a positive correlation between high cholesterol and an increase in the risk for developing Alzheimer's disease statins have been proposed as alternative drugs for its treatment and/or prevention. However, the potential benefits of statins remain controversial.

There are anecdotal reports of significant cognitive decline with statins. There is no strong evidence to support this effect, but there is no strong evidence to exclude it either. Two randomized clinical trials found "cognitive issues," while two did not. A systematic review by the Canadian Working Group Consensus Conference concluded that the available evidence "is not strongly supportive of a major adverse effect of statins." A meta-analysis reported in the *Annals of Internal Medicine* concluded that there is moderate quality evidence of no increase in dementia, mild cognitive impairment or cognitive performance scores, although the strength of the evidence is limited, particularly for high doses. In 2012, in recognition of an increase in anecdotal reports and increasing concerns over the relationship between statins and memory loss (including reports of transient global amnesia), forgetfulness and confusion, the FDA added to its required labeling on statin drugs a warning about possible cognitive impacts. The effects are described as rare, non-serious, and reversible upon cessation of treatment.

However, the 2013 American College of Cardiology/American Heart Association Blood Cholesterol Guidelines stated that *"no evidence* [emphasis added] *is available supporting the conclusion that statins cause an adverse effect on cognition or risk of dementia."*[348] (This is yet another example of how individual professionals and even groups of experts can come to completely opposite conclusions. This is why each reader must weigh the evidence and come to their own conclusions about each topic.)

So, do statins help or hurt when it comes to Alzheimer's disease? Let's explore some of the evidence.

Although they have lipid-lowering properties, statins also have a wide range of biological effects that are unrelated to cholesterol reduction. Mendoza-Oliva and colleagues reviewed the relevant literature in 2014 and concluded that "the effects of statins in the brain are broad and complex and that their use for treating several diseases, including AD, should be carefully analyzed."[349] In other words, their review found potential use in preventing AD, but the authors felt that further research is needed to determine exactly what that potential is. Details of other research follows.

In 2013, researchers from the University of Washington School of Medicine, Seattle, WA, noted, "Statins improve recovery from traumatic brain injury and *show promise in preventing Alzheimer disease.*" They demonstrated in an animal model of AD experiment that oral administration of the statin Zocor (simvastatin) enhances neurogenesis (formation of new nerve cells). They determined that this occurred through a specific pathway, and not through cholesterol. They summarized by stating, *"Collectively, these data add to the growing body of evidence that statins may have therapeutic value for treating certain neurological disorders."*[350]

A type of cholesterol or lipid, LDL (low-density lipoprotein), the so-called "bad cholesterol" is related to heart disease and may be related to Alzheimer's disease as well. LDL metabolism increases free radical formation and reduces plasma antioxidant concentrations, and elevated lipids in mid-life are associated with increased long-term risk of dementia. Although brain cholesterol metabolism is segregated from the systemic circulation, during oxidative stress, plasma LDL and its chemical products could have damaging effects on the function of the blood-brain barrier (the physical barrier between the blood and the brain), and consequently on neurons (brain cells). Researchers have found that "cholesterol-lowering drugs such as *statins may prevent the modifications to LDL in mid-life and might show beneficial effects in later life.*"[351]

The message is clear: if statins are going to be of any benefit, they must be started in mid-life (even when one's cholesterol is within normal limits).

Researchers from the Department of Neurology, Penn State College of Medicine, studied 3069 "cognitively healthy" elderly patients (≥75 years of age). They found that *"statins may slow the rate of cognitive decline and delay the onset of AD and all-cause dementia in cognitively healthy elderly individuals, whereas individuals with MCI [mild cognitive impairment] may not have comparable cognitive protection from these agents."* In participants who initiated statin therapy, lipophilic statins (atorvastatin, fluvastatin, lovastatin, simvastatin) tended to reduce dementia risk more than nonlipophilic agents (pravastatin and rosuvastatin).[352]

Once again, the message is clear: statins may help prevent AD and MCI. They are less effective once MCI is present, and show no clear benefit once AD is present. For example, two recently completed clinical trials indicate that neither atorvastatin nor simvastatin slow the progression of early Alzheimer's disease.[353]

In 2013 researchers conducted what is known as a "meta-analysis" (large review of relevant scientific literature) to estimate any benefit of statins in *preventing* dementia. They concluded, *"The pooled results for all-type dementia suggest that use of statins is associated with a lower risk of dementia when compared to non-statin use. These pooled results suggest that statins may provide a slight benefit in the prevention of AD and all-type dementia."*[354]

In summary, there is evidence that statins may help prevent Alzheimer's disease, if started early enough, and that specific statins may prove more beneficial than others. However, well-designed clinical research studies are needed to more precisely define the potential benefits. Once AD is present, the use of statins, like all other currently available medications, does not improve cognition.

Anti-diabetic Medications

Diabetes[1] is linked to Alzheimer's disease, as described previously. Because of this close link, some medications used to treat diabetes may help prevent AD.

As of 2014, an estimated 387 million people have diabetes worldwide, with type 2 diabetes making up about 90 percent of the cases. This is equal to 8.3 percent of the adult population, with equal rates in both women and men. In the years 2012 to 2014, diabetes is estimated to have resulted in 1.5 to 4.9 million deaths per year in the United States. Diabetes at least doubles the risk of death. The number of people with diabetes world-wide is expected to rise to 592 million by 2035. The global economic cost of diabetes in 2014 was estimated to be $612 billion USD. In the United States, diabetes cost $245 billion in 2012.

Although the brain has been considered an insulin-insensitive organ, recent reports on the location of insulin and its receptors in the brain have introduced new ways of considering this hormone responsible for several functions. The origin of insulin in the brain has been explained from peripheral or central sources, or both. Regardless of whether insu-

---

[1]Diabetes mellitus (DM), commonly referred to as diabetes, is a group of metabolic diseases in which there are high blood sugar levels over a prolonged period. Symptoms of high blood sugar include frequent urination, increased thirst, and increased hunger. If left untreated, diabetes can cause many complications. Acute complications include diabetic ketoacidosis and non-ketotic hyperosmolar coma. Serious long-term complications include cardiovascular disease, stroke, kidney failure, foot ulcers and damage to the eyes. Diabetes is due to either the pancreas not producing enough insulin or the cells of the body not responding properly to the insulin produced.[1] There are two main types of diabetes mellitus:
- Type 1 DM results from the body's failure to produce enough insulin. This form was previously referred to as "insulin-dependent diabetes mellitus" (IDDM) or "juvenile diabetes." The cause is unknown.
- Type 2 DM begins with insulin resistance, a condition in which cells fail to respond to insulin properly. As the disease progresses a lack of insulin may also develop. This form was previously referred to as "non-insulin-dependent diabetes mellitus" (NIDDM) or "adult-onset diabetes." The primary cause is excessive body weight and not enough exercise.

lin is of peripheral origin or produced in the brain, this hormone may act through its own receptors present in the brain. According to a recent report, "The molecular events through which insulin functions in the brain are the same as those operating in the periphery…In addition, *insulin in the brain contributes to the control of nutrient homeostasis, reproduction, cognition, and memory, as well as to neurotrophic, neuromodulatory, and neuroprotective effects.* Alterations of these functional activities may contribute to the manifestation of several clinical entities, such as central insulin resistance, type 2 diabetes mellitus (T2DM), and Alzheimer's disease. A close association between T2DM and AD has been reported, to the extent that AD is twice as frequent in diabetic patients, and some authors have proposed the name "type 3 diabetes" for this association. There are links between AD and T2DM through mitochondrial alterations and oxidative stress, altered energy and glucose metabolism, cholesterol modifications, dysfunctional protein O-GlcNAcylation, formation of amyloid plaques, altered Aβ metabolism, and tau hyperphosphorylation. *Advances in the knowledge of preclinical AD and T2DM may be a major stimulus for the development of treatment for preventing the pathogenic events of these disorders, mainly those focused on reducing brain insulin resistance, which seems to be a common ground for both pathological entities.*[355]

Researchers reviewed some of the recent developments of the common features between T2D and AD, namely on insulin signaling and its participation in the regulation of amyloid β (Aβ) plaque and neurofibrillary tangle formation (the two major neuropathological hallmarks of AD). They note that it is a *"promising field that some anti-T2D drugs may protect against dementia and AD, with a special emphasis on the novel incretin/glucagon-like peptide-1 receptor agonists."*[356]

Other researchers, from Yale-New Haven Hospital, report similar conclusions, "In recent years, there has been a growing interest in the possible links between insulin and Alzheimer's disease. Insulin-induced hypoglycemia causes adaptive changes in the brain, including an improved ability to use alternative fuels. Insulin has been shown to facilitate reduction of intracellular amyloid plaque and downregulation of amyloid-β-derived diffusible ligand-binding sites. Insulin also promotes tau hypophosphorylation, which stabilizes microtubules and promotes tubulin polymerization. Excess exogenous insulin may also play a role in overcoming the decreased utilization and transport of glucose in patients with Alzheimer's disease. Intranasal insulin therapy may have beneficial effects on cognition and function in patients with Alzheimer's disease, as well as having only minor adverse effects, and this route of administration been the focus in clinical trials. *These data support the mechanistic pathways that might link excess exogenous insulin administered to patients with type 1 diabetes mellitus to possible protection from Alzheimer's disease and provide a rationale for using insulin to prevent the disease in high-risk patients.*"[357]

In October 2014, Dr. Hölscher summarized recent developments vis-à-vis type 2 diabetes as a risk factor for Alzheimer's disease and Parkinson's disease (PD). "In the brains of patients with AD and PD, insulin signaling is impaired. This finding has motivated new research that showed good effects using drugs that initially had been developed to treat diabetes. Preclinical studies showed good neuroprotective effects applying insulin or long lasting analogues of incretin peptides. In animal models of AD or PD, analogues of the incretin GLP-1 prevented neurodegenerative processes and improved neuronal and synaptic functionality and reduced the symptoms of the diseases. Amyloid plaque load and synaptic loss as well as cognitive impairment had been prevented in AD mouse models, and dopaminergic loss of transmission and motor function has been reversed in animal models of PD. On the basis of these promising findings, several clinical trials are being conducted with the first encouraging clinical results already published. *In several pilot studies in AD patients, the nasal application of insulin showed encouraging effects on cognition and biomarkers.* A pilot study in PD patients testing a GLP-1 receptor agonist that is currently on the market as a treatment for type 2 diabetes (exendin-4, Byetta) also showed encouraging effects. Several other clinical trials are currently ongoing in AD patients, testing another GLP-1 analogue that is on the market (liraglutide, Victoza). Recently, a third GLP-1 receptor agonist has been brought to the market in Europe (Lixisenatide, Lyxumia), which also shows very promising neuroprotective effects...*GLP-1 analogues show promise in providing novel treatments that may be protec-*

tive or even regenerative in AD and PD, something that no current drug does."[358]

As previously noted, Dr. Claxton and colleagues, reported the results of their research in the January 1, 2015 issue of the *Journal of Alzheimer's Disease*. They studied the effects of intranasal long-lasting insulin detemir) in adults with Alzheimer's disease dementia or amnestic mild cognitive impairment (MCI). "Sixty adults diagnosed with MCI or mild to moderate AD received placebo (n = 20), 20 IU of insulin detemir (n = 21), or 40 IU of insulin detemir (n = 19) for twenty-one days, administered with a nasal drug delivery device. Results revealed a treatment effect for the memory composite for the 40 IU group compared with placebo. *This effect was moderated by APOE status, reflecting improvement for APOE-ε4 carriers, and worsening for non-carriers.* Higher insulin resistance at baseline predicted greater improvement with the 40 IU dose. Significant treatment effects were also apparent for verbal working memory and visuospatial working memory, reflecting improvement for subjects who received the high dose of intranasal insulin detemir. No significant differences were found for daily functioning or executive functioning. In conclusion, *daily treatment with 40 IU insulin detemir modulated cognition for adults with AD or MCI, with APOE-related differences in treatment response for the primary memory composite.*"[359]

As is all too typical in medicine, different experiments sometimes yield conflicting results. For example, in late 2014, researchers conducted a study to measure the safety and efficacy of intranasally delivered rapid acting glulisine insulin in ApoE4 carriers with mild-moderate AD. They found that, *"glulisine was well tolerated but failed to have an acute impact on cognition in ApoE4 carriers with AD. Serum insulin levels acutely dropped following treatment, but peripheral glucose levels remained unchanged. Larger clinical trials of longer duration are necessary to better understand the relationships between RA insulin, ApoE4 carrier status and cognitive performance in AD."*[360]

Metformin

Metformin is an oral antidiabetic drug.. It is one of the first-line drugs of choice for the treatment of type 2 diabetes. It is also used in the treatment of polycystic ovary syndrome, and has been investigated for other diseases where insulin resistance may be an important factor. Metformin works by suppressing glucose (a type of sugar) production by the liver. Limited evidence suggests metformin may prevent the cardiovascular and possibly the cancer complications of diabetes. It helps reduce LDL cholesterol ("bad cholesterol") and triglyceride levels and is not associated with weight gain; in some people, it promotes weight loss. Metformin is one of only two oral antidiabetics in the World Health Organization Model List of Essential Medicines (the other being glibenclamide).

Metformin causes few adverse effects when prescribed appropriately (the most common is gastrointestinal upset) and has been associated with a low risk of hypoglycemia (low blood sugar). Lactic acidosis (a buildup of lactate in the blood) can be a serious concern in overdose and when it is prescribed to people with contraindications, but otherwise, no significant risk exists.

First synthesized and found to reduce blood sugar in the 1920s, metformin was forgotten for the next two decades as research shifted to insulin and other antidiabetic drugs. Interest in metformin was rekindled in the late 1940s after several reports that it could reduce blood sugar levels in people, and in 1957, French physician Jean Sterne published the first clinical trial of metformin as a treatment for diabetes. It was introduced to the United Kingdom in 1958, Canada in 1972, and the United States in 1995. *Metformin is now believed to be the most widely prescribed antidiabetic drug in the world; in the United States alone, more than 48 million prescriptions were filled in 2010 for its generic formulations.*

Metformin has recently been found to extend human life by up to two years (in both diabetics and nondiabetics)! (See the bonus section, Longevity.)

Dr. DiTacchio and colleagues from the Salk Institute for Biological Studies, Molecular Neurobiology Laboratory, La Jolla, CA, reported in 2014 the effects of metformin in an animal model of Alzheimer's disease. They stated, *"Metabolic dysfunction exacerbates Alzheimer's disease incidence and progression...our results show that [the metabolic effects of metformin] increase memory dysfunction in males but is protective in females, suggesting that gender considerations may constitute an important factor in medical intervention of diabetes as well as AD."*[361]

Dr. Moore and over 150 colleagues, reported in 2013 the results of a study to investigate the associations of metformin, serum vitamin B12, calcium supplements, and cognitive impairment in patients with diabetes. Patients with Alzheimer's disease (n=480) or mild cognitive impairment (n=187) and those who were cognitively intact (n=687) were included. Subgroup analyses were performed for participants who had either type 2 diabetes (n=104) or impaired glucose tolerance (n=22). The researchers found that, "Participants with diabetes (n=126) had worse cognitive performance than participants who did not have diabetes (n=1,228). Among participants with diabetes, worse cognitive performance was associated with metformin use. After adjusting for age, sex, level of education, history of depression, serum vitamin B12, and metformin use, participants with diabetes who were taking calcium supplements had better cognitive performance...*Metformin use was associated with impaired cognitive performance. Vitamin B12 and calcium supplements may alleviate metformin-induced vitamin B12 deficiency and were associated with better cognitive outcomes.* Prospective trials are warranted to assess the beneficial effects of vitamin B12 and calcium use on cognition in older people with diabetes who are taking metformin."[362] Metformin can cause a B12 deficiency, which could confound the results of the study.

Dr. Shirazi and colleagues, from the Department of Infectious Diseases, Infection Control and Employee Health, The University of Texas M.D. Anderson Cancer Center, Houston, Texas, reported the results of an intriguing experiment conducted in 2014. The researchers used an experimental model of obesity and hyperglycemia (high blood sugar) in

Drosophila melanogaster (a type of fruit fly) to study the effect of diet modification and administration of metformin on systemic infection with Rhizopus, a common cause of fungal infection in diabetic patients. They found that, *"Survival was significantly decreased in obese flies, while post-infection glucose levels were significantly increased, compared to normal-weight flies. Diet and administration of metformin led to weight loss, normalized glucose levels during infection, and were associated with decreased mortality and tissue fungal burden. In conclusion, diet and metformin help control infection-associated hyperglycemia and improve survival in Drosophila flies with mucormycosis. Fly models of obesity bear intriguing similarities to the pathophysiology of insulin resistance and diabetes in humans, and can provide new insights into the pathogenesis and treatment of infections in obese and diabetic patients."*[363]

Researchers studied the effects of metformin on a cellular model of Alzheimer's disease. They stated, "Currently there is widening recognition that AD is closely associated with impaired insulin signaling and glucose metabolism in brain, suggesting it to be a brain-specific form of diabetes and so also termed as "type 3 diabetes." Hence investigating the role of pharmacological agents that could ameliorate neuronal insulin resistance merit attention in AD therapeutics. In the present study we have determined the effect of metformin on neuronal insulin resistance and AD-associated characteristics." *They found that elevated insulin levels led to development of hallmark AD-associated neuropathological changes, and that treatment with metformin prevented these changes.*[364]

Anti-inflammatory Medications

NSAIDs (nonsteroidal anti-inflammatory drugs: there are many NSAIDs, and only a few are listed here (see wikipedia.org "NSAIDs" for a full description): acetylsalicylic acid (ASA; commonly known as Aspirin), ibuprofen (Advil, Genpril, IBU, Midol, Motrin, Nuprin), naproxin (Aleve, Naprosyn, Anaprox, Naprelan).

PREVENTION

CAUTION: According to an article published by Dr. Risser and colleagues in the journal *American Family Physician:*[365]

> "Nonsteroidal anti-inflammatory drugs (NSAIDs) are commonly used, but have risks associated with their use, including significant upper gastrointestinal tract bleeding. Older persons, persons taking anticoagulants, and persons with a history of upper gastrointestinal tract bleeding associated with NSAIDs are at especially high risk. Although aspirin is cardioprotective, other NSAIDs can worsen congestive heart failure, can increase blood pressure, and are related to adverse cardiovascular events, such as myocardial infarction and ischemia. Cyclooxygenase-2 inhibitors have been associated with increased risk of myocardial infarction; however, the only cyclooxygenase-2 inhibitor still available in the United States, celecoxib, seems to be safer in this regard. Hepatic damage from NSAIDs is rare, but these medications should not be used in persons with cirrhotic liver diseases because bleeding problems and renal failure are more likely. Care should be used when prescribing NSAIDs in persons taking anticoagulants and in those with platelet dysfunction, as well as immediately before surgery. Potential central nervous system effects include aseptic meningitis, psychosis, and tinnitus. Asthma may be induced or exacerbated by NSAIDs. Although most NSAIDs are likely safe in pregnancy, they should be avoided in the last six to eight weeks of pregnancy to prevent prolonged gestation from inhibition of prostaglandin synthesis, premature closure of the ductus arteriosus, and maternal and fetal complications from antiplatelet activity. Ibuprofen, indomethacin, and naproxen are safe in breastfeeding women. Care should be taken to prevent accidental NSAID overdose in children by educating parents about correct dosing and storage in childproof containers."

A new review of the scientific literature, published by the *National Institutes of Health* in December 2014, urged caution with the use of NSAIDs in the possible prevention of Alzheimer's disease. Here is the summary of the article:[366]

> "In the past twenty years, substantial evidence from laboratory and epidemiologic studies have suggested that anti-inflammatory medications could defer or prevent the occurrence of Alzheimer's disease. However, several studies do not corroborate these findings. Objective: To evaluate the association of anti-inflammatory drug use on the incidence of AD. Methods: Pubmed, Embase, and Cochrane Library databases were searched up to March 2014. Studies evaluating the association between use of anti-inflammatory drugs and AD risk were included...Results: *In observational studies, use of non-steroidal anti-inflammatory drugs (NSAIDs) was significantly associated with a reduced risk of AD compared to no use of NSAIDs, especially in long term users; the risks of AD were also lower in both aspirin and non-aspirin NSAID users compared with nonusers*; whereas the use of corticosteroids [powerful anti-inflammatory agents] showed no significant association. In the single randomized controlled trial (RCT), NSAID use showed no significant effect on AD risk among dementia-free individuals. *Conclusion: Observational studies support the use of NSAIDs for prevention of AD, but RCT do not. Well-designed studies and innovative approaches are required to illuminate the exact relationship between NSAID use and AD risk. The appropriate dosage and duration of use to benefit and the safety are also needed to determine.*"

The Alzheimer's Association recently reported that a woman's estimated lifetime risk of developing Alzheimer's at age 65 is 1 in 6, compared to nearly 1 in 11 for a man (ie, female to male ratio 1.8). Several researchers noted in August 2014, "Based on female to male ratio, Alzheimer's disease could well be an autoimmune disorder. Like Alzheimer's, multiple sclerosis, an autoimmune inflammation of the central nervous system, has a female to male ratio of 2.3. Also based on female to male ratio, Alzheimer's resembles the autoimmune inflammatory disease rheumatoid arthritis, which has a female to male ratio of 2.7. The reasons for the female preponderance in autoimmune disease are unclear, but non-steroidal anti-inflammatory drugs (NSAIDs) are widely and successfully employed to treat autoimmune anti-inflammatory disease and dramatically relieve symptoms. Moreover, *oral NSAIDs consistently reduce the risk of [of acquiring] Alzheimer's disease, although they have been totally ineffective as a treatment in multiple failed clinical trials.* A basis for this failure might well be that the brain dose after oral administration is too small and not sufficiently early in the pathogenesis of the disorder. But NSAID brain dose could be significantly increased by delivering the NSAIDs intranasally."[367]

β-Amyloid (Aβ) is a small peptide (protein) that forms amyloid plaques in Alzheimer's disease.. Recent studies suggest that Aβ deposition is deleterious not only in AD, but also in Parkinson's disease (PD) and depression. This Aβ effect is associated with inflammatory processes. Researchers recently used an animal model to explore the impact of Aβ on neurotransmitters and the effect of NSAIDs in preventing damage. They concluded that, *"Our results reveal that Aβ significantly decreased the number of neurons and that anti-inflammatory drugs partially counteracted the Aβ-induced neuronal decline."*[368]

NOSH-Aspirin is a category of new hybrids of aspirin, bearing both nitric oxide (NO)- and hydrogen sulfide (H$_2$S)- releasing areas. Preliminary studies have found that four NOSH variants, evaluated in eleven different human cancer cell lines, were effective in inhibiting the growth of these cell lines. NOSH-1 was also devoid of any cellular toxicity, and was comparable to aspirin in its anti-inflammatory properties.

Dr. Drochioiu and colleagues, in an article in the January 14, 2015 issue of *Medical Hypotheses*, titled NOSH Aspirin May Have a Protective Role In Alzheimer's Disease, reported that, *"We consider NOSH-aspirin a drug of choice for reducing the inflammatory areas in the brain (aspirin moiety), removing the noxious heavy metals from plaques (hydrogen sulfide), and increasing the oxygen supply to neurons since nitrogen oxide is a potent vasodilator and an anti-inflammatory agent.*"[369]

Cromolyn Sodium (disodium cromoglycate)

Cromolyn Sodium is an FDA-approved drug already in use for the treatment of asthma. A team of researchers from Massachusetts General Hospital and Harvard Medical School reported in December 2014 that they had demonstrated, in an animal model of Alzheimer's disease, that "*short-term peripheral (not oral) administration of Cromolyn Sodium decreased the levels of the main peptide (Amyloid β or Aβ peptides) associated with AD by over fifty percent.*" They felt the results of their experimental work clearly warranted further research into the long-term use of this medication for the prevention and/or treatment of AD.[370]

Anti-hypertensive Agents

Hypertension is increasingly recognized as a modifiable risk factor for mild cognitive impairment (MCI), the precursor of dementia. The renin angiotensin aldosterone system (RAAS) is central to blood pressure regulation and *medications targeting RAAS inhibition are associated with reduced rates of both cognitive and functional decline in those with MCI and dementia.* Angiotensin converting enzyme (ACE) inhibitors and angiotensin receptor blockers (ARBs) are widely prescribed anti-hypertensives acting on the RAAS, and there is growing evidence that they act centrally, possibly exerting their effects independent of their blood pressure lowering properties.[371]

Angiotensin Receptor Blockers (ARBs), such as Cozar (losartan) and Diovan (valsartan), also known as Angiotensin II receptor antagonists, are a group of pharmaceuticals that modulate the renin–angiotensin–aldosterone system. Their main uses are in the treatment of hyperten-

PREVENTION

sion (high blood pressure), diabetic nephropathy (kidney damage due to diabetes) and congestive heart failure.

According to an article published in late 2014, "Angiotensin II receptor blockers (ARBs, collectively called sartans) are widely used compounds therapeutically effective in cardiovascular disorders, renal disease, the metabolic syndrome, and diabetes. *It has been more recently recognized that ARBs are neuroprotective and have potential therapeutic use in many brain disorders.* ARBs ameliorate inflammatory and apoptotic (cell death) responses to glutamate, interleukin 1β and bacterial endotoxin in cultured neurons, astrocytes, microglial, and endothelial cerebrovascular cells.

When administered systemically, ARBs enter the brain, protecting cerebral blood flow, maintaining blood brain barrier function and decreasing cerebral hemorrhage, excessive brain inflammation and neuronal injury in animal models of stroke, traumatic brain injury, Alzheimer's and Parkinson's disease and other brain conditions. Epidemiological analyses reported that ARBs reduced the progression of Alzheimer's disease, and clinical studies suggested amelioration of cognitive loss following stroke and aging...However, the complete pharmacological spectrum and therapeutic efficacy of individual ARBs have never been systematically compared, and the neuroprotective efficacy of these compounds has not been rigorously determined in controlled clinical studies. The accumulation of pre-clinical evidence should promote further epidemiological and controlled clinical studies. *Repurposing ARBs for the treatment of brain disorders, currently without effective therapy, may be of immediate and major translational value.*"[372]

Researchers recently summed up the current state of affairs vis-à-vis ARBs and Alzheimer's disease stating, "Because growing evidence suggests that angiotensin II receptor blockers (ARBs) effectively inhibit oxidative stress, amyloid beta protein (Aβ) metabolism, and tau phosphorylation in animal brains, *ARBs are considered to be a potential candidate for the treatment of Alzheimer's disease.* Consistent with such basic studies, *two recent observational studies and a small pro-*

spective, randomized, open-label trial have shown the effectiveness of ARBs in preventing AD and/or slowing its progression. Nonetheless, large clinical trials have not shown their effectiveness, Their results are debatable because of short follow-up durations and heterogeneity of the cognition assessments used in the studies. Because a recent analysis of the Honolulu-Asia Aging study showed that *abnormalities of the serum Aβ level begin approximately fifteen years before the diagnosis of AD*, long-term clinical trials assessing dementia as a primary endpoint with sensitive measurements of cognition and brain imaging techniques will clarify the effectiveness of ARBs in AD treatment."[373]

Angiotensin-converting Enzyme (ACE) Inhibitors

An angiotensin-converting-enzyme inhibitor (ACE inhibitor) is a pharmaceutical drug used primarily for the treatment of hypertension (elevated blood pressure) and congestive heart failure. This group of drugs cause relaxation of blood vessels, as well as a decreased blood volume, which leads to lower blood pressure and decreased oxygen demand from the heart. They inhibit the angiotensin-converting enzyme, an important component of the renin-angiotensin-aldosterone system. Frequently prescribed ACE inhibitors include perindopril (Coversyl/Aceon/Perindo), captopri (Capoten), enalapril (Vasotec/Renitec), lisinopril (Listril/Lopril/Novatec/Prinivil/Zestril), and ramipril (Altace/Prilace/Ramace/Ramiwin/Triatec/Tritace).

Higher angiotensin-converting enzyme (ACE) activity might increase the risk of Alzheimer's disease by increasing blood pressure, and subsequent development of cerebral small vessel disease (CSVD). Yet, it may also decrease this risk, as it functions to degrade amyloid-β, thereby reducing brain atrophy. Researchers, reporting in late 2014, conducted research to examine the associations of serum and cerebrospinal fluid (CSF) ACE protein levels and activity with brain atrophy and CSVD in a memory clinic cohort. They found that, *"Higher CSF ACE activity was associated with a reduced risk of global brain atrophy...These results show that high ACE might have protective effects on the brain. This could suggest that ACE inhibitors, which may lower*

CSF ACE levels, are not preferred as antihypertensive treatment in patients at risk for Alzheimer's disease."[374]

However, a different group of researchers, also reporting in late 2014, came to the opposite conclusion. They stated, "Drug repurposing has provided a new route for AD drug discovery, and medical genetics has shown potential in target-based drug repurposing. We compared AD-associated genes with approved drug targets and found that three [AD-associated genes] are targeted by twenty-three approved drugs. Thus, these drugs may be used to treat AD according to the medical genetic information of the targets. In vitro and in vivo experiments revealed that *four drugs, all of which are angiotensin-converting enzyme (ACE) inhibitors, had potential to treat AD.*"[375]

Calcium-channel Blockers

Calcium channel blockers (CCB), are medications that disrupt the movement of calcium (Ca2+) through calcium channels. Calcium channel blockers are used as antihypertensive drugs, i.e., as medications to decrease blood pressure in patients with hypertension. CCBs are particularly effective against large vessel stiffness, one of the common causes of elevated systolic blood pressure in elderly patients. There are many such agents; some commonly used are: amlodipine (Norvasc), nifedipine (Procardia, Adalat), nilvadipine (Nivadil), and Verapamil (Calan, Isoptin).

Researchers studied the use of nilvadipine (Nivadil) in fifty-five patients with Alzheimer's disease who received nilvadipine 8 mg daily for six weeks compared with thirty non-treated subjects with AD. They found that, "In this open-label trial, among APOE ε4 non-carriers, we observed stabilization of cognition and improvement in executive function among treated individuals compared with non-treated individuals. *Among APOE ε4 carriers, cognitive stabilization was evident for treated individuals whereas a cognitive decline was observed in non-treated individuals.* These findings provide additional evidence for potential therapeutic efficacy of nilvadipine in treating AD and warrant further investigation."[376]

Dr. Paris and colleagues, reporting in the December 5, 2014 issue of the *Journal of Biological Chemistry*, noted that, *"We have previously shown that the L-type calcium channel (LCC) antagonist nilvadipine reduces brain amyloid-β (Aβ) accumulation by affecting both Aβ production and Aβ clearance across the blood-brain barrier (BBB)...A search for the mechanism of action of (-)-nilvadipine revealed that this compound inhibits the spleen tyrosine kinase (Syk). We further validated Syk as a target-regulating Aβ by showing that pharmacological inhibition of Syk or down-regulation of Syk expression reduces Aβ production and increases the clearance of Aβ across the BBB mimicking (-)-nilvadipine effects...Altogether our data highlight Syk as a promising target for preventing both Aβ accumulation and Tau hyperphosphorylation in AD."*[377]

However, researchers conducted a systematic review of calcium channel blocker use in the elderly and cognitive decline/dementia, reporting their results in late 2014. After reviewing 1,968 records and ten articles reporting on nine studies, they concluded that, *"At present, there is no clear evidence to suggest that CCB use increases or decreases risk of cognitive decline or dementia in the very elderly. A robust clinical trial is now required to resolve this."*[378]

Estrogens

Estrogens are a group of compounds named for their importance in both menstrual and estrous reproductive cycles. They are the primary female sex hormones. Natural estrogens are steroid hormones, while some synthetic ones are non-steroidal. Estrogens are used as part of some oral contraceptives, in estrogen replacement therapy for postmenopausal women, and in hormone replacement therapy for trans women. See wikipedia.org for a more comprehensive discussion of estrogens.

PREVENTION

Estrogen has been known to reduce the development of Alzheimer's disease. However, exact mechanisms are not clear. Using an animal model of AD, researchers investigated whether estrogen can increase amyloid-beta (Aβ) degradation and affects Aβ-induced memory impairment in an estrogen deficiency model. Without going into detail of the experiment, the researchers concluded that, *"These results suggest that estrogen may protect memory impairment by stimulating the degradation of Aβ and down-regulate neurogenic inflammation as well as amyloidogenesis."*[379]

Glutamate is the most abundant excitatory brain neurotransmitter that has important functional significance with respect to neurodegenerative conditions. *Glutamate-mediated excitotoxicity and neurodegeneration in Alzheimer's disease has been gradually becoming elucidated recently.* Excessive release of glutamate induces an increase in intracellular Ca(2+) levels, thus triggers a cascade of cellular responses, ultimately leading to neuronal cell death. This type of neuronal damage induced by over-excitation has been proposed to be involved in a number of neuropathological conditions, ranging from acute insults to chronic neurodegenerative disorders, such as AD. Researchers report that, *"Estrogen could be effective in modulating glutamate-induced neurotoxicity and the protective responsivenesses are mostly estrogen receptors (ERs)-dependent...Extensive studies have indicated the neuroprotective effects of ERs against glutamate-induced neurotoxicity."*[380]

However, one case report suggests caution in the chronic use of estrogens:[381]

> "We present a patient with chronic postmenopausal estrogen intake with presence of Kayser-Fleischer ring[1] in the cornea and Alzheimer's disease and discuss the pathophysiological mechanisms of estrogen intake and

---

[1]Kayser–Fleischer rings are dark rings that appear to encircle the iris of the eye. They are due to copper deposition in part of the cornea (Descemet's membrane) as a result of particular liver diseases (especially Wilson's disease). They are named after Dr. Bernhard Kayser and Dr. Bruno Fleischer, the German doctors who first described them in 1902 and 1903.

copy accumulation in various tissues, including the central nervous system. Sonography was compatible with copper accumulation in the basal ganglia, but the patient showed no clinical signs of Wilson's disease[1]. Magnetic resonance imaging and positron emission tomography revealed a typical pattern for Alzheimer's disease. *We propose increased copper levels as a direct effect of estrogen intake* due to an augmented ATP7A-mRNA in the intestine. Moreover, we discuss the impact of elevated free serum copper on accompanying Alzheimer's disease, knowing that copper plays a crucial role in the formation of amyloid plaques and tau aggregation. *This might offer a partial explanation for the observation that postmenopausal estrogen therapy is associated with a higher risk of mild cognitive impairment and Alzheimer's disease.*"

Viagra (sildenafil)

Yes, Viagra may help prevent Alzheimer's disease! Sildenafil, sold as Viagra and other trade names, is a medication used to treat erectile dysfunction and pulmonary arterial hypertension. Since becoming available in 1998, sildenafil has been a common treatment for erectile dysfunction; its primary competitors are tadalafil (Cialis) and vardenafil (Levitra).

In a complicated and detailed experiment conducted in 2014, researchers showed that Viagra improved cognitive (learning and memory) impairments in an animal model of AD, and had profoundly positive effects on numerous enzymes, peptides, and proteins associated with AD. The researchers summarized their results by saying, *"These find-*

---

[1]Wilson's disease or hepatolenticular degeneration is an autosomal recessive genetic disorder in which copper accumulates in tissues; this manifests as neurological or psychiatric symptoms and liver disease. It is treated with medication that reduces copper absorption or removes the excess copper from the body, but occasionally a liver transplant is required.

ings highlight the therapeutic potential of sildenafil in Alzheimer's disease pathogenesis."[382]

Diets

Introduction

Nutrition affects the brain throughout life, with profound implications for cognitive decline and dementia. Epidemiological evidence linking diet, one of the most important modifiable environmental factors, and risk of Alzheimer's disease is rapidly increasing. There are libraries written about diet and health, with many opinions about which is the best diet to follow. Here is not the time or place to analyze each and every one. The Mediterranean diet is generally considered one of the best, and this is discussed below along with several other, perhaps even better, diets (with regard to helping prevent Alzheimer's disease). Most "marketed" diets are geared toward weight loss, but that is not our focus here. *U.S. News* evaluated thirty-five of the most popular diets and identified what they felt were the best ones. See: http://health.usnews.com/best-diet.

Drs. Swaminathan and Jicha, from the Department of Neurology and Sanders-Brown Center on Aging, College of Medicine, University of Kentucky Lexington, KY stated the following in the October 20, 2014 issue of the journal *Frontiers in Aging Neuroscience*:[383]

> "A nutritional approach to prevent, slow, or halt the progression of disease is a promising strategy that has been widely investigated. *Much epidemiologic data suggests that nutritional intake may influence the development and progression of Alzheimer's dementia. Modifiable, environmental causes of AD include potential metabolic derangements caused by dietary insufficiency and/or excess that may be corrected by nutritional supplementation and or dietary modification. Many nutritional*

supplements contain a myriad of health promoting constituents (anti-oxidants, vitamins, trace minerals, flavonoids, lipids, ...etc.) that may have novel mechanisms of action affecting cellular health and regeneration, the aging process itself, or may specifically disrupt pathogenic pathways in the development of AD. Nutritional modifications have the advantage of being cost effective, easy to implement, socially acceptable and generally safe and devoid of significant adverse events in most cases. Many nutritional interventions have been studied and continue to be evaluated in hopes of finding a successful agent, combination of agents, or dietary modifications that can be used for the prevention and/or treatment of AD."

To examine associations between dietary patterns and successful aging, researchers studied 6,308 men and women without a history of major illness at baseline, and aged >70 years at follow-up, or who had died before follow-up but would have been aged >70 at the commencement of follow-up. Their diets were measured in 1990-4, and successful aging in 2003-7. The researchers found that, "Four dietary factors were identified, characterized by higher loadings for (1) vegetables; (2) fruit; (3) feta, legumes, salad, olive oil, and inverse loadings for tea, margarine, cake, sweet biscuits and puddings; (4) meat, white bread, savory pastry dishes and fried foods. In models excluding body size, the second factor 'Fruit' was positively associated with successful aging; while the fourth factor 'Meat/fatty foods' was inversely associated. Factors 1 and 3 did not show significant associations with successful aging...*A dietary pattern including plenty of fruit while limiting meat and fried foods may improve the likelihood of aging successfully.*"[384]

Meat Diet

According to one researcher, *"Dietary epidemiological studies indicate correlations between the consumption of red meat[1] and/or processed meat and cancer of the colon, rectum, stomach, pancreas, bladder, endometrium and ovaries, prostate, breast and lung, heart disease, rheumatoid arthritis, type 2 diabetes and Alzheimer's disease. The correlation of all these major diseases with dietary red meat indicates the presence of factors in red meat that damage biological components. Raw red meat contains several heme proteins. The coordinated heme groups are absorbed and transported by the blood to every organ and tissue. Free heme causes oxidative reactions. Heme-caused oxidations can damage lipids, proteins, DNA and other nucleic acids and various components of biological systems. Biochemical and tissue free radical damage caused by heme catalyzed oxidations is similar to that resulting from ionizing radiation. Oxidative biochemical damage is widespread in diseases."*[385]

According to the same researcher, "It is apparent that decreasing the amount of dietary red meat will limit the level of oxidative catalysts in the tissues of the body. Increasing consumption of vegetables and fruits elevates the levels of antioxidative components, for example, selenium, vitamin E, vitamin C, lycopene, cysteine-glutathione and various phytochemicals."

According to Dr. Koeth and 21 colleagues from the Department of Cellular & Molecular Medicine, Cleveland Clinic, Cleveland, Ohio, *eating red meat leads to the production of a substance that accelerates atherosclerosis ("hardening of the arteries," which is associated with heart disease, stroke, and death)*. For readers interested in the details of their findings:[386]

---

[1]Red meat in traditional culinary terminology is meat which is red when raw and not white when cooked. Red meat also includes the meat of most adult mammals. The meat from mammals such as cows, sheep ,veal calves, lamb, pigs, horses is invariably considered red, while chicken and rabbit meat is invariably considered white.

ALZHEIMER'S DISEASE

"Intestinal microbiota metabolism of choline and phosphatidylcholine produces trimethylamine (TMA), which is further metabolized to a proatherogenic species, trimethylamine-N-oxide (TMAO). We demonstrate here that metabolism by intestinal microbiota of dietary L-carnitine, a trimethylamine abundant in red meat, also produces TMAO and accelerates atherosclerosis in mice. Omnivorous human subjects produced more TMAO than did vegans or vegetarians following ingestion of L-carnitine through a microbiota-dependent mechanism. The presence of specific bacterial taxa in human feces was associated with both plasma TMAO concentration and dietary status. Plasma L-carnitine levels in subjects undergoing cardiac evaluation (n = 2,595) predicted increased risks for both prevalent cardiovascular disease (CVD) and incident major adverse cardiac events (myocardial infarction, stroke or death), but only among subjects with concurrently high TMAO levels. *Chronic dietary L-carnitine supplementation in mice altered cecal microbial composition, markedly enhanced synthesis of TMA and TMAO, and increased atherosclerosis, but this did not occur if intestinal microbiota was concurrently suppressed.* In mice with an intact intestinal microbiota, dietary supplementation with TMAO or either carnitine or choline reduced in vivo reverse cholesterol transport. *Intestinal microbiota may thus contribute to the well-established link between high levels of red meat consumption and CVD risk.*"

According to research published in the January 1, 2015 issue of the *Journal of Alzheimer's Disease,* "Considerable evidence indicates that diet is an important risk-modifying factor for Alzheimer's disease. *Evidence is also mounting that dietary advanced glycation end products (AGEs)[1] are important risk factors for AD*...[in this study] *Meat was*

---

[1]Advanced glycation end products (AGEs), are substances that can be a factor in the development or worsening of many degenerative diseases, such as diabetes, athero-

always the food with the largest amount of AGEs. Other foods with significant AGEs included fish, cheese, vegetables, and vegetable oil. High MeDi [Mediterranean diet] adherence results in lower meat and dairy intake, which possess high AGE content...*we showed that reduced dietary AGE significantly correlates with reduced AD incidence...Dietary AGEs appear to be important risk factors for AD.*"[387]

Mediterranean and DASH Diets

The traditional Mediterranean diet (MeDi) has been recognized by the United Nations Educational Scientific and Cultural Organization as an Intangible Cultural Heritage of Humanity. This dietary pattern is characterized by a high consumption of plant foods (i.e. vegetables, fruits, legumes and cereals), a high intake of olive oil as the main source of fat, a moderate intake of fish, low-to-moderate intake of dairy products and low consumption of meat and poultry, with wine consumed in low-to-moderate amounts during meals. Beyond the well-known association between higher adherence to the MeDi and lower risk of mortality, in particular from cardiovascular disease (CVD) and cancer, new data from large epidemiological studies suggest a relationship between MeDi adherence and cognitive decline or risk of dementia.[388]

Dr. Solfrizzi and colleagues, from the Department of Geriatrics, Center for Aging Brain, Memory Unit, University of Bari, Bari, Italy, summa-

---

sclerosis, chronic renal failure, and Alzheimer's disease. These harmful compounds can affect nearly every type of cell and molecule in the body and are thought to be one factor in aging and in some age-related chronic diseases. AGEs are seen as speeding up oxidative damage to cells and in altering their normal behavior. Smoking is known to elevate the level of AGEs. Barbecued foods are high in AGEs. Dietary AGEs (dAGEs) can be present in some foods (particularly meat, also butter and some vegetable products), and can form in food during cooking, particularly in dry cooking such as frying, roasting and baking, far less so in boiling, stewing, steaming and microwaving. In addition some foods promote glycation within the body. The total state of oxidative and peroxidative stress on the healthy body, with the AGE-related damage to it,[1] is proportional to the dietary intake of exogenous (preformed) AGEs and the consumption of sugars with a propensity towards glycation such as fructose and galactose. See wikipedia.org for more information.

rized the literature (as of 2011) on elements of the Mediterranean diet:[389]

> "Elevated saturated fatty acids could have negative effects on age-related cognitive decline and mild cognitive impairment (MCI). Furthermore, at present, epidemiological evidence suggests a possible association between fish consumption, monounsaturated fatty acids and polyunsaturated fatty acids (PUFA; in particular, n-3 PUFA) and a reduced risk of cognitive decline and dementia.
>
> Poorer cognitive function and an increased risk of vascular dementia (VaD) were found to be associated with a lower consumption of milk or dairy products. However, the consumption of whole-fat dairy products may be associated with cognitive decline in the elderly.
>
> Light-to-moderate alcohol use may be associated with a reduced risk of incident dementia and AD, while for VaD, cognitive decline and predementia syndromes, the current evidence is only suggestive of a protective effect.
>
> The limited epidemiological evidence available on fruit and vegetable consumption and cognition generally supports a protective role of these macronutrients against cognitive decline, dementia and AD. Only recently, higher adherence to a Mediterranean-type diet was associated with decreased cognitive decline, although the Mediterranean diet (MeDi) combines several foods, micro- and macro-nutrients already separately proposed as potential protective factors against dementia and predementia syndromes. In fact, *recent prospective studies provided evidence that higher adherence to a Mediterranean-type diet could be associated with slower cognitive decline, reduced risk of progression from MCI*

to AD, reduced risk of AD and a decreased all-cause mortality in AD patients. These findings suggested that adherence to the MeDi may affect not only the risk of AD, but also of predementia syndromes and their progression to overt dementia. Based on the current evidence concerning these factors, no definitive dietary recommendations are possible. However, following dietary advice for lowering the risk of cardiovascular and metabolic disorders, high levels of consumption of fats from fish, vegetable oils, non-starchy vegetables, low glycemic index fruits and a diet low in foods with added sugars and with moderate wine intake should be encouraged. Hopefully this will open new opportunities for the prevention and management of dementia and AD."

Dr. Olsson and colleagues published the results of their research on the relationship between a Mediterranean-like diet (mMDS) or a low carbohydrate high protein diet and Alzheimer's disease in the July 25, 2014 issue of the *Journal of Alzheimer's Disease*. The researchers reported that, "During a mean follow-up of twelve years, 84, 143, and 198 men developed AD, all-type dementia, and all-type cognitive impairment, respectively... *mMDS was not associated with dementia diagnosis*...We found no strong associations with development of cognitive dysfunction for any of the dietary patterns investigated. However, *there was a potentially beneficial association for a Mediterranean-like diet on the development of cognitive dysfunction in the subpopulation.*"[390]

Several studies have shown that higher adherence to a Mediterranean diet (MeDi) is associated with reduced risk of AD. In 2014, Dr. Mosconi and colleagues studied the associations between high vs. lower adherence to a MeDi and structural MRI-based brain atrophy in key regions for AD in 52 cognitively normal (NL) individuals with and without risk factors for AD. "Of the 52 participants, 20 (39 percent) showed higher MeDi adherence (MeDi+) and 32 (61 percent) showed lower adherence (MeDi-)...*NL individuals showing lower adherence to the MeDi had cortical thinning in the same brain regions as clinical*

AD patients compared to those showing higher adherence. These data indicate that the MeDi may have a protective effect against tissue loss, and suggest that dietary interventions may play a role in the prevention of AD."[391]

A different group of researchers examined associations between Dietary Approaches to Stop Hypertension (DASH)[1]- and Mediterranean-style dietary patterns and age-related cognitive change. To do so, they followed 3,831 men and women ≥65 y of age. Without discussing the specifics of the study, the researchers concluded that, *"Higher levels of accordance with both the DASH and Mediterranean dietary patterns were associated with consistently higher levels of cognitive function in elderly men and women over an 11-year period. Whole grains and nuts and legumes[2] were positively associated with higher cognitive functions and may be core neuroprotective foods common to various healthy plant-centered diets around the globe."*[392]

Dr. Tangney and colleagues, reporting in the October 14, 2014 issue of the journal *Neurology*, examined whether adherence to the DASH (Dietary Approach to Stop Hypertension) and Mediterranean diets is associated with slower cognitive decline in a group of 826 individuals (aged 81.5 ± 7.1 years), who were followed for 4.1 years. The researchers concluded that, *"These findings support the hypothesis that both the DASH and Mediterranean diet patterns are associated with slower rates of cognitive decline in a group of older persons."*[393]

---

[1]The DASH diet (Dietary Approaches to Stop Hypertension) is a dietary pattern promoted by the U.S.-based National Heart, Lung, and Blood Institute (part of the National Institutes of Health, an agency of the United States Department of Health and Human Services) to prevent and control hypertension. The DASH diet is rich in fruits, vegetables, whole grains, and low-fat dairy foods; includes meat, fish, poultry, nuts, and beans; and is limited in sugar-sweetened foods and beverages, red meat, and added fats. In addition to its effect on blood pressure, it is designed to be a well-balanced approach to eating for the general public. DASH is recommended by the United States Department of Agriculture (USDA) as one of its ideal eating plans for all Americans.

[2]Well-known legumes include alfalfa, clover, peas, beans, lentils, lupins, mesquite, carob, soybeans, peanuts, tamarind, and the woody climbing vine wisteria.

Another group of researchers examined the association between dietary habits, cognitive functioning and brain volumes in older individuals. In order to do so, they followed 194 cognitively healthy individuals for five years. "At age 70, participants kept diaries of their food intake for one week. These records were used to calculate a Mediterranean diet (MeDi) score (comprising dietary habits traditionally found in Mediterranean countries, e.g. high intake of fruits and low intake of meat), with higher scores indicating more pronounced MeDi-like dietary habits. Five years later, participants' cognitive capabilities were examined by the seven minute screening (7MS) (a cognitive test battery used by clinicians to screen for dementia), and their brain volumes were measured by volumetric magnetic resonance imaging (MRIs)...*a low consumption of meat and meat products was linked to a better performance on the 7MS test and greater total brain volume...Integrating all dietary features into the total MeDi score explained less variance in cognitive functioning and brain volumes than its single dietary component meat intake. These observational findings suggest that keeping to a low meat intake could prove to be an impact-driven public health policy* to support healthy cognitive aging, when confirmed by longitudinal studies."[394]

Previous to the above research, other investigators came to a similar conclusion. They noted that *diets "...characterized by higher intake of fruits, vegetables, fish, nuts and legumes, and lower intake of meats, high fat dairy, and sweets seemed to be associated with lower odds of cognitive deficits or reduced risk of AD."*[395]

Paleo Diet

The term Paleolithic describes a cultural period circa 2 million BC and 10,000 BC characterized by the use of flint, stone, and bone tools, hunting, fishing, and the gathering of plant foods. The term was coined by archaeologist John Lubbock in 1865. The terms *caveman diet* and *stone-age diet* are also used, with paleo diet used by 2002. Loren Cordain trademarked the term "Paleo Diet."

The paleolithic diet, also known as the paleo diet or caveman diet, is based on the food humans' ancient ancestors might likely have eaten, such as lean meat, nuts and berries. The diet is based on several premises. Proponents of the diet posit that during the Paleolithic era — a period lasting around 2.5 million years that ended about 10,000 years ago with the advent of agriculture and domestication of animals — humans evolved nutritional needs specific to the foods available at that time, and that the nutritional needs of modern humans remain best adapted to the diet of their Paleolithic ancestors. Proponents claim that human metabolism has been unable to adapt fast enough to handle many of the foods that have become available since the advent of agriculture. Thus, modern humans are said to be maladapted to eating foods such as grain, legumes, and dairy, and in particular the high-calorie processed foods that are a staple of most modern diets. Proponents claim that modern humans' inability to properly metabolize these comparatively new types of food has led to modern-day problems such as obesity, heart disease, and diabetes. They claim that followers of the Paleolithic diet may enjoy a longer, healthier, more active life.

Critics of the Paleolithic diet have pointed out a number of flaws with its underlying logic, including the fact that there is abundant evidence that paleolithic humans did in fact eat grains and legumes, that humans are much more nutritionally flexible than previously thought, that the hypothesis that Paleolithic humans were genetically adapted to specific local diets remains to be proven, that the Paleolithic period was extremely long and saw a variety of forms of human settlement and subsistence in a wide variety of changing nutritional landscapes, and that currently very little is known for certain about what Paleolithic humans ate.

Paleolithic life expectancies were much shorter than modern life expectancies, and food and diet composition are among the main reasons for this change

While there is no research with regard to the Paleo diet and Alzheimer's disease, there is scientific research showing some of the benefits of adhering to the Paleo diet. For example, Dr. Carter and colleagues conducted a systematic review of the scientific literature aiming to determine the effects of a Mediterranean diet compared to other dietary interventions on glycemic control irrespective of weight loss, and published the results of their research in 2014. Without going into the details of their findings, they concluded that, "None of the interventions were significantly better than the others in lowering glucose parameters. *The Mediterranean diet reduced HbA1c[1] significantly compared to usual care but not compared to the Paleolithic diet [e.g., the Paleo diet reduced blood sugar the most in this analysis]*."[396]

Epigenetic Diet

The pronounced effects of the epigenetic[2] diet (ED) and caloric restriction (CR) have on epigenetic gene regulation have been documented in many pre-clinical and clinical studies. Understanding epigenetics is of high importance because of the concept that external factors such as nutrition and diet may possess the ability to alter gene expression without modifying the DNA sequence. *The ED introduces bioactive medicinal chemistry compounds such as sulforaphane (SFN), curcumin (CCM), epigallocatechin gallate (EGCG) and resveratrol (RSV) that are thought to aid in extending the human lifespan.* CR, although similar to ED in the target of longevity, mildly reduces the total daily calorie intake while concurrently providing all beneficial nutrients. Both CR and ED may act as epigenetic modifiers to slow the aging process through histone modification, DNA methylation, and by modulating

---

[1]Glycated hemoglobin (*hemoglobin A1c, HbA$_{1c}$, A1C*, or *Hb$_{1c}$*; sometimes also HbA1c or HGBA1C) is a form of hemoglobin that is measured primarily to identify the average plasma glucose concentration over prolonged periods of time. This serves as a marker for average blood glucose levels over the previous three months prior to the measurement as this is the half-life of red blood cells.

[2]In biology, epigenetics is the study of cellular and physiological trait variations that are *not* caused by changes in the DNA sequence; epigenetics describes the study of dynamic alterations in the transcriptional potential of a cell. These alterations may or may not be heritable, although the use of the term epigenetic to describe processes that are not heritable is controversial. Unlike genetics based on changes to the DNA sequence (the genotype), the changes in gene expression or cellular phenotype of epigenetics have other causes.

microRNA expression. *CR and ED have been proposed as two important mechanisms that modulate and potentially slow the progression of age-related diseases such as cardiovascular disease (CVD), cancer, obesity, Alzheimer's and osteoporosis to name a few.*[397]

According to other researchers, also writing in 2014, "*Various epigenetic mechanisms are linked to pathogenesis of AD.* Epigenetic alterations may occur through external factors and are known for their reversibility. *Dietary factors can influence epigenetic mechanisms. Several neuroprotective nutrients have been shown to enhance cognition, memory and other impaired functions seen in AD.* Within recent years neuroprotective nutrients have gained more attention in the field of epigenetics. *A growing body of evidence suggest that epigenetic changes triggered by dietary nutrients have an important role in health and in prevention of some diseases, especially neurodegenerative disorders [such as Alzheimer's disease]. Several studies have shown that folic acid, vitamin B12, choline, zinc, selenium, dietary polyphenols are capable of interacting with epigenetic mechanisms and ultimately gene expression. Epigenetic mechanisms resulting in neuronal dysfunction may be modified by diet.* Therefore manipulation of epigenetic mechanisms via dietary nutrients may affect or influence the vulnerability of neurons to degeneration which is seen in AD."[398]

Other researchers also underscore the importance of the interaction between nutrition and epigenetics:[399]

> "Nutrition affects the brain throughout life, with profound implications for cognitive decline and dementia. These effects are mediated by changes in expression of multiple genes, and responses to nutrition are in turn affected by individual genetic variability. *An important layer of regulation is provided by the epigenome: nutrition is one of the many epigenetic regulators that modify gene expression without changes in DNA sequence.* Epigenetic mechanisms are central to brain development, structure and function, and include DNA methylation, histone modifications and non-protein-coding RNAs.

They enable cell-specific and age-related gene expression. Although epigenetic events can be highly stable, they can also be reversible, highlighting a critical role for nutrition in prevention and treatment of disease. Moreover, they suggest key mechanisms by which nutrition is involved in the pathogenesis of age-related cognitive decline: many nutrients, foods and diets have both immediate and long-term effects on the epigenome, including energy status, that is, energy intake, physical activity, energy metabolism and related changes in body composition, and micronutrients involved in DNA methylation, for example, folate, vitamins B6 and B12, choline, methionine. *Optimal brain function results from highly complex interactions between numerous genetic and environmental factors, including food intake, physical activity, age and stress.*"

Whole-food Diet

Life is sometimes complicated. Dr. Parrott and colleagues, reported in the August 16, 2014 issue of the journal *Neurobiology of Aging* the paradoxical results of their research, where they hypothesized that a combination whole-food diet containing freeze-dried fish, vegetables, and fruits would improve cognitive function in an animal model of Alzheimer's disease, by modulating brain insulin signaling and neuroinflammation. "*Unexpectedly, the animals fed the whole-food diet exhibited even worse cognitive function than their counterparts fed the control diet.* These results indicate that a dietary profile identified from epidemiologic studies exacerbated cognitive dysfunction and neuroinflammation in a mouse model of familial Alzheimer's disease. *We suggest that normally adaptive cellular responses to dietary phytochemicals were impaired by amyloid-beta deposition leading to increased oxidative stress, neuroinflammation, and behavioral deficits.*"[400] Once again, this indicates that once Alzheimer's disease is present, there is nothing that can help or reverse it.

Ketogenic Diet

According to a review of the ketogenic diet[1] published in 2014, *"An increasing number of data demonstrate the utility of ketogenic diets in a variety of metabolic diseases as obesity, metabolic syndrome, and diabetes. In regard to neurological disorders, ketogenic diet is recognized as an effective treatment for pharmaco-resistant epilepsy but emerging data suggests that ketogenic diet could be also useful in amyotrophic lateral sclerosis, Alzheimer, Parkinson's disease, and some mitochondriopathies. Although these diseases have different pathogenesis and features, there are some common mechanisms that could explain the effects of ketogenic diets. These mechanisms are to provide an efficient source of energy for the treatment of certain types of neurodegenerative diseases characterized by focal brain hypo-metabolism; to decrease the oxidative damage associated with various kinds of metabolic stress; to increase the mitochondrial biogenesis pathways; and to take advantage of the capacity of ketones to bypass the defect in complex I activity implicated in some neurological diseases."*[401]

Fish Diet

In the October 2014 issue of the *American Journal of Preventive Medicine*, Dr. Raji and colleagues, published the results of their research to determine whether or not dietary fish consumption is related to brain structural integrity among cognitively normal elders. Without going into the details of their research, they concluded that, *"Dietary consumption of baked or broiled fish is related to larger gray matter volumes independent of omega-3 fatty acid content. These findings suggest that a confluence of lifestyle factors influence brain health, adding to*

---

[1] The ketogenic diet is a high-fat, adequate-protein, low-carbohydrate diet that is used primarily to treat difficult-to-control (refractory) epilepsy in children. The diet forces the body to burn fats rather than carbohydrates. Normally, the carbohydrates contained in food are converted into glucose, which is then transported around the body and is particularly important in fueling brain function. However, if there is very little carbohydrate in the diet, the liver converts fat into fatty acids and ketone bodies. The ketone bodies pass into the brain and replace glucose as an energy source.

the growing body of evidence that prevention strategies for late-life brain health need to begin decades earlier."[402]

Anti-Alzheimer's Diet

Dr. Morris and colleagues, published the results of their study of the relationship between three diets and Alzheimer's disease, in the February 11, 2015 issue of the journal *Alzheimer's Dementia*. They followed 923 participants, ages 58 to 98 years, an average 4.5 years. They studied the "MIND[1]," the "DASH," and the Mediterranean diets. They found that, *"High adherence to all three diets may reduce AD risk. Moderate adherence to the MIND diet may also decrease AD risk."*[403]

According to an article discussing these findings:[404]

> "Developed by nutritional epidemiologist Martha Clare Morris, PhD, and colleagues at Rush University Medical Center in Chicago, the MIND diet is a hybrid of the Mediterranean and DASH (Dietary Approaches to Stop Hypertension) diets, both of which have been found to reduce the risk of cardiovascular conditions, like hypertension, heart attack, and stroke. Some researchers have found that these two older diets provide protection against dementia as well.
>
> In the latest study, the MIND diet was compared with the two earlier diets. People with high adherence to the DASH and Mediterranean diets also had reductions in AD — 39 percent with the DASH diet and 54 percent with the Mediterranean diet — but got negligible benefits from moderate adherence to either of the two other diets.

---

[1]The MIND diet is a hybrid of the Mediterranean and DASH (Dietary Approaches to Stop Hypertension) diets, both of which have been found to reduce the risk of cardiovascular conditions, like hypertension, heart attack, and stroke.

The MIND diet is also easier to follow than, say, the Mediterranean diet, which calls for daily consumption of fish and three to four daily servings of each of fruits and vegetables, Morris said.

The MIND diet has fifteen dietary components, including ten "brain-healthy food groups" — green leafy vegetables, other vegetables, nuts, berries, beans, whole grains, fish, poultry, olive oil and wine — and (because it was tracking what people actually eat, rather than what they should) five unhealthy groups that comprise red meats, butter and stick margarine, cheese, pastries and sweets, and fried or fast food.

The MIND diet includes at least three servings of whole grains, a salad and one other vegetable every day — along with a glass of wine. It also involves snacking most days on nuts and eating beans every other day or so, poultry and berries at least twice a week and fish at least once a week. *Dieters must limit eating the designated unhealthy foods, especially butter (less than 1 tablespoon a day), cheese, and fried or fast food (less than a serving a week for any of the three), to have a real shot at avoiding the devastating effects of Alzheimer's, according to the study.*

Berries are the only fruit specifically to make the MIND diet. *"Blueberries are one of the more potent foods in terms of protecting the brain,"* Morris said, *and strawberries have also performed well in past studies of the effect of food on cognitive function.*

Participants in study were assigned points if they ate brain-healthy foods frequently and avoided unhealthy foods. The one exception was that participants got one point if they said olive oil was the primary oil used in their homes.

Food more important than genetic risk factors

"With late-onset AD, with that older group of people, genetic risk factors are a small piece of the picture," she said. *Past studies have yielded evidence that suggests that what we eat may play a significant role in determining who gets AD and who doesn't*, Morris said.

When the researchers in the new study left out of the analyses those participants who changed their diets somewhere along the line — say, on a doctor's orders after a stroke — they found that "the association became stronger between the MIND diet and [favorable] outcomes" in terms of AD, Morris said. "That probably means that people who eat this diet consistently over the years get the best protection."

In other words, it looks *like the longer a person eats the MIND diet, the less risk that person will have of developing AD*, Morris said. As is the case with many health-related habits, including physical exercise, she said, *"You'll be healthier if you've been doing the right thing for a long time."*

The study was funded by the National Institute on Aging.

Healthy Lifestyle

In late 2014, results of a study of the relationship between lifestyle and Alzheimer's disease were published. Dr. Willam examined whether or not exercise, diet, or statins affect AD mortality in 153,536 participants of the National Runners' and Walkers' Health Studies. "The National Death Index identified 175 subjects who died with AD listed as an underlying (n = 116) or contributing (n = 59) cause of death during an 11.6-year average follow up. Relative to exercising, AD mortality was

6.0 percent lower for 1.07 to 1.8 MET[1]-hours/d, 24.8 percent lower for 1.8 to 3.6 MET-hours/d, and 40.1 percent lower for ≥3.6 MET-hours/d. Relative to non-use, statin use was associated with 61 percent lower AD mortality, whereas use of other cholesterol-lowering medications was not. Relative to <1 piece of fruit/day, consuming 2 to 3 pieces daily was associated with 39.7 percent lower AD mortality and ≥3 pieces/day with 60.7 percent lower AD mortality. *Conclusions: Exercise, statin, and fruit intake were associated with lower risk for AD mortality.*"[405]

Life Space

From the Department of Internal Medicine, Rush University Medical Center, Chicago, IL, Dr. James and colleagues report that a smaller "life space" is associated with an increased risk of Alzheimer's dementia. To test the hypothesis that a constricted life space, the extent of movement through the environment covered during daily functioning, is associated with an increased risk of Alzheimer disease, increased risk of mild cognitive impairment, and more rapid cognitive decline in older adults, the researchers studied 1,294 community-dwelling elders without baseline clinical dementia for an average of 4.4 years. During that time, 180 persons developed AD.

A person with a life space constricted to their home was almost twice as likely to develop AD than a person with the largest life space (out of town). The association did not vary along demographic lines and persisted even after adjustments for performance-based physical function, disability, depressive symptoms, social network size, vascular disease burden, and vascular risk factors. A constricted life space was also associated with an increased risk of MCI, and a more rapid rate of global

---

[1]The Metabolic Equivalent of Task (MET), or simply metabolic equivalent, is a physiological measure expressing the energy cost of physical activities and is defined as the ratio of metabolic rate (and therefore the rate of energy consumption) during a specific physical activity to a reference metabolic rate. 1 MET is also defined as 58.2 W/m^2 (18.4 $Btu/h \cdot ft^2$), which is equal to the rate of energy produced per unit surface area of an average person seated at rest.

cognitive decline. The authors concluded that, *"A constricted life space is associated with increased risk of AD, MCI, and cognitive decline among older persons."*[406]

Mental Activities

Cognitive Training/Activity

Cognitive training is an approach that has received increased attention in recent years as a non-pharmacological, cost-effective intervention for Alzheimer's disease. There has been increasing behavioral evidence regarding training-related improvement in cognitive performance in early stages of AD. Dr. Hosseini and colleagues, published the results of their research on this topic in the August 26, 2014 issue of the journal *Frontiers of Aging Neuroscience*. "In this study, we reviewed the existing neuroimaging studies on cognitive training in persons at risk of developing AD to provide an overview of the overlap between neural networks rehabilitated by the current training methods and those affected in AD. *The data suggest a consistent training-related increase in brain activity in medial temporal, prefrontal, and posterior default mode networks, as well as increase in gray matter structure in frontoparietal and entorhinal regions.* This pattern differs from the observed pattern in healthy older adults that shows a combination of increased and decreased activity in response to training. *Detailed investigation of the data suggests that training in persons at risk of developing AD mainly improves compensatory mechanisms and partly restores the affected functions."*[407]

To test the hypothesis that frequent participation in cognitive activities is associated with a reduced risk of Alzheimer's disease, another group of researchers followed 801 older Catholic nuns, priests, and brothers without dementia at enrollment, recruited from forty groups across the United States. "During an average of 4.5 years of follow-up, 111 persons developed AD...*These results suggest that frequent participation in cognitively stimulating activities is associated with reduced risk of AD.*"[408]

Early life education and participation in cognitively stimulating leisure activities later in life are two factors thought to reflect cognitive reserve, which may delay the onset of the memory decline in the preclinical stages of dementia. To test these relationships, researchers followed 488 initially cognitively intact community residing individuals. "We assessed the influence of self-reported participation in cognitively stimulating leisure activities on the onset of accelerated memory decline as measured by the Buschke Selective Reminding Test in 101 individuals who developed incident dementia using a change point model. *Each additional self-reported day of cognitive activity at baseline delayed the onset of accelerated memory decline by 0.18 years. Higher baseline levels of cognitive activity were associated with more rapid memory decline after that onset. Inclusion of education did not significantly add to the fit of the model beyond the effect of cognitive activities. Our findings show that late life cognitive activities influence cognitive reserve independently of education.* The effect of early life education on cognitive reserve may be mediated by cognitive activity later in life. Alternatively, early life education may be a determinant of cognitive reserve, and individuals with more education may choose to participate in cognitive activities without influencing reserve."[409]

Publishing their results of their research in the October 31, 2014 issue of *Brain Imaging & Behavior,* Dr Schultz and colleagues, from the Geriatric Research Education and Clinical Center, William S. Middleton Memorial Veterans Hospital, Madison, WI, tested the hypothesis that frequent participation in cognitively-stimulating activities, specifically those related to playing games and puzzles, is beneficial to brain health and cognition among middle-aged adults at increased risk for Alzheimer's disease. They followed 329 cognitively normal, middle-aged adults (age range, 43.2-73.8 years), who reported their current engagement in cognitive activities, underwent a structural MRI scan, and completed a comprehensive cognitive battery. The researchers concluded that, "*For some individuals, participation in cognitive activities pertinent to game playing may help prevent AD by preserving brain structures and cognitive functions vulnerable to AD pathophysiology.*"[410]

Higher Education

Epidemiological studies have reported that higher education (HE) is associated with a reduced risk of incident Alzheimer's disease. However, after the clinical onset of AD, patients with HE levels show more rapid cognitive decline than patients with lower education (LE) levels. In 2014, researchers studied the relationship between education level and cortical decline in patients with AD. "The aim of this study was to compare the topography of cortical [brain] atrophy longitudinally between AD patients with HE (HE-AD) and AD patients with LE (LE-AD). We recruited thirty-six patients with early-stage AD and fourteen normal controls. The patients were classified into two groups according to educational level, 23 HE-AD (>9 years) and 13 LE-AD (≤9 years). As AD progressed over the 5-year longitudinal follow-ups, the HE-AD showed a significant group-by-time interaction in the right dorsolateral frontal and precuneus, and the left parahippocampal regions compared to the LE-AD. Conclusion: *Our study reveals that the preliminary longitudinal effect of HE accelerates cortical atrophy in AD patients over time*, which underlines the importance of education level for predicting prognosis."[411]

Several other studies, conducted by different research groups, came to the very same conclusions.[412, 413]

To evaluate the effects of vascular conditions and education quality on cognition over time in White and African American (AA) older adults, researchers investigated cross-sectional and longitudinal racial differences in executive functioning (EF) and memory composites among Whites (n = 461) and AAs (n = 118) enrolled in a study. "We examined whether cerebrovascular risk factors and Shipley Vocabulary scores (a proxy for education quality) accounted for racial differences. On average, AAs had lower quality of education and more cerebrovascular risk factors including hypertension, diabetes, and obesity. AAs had lower mean EF and memory at baseline, but there were no group differences in rates of decline...*Quality of education appears to be more important than cerebrovascular risk factors in explaining cross-sectional differences in memory and EF performance between White and AA older adults.*"[414]

Learning a Language

Studies have shown that knowing a second language may be helpful in delaying the onset of Alzheimer's disease. To further investigate this relationship, researchers reviewed the case records of 648 patients with dementia (391 of them bilingual). The age at onset of first symptoms was compared between monolingual and bilingual groups. The influence of number of languages spoken, education, occupation, and other potentially interacting variables was examined. The researchers found that, "*Overall, bilingual patients developed dementia 4.5 years later than the monolingual ones.* A significant difference in age at onset was found across Alzheimer disease dementia as well as frontotemporal dementia and vascular dementia, and was also observed in illiterate patients. *There was no additional benefit to speaking more than two languages.* The bilingual effect on age at dementia onset was shown independently of other potential confounding factors such as education, sex, occupation, and urban vs rural dwelling of subjects. This is the largest study so far documenting a delayed onset of dementia in bilingual patients and the first one to show it separately in different dementia subtypes. *It is the first study reporting a bilingual advantage in those who are illiterate, suggesting that education is not a sufficient explanation for the observed difference.*"[415]

Other researchers have also stated, "... *research shows that being bilingual enhances mental performance and may protect from Alzheimer's disease.*"[416]

Meditation

According to wikipedia.org, "Meditation is a practice in which an individual trains the mind or induces a mode of consciousness, either to realize some benefit or for the mind to simply acknowledge its content without becoming identified with that content, or as an end in itself." See wikipedia.org for a more complete explanations.

Meditation is often used to decrease stress, which we know is a good thing, vis-à-vis minimizing our risk of Alzheimer's disease.

According to Dr. Newberg and colleagues, from the Jefferson Myrna Brind Center of Integrative Medicine, Thomas Jefferson University, Philadelphia, Pennsylvania, who reported the results of their literature review in the January 2014 issue of the journal the *Annals of the New York Academy of Sciences*, "Meditation techniques present an interesting potential adjuvant [additional] treatment for patients with neurodegenerative diseases and have the advantage of being inexpensive, and easy to teach and perform. *There is increasing research evidence to support the application of meditation techniques to help improve cognition and memory in patients with neurodegenerative diseases.*"[417]

Meditation has been shown to have many health benefits. An article published in February 2015 explains some of the benefits with regard to brain health:[418]

> "Forever young: Meditation might slow the age-related loss of gray matter in the brain.
>
> Since 1970, life expectancy around the world has risen dramatically, with people living more than ten years longer. That's the good news. The bad news is that starting when people are in their mid-to-late-20s, the brain begins to wither—its volume and weight begin to decrease. As this occurs, the brain can begin to lose some of its functional abilities.

ALZHEIMER'S DISEASE

So although people might be living longer, the years they gain often come with increased risks for mental illness and neurodegenerative disease [such as Alzheimer's disease]. Fortunately, *a new study shows meditation could be one way to minimize those risks.*

Building on their earlier work that suggested people who meditate have less age-related atrophy in the brain's white matter, a new study by UCLA researchers found that meditation appeared to help preserve the brain's gray matter, the tissue that contains neurons.

The scientists looked specifically at the association between age and gray matter. They compared fifty people who had mediated for years and fifty who didn't. *People in both groups showed a loss of gray matter as they aged. But the researchers found among those who meditated, the volume of gray matter did not decline as much as it did among those who didn't.*

The article appears in the current online edition of the journal *Frontiers in Psychology*. Dr. Florian Kurth, a co-author of the study and postdoctoral fellow at the UCLA Brain Mapping Center, said the researchers were surprised by the magnitude of the difference. "We expected rather small and distinct effects located in some of the regions that had previously been associated with meditating," he said. "Instead, *what we actually observed was a widespread effect of meditation that encompassed regions throughout the entire brain.*"

Each group in the study was made up of twenty-eight men and twenty-two women ranging in age from twenty-four to seventy-seven. Those who meditated had been doing so for four to forty-six years, with an average of twenty years. The participants' brains were scanned using high-resolution magnetic resonance imaging [MRI].

Although the researchers found a negative correlation between gray matter and age in both groups of people—suggesting a loss of brain tissue with increasing age—they also found that large parts of the gray matter in the brains of those who meditated seemed to be better preserved, Kurth said.

Mindfulness

Mindfulness is a popular method to handle emotions by paying attention to them. It is derived from the Buddhist concept Sati. Mindfulness means maintaining a moment-by-moment awareness of our thoughts, feelings, bodily sensations, and surrounding environment.

Mindfulness also involves acceptance, meaning that we pay attention to our thoughts and feelings without judging them—without believing, for instance, that there's a "right" or "wrong" way to think or feel in a given moment. When we practice mindfulness, our thoughts tune into what we're sensing in the present moment rather than rehashing the past or imagining the future.

Though it has its roots in Buddhist meditation, a secular practice of mindfulness has entered the American mainstream in recent years, in part through the work of Jon Kabat-Zinn and his Mindfulness-Based Stress Reduction (MBSR) program, which he launched at the University of Massachusetts Medical School in 1979. Since that time, thousands of studies have documented the physical and mental health benefits of mindfulness in general and MBSR in particular.

According to one group of researchers, "*Those with high baseline stress levels are more likely to develop mild cognitive impairment (MCI) and Alzheimer's Disease.*" Using functional MRI (fMRI), they studied fourteen adults with MCI to determine whether Mindfulness Based Stress Reduction (MBSR) would be beneficial. Without discussing their experiment in detail here, the researchers concluded that, "*These preliminary results indicate that in adults with MCI, MBSR may have a positive impact on the regions of the brain most related to MCI and AD.*"[419]

Physical Activity

Without a doubt, greater physical activity is related to improved overall health and a decreased risk of Alzheimer's disease. Recent epidemiological evidence suggests that modifying lifestyle by increasing physical activity could be a non-pharmacological approach to improving symptoms and slowing disease progression in Alzheimer's disease. Researchers reported in 2014 that, *"Regular physical activity is protective against and beneficial for Mild Cognitive Impairment (MCI), dementia, and Alzheimer's disease."*[420]

According to Drs. Watson and Baar, from the Department of Neurobiology, Physiology, and Behavior, University of California Davis, reporting in December 2014:[421]

> "Exercise is the greatest physiological stress that our bodies experience. For example, during maximal endurance exercise in elite athlete's cardiac output can increase up to 8-fold and the working muscles receive twenty-one times more blood each minute than at rest. Given the physiological stress associated with exercise and the adaptations that occur to handle this stress, *it is not surprising that exercise training is known to prevent or effectively treat a multitude of degenerative conditions including cardiovascular disease, cancer, diabetes, depression, Alzheimer's disease, Parkinson's disease, and many others.* Many of the health benefits of exercise are mediated by the mammalian/mechanistic target of rapamycin (mTOR)[1], either in complex one or two, not

---

[1]The mechanistic target of rapamycin, also known as mammalian target of rapamycin (mTOR) is a protein that in humans is encoded by the MTOR gene. MTOR is a serine/threonine protein kinase that regulates cell growth, cell proliferation, cell motility, cell survival, protein synthesis, and transcription.

only within the working muscle, but also in distant tissues such as fat, liver, and brain. This review will discuss how *exercise activates mTOR in diverse tissues and the ways that mTOR is important in the adaptive response that makes us bigger, stronger, and healthier as a result of exercise.*"

The positive effects of physical activity helping prevent Alzheimer's disease have been known for years. For example, in 2001, researchers published the results of their study of 9,008 randomly selected men and women 65 years or older, who were evaluated in the 1991-1992 Canadian Study of Health and Aging. "Of the 6,434 eligible subjects who were cognitively normal at baseline, 4,615 completed a 5-year follow-up. In 1996-1997, 3,894 remained without cognitive impairment, 436 were diagnosed as having cognitive impairment-no dementia, and 285 were diagnosed as having dementia. Compared with no exercise, physical activity was associated with lower risks of cognitive impairment, Alzheimer disease, and dementia of any type. Significant trends for increased protection with greater physical activity were observed. High levels of physical activity were associated with reduced risks of cognitive impairment, Alzheimer disease, and dementia of any type. *Regular physical activity could represent an important and potent protective factor for cognitive decline and dementia in elderly persons.*"[422]

In 2006, researchers studied this relationship by following 2,288 persons sixty-five years and older without dementia. Patients were enrolled from 1994 to 1996 and followed up through October 2003. The researchers found that, "During follow-up 319 participants developed dementia (221 had AD). The age-specific incidence rate of dementia was 53.1 per 1000 person-years for participants who scored lower on a performance-based physical function test at baseline compared with 17.4 per 1000 person-years for those who scored higher. A 1-point lower performance-based physical function score was associated with an increased risk of dementia, an increased risk of Alzheimer's disease, and an increased rate of decline in the Cognitive Ability Screening Instrument scores after adjusting for age, sex, years of education, baseline cognitive function, APOE epsilon4 allele, family history of AD, depression, coronary heart disease, and cerebrovascular disease. Lower levels of physical performance were associated with an increased risk of dementia and AD. *The study suggests that poor physical function may precede the onset of dementia and AD and higher levels of physical function may be associated with a delayed onset.*"[423]

In 2014, researchers reviewed the relevant literature on the association between cognition and physical function, as well as roles of muscle and brain structure in this relationship. The researchers found that, "...there is evidence that *gait speed is positively associated with whole brain volume*; this relationship may be driven by total WM [white matter] volume or regional GM [gray matter] volumes, specifically the hippocampus [memory area]. *Markers of brain aging, that is brain atrophy and greater accumulation of white matter hyperintensities (WMH), were associated with grip strength and gait speed.* The location of WMH is important for gait speed; periventricular hyperintensities and brainstem WMH are associated with gait speed but subcortical WMH play less of a role. Cognitive function does not appear to be associated with muscle size...*Conclusion: There is evidence that brain structure is associated with muscle structure and function.*"[424]

Dr. Boyle and colleagues, reported in the August 27, 2014 issue of the *Neurobiology of Aging,* their findings about the associations between physical activity (PA), body mass index (BMI)[1], and brain structure in normal aging, mild cognitive impairment, and Alzheimer's dementia. To do so, they studied 963 participants (mean age: 74.1) from the multisite Cardiovascular Health Study including healthy controls (n = 724), Alzheimer's dementia patients (n = 104), and people with mild cognitive impairment (n = 135). They found that, "physical activity was independently associated with greater whole brain and regional brain volumes and reduced ventricular dilation [brain atrophy]. *People with*

---

[1]Body mass index (BMI): is a measure of relative size based on the mass and height of an individual. The BMI for a person is defined as their body mass divided by the square of their height—with the value universally being given in units of kg/m^2. So if the weight is in kilograms and the height in meters, the result is immediate, if pounds and inches are used, a conversion factor of 703 $(kg/m^2)/(lb/in^2)$ must be applied.

higher BMI had lower whole brain and regional brain volumes. A PA-BMI conjunction analysis showed brain preservation with PA and volume loss with increased BMI in overlapping brain regions. In one of the largest studies to date, PA and lower BMI may be beneficial to the brain across the spectrum of aging and neurodegeneration."[425] Bottom line: greater physical activity, and lower weight are associated with bigger brains.

Accumulating evidence suggests that some dietary patterns, specifically high fat diet (HFD), increase the risk of developing sporadic (e.g., not genetically related) Alzheimer's disease. Thus, interventions targeting HFD-induced metabolic dysfunctions may be effective in preventing the development of AD. Researchers previously demonstrated that amyloid precursor protein (APP)-overexpressing mice fed HFD showed worsening of cognitive function when compared with control APP mice on a normal diet. They also reported that voluntary exercise ameliorates HFD-induced memory impairment and β-amyloid (Aβ) deposition. "In the present study, we conducted diet control to ameliorate the metabolic abnormality caused by HFD on APP transgenic mice and compared the effect of diet control on cognitive function with that of voluntary exercise as well as that of combined (diet control plus exercise) treatment. Surprisingly, we found that exercise was more effective than diet control, although both exercise and diet control ameliorated HFD-induced memory deficit and Aβ deposition. The production of Aβ was not different between the exercise- and the diet control-treated mice. On the other hand, exercise specifically strengthened the activity of neprilysin, the Aβ-degrading enzyme, the level of which was significantly correlated with that of deposited Aβ in our mice. *Notably, the effect of the combination treatment (exercise and diet control) on memory and amyloid pathology was not significantly different from that of exercise alone. These studies provide solid evidence that exercise is a useful intervention to rescue HFD-induced aggravation of cognitive decline in a mice model of AD.*" In summary, exercise was more effective than diet in ameliorating a high-fat diet-induced memory deficit and Aβ deposition in an animal of AD.[426]

Recall that one hypothesis of the cause of Alzheimer's disease is "tau" pathology. Previous studies have shown that exercise reduces tau hyperphosphorylation, which is thought to be part of the abnormality in AD. In order to study this further, researchers studied the relationship between tau pathology and exercise in an animal model of AD. In this study, animals were subjected to 12-weeks of forced treadmill exercise and evaluated for effects on motor function and tau pathology at ten months of age. Without going into the specifics of the research, the researchers reported that, "Our results suggest that forced treadmill exercise differently affects the brain and spinal cord of mice, with greater benefits observed in the spinal cord versus the brain. *Our work adds to the growing body of evidence that exercise is beneficial in tauopathy, however these benefits may be more limited at later stages of disease.*"[427]

Physical exercise interventions and cognitive training programs have individually been reported to improve cognition in the healthy elderly population; however, the clinical significance of using a combined approach is currently lacking. In order to study whether or not physical activity (PA), computerized cognitive training and/or a combination of both could improve cognition, Dr. Shah and colleagues, reported their results in December 2014. They studied 224 healthy community-dwelling older adults (60-85 years), who were assigned to sixteen weeks home-based PA (n=64), computerized cognitive stimulation (n=62), a combination of both (combined, n=51) or a control group (n=47). "A subset (total n=45) of participants underwent [(18)F] fluorodeoxyglucose positron emission tomography [PET] scans at sixteen weeks (post-intervention)...Compared with the control group, the combined group showed improved verbal episodic memory and significantly higher brain glucose...The higher cerebral glucose metabolism in this brain region was positively associated with improved verbal memory seen in the combined group only. *Our study provides evidence that a specific combination of physical and mental exercises for sixteen weeks can improve cognition and increase cerebral glucose metabolism in cognitively intact healthy older adults.*"[428]

PREVENTION

Dr. Boots and colleagues, reporting in the October 16, 2014 issue of *Brain Imaging and Behavior,* note that:

> "Cardiorespiratory fitness (CRF) is an objective measure of habitual physical activity (PA), and has been linked to increased brain structure and cognition. The gold standard method for measuring CRF is graded exercise testing (GXT), but GXT is not feasible in many settings. The objective of this study was to examine whether a non-exercise estimate of CRF is related to gray matter (GM) volumes, white matter hyperintensities (WMH), cognition, objective and subjective memory function, and mood in a middle-aged group at risk for Alzheimer's disease. Three hundred and fifteen cognitively healthy adults (mean age =58.58 years) enrolled in the Wisconsin Registry for Alzheimer's Prevention underwent structural MRI scanning, cognitive testing, anthropometric assessment, venipuncture for laboratory tests, and completed a self-reported PA questionnaire. A subset (n = 85) underwent maximal GXT. CRF was estimated using a previously validated equation incorporating sex, age, body-mass index, resting heart rate, and self-reported PA. *Results indicated that the CRF estimate was significantly associated with GXT-derived peak oxygen consumption, validating its use as a non-exercise CRF measure in our sample.*
>
> Support for this finding was seen in significant associations between the CRF estimate and several cardiovascular risk factors. Higher CRF was associated with greater GM volumes in several AD-relevant brain regions including the hippocampus, amygdala, precuneus, supramarginal gyrus, and rostral middle frontal gyrus. Increased CRF was also associated with lower WMH and better cognitive performance in Verbal Learning and Memory, Speed and Flexibility, and Visuospatial Abil-

ity. Lastly, CRF was negatively correlated with self- and informant-reported memory complaints, and depressive symptoms. *Together, these findings suggest that habitual participation in physical activity may provide protection for brain structure and cognitive function, thereby decreasing future risk for AD.*"[429]

Brown and colleagues, reporting in the October 7, 2014 issue of *Neurology*, reported their findings between "...the association between habitual physical activity levels and brain temporal lobe volumes, and the interaction with the brain-derived neurotrophic factor (BDNF) Val66Met polymorphism [e.g. genetic variation]. This study is a cross-sectional analysis of 114 cognitively healthy men and women aged sixty years and older. Brain volumes quantified by MRI were correlated with self-reported physical activity levels. The effect of the interaction between physical activity and the BDNF Val66Met polymorphism on brain structure volumes was assessed. The BDNF Val66Met polymorphism interacted with physical activity to be associated with hippocampal ($\beta = -0.22$, $p = 0.02$) and temporal lobe ($\beta = -0.28$, $p = 0.003$) volumes [e.g., lower brain volumes]. *In Val/Val homozygotes, higher levels of physical activity were associated with larger hippocampal [where memories are formed] and temporal lobe volumes, whereas in Met carriers, higher levels of physical activity were associated with smaller temporal lobe volume.*" So, depending on your genetic status, with regard to brain-derived neurotrophic factor (BDNF) Val66Met, exercise either increased or decreased your brain size in specific areas.[430]

Cardiovascular activity has been shown to be positively associated with gray and white matter volume of, amongst others, frontal and temporal brain regions in older adults. This is particularly true for the hippocampus, a brain structure that plays an important role in learning and memory, and whose decline has been related to the development of Alzheimer's disease. Researchers, who reported their findings in 2014, were interested in whether not only cardiovascular activity but also other types of physical activity, i.e., coordination training, were also positively associated with the volume of the hippocampus in older adults. For this purpose they first collected cross-sectional data on "metabolic fitness" (cardiovascular fitness and muscular strength) and "motor fitness" (e.g., balance, movement speed, fine coordination). Second, they performed a 12-month randomized controlled trial. They concluded that, *"After the 12-month intervention period, both cardiovascular and coordination training led to increases in hippocampal volume. Our findings suggest that a high motor fitness level as well as different types of physical activity were beneficial to diminish age-related hippocampal volume shrinkage or even increase hippocampal volume."*[431]

Leisure activities have been associated with a decreased risk of dementia. Dr. Yang and colleagues, reporting in late 2014, studied the relationships between dementia risk, apolipoprotein E (ApoE) e4 status, vascular risk factors, and leisure activities. They recruited patients (age ≥ 60 years) with Alzheimer's disease (AD; n = 292) and vascular dementia (VaD; n = 144) and healthy controls (n = 506). Information on patient's leisure activities were obtained through a questionnaire. They discovered that, *"High-frequency physical activity was associated with a decreased risk of AD, and the results become more evident among ApoE e4 carriers with AD and VaD. Similar findings were observed for cognitive and social activities for AD.* High-frequency physical, cognitive, and social activities were associated with a decreased risk of VaD. Physical and social activities significantly interacted with each other on the risk of VaD. *Physical activity consistently protects against AD and VaD. Significant interactions were identified across different types of leisure activities in lowering dementia risk."*[432]

Also in 2014, another group of researchers studied the effects of high intensity progressive resistance training with or without cognitive training (computerized, multi-domain cognitive training) on 100 adults with mild cognitive impairment (MCI) [70.1 years; 68 percent women]. The researchers found that, *"Resistance training [alone] significantly improved global cognitive function, with maintenance of executive and global benefits over eighteen months."*[433]

In order to identify and characterize the scientific literature on the effects of exercise on Alzheimer's disease, researchers conducted a literature search. They concluded that, *"Given the results discussed here, exercise may be important for the improvement of functionality and performance of daily life activities, neuropsychiatric disturbances, cardiovascular and cardiorespiratory fitness, functional capacity components (flexibility, agility, balance, strength), and improves some cognitive components such as sustained attention, visual memory and frontal cognitive function in patients with Alzheimer's disease."*[434]

Dr. Okonkwo and seventeen colleagues, reported the results of their research in the November 4, 2014 issue of *Neurology* on whether or not engagement in physical activity might favorably alter the age-dependent evolution of Alzheimer's disease-related brain and cognitive changes in a group of at-risk, late-middle-aged adults. They followed 317 individuals who underwent PET scanning. Participants' responses on a self-report measure of current physical activity were used to classify them as either physically active or physically inactive based on American Heart Association guidelines. They found that, "There were significant age × physical activity interactions for β-amyloid burden, glucose metabolism, and hippocampal volume such that, *with advancing age, physically active individuals exhibited a lesser degree of biomarker alterations compared with the physically inactive. Similar age × physical activity interactions were also observed on cognitive domains of Immediate Memory and Visuospatial Ability. In addition, the physically active group had higher scores on Speed and Flexibility compared with the inactive group...In a middle-aged, at-risk group, a physically active lifestyle is associated with an attenuation of the deleterious influence of age on key biomarkers of AD pathophysiology."*[435]

Researchers studied the effects of an 8-week exercise-intervention on cognition and related serum biochemical markers in nonagenarians[1]. The intervention focused on supervised, light-to-moderate-intensity aerobic and resistance exercises (mainly leg press), and included three weekly sessions. "Cognitive status was determined by the mini-mental

---

[1]Nonagenarian: a person who is from 90 to 99 years old.

state examination and geriatric depression scale. We analyzed proteins with reported relation with mechanisms behind cognition changes such as serum levels of angiotensin converting enzyme, amyloid-precursor protein, epidermal growth factor, brain-derived neural factor and tumor necrosis factor. No significant change in any of the variables studied was found following the exercise intervention compared with the standard-care group. Overall changes after the exercise intervention in serum biomarkers were not associated with changes in functional capacity and cognitive measures. *An 8-week exercise intervention focusing on resistance exercises neither benefits cognitive function nor affects the levels of the serum proteins analyzed in nonagenarians.*"[436] This once again shows that short-term interventions in the elderly are unlikely to result in significant improvements in any area.

Researchers studied fourteen individuals with mild Alzheimer's disease to further the understanding of how people with mild AD reason about physical activity as part of everyday life, with a specific focus on the meanings attached to such activity. "The analysis revealed three sub-themes reflecting interrelated perspectives on how people with mild AD reason about physical activity: (1) striving to be physically active, mirrors the concrete approaches used for handling the consequences of having AD in relation to being active; (2) perceptions of physical activity, reflect how their thoughts and beliefs regarding written and tacit norms encouraged them to remain physically active, and (3) physical activity as a means to well-being, alludes to feelings and emotions related to the performance of physical activity. Interpretation of the underlying patterns in these sub-themes revealed one overarching theme: Physical activity as a means to selfhood maintenance, which suggests that physical activity can help to shift the focus from the dementia diagnosis (i.e. ill health) to a more healthy and able self. *Conclusion: The findings suggest that physical activity, apart from maintaining body functions, can be a way to sustain well-being and selfhood in mild AD.*"[437]

Researchers reviewed the literature vis-à-vis exercise and cardiovascular health and longevity, noting the following in 2014: "The question is not whether exercise is or isn't one of the very best strategies for improving quality of life, cardiovascular (CV) health and longevity-it is. And there is no debate as to whether or not strenuous high-intensity endurance training produces an amazingly efficient, compliant, and powerful pump [heart]-it does. The essence of the controversy centers on what exactly is the ideal pattern of long-term physical activity (PA) for conferring robust and enduring CV health, while also optimizing life expectancy. With that goal in mind, this review will focus on the question: 'Is more always better when it comes to exercise?' And if a dose-response curve exists for the therapeutic effects of PA, where is the upper threshold at which point further training begins to detract from the health and longevity benefits noted with moderate exercise? *The emerging picture from the cumulative data on this hotly debated topic is that moderate exercise appears to be the sweet spot for bestowing lasting CV health and longevity.* However, the specific definition of moderate in this context is not clear yet."[438]

And finally, a word of caution about exercise and weight loss. Dr. Malhotra and colleagues, published an editorial in the April 22, 2015 issue of the *British Journal of Sports Medicine*, where they noted the following:[439]

> A recent report from the UK's Academy of Medical Royal Colleges described 'the miracle cure' of performing thirty minutes of moderate exercise five times a week as more powerful than many drugs administered for chronic disease prevention and management. *Regular physical activity reduces the risk of developing cardiovascular disease, type 2 diabetes, dementia and some cancers by at least 30 percent. However, physical activity does not promote weight loss.*
>
> In the past thirty years, as obesity has rocketed, there has been little change in physical activity levels in the Western population. *This places the blame for our expanding waist lines directly on the type and amount of calories consumed.* However, the obesity epidemic represents only the tip of a much larger iceberg of the adverse

health consequences of poor diet. According to the *Lancet* global burden of disease reports, *poor diet now generates more disease than physical inactivity, alcohol and smoking combined. Up to 40 percent of those with a normal body mass index [BMI] will harbor metabolic abnormalities typically associated with obesity...*"

Physical Activity Trackers

Using an "activity tracker" can help people focus on their activity levels, among other things. From wikipedia.org:

"An activity tracker is a device or application for monitoring and tracking fitness-related metrics such as distance walked or run, calorie consumption, and in some cases heartbeat and quality of sleep. The term is now primarily used for dedicated electronic monitoring devices that are synced, in many cases wirelessly, to a computer or smartphone for long-term data tracking, an example of wearable technology. There are also independent smartphone and Facebook apps.

The term "activity trackers" now primarily refers to wearable devices that monitor and record a person's fitness activity. Electronic activity trackers are fundamentally upgraded versions of pedometers; in addition to counting steps, they use accelerometers and altimeters to calculate mileage, graph overall physical activity, calculate calorie expenditure, and in some cases also monitor and graph heart rate and quality of sleep. Some also include a silent alarm. Some newer models approach the U.S. definition of a Class II medical monitor, and some manufacturers hope to eventually make them capable of alerting to a medical problem, although FDA approval would be required.

Early versions such as the original Fitbit (2009), were worn clipped to the waist; formats have since diversified to include wristbands and armbands (smart bands) and smaller devices that can be clipped wherever preferred. Apple and Nike together developed the Nike+iPod, a sensor-equipped shoe that worked with an iPod Nano. In addition, logging apps exist for smartphones and Facebook; the Nike+ system now works without the shoe sensor, through the GPS unit in the phone. The forthcoming Apple Watch and some other smart watches offer activity tracker functions. In the U.S., BodyMedia has developed a disposable activity tracker to be worn for a week, which is aimed at medical and insurance providers and employers seeking to measure employees' fitness, and Jawbone's UP for Groups aggregates and anonymizes data from the company's wearable activity trackers and apps for employers. Other activity trackers are intended to monitor vital signs in the elderly, epileptics, and people with sleep disorders and alert a caregiver to a problem.

Earbuds and headphones are a better location for measuring some data, including core body temperature; Valencell has developed sensor technology for new activity trackers that take their readings at the ear rather than the wrist, arm, or waist.

Much of the appeal of activity trackers that makes them effective tools in increasing personal fitness comes from their making it into a game, and from the social dimension of sharing via social media and resulting rivalry. The device can serve as a means of identification with a community, which extends to broader participation.

Some users and reviewers remain ambivalent toward the technology, making the point that in such a "mirror" displaying one's identity, misrepresentations are problematic. All forms of life-logging also carry privacy implications. Social networks associated with activity trackers have led to breaches of privacy such as involuntary publication of sexual activity, and the potential for advertisers and health insurers to access private health data through the devices is a concern."

Current Producers and products:

- Basis (owned by Intel) - Basis Carbon Steel Edition
- Bomdic - Gomore
- Fitbit - Fitbit Flex, Fitbit One, Fitbit Zip, Fitbit Surge, Fitbit Charge (replacement for Fitbit Force, which was recalled because some users experienced skin irritation), Fitbit Charge HR
- Garmin - Garmin Vivofit
- Huawei - Huawei Talkband B1
- Jawbone - Jawbone UP, Jawbone UP24, Jawbone UP3
- LG Electronics - LifeBand Touch and heart-monitoring headphones
- Microsoft - Microsoft Band
- Misfit Wearables - Misfit Shine, Misfit Flash
- Nike - Nike+ FuelBand and Nike+ FuelBand SE
- Pivotal Corporation - Pivotal Tracker 1
- Polar Electro - Polar Loop
- Runtastic
- Samsung - Samsung Gear Fit
- Sony - Sony SmartBand SWR10, Sony SmartBand Talk SWR30
- Spire - Spire
- Withings - Withings Pulse O_2, Withings Pulse
- Nudge: an app dashboard for activity trackers
- Xiaomi: Xiaomi Mi Band

See this reference for an excellent review of fitness trackers by Joanna Stern of the *Wall Street Journal*:[440] *Review: Best Fitness Trackers to*

Get You Up Off the Couch. http://www.wsj.com/articles/review-best-fitness-trackers-to-get-you-up-off-the-couch-1418760813?mod=ST1.

Or, see this reference by Jill Duffy of *PC Magazine* for another review of fitness trackers:[441] *The Best Activity Trackers for Fitness.* http://www.pcmag.com/article2/0,2817,2404445,00.asp.

Supplements, Antioxidants, and Micronutrients

NOTE: It is important to get the right amount (not too little, and not too much), and it is worth mentioning that healthcare providers generally don't test blood or serum levels for most of the nutrients or medications discussed.

A 2013 study from the Canadian Institutes of Health Research estimated there are about 65,000 dietary supplements on the market consumed by more than 150 million Americans.

Before we discuss the particulars of supplements, antioxidants and micronutrients, please take a minute and review the two cautions listed below. The bottom line is: use common sense, and discuss any potential concerns with your healthcare provider. Let the buyer beware!

Caution 1

Supplements, Meds Can Be Dangerous Mix, according to a U.S. Food and Drug Administration (FDA), news release, Oct. 27, 2014:[442]

> "Taking vitamins or other dietary supplements along with medication can be dangerous, the U.S. Food and Drug Administration warns. Dietary supplements can alter the absorption and metabolism of prescription and over-the-counter medications, the FDA said. "Some dietary supplements may increase the effect of your medication, and other dietary supplements may decrease it," Robert Mozersky, a medical officer at the FDA, ex-

plained in an agency news release. For example, the supplement St. John's Wort can make birth control pills less effective, the FDA reported. Both the herbal supplement ginkgo biloba and vitamin E can thin blood. Mixing either supplement with the prescription blood thinner warfarin or aspirin could increase the risk of internal bleeding or stroke, the report said.

Dietary supplements are widely used in the United States. The U.S. Centers for Disease Control and Prevention's 2005-2008 National Health and Nutrition Examination Survey found that roughly 72 million people in the United States who are on a prescription medication also took some type of dietary supplement. Although many people take supplements to make sure they get proper nutrition, the FDA said there is no substitute for eating a healthy diet, and products labeled as "natural" or "herbal" are not necessarily harmless. "Natural does not always mean safe," Mozersky said. "This is particularly true for children," he added.

"Parents should know that children's metabolisms are so unique, that at different ages they metabolize substances at different rates. For kids, ingesting dietary supplements together with other medications make adverse events a real possibility," Mozersky explained.

People planning to have surgery should inform their doctor of every medication and supplement they use. It may be necessary to stop taking supplements a few weeks before an operation to avoid potentially serious changes in heart rate, blood pressure or bleeding risk, the FDA said.

Women who are pregnant or breast-feeding should also talk to their doctor about any supplements they take.

"The bottom line is, before you take any dietary supplement or medication – over-the-counter or prescription – discuss it with your health care professional," Mozersky said. The FDA added the following tips for consumers:

- Every time you visit the doctor, bring a list of all the dietary supplements and medications you take. This list should include dosages and frequency.

- Tell your doctor if your health has changed, including any recent illnesses, surgeries or other procedures. You should also tell your doctor if you are pregnant or breast-feeding."

Finding specific interactions can be difficult, however. In one instance, researchers reviewed the scientific literature for possible interactions that may occur between warfarin and fruit products. They concluded that, *"Although a number of case reports have been published that suggest warfarin has the potential to interact with several fruit products, it is difficult to determine their relevance, as scientific evidence is scarce.* Until further information is available, clinicians may want to encourage patients to consume cranberry products and grapefruit juice in small to moderate quantities and to inquire about the recent consumption of mangos, pomegranate juice, and avocados when taking a dietary history."[443]

Another researcher recently reported that, "The area of fruit juice-drug interaction has received wide attention with numerous scientific and clinical investigations performed and reported for scores of drugs metabolized by CYP3A4/CYP2C9 [specific liver enzymes that metabolize specific chemicals]. While grapefruit juice has been extensively studied with respect to its drug-drug interaction potential, numerous other fruit juices such as cranberry juice, orange juice, grape juice, pineapple juice and pomegranate juice have also been investigated for its potential to show drug-drug interaction of any clinical relevance. This review focuses on establishing any relevance for clinical drug-drug interaction potential with pomegranate juice, which has been shown to produce therapeutic benefits over a wide range of disease areas…In vitro and animal pharmacokinetic data support the possibility of CYP3A4/CYP2C9 inhibition by pomegranate juice; *however, the human relevance for drug-drug interaction was not established based on the limited case studies.*"[444]

Caution 2

According to an article posted February 3, 2015:[445]

> "Numerous store brand supplements aren't what their labels claim to be, an ongoing investigation of popular herbal supplements subjected to DNA testing has found, New York state's top law enforcement official said Tuesday. GNC, Target, Walmart and Walgreen Co. sold supplements that either couldn't be verified to contain the labeled substance or that contained ingredients not listed on the label, Attorney General Eric Schneiderman's office said.
>
> The supplements, including echinacea, ginseng, St. John's wort, garlic, ginkgo biloba and saw palmetto, were contaminated with substances including rice, beans, pine, citrus, asparagus, primrose, wheat, houseplant and wild carrot. In many cases, unlisted contaminants were the only plant material found in the product samples.
>
> *Overall, 21 percent of the test results from store brand herbal supplements contained DNA from the plants listed on the labels. The retailer with the poorest showing was Walmart, where 4 percent of the products tested showed DNA from the plants listed on the labels.*
>
> "This investigation makes one thing abundantly clear: The old adage 'buyer beware' may be especially true for consumers of herbal supplements," Schneiderman said.

Walmart spokesman, Brian Nick, said the company is immediately reaching out to suppliers and will take appropriate action. Walgreen and GNC pledged to cooperate with the attorney general. Target didn't initially respond to a request for comment. "We stand by the quality, purity and potency of all ingredients listed on the labels of our private label products," said GNC spokeswoman Laura Brophy.

The U.S. Food and Drug Administration (FDA) requires companies to verify their products are safe and properly labeled. But supplements aren't subjected to the rigorous evaluation process used for drugs. If a manufacturer fails to identify all the ingredients on an herbal product's label, a consumer with allergies or who is taking medication for an unrelated illness could risk serious health issues every time a contaminated herbal supplement is ingested.

Using DNA barcoding technology to examine the contents of herbal supplements, the attorney general's investigation is focused on what appears to be the practice of substituting contaminants and fillers in the place of authentic product, his office says. The investigation looked at six different herbal supplements sold at the four major retail companies in thirteen regions across the state, including Binghamton, Brooklyn, Buffalo, Harlem, Nassau County, Plattsburgh, Poughkeepsie, Rochester, Suffolk County, Syracuse, Utica, Watertown, and Westchester County.

The testing revealed that all of the retailers were selling a large percentage of supplements for which modern DNA barcode technology could not detect the labeled botanical substance. The DNA tests were performed on three to four samples of each of the six herbal supplements purchased from the New York stores. Each sample was tested with five distinct sequence runs, meaning each sample was tested five times. Three hundred and ninety tests involving 78 samples were performed overall.

Here are details on the tests for the four major retail companies:

GNC:

- Six "Herbal Plus" brand herbal supplements per store were purchased and analyzed: Gingko Biloba, St. John's Wort, Ginseng, Garlic, Echinacea, and Saw Palmetto. Purchased from four locations with representative stores in Binghamton, Harlem, Plattsburgh & Suffolk.
- Only one supplement consistently tested for its labeled contents: Garlic. One bottle of Saw Palmetto tested positive for containing DNA from the saw palmetto plant, while three others did not. The remaining four supplement types yielded mixed results, but none revealed DNA from the labeled herb.
- Of 120 DNA tests run on twenty-four bottles of the herbal products purchased, DNA matched label identification 22 percent of the time.
- Contaminants identified included asparagus, rice, primrose, alfalfa/clover, spruce, ranuncula, houseplant, allium, legume, saw palmetto, and Echinacea.

Target:

- Six "Up & Up" brand herbal supplements per store were purchased and analyzed: Gingko Biloba, St. John's Wort, Valerian Root, Garlic, Echinacea, and Saw Palmetto. Purchased from three locations with representative stores in Nassau County, Poughkeepsie, and Syracuse.
- Three supplements showed nearly consistent presence of the labeled contents: Echinacea (with one sample identifying

rice), Garlic, and Saw Palmetto. The remaining three supplements did not reveal DNA from the labeled herb.
- Of 90 DNA tests run on eighteen bottles of the herbal products purchased, DNA matched label identification 41 percent of the time.
- Contaminants identified included allium, French bean, asparagus, pea, wild carrot and saw palmetto.

Walgreens:

- Six "Finest Nutrition" brand herbal supplements per store were purchased and analyzed: Gingko Biloba, St. John's Wort, Ginseng, Garlic, Echinacea, and Saw Palmetto. Purchased from three locations with representative stores in Brooklyn, Rochester and Watertown.
- Only one supplement consistently tested for its labeled contents: Saw Palmetto. The remaining five supplements yielded mixed results, with one sample of garlic showing appropriate DNA. The other bottles yielded no DNA from the labeled herb.
- Of the 90 DNA test run on eighteen bottles of herbal products purchased, DNA matched label representation 18 percent of the time.
- Contaminants identified included allium, rice, wheat, palm, daisy, and dracaena (houseplant).

Walmart:

- Six "Spring Valley" brand herbal supplements per store were purchased and analyzed: Gingko Biloba, St. John's Wort, Ginseng, Garlic, Echinacea, and Saw Palmetto. Purchased from three geographic locations with representative stores in Buffalo, Utica and Westchester.
- None of the supplements tested consistently revealed DNA from the labeled herb. One bottle of garlic had a minimal showing of garlic DNA, as did one bottle of Saw Palmetto.

PREVENTION

> All remaining bottles failed to produce DNA verifying the labeled herb.
> - Of the 90 DNA test run on eighteen bottles of herbal products purchased, DNA matched label representation 4 percent of the time.
> - Contaminants identified included allium, pine, wheat/grass, rice mustard, citrus, dracaena (houseplant), and cassava (tropical tree root).
>
> U.S. Pharmacopeia provides independent third-party certification to drug and supplement manufacturers, who can then use the certification to assure consumers their products are genuine. But John Atwater, director of verification programs for the organization, said *less than one percent of herbal supplements carry the USP mark.*"

Following the above revelation, numerous state attorneys general have taken further action, as reported on April 2, 2015:[446]

> "GNC is one of several retail stores that are selling herbal products that do not contain the herbs listed on their labels. New York Attorney General Eric Schneiderman, who announced just this week that his office had reached a ground-breaking deal that calls for retail giant GNC to adopt tough new testing standards for its herbal products, isn't letting up on the supplement industry.
>
> Schneiderman and thirteen other attorneys generals sent a letter Thursday to congressional leaders asking for a "comprehensive inquiry" into the still largely unregulated industry. The letter also asked lawmakers to consider "a more robust oversight role" for the U.S. Food and Drug Administration.
>
> "When consumers take an herbal product, they should be able to do so with full knowledge of what is in that

product and confidence that every precaution was taken to ensure its authenticity and purity," Schneiderman said.

The letter from the bipartisan group, led by Schneiderman and Indiana's Republican Attorney General Greg Zoeller, cited a recent investigation conducted by the New York attorney general's office that concluded 80 percent of the herbal products it obtained from GNC, Target, Walgreens and Walmart did not contain any of the herbs listed on their labels. Many of the products, Schneiderman said, contained wheat, legumes and other ingredients dangerous to consumers with allergies. His office sent a letter to the retailers in early February demanding that they pull scores of herbal products from their shelves.

"The multi-billion dollar herbal supplements industry is built on the promise that its products will improve the health and well-being of those who use them," Schneiderman, Zoeller and the other attorneys general wrote in the letter to Sen. Jerry Moran (R-Kansas), the chairman of the Senate Commerce subcommittee responsible for consumer protection issues, Rep. Joe Pitts, chairman of the House Energy and Commerce health subcommittee, and other lawmakers. "Yet a current state investigation has raised serious concerns about the marketing and safety of the herbal supplements regularly consumed by millions of Americans."

Consumer advocates and other critics have called for greater regulation of the $33 billion-a-year supplement industry ever since Congress passed the Dietary Supplement Health and Education Act in 1994, which exempts manufacturers from the strict approval process the FDA requires for prescription drugs. DSHEA has given unscrupulous manufacturers the green light to sell adulterated and mislabeled products, the critics say.

Many athletes have blamed positive drug tests for steroids and other banned substances on tainted supplements, and while some of those claims are undoubtedly false, sports physicians and anti-doping experts say many of those positive tests were triggered by mislabeled or adulterated products. The heat stroke deaths of Baltimore Orioles pitcher Steve Bechler and Korey Stringer of the Minnesota Vikings were also linked to ephedra, an herbal product athletes used to boost energy and lose weight.

The AGs' letter said researchers have found high levels of mercury, lead, arsenic and other heavy metals in supplements.

"Products falsely identified as black cohosh — an herb commonly taken to reduce menopause symptoms — may have caused severe liver damage in certain women. And media reports have uncovered over-the-counter supplements, including those purporting to build muscle, aid weight loss, and reduce anxiety, that were secretly laced with dangerous prescription medications," the letter added.

Supplement-industry leaders ripped Schneiderman's testing method, claiming the DNA bar-code testing his office used was questionable. Many of the products tested are extracts that would not be expected to contain DNA from parent materials; DNA can also be damaged by heat during the manufacturing process, they said."

And the response from the companies involved in the investigation:[447]

"New York Attorney General Eric Schneiderman and thirteen other attorneys general sent a letter to congressional leaders Thursday asking for a "comprehensive inquiry" into the supplement industry. The request for a congressional investigation, first reported by the Daily News, also asked lawmakers to consider a "more robust oversight role" for the U.S. Food and Drug Administration, which oversees the industry.

Supplement industry leaders, not surprisingly, are unhappy. "This is just harassment at this point," Daniel Fabricant, chief executive officer of the Natural Products Alliance, told Nutra-Ingredients-USA. Steve Mister, of the Council for Responsible Nutrition, also issued a statement criticizing the letter and Schneiderman's ongoing focus on the supplement industry.

"It is unfortunate that the New York State Attorney General (NY AG) has spearheaded a request for Congress to spend taxpayers' money to 'launch a comprehensive congressional inquiry into the herbal supplements industry' when the industry is already amply regulated on a federal level by FDA and FTC. In fact, concerns raised in that letter about alleged widespread safety issues are not true, based on government's post-market surveillance system which demonstrates relatively few safety issues for these products, particularly in comparison to other industries regulated by FDA," Mister said.

Consumer advocates and other critics have called for greater regulation of the $33 billion-a-year supplement industry ever since Congress passed the Dietary Supplement Health and Education Act in 1994, which exempts manufacturers from the strict approval process the FDA requires for prescription drugs. DSHEA has given unscrupulous manufacturers the green light to sell adulterated and mislabeled products, the critics say.

The letter from the bipartisan group of attorneys general led by Schneiderman and Indiana's Republican Attorney General Greg Zoeller, cited a recent investigation conducted by the New York attorney general's office that concluded 80 percent of the herbal products it obtained from GNC, Target, Walgreens and Walmart did not contain any of the herbs listed on their labels. Many of the products, Schneiderman said, contained wheat, legumes and other ingredients dangerous to consumers with allergies. His office sent a letter to the retailers in early February demanding that they pull scores of herbal products from their shelves.

GNC infuriated industry leaders earlier this week by agreeing to a strict testing regimen on its herbal products. GNC's decision to agree to more intense testing that would be administered by the AG's office sets a bad precedent, supplement industry leaders say.

Supplement-industry leaders ripped Schneiderman's testing method, claiming the DNA bar-code testing his office used was questionable. Many of the products tested are extracts that would not be expected to contain DNA from parent materials; DNA can also be damaged by heat during the manufacturing process, they said. The industry executives have called on Schneiderman to release his test results and methodology."

Introduction

According to an article by Drs. Swaminathan and Jicha, published in the October 20, 2014 issue of the journal *Frontiers in Aging Neuroscience*, "A nutritional approach to prevent, slow, or halt the progression of disease is a promising strategy that has been widely investigated. *Much epidemiologic data suggests that nutritional intake may influence the development and progression of Alzheimer's dementia.* Modifiable, environmental causes of AD include potential metabolic derangements caused by dietary insufficiency and/or excess that may be corrected by nutritional supplementation and/or dietary modification. *Many nutritional supplements contain a myriad of health promoting constituents (anti-oxidants, vitamins, trace minerals, flavonoids, lipids, ...etc.) that may have novel mechanisms of action affecting cellular health and regeneration, the aging process itself, or may specifically disrupt pathogenic pathways in the development of AD.* Nutritional modifications have the advantage of being cost effective, easy to implement, socially acceptable and generally safe and devoid of significant adverse events in most cases."[448]

Reporting in the July 2014 issue of *Alzheimer's Dementia*, researchers noted their findings of a comprehensive review of the scientific literature on the nutrient status of patients with Alzheimer's disease compared to "normal controls." They concluded that, "Analysis showed significantly lower plasma [blood] levels of folate and vitamin A, vitamin B12, vitamin C, and vitamin E. No significant differences were observed for plasma levels of copper and iron...The lower plasma nutrient levels indicate that patients with AD have impaired systemic availability of several nutrients...*Given the potential role of nutrients in the pathophysiological processes of AD, the utility of nutrition may currently be underappreciated and offer potential in AD management*."[449]

In 2014, Dr. Olde Rikkert and colleagues, reported in the *Journal of Alzheimer's Disease* the results of their research comparing the nutritional status between mild Alzheimer's disease outpatients and healthy controls. They concluded that, "*In non-malnourished patients with very mild AD, lower levels of some micronutrients, a different fatty acid profile in erythrocyte [red blood cell] membranes and a slightly but significantly lower MNA [Mini Nutritional Assessment] screening score were observed. This suggests that subtle differences in nutrient status are present already in a very early stage of AD and in the absence of protein/energy malnutrition."*[450]

A link between Alzheimer's disease and an excess presence of oxygen free radicals[1] in the brain has frequently been reported. It is generally assumed that such oxidative stress and related cellular damage is caused by inflammatory changes in the brain and is consequent to amyloid deposition. A group of researchers report, *"Elevated oxidative stress in AD is an early causal event in the initiation and advancement of this disease. Oxidative stress can be decreased by enhancing antioxidant enzymes...and by dietary antioxidant chemicals."*[451] The researchers pointed out that studying the effects of individual antioxidants has limitations, and that studying combinations of antioxidants might be more appropriate.

Also in 2014, researchers noted that:[452]

> "Alzheimer's disease is a progressive neurodegenerative disorder, characterized by deposition of amyloid beta, neurofibrillary tangles, astrogliosis and microgliosis [inflammatory nerve cells], leading to neuronal dysfunction and loss in the brain. Bio- and histochemical evidence suggests a pivotal role of central and peripheral inflammation in its etiopathology, linked to the production of free radicals.
>
> *Numerous epidemiological studies support that the long-term use of non-steroidal anti-inflammatory drugs [NSAIDs, such as Aspirin and ibuprofen] is preventive*

---

[1]Free radicals play an important role in a number of biological processes. Many of these are necessary for life, such as the killing of bacteria by white blood cells. However, because of their reactivity, these same free radicals can participate in unwanted side reactions resulting in cell damage. Excessive amounts of these free radicals can lead to cell injury and death, which may contribute to many diseases such as cancer, stroke, myocardial infarction, diabetes, neurodegenerative disorders (e.g., Alzheimer's disease, Parkinson's disease, and so forth), and other diseases.

against AD, but these medications do not slow down the progression of the disease in already diagnosed patients. There are a number of studies focusing on traditional herbal medicines and small molecules (usually plant secondary metabolites) as potential anti-inflammatory drugs, particularly in respect to cytokine [inflammatory chemical] suppression. For instance, ω-3 polyunsaturated fatty acids and a number of polyphenolic phytochemicals have been shown to be effective against inflammation in animal and cell models. Some of these plant secondary metabolites have also been shown to possess antioxidant, anti-inflammatory, anti-amyloidogenic, neuroprotective, and cognition-enhancing effects. This review will provide an overview of the effects of catechins/proanthocyanidins from green tea, curcumin from turmeric, extracts enriched in bacosides from Brahmi (Bacopa monnieri), flavone glycosides from Ginkgo biloba, and ω-3 polyunsaturated fatty acids.

They do not only counteract one pathophysiological aspect of AD in numerous in vitro and in vivo studies of models of AD, but also ameliorate several of the above mentioned pathologies. The evidence suggests that increased consumption of these compounds might lead to a safe strategy to delay the onset of AD. The continuing investigation of the potential of these substances is necessary as they are promising to yield a possible remedy for this pervasive disease."

As is almost always the case in medical research, different researchers often find conflicting results. For example, reporting in 2014 in the journal *Aging* (Albany NY), a different group of researchers evaluated the effects of multiple antioxidants on cardiovascular health:[453]

"Dietary supplements are widely used for health purposes. However, little is known about the metabolic and cardiovascular effects of combinations of popular over-the-counter supplements, each of which has been shown to have anti-oxidant, anti-inflammatory and pro-longevity properties in cell culture or animal studies. This study was a 6-month randomized, single-blind controlled trial, in which fifty-six non-obese men and women, aged thirty-eight to fifty-five yrs., were assigned to a dietary supplement (SUP) group or control (CON) group, with a 6-month follow-up. The SUP group took ten dietary supplements each day (100 mg of resveratrol, a complex of 800 mg each of green, black, and white tea extract, 250 mg of pomegranate extract, 650 mg of quercetin, 500 mg of acetyl-l-carnitine, 600 mg of lipoic acid, 900 mg of curcumin, 1 g of sesamin, 1.7 g of cinnamon bark extract, and 1.0 g fish oil). Both the SUP and CON groups took a daily multivitamin/mineral supplement. The main outcome measures were arterial stiffness, endothelial [blood vessel wall] function, biomarkers of inflammation and oxidative stress, and cardiometabolic risk factors.

Twenty-four weeks of daily supplementation with ten dietary supplements did not affect arterial stiffness or endothelial function in non-obese individuals. These compounds also did not alter body fat measured by DEXA, blood pressure, plasma lipids, glucose, insulin, IGF-1, and markers of inflammation and oxidative stress. In summary, supplementation with a combination of popular dietary supplements has no cardiovascular or metabolic effects in non-obese relatively healthy individuals [after 6-months use]."

This study, once again, demonstrates that short-term use of most medications, nutrients, or supplements has no clear beneficial effects. However, these authors, as many researchers do, jump to the conclusion that the agents studied have no benefit whatsoever. What about the beneficial effects after ten or twenty years? No one studies that!

More words of caution from a different group of researchers:[454]

"Alzheimer's disease has become a health problem to societies worldwide affecting millions of people. AD normally ensues in middle and late life but its specific cause remains unknown. Besides amyloid-β deposition and hyperphosphorylated tau protein, increased production of reactive species (RS)[1] has also been described to be a hallmark in early steps of this disorder. Antioxidant therapy has received considerable attention over the last years as a promising approach to delay or slow the neurodegeneration progression in AD either by boosting the pool of endogenous [naturally occurring in the body] antioxidants (e.g. vitamins, coenzyme Q10 or melatonin) or by the intake of dietary antioxidants, such as phenolic compounds of flavonoid or non-flavonoid type. However, the majority of antioxidants studied so far have limited success in clinical trials, a fact that could be related to their poor distribution and with the inherent difficulties to cross the blood brain barrier and attain the target sites. Despite the evidence that different classes of antioxidants are neuroprotectants in vitro, the clinical data is not consistent. *Alzheimer's disease and antioxidant therapy is still an open question*: the research is far from the end but the success may not be so time-consuming if the data obtained so far are gathered and rationally analyzed either by checking new targets or by the development of new and effective compounds, for instance by the rational modification of the previous ones."

---

[1]Reactive oxygen species (ROS) are chemically reactive molecules containing oxygen. Examples include oxygen ions and peroxides. ROS are formed as a natural by-product of the normal metabolism of oxygen and have important roles in cell signaling and homeostasis. However, during times of environmental stress (e.g., UV or heat exposure), ROS levels can increase dramatically. This may result in significant damage to cell structures. Cumulatively, this is known as oxidative stress.

And, from study reported in 2012, researchers studied sixty-six individuals with mild to moderate Alzheimer's disease in order to evaluate whether antioxidant supplements presumed to target specific cellular compartments affected cerebrospinal fluid (CSF) biomarkers. They were random assignment to treatment for sixteen weeks with 800 IU/d of vitamin E (α-tocopherol) plus 500 mg/d of vitamin C plus 900 mg/d of α-lipoic acid (E/C/ALA); 400 mg of coenzyme Q 3 times/d; or placebo. The researchers found that, *"Study drugs were well tolerated, but accelerated decline in Mini-Mental State Examination [MMSE] scores occurred in the E/C/ALA group, a potential safety concern.* Changes in CSF Aβ42, tau, and P-tau(181) levels did not differ between the three groups. Cerebrospinal fluid F2-isoprostane levels, an oxidative stress biomarker, decreased on average by 19 percent from baseline to week sixteen in the E/C/ALA group but were unchanged in the other groups. Antioxidants did not influence CSF biomarkers related to amyloid or tau pathology. *Lowering of CSF F2-isoprostane levels in the E/C/ALA group suggests reduction of oxidative stress in the brain. However, this treatment raised the caution of faster cognitive decline, which would need careful assessment if longer-term clinical trials are conducted."*[455]

Still another group of researchers, reported the results of their systemic literature review of the evidence for an association between habitual dietary intake of antioxidants and cognition. They found that, "There were mixed findings for the association between antioxidant intake, cognition and risk of dementia and Alzheimer's disease...*Overall, findings do not consistently show habitual intakes of dietary antioxidants are associated with better cognitive performance or a reduced risk for dementia.* Future intervention trials are warranted to elucidate the effects of a high intake of dietary antioxidants on cognitive functioning, and to explore effects within a whole dietary pattern."[456]

However, reporting in the July 2014 issue of *Alzheimer's Dementia*, Dr. Lopes da Silva and colleagues reviewed the literature on the nutritional status of individuals with Alzheimer's disease. They found that, "*...analysis showed significantly lower plasma [blood] levels of folate and vitamin A, vitamin B12, vitamin C, and vitamin E,* whereas non-significantly lower levels of zinc and vitamin D were found in AD patients. No significant differences were observed for plasma levels of copper and iron...The lower plasma nutrient levels indicate that *patients with AD have impaired systemic availability of several nutrients.* This difference appears to be unrelated to the classic malnourishment that is well known to be common in AD, suggesting that compromised micronutrient status may precede protein and energy malnutrition. Contributing factors might be AD-related alterations in feeding behavior and intake, nutrient absorption, alterations in metabolism, and increased utilization of nutrients for AD pathology-related processes. Given the potential role of nutrients in the pathophysiological processes of AD, the utility of nutrition may currently be underappreciated and offer potential in AD management."[457]

And, in 2014, Dr. Mosconi and colleagues reported their findings examining the relationship between dietary nutrients and brain biomarkers of AD in cognitively normal individuals (NL) with and without AD risk factors. They studied forty-nine NL individuals (age 25-72 years, 69 percent women) with dietary information and PET scans. They found that, "...*higher intake of vitamin B12, vitamin D and ω-3 polyunsaturated fatty acid (PUFA) was associated with lower Aβ load in AD regions on PET...The identified nutrient combination was associated with higher intake of vegetables, fruit, whole grains, fish and legumes, and lower intake of high-fat dairies, meat and sweets. Our data provide a potential pathophysiological mechanism for epidemiological findings showing that dietary interventions may play a role in the prevention of AD.*"[458]

In 2014, researchers noted that, "In recent times, there have been major advancements in our understanding of various neurodegenerative disease [NDDs] states that have revealed common pathologic features or mechanisms. The many mechanistic parallels discovered between various neurodegenerative diseases [including Alzheimer's disease] suggest that a single therapeutic approach may be used to treat multiple disease conditions. *Of late, natural compounds and supplemental substances have become an increasingly attractive option to treat NDDs because there is growing evidence that these nutritional constituents*

PREVENTION

have potential adjunctive therapeutic effects (be it protective or restorative) on various neurodegenerative diseases. Here we review relevant experimental and clinical data on *supplemental substances (i.e., curcuminoids, rosmarinic acid, resveratrol, acetyl-L-carnitine, and ω-3 (n-3) polyunsaturated fatty acids) that have demonstrated encouraging therapeutic effects on chronic diseases, such as Alzheimer's disease* and neurodegeneration resulting from acute adverse events, such as traumatic brain injury."[459]

Remington and colleagues, reporting in the January 1, 2015 issue of the *Journal of Alzheimer's Disease*, note that, *"Increasing evidence points toward the efficacy of nutritional modifications in delaying cognitive decline and mood/behavioral difficulties in Alzheimer's disease. Nutritional supplementation with individual agents has shown varied results suggesting the need for combinatorial intervention.* We set out to determine whether nutritional intervention could positively impact cognitive performance and behavioral difficulties for individuals diagnosed with AD. A double-blind, multi-site, phase II study (ClinicalTrials.gov NCT01320527; Alzheimer's Association Trialmatch) was conducted in which 106 individuals with AD were randomized to a nutraceutical formulation (NF; folate, alpha-tocopherol, B12, S-adenosyl methioinine, N-acetyl cysteine, acetyl-L-carnitine) or placebo for three or six months, followed by an open-label extension where participants received NF for six additional months. The NF cohort improved versus the placebo cohort within three months...These findings extend phase I studies where *NF maintained or improved cognitive performance and mood/behavior.*"[460]

With regard to mitochondrial dysfunction and biogenesis, it was recently noted that:[461]

> "...mitochondrial biogenesis is not only produced in association with cell division. It can be produced in response to an oxidative stimulus, to an increase in the energy requirements of the cells, to exercise training, to electrical stimulation, to hormones, during development, in certain mitochondrial diseases, etc. Mitochondrial bi-

ogenesis is therefore defined as the process via which cells increase their individual mitochondrial mass. Recent discoveries have raised attention to mitochondrial biogenesis as a potential target to treat diseases which up to date do not have an efficient cure.

Mitochondria, as the major ROS [reactive oxygen species] producer and the major antioxidant producer exert a crucial role within the cell mediating processes such as apoptosis [cell death], detoxification, Ca2+ buffering, etc. This pivotal role makes mitochondria a potential target to treat a great variety of diseases. Mitochondrial biogenesis can be pharmacologically manipulated...other diseases in which mitochondrial dysfunction plays a very important role include neurodegenerative diseases [such as Alzheimer's disease], diabetes or cancer...Several pharmacological strategies...are the use of Sirt1 agonists [stimulators] such as quercetin or resveratrol. Other strategies currently used include the addition of antioxidant supplements to the diet (dietary supplementation with antioxidants) such as L-carnitine, coenzyme Q10, MitoQ10 and other mitochondria-targeted antioxidants, N-acetylcysteine (NAC), vitamin C, vitamin E, vitamin K1, vitamin B, sodium pyruvate or -lipoic acid.

As aforementioned, other diseases do not have exclusively a mitochondrial origin but they might have an important mitochondrial component both on their onset and on their development. This is the case of type 2 diabetes or neurodegenerative diseases. Type 2 diabetes is characterized by a peripheral insulin resistance accompanied by an increased secretion of insulin as a compensatory system. Among the explanations about the origin of insulin resistance...consider the hypothesis that mitochondrial dysfunction, e.g. impaired (mitochondrial) oxidative capacity of the cell or tissue, is one of the main underlying causes of insulin resistance and type 2 diabetes. Although this hypothesis is not free of controversy due to the uncertainty on the sequence of events during type 2 diabetes onset, e.g. whether mitochondrial dysfunction is the cause or the consequence of insulin resistance, it has been widely observed that improving mitochondrial function also improves insulin sensitivity and prevents type 2 diabetes.

Thus restoring oxidative capacity by increasing mitochondrial mass appears as a suitable strategy to treat insulin resistance. The effort made by researchers trying to understand the signaling pathways mediating mitochondrial biogenesis has uncovered new potential pharmacological targets and opens the perspectives for the design of suitable treatments for insulin resistance. In addition some of the currently used strategies could be used to treat insulin resistance, such as lifestyle interventions (caloric restriction and endurance exercise) and pharmacological interventions (thiazolidinediones and other PPAR agonists, resveratrol and other calorie restriction mimetics, AMPK activators, ERR activators).

Mitochondrial biogenesis is of special importance in modern neurochemistry because of the broad spectrum of human diseases arising from defects in mitochondrial ion and ROS homeostasis, energy production and morphology...Among them creatine, Coenzyme Q10 and mitochondrial targeted antioxidants/peptides are reported to have the most remarkable effects in clinical trials.

A common hallmark of several neurodegenerative diseases (Huntington's Disease, Alzheimer's Disease and Parkinson's Disease) is the impaired function or expression of PGC-1α, the master regulator of mitochondrial biogenesis. Among the promising strategies to ameliorate mitochondrial-based diseases these authors highlight the induction of PGC-1α via activation of PPAR receptors (rosiglitazone[1], bezafibrate[2]) or modulating its activity by AMPK (AICAR, metformin, resveratrol) or SIRT1 (SRT1720 and several isoflavone-derived compounds)."

In a brain cell experiment mimicking the conditions observed in neurodegenerative disorders, such as Alzheimer's disease, researchers found that, "...The latter effect, as well *as tau hyperphosphorylation [found in some neurodegenerative disorders, including AD], was prevented both by a mixture of antioxidant drugs (100 µM ascorbic acid [vitamin C], 10 µM trolox [vitamin E], 100 µM glutathione) and by the anti-Alzheimer drug, memantine, 20 µM.* ...The neurotoxic treatment depressed the neurosecretory function and *the mixture of antioxidant drugs, as well as memantine, were able to restore it.* The neuronal damage induced by the in vitro protocol adopted in the present work displays peculiarities of neurodegenerative disorders, e.g. Alzheimer's disease, *underlining the role of mitochondrial failure and oxidative*

---

[1]Rosiglitazone (Avandia), is an antidiabetic drug. It works as an insulin sensitizer, by binding to the PPAR receptors in fat cells and making the cells more responsive to insulin. It is marketed by the pharmaceutical company GlaxoSmithKline (GSK) as a stand-alone drug or for use in combination with metformin or with glimepiride. First released in 1999, annual sales peaked at approximately $2.5-billion in 2006; however, following a meta-analysis published in the New England Journal of Medicine in 2007 that linked the drug's use to an increased risk of heart attack, sales plummeted to just $9.5-million in 2012. The drug's patent expired in 2012. Despite rosiglitazone's effectiveness at decreasing blood sugar in type 2 diabetes mellitus, its use decreased dramatically as studies showed apparent associations with increased risks of heart attacks and death. Adverse effects alleged to be caused by rosiglitazone were the subject of over 13,000 lawsuits against GSK; as of July 2010, GSK had agreed to settlements on more than 11,500 of these suits.

[2]Bezafibrate (marketed as Bezalip and various other brand names) is a fibrate drug used for the treatment of hyperlipidemia. It helps to lower LDL cholesterol and triglyceride in the blood, and increase HDL. Studies show that in patients with impaired glucose tolerance, bezafibrate may delay progress to diabetes. Bezafibrate has been shown to reduce tau protein hyperphosphorylation [found in Alzheimer's disease] and other signs of tauopathy in transgenic mice having human tau mutation.

stress, which appear to occur upstream the neurodegenerative process."[462]

A (Vitamin A; Retinol; Retinal; and Retinoic Acid; and β-carotene)

Vitamin A is a group of unsaturated nutritional organic compounds, that includes retinol, retinal, retinoic acid, and several provitamin A carotenoids, among which beta-carotene is the most important. Vitamin A has multiple functions: it is important for growth and development, for the maintenance of the immune system and good vision. Vitamin A is needed by the retina of the eye in the form of retinal, which combines with protein opsin to form rhodopsin, the light-absorbing molecule necessary for both low-light (scotopic vision) and color vision. Vitamin A also functions in a very different role as retinoic acid (an irreversibly oxidized form of retinol), which is an important hormone-like growth factor for epithelial and other cells.

The deposition of amyloid β-protein (Aβ) in the brain is an invariant feature of Alzheimer's disease (AD). Vitamin A, which has been traditionally considered an anti-oxidant compound, plays a role in maintaining higher function in the central nervous system. *"Plasma or cerebrospinal fluid concentrations of vitamin A and β-carotene have been reported to be lower in AD patients, and these vitamins have been clinically shown to slow the progression of dementia. Vitamin A (retinol, retinal and retinoic acid) and β-carotene have been shown in in vitro studies to inhibit the formation, extension and destabilizing effects of β-amyloid fibrils.* Recently, the inhibition of the oligomerization of Aβ has been suggested as a possible therapeutic target for the treatment of AD. We have recently shown the inhibitory effects of vitamin A and β-carotene on the oligomerization of Aβ40 and Aβ42 in vitro. In previous in vivo studies, intraperitoneal injections of vitamin A decreased brain Aβ deposition and tau phosphorylation in transgenic mouse models of AD, attenuated neuronal degeneration, and improved spatial learning and memory. *Thus, vitamin A and β-carotene could be key molecules for the prevention and therapy of AD.*"[463]

ALZHEIMER'S DISEASE

Dr. Lerner and colleagues, from the Department of Neurology, University Hospitals Case Medical Center, Cleveland, OH, note that, "Retinoids are Vitamin A derivatives involved in cellular regulatory processes including cell differentiation, neurite [nerve cell] outgrowth and defense against oxidative stress. Retinoids may also influence Amyloid beta processing upregulation of alpha secretase via ADAM10. *Vitamin A and other retinoids also directly inhibit formation of Amyloid fibrils in vivo.* These properties of retinoids are relevant to theories of Alzheimer's disease pathogenesis. Retinoids are already used in treatment of acne vulgaris, psoriasis, neuroblastoma and acute promyelocytic leukemia. Clinical studies involving in cognitively impaired older adults with Alzheimer's disease are beginning with a variety of retinoids. These studies need to address safety issues of retinoids in older populations, and hold hope for demonstrating efficacy in translating these basic mechanisms to treatment of a widespread dementing illness."[464]

Recent studies have revealed that disruption of vitamin A signaling observed in Alzheimer's disease leads to beta-amyloid (Abeta) accumulation and memory deficits in rodents. In order to study this phenomenon further, Dr. Ding and colleagues, reporting in *The Journal of Neuroscience*, noted that, "The aim of the present study was to evaluate the therapeutic effect of all-trans retinoic acid (ATRA), an active metabolite of vitamin A, on the neuropathology and deficits of spatial learning and memory in amyloid precursor protein (APP) and presenilin 1 (PS1) double-transgenic mice, a well-established AD mouse model...*These results support ATRA as an effective therapeutic agent for the prevention and treatment of AD.* "[465]

In 2014, researchers noted that "Vitamin A and its derivatives, the retinoids, modulate several physiological and pathological processes through their interactions with nuclear retinoid receptor proteins termed as retinoic acid receptors (RARs) and retinoid X receptors (RXRs). An increasing body of evidence signifies the existence of retinoid signaling in diverse brain areas including cortex, amygdala, hypothalamus, hippocampus, and striatum suggesting its involvement in adult brain functions. *Defective retinoid signaling has been evidenced in the pathology of Alzheimer's disease.* Reports demonstrate that vitamin A deprived mice exhibit serious defects in spatial learning and memory signifying its importance in the maintenance of memory functions. *Retinoid signaling impacts the development of AD pathology through multiple pathways.* Ligand activation of RAR and RXR in APP/PS1 transgenic mice *ameliorated the symptoms of AD and reduced amyloid accumulation and tau hyperphosphorylation...*Through this review we summarize the biology of retinoids, *emphasizing their probable neuroprotective mechanisms that will help to elucidate the pivotal role of these receptors in AD pathology.*"[466]

Acetyl-L-carnitine

Age-related dementias such as Alzheimer's disease have been linked to vascular disorders like hypertension, diabetes and atherosclerosis. These risk factors cause ischemia, inflammation, and oxidative damage, which is largely due to reactive oxygen species (ROS) that are believed to induce mitochondrial damage. At higher concentrations, ROS can cause cell injury and death which occurs during the aging process, where oxidative stress is incremented due to an accelerated generation of ROS and a gradual decline in cellular antioxidant defense mechanisms. Neuronal mitochondria are especially vulnerable to oxidative stress due to their role in energy supply and use, causing a cascade of debilitating factors such as the production of giant and/or vulnerable young mitochondrion whose DNA has been compromised. *"Therefore, mitochondria specific antioxidants such as acetyl-L-carnitine and R-alphalipoic acid seem to be potential treatments for AD. They target the factors that damage mitochondria and reverse its effect, thus eliminating the imbalance seen in energy production and amyloid beta oxidation and making these antioxidants very powerful alternate strategies for the treatment of AD."*[467]

Researchers studied the efficacy, safety and tolerability of acetyl-L-carnitine (ALC) during a 12-week trial in patients with mild dementia caused by the Alzheimer's disease (AD) and vascular dementia (VD). ALC was administered in doses from 2250 to 3000 mg per day. The researchers found that, "The treatment effect of ALC was 2.8 times higher than in placebo-treated patients. The clinical improvement by CGI scores was significantly better in AD patients compared to VD and did not depend on the severity of baseline cognitive deficit. The drug was well-tolerated. *ALC can be recommended in the above mentioned doses for treatment of early stages of AD and VD.*"[468]

Alpha-lipoic Acid

Alpha-lipoic acid is a naturally occurring substance, essential for the function of different enzymes that take part in mitochondria's oxidative metabolism. It is believed that alpha-lipoic acid has many other biochemical functions as well. These actions have been shown in experimental studies emphasizing the use of alpha-lipoic acid as a potential therapeutic agent for many chronic diseases such as brain diseases and cognitive dysfunctions like Alzheimer's disease, obesity, nonalcoholic fatty liver disease, burning mouth syndrome, cardiovascular disease, hypertension, some types of cancer, glaucoma and osteoporosis. Many conflicting data have been found concerning the clinical use of alpha-lipoic acid in the treatment of diabetes and of diabetes-related chronic complications.[469]

Several clinical studies have shown Alzheimer's disease to be associated with disturbances in glucose metabolism, especially low brain glucose or hypometabolism. As reported in 2014, in the *Journal of Cerebral Blood Flow Metabolism*, researchers demonstrated that this hypometabolism can be partially or completely restored by lipoic acid feeding. The researchers concluded that, *"The ability of lipoic acid to restore glucose metabolism further substantiates its role in overcoming the hypometabolic state inherent in early stages of Alzheimer's disease."*[470]

Shinto and colleagues reported in 2014, in the *Journal Alzheimer's Disease,* on their research on the association of fish consumption and alpha lipoic acid and AD. They studied the effects of supplementation with omega-3 fatty acids alone (ω-3) or omega-3 plus alpha lipoic acid.

Thirty-nine AD subjects were randomized to one of three groups: 1) placebo, 2) ω-3, or 3) ω-3 + LA for a treatment duration of twelve months. They found that, *"The combination of ω-3 + LA slowed cognitive and functional decline in AD over 12 months.* Because the results were generated from a small sample size, further evaluation of the combination of omega-3 fatty acids plus alpha-lipoic acid as a potential treatment in AD is warranted."[471]

In another animal model of AD, researchers studied the concentrations of lipoic acid and related compounds in brain tissue. The concluded that, "This study is consonant with the notion that *lipoic acid supplementation could be a potential treatment for the observed loss of cellular energetics in AD and potentiate the antioxidant defense system to prevent or delay the oxidative stress in and progression of this devastating dementing disorder.*"[472]

Ascorbic Acid (Vitamin C)

Ascorbic acid is a naturally occurring organic compound with antioxidant properties. Because it is derived from glucose, many animals are able to produce it, but humans require it as part of their nutrition. From the middle of the 18th century, it was noted that lemon and lime juice could help prevent sailors from developing scurvy. The newly discovered food-factor was eventually called vitamin C.

According to Dr. Heo and colleagues, "Oxidative stress is suggested to play a major role in the pathogenesis of Alzheimer's disease. Among the antioxidants, vitamin C has been regarded as the most important one in neural tissue. It also decreases β-amyloid generation and acetylcholinesterase activity and prevents endothelial dysfunction by regulating nitric oxide, a newly discovered factor in the pathogenesis and progression of AD. However, *clinical trials using antioxidants, including vitamin C, in patients with AD yielded equivocal results.*"[473]

Clinical trials using antioxidants, including vitamin C, in patients with AD yielded equivocal (some positive, some negative) results. For example, researchers studied the effects of vitamin C (1,000 mg/day) and E (400 I.U./day) in patients with AD, over a period of one year. While the researchers were able to demonstrate a "significant" increase in these vitamins in the cerebrospinal fluid (CSF), *"The clinical course of AD did not significantly differ between the vitamin and the control group. We conclude that supplementation with vitamins E and C did not have a significant effect on the course of AD over one year despite of a limited antioxidant effect that could be observed in CSF."*[474] This is more evidence that prevention is much more effective and powerful than attempts at curing the disease, through the use of medications, vitamins, nutrition, or supplements.

However, in 2014 and for the first time, in a unique animal model of Alzheimer's disease, researchers were able to demonstrate the powerful protective effects of vitamin C against Alzheimer's disease pathology. They studied both low and high dose administration of vitamin C. They report, "Blood-brain barrier (BBB) breakdown and mitochondrial dysfunction have been implicated in the pathogenesis of AD. Besides vitamin C being one of the important antioxidants, recently, it has also been reported as a modulator of BBB integrity and mitochondria morphology. Plasma levels of vitamin C are decreased in AD patients, which can affect disease progression. *We found that the higher supplementation of vitamin C had reduced amyloid plaque burden in the brain, resulting in amelioration of BBB disruption and mitochondrial alteration. These results suggest that intake of a larger amount of vitamin C could be protective against AD-like pathologies."*[475]

Ashwagandha (Withania somnifera)

According to wikipedia.com: *Withania somnifera*, known commonly as *ashwagandha*, Indian ginseng, poison gooseberry, or winter cherry, is a plant in the Solanaceae or nightshade family. It is used as an herb in Ayurvedic medicine. In Ayurveda, the berries and leaves are applied externally to tumors, tubercular glands, carbuncles, and ulcers. The roots are used to prepare the herbal remedy *ashwagandha*, which has been traditionally used for various symptoms and conditions. Double-blind, placebo-controlled studies on humans have found the remedy to be effective at a number of health-related uses, including anxiety treatment, neuroprotection, long-term memory, anaerobic running endurance, and bodily regulation of cholesterol, cortisol, and C-reactive protein. Benefits were seen in healthy as well as non-healthy patients.

Dr. Kuboyanna and colleagues, reporting in 2014 in the journal *Biological & Pharmaceutical Bulletin,* note that, "Neurodegenerative diseases commonly induce irreversible destruction of central nervous system (CNS) neuronal networks, resulting in permanent functional impairments. Effective medications against neurodegenerative diseases are currently lacking. Ashwagandha (roots of Withania somnifera Dunal) is used in traditional Indian medicine (Ayurveda) for general debility, consumption, nervous exhaustion, insomnia, and loss of memory."[476]

Dr. Vareed and colleagues, from the Department of Biochemistry and Molecular Biology and Cancer Center, Medical College of Georgia, Augusta, GA, reported in August 2014 issue of *Phytotherapy Research* that, "The neuroprotective effect of Withania somnifera L. Dunal fruit extract, in rodent models, is known. Withanamides, the primary active constituents in W.somnifera fruit extract exhibited neuroprotective effects against β-amyloid-induced cytotoxicity in neuronal cell culture studies."[477]

Dr. Sehgal and colleagues, from the Division of Molecular and Cellular Neuroscience, National Brain Research Centre, Nainwal Mode, Manesar, Haryana, India, reported the results of their research on the effects of Ashwagandha in an animal model of Alzheimer's disease, in the *Proceedings of the National Academy of Sciences (USA)*. The researchers found that:[478]

> "A 30-d course of oral administration of a semi-purified extract of the root of Withania somnifera consisting predominantly of withanolides and withanosides reversed behavioral deficits, plaque pathology, accumulation of β-amyloid peptides (Aβ) and oligomers in the brains of middle-aged and old APP/PS1 Alzheimer's disease

transgenic mice. It was similarly effective in reversing behavioral deficits and plaque load in APPSwInd mice (line J20). The temporal sequence involved an increase in plasma Aβ and a decrease in brain Aβ monomer after 7 d, indicating increased transport of Aβ from the brain to the periphery. Enhanced expression of low-density lipoprotein receptor-related protein (LRP) in brain micro-vessels and the Aβ-degrading protease neprilysin (NEP) occurred 14-21 d after a substantial decrease in brain Aβ levels. However, significant increase in liver LRP and NEP occurred much earlier, at 7 d, and were accompanied by a rise in plasma sLRP, a peripheral sink for brain Aβ. In WT mice, the extract induced liver, but not brain, LRP and NEP and decreased plasma and brain Aβ, indicating that increase in liver LRP and sLRP occurring independent of Aβ concentration could result in clearance of Aβ...*The remarkable therapeutic effect of W. somnifera mediated through up-regulation of liver LRP indicates that targeting the periphery offers a unique mechanism for Aβ clearance and reverses the behavioral deficits and pathology seen in Alzheimer's disease models."*

Researchers, reported in *The Journal of Biomolecular Structure and Dynamics*:[479]

"Alzheimer's disease, a neurodegenerative disorder, is the most common cause of dementia. So far only five drugs have been approved by U.S. FDA that temporarily slow worsening of symptoms for about six to twelve months. The limited number of therapeutic options for AD drives the exploration of new drugs. Enhancement of the central cholinergic function by the inhibition of acetylcholinesterase is a prominent clinically effective approach for the treatment of AD. *Recently withanolide A, a secondary metabolite from the ayurvedic plant Withania somnifera has shown substantial neuro-*

protective ability. The present study is an attempt to elucidate the cholinesterase inhibition potential of withanolide A along with the associated binding mechanism...The study provides evidence for consideration of withanolide A as a valuable small ligand molecule in treatment and prevention of AD associated pathology."

Dr. Jayaprakasam and colleagues, from the Bioactive Natural Products and Phytoceuticals, Department of Horticulture and National Food Safety and Toxicology Center, Michigan State University, East Lansing, Michigan, reporting in the journal *Phytotherapy Research*, note that:[480]

"Alzheimer's disease is an irreversible neurodegenerative disorder with symptoms of confusion, memory loss, and mood swings. The beta-amyloid peptide, with 39-42 amino acid residues (BAP), plays a significant role in the development of AD. Although there is no cure for AD, it can be managed with available drugs to some degree. Several studies have revealed that natural antioxidants, such as vitamin E, vitamin C and beta-carotene, may help in scavenging free radicals generated during the initiation and progression of this disease. Therefore, there has been considerable interest in plant phytochemicals with antioxidant property as potential agents to prevent the progression of AD.

Our earlier investigations of the Withania somnifera fruit afforded lipid peroxidation inhibitory withanamides that are more potent than the commercial antioxidants. In this study, we have tested two major withanamides A (WA) and C (WC) for their ability to protect the PC-12 cells, rat neuronal cells, from beta-amyloid induced cell damage. *The cell death caused by beta-amyloid was negated by withanamide treatment. Molecular modeling studies showed that withanamides A and C uniquely bind to the active motif of beta-*

amyloid (25-35) and suggest that withanamides have the ability to prevent the fibril formation."

B Vitamins

Despite B vitamin supplementation playing an important role in cognitive function, the exact effect remains unknown. In order to shed light on this question, Li and colleagues reviewed the scientific literature in 2014, with the aim of understanding the effectiveness of treatment with vitamins B supplementation in slowing the rate of cognitive, behavioral, functional and global decline in individuals with mild cognitive impairment (MCI) or Alzheimer's disease (AD). *The analysis showed a moderate beneficial effect of vitamins B supplementation on memory, but no significant benefit on general cognitive function, executive function and attention were found in MCI patients.* In addition, no significantly cognitive benefits were observed in AD patients. The authors concluded, "Collectively, weak evidence of benefits was observed for the domains of memory in patients with MCI. Nevertheless, future standard clinical trials are still needed to determine whether it was still significant in larger populations. However, the data does not yet provide adequate evidence of an effect of vitamins B on general cognitive function, executive function and attention in people with MCI. Similarly, folic acid alone or vitamins B in combination are unable to stabilize or slow decline in cognition, function, behavior, and global change of AD patients."[481]

A significant portion of our risk for dementia in old age is associated with lifestyle factors (diet, exercise, and cardiovascular health) that are modifiable, at least in principle. One such risk factor, high-*homocysteine levels* in the blood, is known to increase risk for Alzheimer's disease and vascular disorders. Homocysteine has been associated with cognitive impairment and various psychiatric symptoms. It is a non-protein α-amino acid. Homocysteine can be changed into methionine or converted into cysteine with the aid of certain B-vitamins. A high level of homocysteine in the blood (hyperhomocysteinemia) makes a person more prone to endothelial cell (cells which line the walls of blood vessels) injury, which leads to inflammation in the blood vessels, which in turn may lead to atherogenesis, which can result in ischemic injury. Hyperhomocysteinemia is therefore a possible risk factor for coronary artery disease and/or dementia. It appears that there is a critical level of brain shrinkage, possibly mediated by elevated homocysteine, which when reached, results in cognitive decline, especially in episodic memory performance.[482]

Epidemiological and clinical studies indicate that elevated circulating level of homocysteine is a risk factor for developing Alzheimer's disease. *Dietary deficiency of folate, vitamin B6 and B12 results in a significant increase of homocysteine levels.* Researchers used an animal model of AD to study the relationship between B vitamins and folate levels and the pathology associated with AD. They found that animals who received the diet deficient for folate, B6 and B12 developed increase of homocysteine levels. This condition was associated with a significant increase in Abeta levels and deposits in specific areas of the brain associated with memory. The authors concluded that, *"Our findings further support the concept that dietary factors can contribute to the development of AD neuropathology."*[483]

In order to clarify whether a relationship exists between the serum levels of homocysteine and the behavioral and psychological symptoms of dementia, researchers studied patients with Alzheimer's disease (n=77) and control subjects (n=37). The patients' serum homocysteine, folate, and vitamin B12 levels were measured. *"Patients with Alzheimer's disease had statistically significantly higher serum homocysteine levels compared to the control subjects. Mean serum folate and vitamin B12 concentration were significantly lower in patients with Alzheimer's disease compared to control subjects."*[484]

In late 2014, Dr. Madsen and colleagues from the Department of Neurology, Imaging Genetics Center, Institute for Neuroimaging and Informatics, Keck School of Medicine, University of Southern California, Los Angeles, CA, reported on the results of brain magnetic resonance imaging (MRI) in 803 elderly subjects from the Alzheimer's disease Neuroimaging Initiative data set. They wanted to understand how homocysteine levels relate to cortical gray matter distribution (thickness, volume, and surface area). They found that *individuals with higher blood levels of homocysteine had lower gray matter thickness in multiple areas, as well as lower gray matter volumes* after controlling for diagnosis, age, and sex. They concluded that, "These regional differences in gray matter structure may be useful biomarkers to assess the effectiveness of interventions, such as vitamin B supplements, that aim to prevent homocysteine-related brain atrophy by normalizing homocysteine levels."[485]

Researchers conducted a two-year study of 266 individuals, aged 70 or older, with mild cognitive impairment (MCI). One half received a daily dose of 0.8 mg folic acid, 0.5 mg vitamin B_{12} and 20 mg vitamin B_6. *The researchers previously showed that homocysteine-lowering treatment with B vitamins slows the rate of brain atrophy in mild cognitive impairment (MCI).* Here they report the effect of B vitamins on cognitive and clinical decline in the same study. They found that the average blood homocysteine level was 30 percent lower in those treated with B vitamins relative to placebo. They concluded, "In this small intervention trial, *B vitamins appear to slow cognitive and clinical decline in people with MCI, in particular in those with elevated homocysteine.* Further trials are needed to see if this treatment will slow or prevent conversion from MCI to dementia."[486]

B12 (Vitamin B12)

The term B_{12} may be properly used to refer to cyanocobalamin, the principal B_{12} form used for foods and in nutritional supplements.

Vitamin B_{12}, also called cobalamin, is a water-soluble vitamin with a key role in the normal functioning of the brain and nervous system, and for the formation of blood. It is one of the eight B vitamins. It is normally involved in the metabolism of every cell of the human body, especially affecting DNA synthesis and regulation, but also fatty acid metabolism and amino acid metabolism. Neither fungi, plants, nor animals are capable of producing vitamin B_{12}. Only bacteria and archaea have the enzymes required for its synthesis, although many foods are a natural source of B_{12} because of bacterial symbiosis. The vitamin is the largest and most structurally complicated vitamin and can be produced industrially only through bacterial fermentation-synthesis.

The dietary reference intake for an adult ranges from 2 to 3 µg per day (US), and 1.5 µg per day (UK). But according to a new study, the DRI should be 4 to 7 µg per day. The Center for Food Safety and Applied Nutrition recommends 6 µg per day, based on a caloric intake of 2,000 calories, for adults and children four or more years of age.

Vitamin B_{12} is believed to be safe when used orally in amounts that do not exceed the recommended dietary allowance (RDA). There have been studies that showed no adverse consequences of doses above the RDA. The RDA for vitamin B_{12} in pregnant women is 2.6 µg per day and 2.8 µg during lactation periods. There is insufficient reliable information available about the safety of consuming greater amounts of vitamin B_{12} during pregnancy.

Vitamin B_{12} is found in most animal derived foods, including fish and shellfish, meat (especially liver), poultry, eggs, milk, and milk products. However, the binding capacity of egg yolks and egg whites is markedly diminished after heat treatment.

The Institute of Medicine states that because 10 to 30 percent of older people may be unable to absorb naturally occurring vitamin B_{12} in foods, it is advisable for those 51 years old and older to consume B_{12}-fortified foods or B_{12} supplements to meet the recommended intake.

Vitamin B_{12} deficiency can potentially cause severe and irreversible damage, especially to the brain and nervous system. At levels only slightly lower than normal, a range of symptoms such as fatigue, depression, and poor memory may be experienced. Vitamin B_{12} deficiency can also cause symptoms of mania and psychosis.

Vitamin B_{12} has extremely low toxicity, and even taking enormous doses does not appear to be harmful to healthy individuals.

- H$_2$-receptor antagonists: include cimetidine (Tagamet), famotidine (Pepcid), nizatidine (Axid), and ranitidine (Zantac). Reduced secretion of gastric acid and pepsin produced by H$_2$ blockers can reduce absorption of protein-bound (dietary) vitamin B$_{12}$, but not of supplemental vitamin B$_{12}$. Gastric acid is needed to release vitamin B$_{12}$ from protein for absorption. Clinically significant vitamin B$_{12}$ deficiency and megaloblastic anemia are unlikely, unless H$_2$ blocker therapy is prolonged (two years or more), or the person's diet is poor. It is also more likely if the person is rendered achlorhydric (with complete absence of gastric acid secretion), which occurs more frequently with proton pump inhibitors than H$_2$ blockers. Vitamin B$_{12}$ levels should be monitored in people taking high doses of H$_2$ blockers for prolonged periods.

- Metformin (Glucophage): Metformin may reduce serum folic acid and vitamin B$_{12}$ levels. Long-term use of metformin substantially increases the risk of B$_{12}$ deficiency and (in those patients who become deficient) hyperhomocysteinemia, which is "an independent risk factor for cardiovascular disease, especially among individuals with type 2 diabetes." There are also rare reports of megaloblastic anemia in people who have taken metformin for five years or more. Reduced serum levels of vitamin B$_{12}$ occur in up to 30 percent of people taking metformin chronically. However, clinically significant deficiency is not likely to develop if dietary intake of vitamin B$_{12}$ is adequate. Deficiency can be corrected with vitamin B$_{12}$ supplements even if metformin is continued. The metformin-induced malabsorption of vitamin B$_{12}$ is reversible by oral calcium supplementation. The general clinical significance of metformin upon B$_{12}$ levels is as yet unknown..

- Proton pump inhibitors (PPIs): The PPIs include omeprazole (Prilosec, Losec), lansoprazole (Prevacid), rabeprazole (Aciphex), pantoprazole (Protonix, Pantoloc), and esomeprazole (Nexium). The reduced secretion of gastric acid and pepsin produced by PPIs can reduce absorption of protein-bound (dietary) vitamin B_{12}, but not supplemental vitamin B_{12}. Gastric acid is needed to release vitamin B_{12} from protein for absorption. Reduced vitamin B_{12} levels may be more common with PPIs than with H2-blockers, because they are more likely to produce achlorhydria (complete absence of gastric acid secretion). However, clinically significant vitamin B_{12} deficiency is unlikely, unless PPI therapy is prolonged (two years or more) or dietary vitamin intake is low. Vitamin B_{12} levels should be monitored in people taking high doses of PPIs for prolonged periods.

Getting B12 shots in California is all the rage now, especially in dermatologist's offices and spas. No appointment necessary, just walk in and request a shot. Advertised for weight loss and energy, and much more. Or, just go to TheShotBar.com, with physical locations in southern California. While we don't recommend B12 shots (or any other injections for general health), we do recommend taking supplemental oral B12. Let's see why...

According to one group of researchers, "Vitamin B12 is a cofactor of methionine synthase in the synthesis of methionine, the precursor of the universal methyl donor S-Adenosylmethionine (SAMe), which is involved in different epigenomic regulatory mechanisms and especially in brain development. A Vitamin B12 deficiency expresses itself by a wide variety of neurological manifestations such as paresthesias, skin numbness, coordination disorders and reduced nerve conduction velocity. *In elderly people, a latent Vitamin B12 deficiency can be associated with a progressive brain atrophy. Moderately elevated concentrations of homocysteine (>10 μmol/L) have been associated with an increased risk of dementia, notably Alzheimer's disease, in many cross-sectional and prospective studies.* Raised plasma concentrations of homocysteine is also associated with both regional and whole brain atrophy, not only in Alzheimer's disease but also in healthy elderly people. *Clinician awareness should be raised to accurately diagnose and treat early Vitamin B12 deficiency to prevent irreversible structural brain damage".*[487]

Other researchers report, "The advent of sensitive diagnostic tests, including homocysteine and methylmalonic acid assays, has revealed *a surprisingly high prevalence of a more subtle 'subclinical' form of B12 deficiency, particularly within the elderly. This is often associated with cognitive impairment and dementia, including Alzheimer's disease.* Metabolic evidence of B12 deficiency is also reported in association with other neurodegenerative disorders including vascular dementia, Parkinson's disease and multiple sclerosis. These conditions are all associated with chronic neuro-inflammation and oxidative stress. It is possible that these clinical associations reflect compromised vitamin B12 metabolism due to such stress."[488]

Reporting in 2014 in the *Journal of Alzheimer's Disease*, Dr. Moore and colleagues note that, *"Folate fortification of food aims to reduce the number of babies born with neural tube defects[1], but has been associated with cognitive impairment when vitamin B12 levels are deficient.* Given the prevalence of low vitamin B12 levels among the elderly, and the global deployment of food fortification programs, investigation of the associations between cognitive impairment, vitamin B12, and folate are needed. To investigate the associations of serum vitamin B12, red cell folate, and cognitive impairment, data were collected on 1,354 subjects in two studies investigating cognitive impairment. Subjects with stroke or neurodegenerative diseases other than Alzheimer's disease were excluded. Participants with low serum vitamin B12 (<250 pmol/L) and high red cell folate (>1,594 nmol/L) levels were more likely to have impaired cognitive performance when compared to participants with biochemical measurements that were within the normal

---

[1]Neural tube defects (NTDs) is an opening in the spinal cord or brain that occurs very early in human development. In the 3rd week of pregnancy called gastrulation, specialized cells on the dorsal side of the fetus begin to change shape and form the neural tube. When the neural tube does not close completely, an NTD develops. NTDs are one of the most common birth defects, affecting over 300,000 births globally each year. For example, **spina bifida** affects approximately 1,500 births annually in the USA, or about 3.5 in every 10,000 (0.035 percent of US births), which has decreased from around 5 per 10,000 (0.05 percent of U.S. births) since folate fortification was instituted.

ranges. *Participants with high folate levels, but normal serum vitamin B12, were also more likely to have impaired cognitive performance. High folate or folic acid supplements may be detrimental to cognition in older people with low vitamin B12 levels.*"[489]

In a study by Dr. Aisen and colleagues, reported in *the Journal of the American Medical Association (JAMA)*, the authors note, "Blood levels of homocysteine may be increased in Alzheimer disease (AD) and hyperhomocysteinemia may contribute to disease pathophysiology by vascular and direct neurotoxic mechanisms. Even in the absence of vitamin deficiency, homocysteine levels can be reduced by administration of high-dose supplements of folic acid and vitamins B(6) and B(12). To determine the efficacy and safety of B vitamin supplementation in the treatment of AD, a multicenter, randomized, double-blind controlled clinical trial of high-dose folate, vitamin B(6), and vitamin B(12) supplementation in 409 individuals with mild to moderate AD and normal folic acid, vitamin B(12), and homocysteine levels was conducted. Participants were randomly assigned to two groups of unequal size to increase enrollment (60 percent treated with high-dose supplements [5 mg/d of folate, 25 mg/d of vitamin B(6), 1 mg/d of vitamin B(12)] and 40 percent treated with identical placebo); duration of treatment was eighteen months. Although the vitamin supplement regimen was effective in reducing homocysteine levels in the active treatment group vs in the placebo group, it had no beneficial effect on the primary cognitive measure. A higher quantity of adverse events involving depression was observed in the group treated with vitamin supplements. *This regimen of high-dose B vitamin supplements does not slow cognitive decline in individuals with mild to moderate AD.*"[490] This study once again demonstrates that once AD is present, few interventions are beneficial. An ounce of prevention is worth a pound of cure.

Dr. Moore and colleagues reviewed the literature on the associations between low vitamin B12 levels, neurodegenerative disease, and cognitive impairment. The potential impact of comorbidities and medications associated with vitamin B12 derangements were also investigated. In addition, the researchers also reviewed the evidence as to whether vitamin B12 therapy is efficacious for cognitive impairment and dementia. They found that, *"Vitamin B12 levels in the subclinical low-normal range (<250 pmol/L) are associated with Alzheimer's disease, vascular dementia, and Parkinson's disease. Vegetarianism and metformin use contribute to depressed vitamin B12 levels and may independently increase the risk for cognitive impairment. Vitamin B12 deficiency (<150 pmol/L) is associated with cognitive impairment. Vitamin B12 supplements administered orally or parenterally at high dose (1 mg daily) were effective in correcting biochemical deficiency, but improved cognition only in patients with pre-existing vitamin B12 deficiency (serum vitamin B12 levels <150 pmol/L or serum homocysteine levels >19.9 µmol/L)."*[491]

Berberine

As a Chinese traditional medicine or dietary supplement, berberine has shown some activity against fungal infections, *Candida albicans*, yeast, parasites, and bacterial/viral infections. Berberine seems to exert synergistic effects with fluconazole even in drug-resistant *C. albicans* infections. Some research has been undertaken into possible use against MRSA infection. Berberine is considered an antibiotic. When applied *in vitro* and in combination with methoxyhydnocarpin, an inhibitor of multidrug resistance pumps, berberine inhibits growth of *Staphylococcus aureus* and *Microcystis aeruginosa*. Berberine prevents and suppresses proinflammatory cytokines, E-selectin, and genes, and increases adiponectin expression, which partly explains its versatile health effects.

Berberine seems to act as an herbal antidepressant and a neuroprotector against neurodegenerative disorders (including Alzheimer's disease). As berberine is a natural compound that has been safely administered to humans, preliminary results suggest the initiation of clinical trials in patients with depression, bipolar affective disorder, schizophrenia, or related diseases in which cognitive capabilities are affected, with either the extract or pure berberine.

PREVENTION

New experimental results suggest berberine may have a potential for inhibition and prevention of Alzheimer's disease, mainly through both cholinesterase (ChEs) inhibitory and β-amyloids pathways, and additionally through antioxidant capacities.

Studies have shown berberine to increase noradrenaline and serotonin levels in the brain (rats) while inhibiting dopaminergic activity. The half-life of berberine *in vivo* seems to be three to four hours, thus suggesting administration three times a day if steady levels are to be achieved.

According to a research report published in 2014, "Berberine is a primary component of the most functional extracts of Coptidis rhizome used in traditional Chinese medicine for centuries. *Recent reports indicate that Berberine has the potential to prevent and treat Alzheimer's disease*. Without discussing the details of the research, the authors concluded that, *"Our findings also suggest that Berberine may be a potential therapeutic drug for AD."*[492]

Dr. Jia and colleagues summarized the results of their research on the potential benefits of Berberine in Alzheimer's disease, in the *Journal of Pharmacy and Pharmacology* by stating, "The neuroinflammation induced by amyloid-beta peptide (Aβ) is one of the key events in Alzheimer's disease progress in which microglia are the main cells involved. Berberine, one of the major constituents of Chinese herb Rhizoma coptidis, is known for its anti-inflammatory, anti-oxidative and anti-microbial activity. In this study, we examined the effects and possible underlying mechanisms of berberine in Aβ-induced neuroinflammation...*Our data indicated berberine is a potent suppressor of neuroinflammation,* presumably through inhibition of NF-κB activation, *and suggested berberine has therapeutic potential for the treatment of neuroinflammation that is involved in neurological diseases such as AD."*[493]

Berberine also has some powerful longevity properties. See the section below, Longevity: Berberine.

Black Pepper

Black pepper (*Piper nigrum*) is a flowering vine in the family Piperaceae, cultivated for its fruit, which is usually dried and used as a spice and seasoning. The fruit, known as a peppercorn when dried, is approximately 5 millimeters (0.20 in) in diameter, dark red when fully mature, and, like all drupes, contains a single seed. Peppercorns, and the ground pepper derived from them, may be described simply as pepper, or more precisely as black pepper (cooked and dried unripe fruit), green pepper (dried unripe fruit) and white pepper (ripe fruit seeds).

Black pepper is native to south India, and is extensively cultivated there and elsewhere in tropical regions. Currently Vietnam is the world's largest producer and exporter of pepper, producing 34 percent of the world's *Piper nigrum* crop as of 2008. Dried ground pepper has been used since antiquity for both its flavor and as a traditional medicine. Black pepper is the world's most traded spice.

Researchers studied the effect of piperine, a main active alkaloid in fruit of Piper nigrum, on memory performance and neurodegeneration in an animal model of Alzheimer's disease. The researchers noted, "Results showed that *piperine at all dosage range used in this study significantly improved memory impairment and neurodegeneration in [the] hippocampus.* The possible underlying mechanisms might be partly associated with the decreased lipid peroxidation and acetylcholinesterase enzyme."[494]

Carotenoids (Including Lycopene, Lutein and Zeaxanthin)

Carotenoids are organic pigments that are found in the chloroplasts and chromoplasts of plants and some other photosynthetic organisms, including some bacteria and some fungi. There are over 600 known carotenoids. In humans, three carotenoids (beta-carotene, alpha-carotene, and beta-cryptoxanthin) have vitamin A activity (meaning that they can be converted to retinal), and these and other carotenoids can also act as antioxidants.

Lycopene from the neo-Latin *lycopersicum*, the tomato species, is a bright red carotene and carotenoid pigment and phytochemical found in tomatoes and other red fruits and vegetables, such as red carrots, watermelons, gac, and papayas, although not in strawberries, red bell peppers, or cherries. Although lycopene is chemically a carotene, it has no vitamin A activity. Foods that are not red may also contain lycopene, such as brown beans or parsley.

Lutein from Latin *luteus* meaning "yellow") is a xanthophyll and one of 600 known naturally occurring carotenoids. Lutein is synthesized only by plants and like other xanthophylls is found in high quantities in green leafy vegetables such as spinach, kale and yellow carrots.

Lutein is obtained by animals directly or indirectly, from plants. Lutein is apparently employed by animals as an antioxidant and for blue light absorption. Lutein is found in egg yolks and animal fats. In addition to coloring yolks, lutein causes the yellow color of chicken skin and fat, and is used in chicken feed for this purpose. The human retina accumulates lutein and zeaxanthin. The latter predominates at the macula lutea while lutein predominates elsewhere in the retina. There, it may serve as a photo-protectant for the retina from the damaging effects of free radicals produced by blue light. Lutein is isomeric with zeaxanthin, differing only in the placement of one double bond.

Zeaxanthin is one of the most common carotenoid alcohols found in nature. It is important in the xanthophyll cycle. Synthesized in plants and some micro-organisms, it is the pigment that gives paprika (made from bell peppers), corn, saffron, wolfberries, and many other plants and microbes their characteristic color.

The name (pronounced *zee-uh-zan'-thin*) is derived from *Zea mays* (common yellow maize corn, in which zeaxanthin provides the primary yellow pigment), plus *xanthos*, the Greek word for "yellow."

Xanthophylls such as zeaxanthin are found in highest quantity in the leaves of most green plants.

Animals derive zeaxanthin from a plant diet. Zeaxanthin is one of the two primary xanthophyll carotenoids contained within the retina of the eye. Within the central macula, zeaxanthin is the dominant component, whereas in the peripheral retina, lutein predominates.

Reporting in the November 2014 issue of the journal *Neuropharmacology*, Dr. Yin and colleagues reported that, *"Fructose[1] intake is linked with the increasing prevalence of insulin resistance, and insulin resistance links Alzheimer's disease with impaired insulin signaling, oxidative damage, neuroinflammation, and cognitive impairment. As a member of the carotenoid family of phytochemicals, lycopene is used as a potent free scavenger, and has been demonstrated to be effective in anti-oxidative stress and anti-inflammatory reaction in the models of AD and other neurodegenerative diseases. Here, we investigated the effect of lycopene on learning and memory impairment and the possible underlying molecular events in fructose-drinking insulin resistant rats. We found that long-term fructose-drinking causes insulin resistance, impaired insulin signaling, oxidative stress, neuroinflammation, down-regulated activity of cholinergic system, and cognitive impairment, which could be significantly ameliorated by oral lycopene administration. The results from this study provide experimental evidence for using lycopene in the treatment of brain damage caused by fructose-drinking insulin resistance."*[495]

---

[1]Fructose, or fruit sugar, is a simple ketonic monosaccharide found in many plants, where it is often bonded to glucose to form the disaccharide sucrose. It is one of the three dietary monosaccharides, along with glucose and galactose, that are absorbed directly into the bloodstream during digestion. Fructose is found in honey, tree and vine fruits, flowers, berries, and most root vegetables. Commercially, fructose is frequently derived from sugar cane, sugar beets, and corn. High-fructose corn syrup (HFCS) is a mixture of glucose and fructose as monosaccharides. All forms of fructose, including fruits and juices, are commonly added to foods and drinks for palatability and taste enhancement, and for browning of some foods, such as baked goods.

Reporting in 2014, researchers investigated whether or not serum levels of carotenoids were associated with the risk of Alzheimer's disease mortality in a nationally representative sample of U.S. adults. The researchers studied data from the Third Nutrition and Health Examination Survey (NHANES III) database and the NHANES III Linked Mortality File. A total of 6,958 participants aged older than fifty years were included in this study. They reported that, *"We found that high serum levels of lycopene and lutein+zeaxanthin at baseline were associated with a lower risk of AD mortality* after adjustment for potential covariates. *The reduction in the mortality risk was progressively raised by increasing serum lycopene and lutein+zeaxanthin levels. In contrast, no associations with AD mortality were observed for other serum carotenoids, including alpha-carotene, beta-carotene, and beta-cryptoxanthin. High serum levels of lycopene and lutein+zeaxanthin are associated with a lower risk of AD mortality in adults. Our findings suggest that a high intake of lycopene- or lutein+zeaxanthin-rich food may be important for reducing the AD mortality risk."*[496]

People consuming diets rich in carotenoids from natural foods, such as fruits and vegetables, are healthier and have lower mortality from a number of chronic illnesses. Although *a recent meta-analysis of 68 reliable antioxidant supplementation experiments involving a total of 232,606 individuals concluded additional β-carotene from supplements is unlikely to be beneficial and may actually be harmful*, this may be due to the inclusion of studies involving smokers - β-carotene under intense oxidative stress (e.g. induced by heavy smoking) gives breakdown products that reduce plasma vitamin A and worsen the lung cell proliferation induced by smoke. With the notable exception of the gac fruit and crude palm oil, most carotenoid-rich fruits and vegetables are low in lipids. Since dietary lipids have been hypothesized to be an important factor for carotenoid bioavailability, a 2005 study investigated whether addition of avocado fruit or oil, as lipid sources, would enhance carotenoid absorption in humans. The study found that the addition of either avocado fruit or oil significantly enhanced the subjects' absorption of all carotenoids tested (α-carotene, β-carotene, lycopene, and lutein).

Another group of researchers investigated whether serum levels of carotenoids were associated with the risk of AD mortality in a nationally representative sample of U.S. adults. They studied 6,958 participants, fifty years or older, from the Third Nutrition and Health Examination Survey (NHANES III). They found that *"high serum levels of lycopene and lutein+zeaxanthin at baseline were associated with a lower risk of AD mortality (death). In contrast, no associations with AD mortality were observed for other serum carotenoids, including alpha-carotene, beta-carotene, and beta-cryptoxanthin. Our findings suggest that a high intake of lycopene- or lutein+zeaxanthin-rich food may be important for reducing the AD mortality risk."*[497]

Chia (*Salvia hispanica*)

Although no studies have been done with Chia and Alzheimer's disease, it is included here because of its other beneficial effects, including its positive effects on obesity, inflammation, and hypertension. Chia, is a species of flowering plant in the mint family, Lamiaceae, native to central and southern Mexico and Guatemala. The 16th-century *Codex Mendoza* provides evidence that it was cultivated by the Aztec in pre-Columbian times; economic historians have suggested it was as important as maize as a food crop. Ground or whole chia seeds are still used in Paraguay, Bolivia, Argentina, Mexico and Guatemala for nutritious drinks and as a food source.

Chia is grown commercially for its seed, a food that is rich in omega-3 fatty acids, since the seeds yield 25–30 percent extractable oil, including α-linolenic acid (ALA). Of total fat, the composition of the oil can be 55 percent ω-3, 18 omega ω-6, 6 percent ω-9, and 10 percent saturated fat.

A 100 gram serving of chia seeds is a rich source (54% and 59%, respectively) of the Daily value, DV) of the B vitamins thiamine and niacin, and a good source (14 and 12%, respectively) of the B vitamins riboflavin and folate. The same amount of chia seeds is also a rich source (>20% DV) of the dietary minerals calcium, iron, magnesium, manganese, phosphorus, and zinc.

In 2009, the European Union approved chia seeds as a novel food, allowing up to 5 percent of a bread product's total matter. Chia seeds may be added to other foods as a topping or put into smoothies, breakfast cereals, energy bars, granola bars, yogurt, tortillas, bread, made into a gelatin-like substance or consumed raw. The gel can be used to replace as much as 2 percent of egg content and oil in cakes while providing other nutrients.

In the May 2015 issue of the journal *Nutrition*, Drs. Marineli and colleagues reported the results of their research studying the protective effects of Chia in an animal model of metabolically-induced diabetes. Without going into the details of their research, the authors found that, "Chia oil restored the antioxidant system and induced the expression of a higher number of proteins than chia seed. *The present study demonstrated new properties and molecular mechanisms associated with the beneficial effects of chia seed and chia oil consumption in diet-induced obese rats.*"[500]

Reporting in the December 2014 issue of the journal *Plant Foods for Human Nutrition*, Dr. Toscano and colleagues reported the results of their study "...to investigate the effect of chia supplementation (Salvia hispanica L.) on blood pressure (BP) and its associated cardiometabolic factors in treated and untreated hypertensive individuals." Without going into the details of their research, the authors concluded that, *"Chia flour has the ability to reduce ambulatory and clinical BP in both treated and untreated hypertensive individuals."*[501]

Another group of researchers noted the following, "Despite strong correlations linking whole-grain consumption to reductions in heart disease, the physiological mechanisms involved remain ambiguous. We assessed whether Salba (Salvia Hispanica L.) whole grain reduces postprandial glycemia in healthy subjects, as a possible explanation for its cardioprotective effects observed in individuals with diabetes...*Appetite ratings were decreased at 60 min after high, 90 min after high and intermediate and at 120 min after all treatments. Decrease in postprandial glycemia provides a potential explanation for improvements in blood pressure, coagulation and inflammatory markers previously observed after 12-week Salba supplementation in type II diabetes.*"[502]

Chinese Herbal Preparations

The *Shen Nong Ben Cao Jing* is the oldest known compendium of Chinese herbal medicines that were believed to exert neither fast acting pharmacological effects nor discernible toxicity, but to promote general health and longevity. In modern terms, these herbal medicines could be considered as complementary health care products for prevention rather than treatment of diseases. Using certain tests and cell cultures, a group of researchers examined whether a selection of thirteen such herbal medicines exhibit neuroprotective activity. The researchers found that,[503]

> "*Most of the herbal extracts showed negligible toxic effects* at 100 µg/ml. However, Polygonum multiflorum and Rhodiola rosea exhibited some neurotoxicity at this concentration. Extracts of Ganoderma lucidum, Glycyrrhiza glabra, Schizandra chinensis, and Polygonum cuspidatum inhibited staurosporine-induced apoptosis [cell death] by 30 - 50 percent in a dose-dependent manner.
>
> *The neuroprotective effects of Polygonum cuspidatum were predominantly due to its major ingredient, resveratrol.* The effective herbal extracts showed various levels of reactive oxygen species (ROS) scavenging capacity, which was significantly correlated with their neuroprotective activity. However, P. multiflorum and R. rosea extracts proved to be the exception as they exhibited a high level of antioxidant capacity, but did not exhibit neuroprotective effects in cell-based assay. *This in*

vitro study provides evidence for neuroprotective activity of some Chinese herbal medicines traditionally used to promote healthy aging and longevity. Our results provide a justification for further study of these herbal extracts in neurodegenerative animal models to assess their safety and effectiveness as a basis for subsequent clinical trials. These herbal medicines might potentially offer a novel preemptive neuroprotective approach in neurodegenerative diseases and might be developed for use in persons at risk."

Dr. Hou, from the State Key Laboratory of Cell Biology, Institute of Biochemistry and Cell Biology, Shanghai Institutes for Biological Sciences, Graduate School of the Chinese Academy of Sciences, Chinese Academy of Sciences, Shanghai, China, and colleagues published the results of their research in the November 11, 2014 issue of *Plos One*. They studied the effects of Smart Soup (SS), a Chinese medicinal formula composed of Rhizoma Acori Tatarinowii (AT), Poria cum Radix Pini (PRP), and Radix Polygalae (RP), which is a typical prescription against memory deficits. They studied smart soup on an animal model of Alzheimer's disease. Without discussing the details of their experiment, they concluded that, *"Taken together, our study indicates that SS could be effective against AD, providing a practical therapeutic strategy against the disease.*[504]

Yizhijiannao granules have been shown to improve cognitive function in Alzheimer's disease patients. Using an animal model, another group of researchers sought to explore the mechanisms involved in the cognitive enhancing effects of Yizhijiannao granule. They found that, "Thirty-seven differential protein spots were found in the temporal lobe area of both groups. ...Among other functions, these proteins are separately involved in the regulation of amyloid beta production, oxidative stress, neuroinflammation, regulation of tau phosphorylation, and regulation of neuronal apoptosis. *Our results revealed that Yizhijiannao granule can regulate the expression of various proteins in the temporal lobe of senescence-accelerated mouse prone eight mice, and may be therapeutically beneficial for the treatment of Alzheimer's disease.*"[505]

Coconut

Virgin coconut oil, which is rich in polyphenols and medium-chain fatty acids, has been consumed worldwide for various health-related reasons and some of its benefits have been scientifically evaluated. Recently, virgin coconut oil has been growing in popularity due to its potential cardiovascular benefits.[506]

Coconut oil and juice are all the rage currently in the U.S., in terms of use to promote health. For example, in 2015 it is only the only juice available in the well-known health store, GNC.

Studies in a classic animal model of stress, completed in 2015, revealed that virgin coconut oil has clear antistress and antioxidant properties. Its use increased brain antioxidants, lowered blood cholesterol, triglyceride, glucose, and corticosterone (the main stress hormone) levels. In conclusion, the authors wrote, "These results suggest the potential value of virgin coconut oil as an antistress functional oil.[507]

Dietary supplementation with coconut oil has been studied as an approach to ameliorating deficits associated with aging and neurodegeneration. Last year, researchers used nerve cell cultures to investigate the potential of coconut oil supplementation to protect against damage from amyloid-β (Aβ) peptide, the peptide associated with Alzheimer's disease. The researchers found that *coconut oil was indeed protective against this toxin, protecting not only the nerve cells directly, but also attenuates Aβ-induced mitochondrial alterations.*[508]

Researchers studied the potential benefit of young coconut juice in a menopausal animal model of Alzheimer's disease. Preliminary studies on young coconut juice have reported the presence of estrogen-like components in it. Aβ deposition, characteristic of AD, was significantly reduced in the group treated with young coconut juice, and there were other positive cellular and sub-cellular changes as well. The researchers concluded, "This is a novel study demonstrating that *young coconut juice could have positive future implications in the prevention and treatment of AD in menopausal women.*"[509]

Coffee

Recent epidemiologic studies suggest that caffeine may be protective against Alzheimer's disease. Supportive of this premise, prior studies have shown that moderate caffeine administration protects/restores cognitive function and suppresses brain amyloid-beta (Abeta) production in an animal model of AD. Researchers from the Byrd Alzheimer's Center & Research Institute, Tampa, FL, found that acute caffeine administration to both young adult and aged AD mice rapidly reduces Abeta levels in both brain fluid and plasma (blood). Long-term oral caffeine treatment to aged AD mice provided not only sustained reductions in plasma Abeta, but also decreases in specific areas of the brain associated with learning and memory. The researchers concluded that, in their animal model of AD, *"both plasma and brain Abeta levels are reduced by acute or chronic caffeine administration...indicating a therapeutic value of caffeine against AD."*[510]

While animal data suggest a protective effect of caffeine on cognition, studies in humans remain inconsistent. To further define the effects of coffee and caffeine intake on cognitive impairment in aging males, researchers studied the 3,494 men in the Honolulu-Asia Aging Study, including 418 decedents who underwent brain autopsy. Dementia was diagnosed in 226 men (including 118 with Alzheimer's dementia, and 80 with vascular dementia), and cognitive impairment in 347. *"There were no significant associations between coffee or caffeine intake and risk of cognitive impairment or either type of dementia."*[511]

However, researchers who reviewed the literature vis-à-vis coffee/caffeine and Alzheimer's disease, found that, "Although the underlying mechanisms are not fully understood, when comparing coffee drinkers with non-drinkers, *moderate doses of caffeine showed protective effects against Alzheimer's disease (AD) and cardiovascular disease CVD. We hypothesized that caffeine may be a novel therapy to treat CVD and dementia/AD.*"[512]

Coenzyme Q_{10} (CoQ10)

Warning: Coenzyme Q10 has potential to inhibit the effects of warfarin (Coumadin), a potent anticoagulant. The structure of coenzyme Q10 is very much similar to the structure of vitamin K, which competes with and counteracts warfarin's anticoagulation effects. *Coenzyme Q10 should be avoided in patients currently taking warfarin due to the increased risk of clotting.*

Coenzyme Q_{10}, also known as ubiquinone, ubidecarenone, coenzyme Q, is a 1,4-benzoquinone, where Q refers to the quinone chemical group, and ten refers to the number of isoprenyl chemical subunits in its tail. Enough said!

This vitamin-like substance is present in most cells, primarily in the mitochondria. It is a component of the electron transport chain and participates in aerobic cellular respiration, generating energy in the form of ATP. Ninety-five percent of the human body's energy is generated this way. The capacity of this molecule to exist in a completely oxidized form and a completely reduced form enables it to perform its functions in the electron transport chain, and as an antioxidant, respectively.

Coenzyme Q10 is not approved by the U.S. Food and Drug Administration (FDA) for the treatment of any medical condition. It is sold as a dietary supplement. In the U.S. supplements are not regulated as drugs but as foods. How CoQ10 is manufactured is not regulated and different batches and brands may vary significantly.

A 2004 laboratory analysis by ConsumerLab.com found CoQ10 supplements on the market did not all contain the quantity identified on the product label. Amounts varied from "no detectable CoQ10" to 75 percent of stated dose up to a 75 percent excess. Tod Cooperman president of ConsumerLab.com stated, "When a patient can go from zero dose to 175 percent of dose just by switching brands, there is potential for a real problem..." Because of this potential problem, it is probably wise to stick with one brand.

PREVENTION

Coenzyme Q10 is generally well tolerated. The most common side effects are gastrointestinal symptoms (nausea, vomiting, appetite suppression and stomachache), rash and headache.

CoQ_{10} shares a biosynthetic pathway with cholesterol. The synthesis of an intermediary precursor of CoQ_{10}, mevalonate, is inhibited by some beta blockers, blood pressure-lowering medications, and statins, a class of cholesterol-lowering drugs. Statins can reduce serum levels of CoQ_{10} by up to 40 percent. Some research suggests the logical option of supplementation with CoQ_{10} as a routine adjunct to any treatment that may reduce endogenous production of CoQ_{10}, based on a balance of likely benefit against very small risk.

In addition to their lipid-lowering effect, statins have other beneficial effects that may extend their use to the treatment and prevention of various other diseases such as cancer, osteoporosis, multiple sclerosis, rheumatoid arthritis, Type II diabetes, and Alzheimer's disease. Consequently, the number of patients taking statins is expected to increase.

The side effect of statins, statin-induced myopathy (muscle damage), which may result from reduced muscular coenzyme Q10 levels, limits their use. In order to determine if coadministration of CoQ10 could modify or prevent this damage, researchers used an animal model wherein CoQ10 and a common statin, Lipitor (atorvastatin) where coadministered. The results showed that the use of Lipitor caused significant, even striking, and varied muscle damage, but that this was prevented when CoQ10 was added as a supplement. The authors concluded by stating, "Conclusion: *Co Q10 may ameliorate atorvastatin induced skeletal muscle injury.*"[513]

Dr. Mitilineos and colleagues just published the interesting results of their research in the *American Journal of Alzheimer's Disease and Other Dementias*. The researchers found abnormalities in early cases of AD in specific areas of the brain associated with learning and memory, the hypothalamus. This finding is not new. What is very interesting, however, is that although they found a variety of abnormalities of nerve cells, the characteristic lesions of Alzheimer's disease were minimal.

What they did find with the use of electron microscopy were *mitochondrial abnormalities* in the nerve cells.[514] So, *the earliest lesions in incipient AD, at least in this study, were mitochondrial abnormalities, not the characteristic plaques of AD*. This implies that early administration of CoQ10 might help prevent Alzheimer's disease.

Dr. Durán-Prado and nine colleagues in late 2014 published the results of very interesting research which showed that ß-amyloid peptides, characteristic of the pathology associated with AD, severely damage endothelial cells (the cells that line the inside of blood vessels) in the brain. Using a variety of techniques, they were able to show that pretreatment with CoQ10 was able to prevent the many abnormalities previously caused by ß-amyloid peptides. They concluded that, *"CoQ protected endothelial cells from Aß-induced injury in human plasma after oral CoQ supplementation and thus could be a promising molecule to protect endothelial cells against amyloid angiopathy (e.g., the damage caused by ß-amyloid peptides)."*[515] This is very exciting because small-blood-vessel damage is part-and-parcel of the abnormalities found in Alzheimer's disease.

Finally, Dr. Shetty and others, from the Department of Pharmacology and Neuroscience, University of North Texas Health Science Center at Fort Worth, Fort Worth, TX recently published a report of their research involving the use of vitamin E and CoQ10 in an animal model of Alzheimer's disease. Although the use of α-tocopherol (one form of vitamin E) in the prevention and/or treatment of AD has had mixed reviews over the years, this research found that its use was protective of cognitive decline in aged mice. Similar results were found with supplementation with CoQ10. They authors concluded by stating, *"Protein damage was decreased especially when the mice received vitamin E + CoQ10 combination. Overall, these results suggest that, vitamin E and CoQ supplementation can ameliorate age-related impairment and reduce protein oxidation. Moreover, concurrent supplementation of CoQ10 and vitamin E may be more effective than either antioxidant alone."*[516]

Curcumin (Turmeric)

Curcumin is the principal curcuminoid of turmeric, which is a member of the ginger family (*Zingiberaceae*). Turmeric's other two curcuminoids are desmethoxycurcumin and bis-desmethoxycurcumin. The curcuminoids are natural phenols that are responsible for the yellow color of turmeric. Curcumin is known as the curry spice turmeric (yellow curry). Curcumin is widely used in traditional Asian kitchen as a cooking ingredient. Despite its low bioavailability, epidemiological data, on low cancer incidence in Asia, suggest beneficial health effects of this compound.[517]

It is generally believed that curcumin is the most important constituent of the curcuminoid mixture that contributes to the pharmacological profile of parent curcuminoid mixture or turmeric. A careful literature study reveals that the other two constituents of the curcuminoid mixture also contribute significantly to the effectiveness of curcuminoids in AD. Therefore, it is emphasized that each component of the curcuminoid mixture plays a distinct role in making curcuminoid mixture useful in AD, and hence, the curcuminoid mixture represents turmeric in its medicinal value better than curcumin alone.[518]

Turmeric has been demonstrated to have antioxidant and anti-inflammatory effects as well as effects on reducing beta-amyloid aggregation. It reduces pathology in animal models of Alzheimer's disease and is a promising candidate for treating human AD.

So-called "heat shock proteins" play a crucial role in a variety of cellular processes, including the removal of damaged, toxic, or misformed proteins, like β-amyloid peptide (Aβ), which is strongly associated with Alzheimer's disease pathology. Natural products that can modulate heat shock proteins are considered promising for treating neurodegenerative diseases, such as AD. *Curcumin has been shown to augment expression or function of heat shock proteins in the cell.*[519]

Research is ongoing in many areas in an attempt to find more potent anti-Alzheimer's disease compounds. This is true for resveratrol as well as curcumin. One group of researchers reported discovering an analog of curcumin that is not only more potent than curcumin in inhibiting amyloid β peptide, but is 160 times more water soluble, which increases its effectiveness.[520]

In 2014, another group of researchers found a different curcumin derivative, dubbed FMeC1, that not only reduced deposits of amyloid β (Aβ) in the brain, but it also significantly reduced the cell toxicity of Aβ, something that curcumin did not do. *The researchers concluded that, "These results indicate that FMeC1 may have potential for preventing AD."*[521]

Researchers from the Department of Emergency Medicine, Brain Research Laboratory, Emory University, Atlanta, GA, reported that, "Recent evidence indicates that curcumin, the principal curcuminoid of turmeric, exhibits antioxidant potential and protects the brain against various oxidative stressors. They used an animal model to determine the protective effects of curcumin against a toxic substance on brain function. The results showed a number of positive effects on numerous cellular activities, processes, and enzymes. They summarized by saying, *"The study suggests that curcumin is effective in preventing cognitive deficits, and might be beneficial for the treatment of sporadic dementia of Alzheimer's type (SDAT)."*[522]

Researchers reported on three patients in India with the Alzheimer's disease, whose behavioral symptoms were improved remarkably as a result of the turmeric treatment, which is a traditional Indian medicine. Their cognitive decline and behavioral symptoms were very severe. All three patients exhibited irritability, agitation, anxiety, apathy, and two patients suffered from urinary incontinence and wandering. They were prescribed turmeric powder capsules and started recovering from these symptoms without any adverse reactions. The authors reported that one patient's cognition actually improved, and the other two patients were able to recognize family members after one year of treatment. All three had a significant improvement of the behavioral symptoms with the turmeric treatment.[523]

In another, larger study of the use of turmeric, researchers studied thirty-six people with mild-to-moderate AD, who were followed for up to forty-eight weeks. The average age of those completing the study (n = 30) was 73.5 years. The researchers concluded that, "Curcumin was generally well-tolerated although three subjects on curcumin withdrew due to gastrointestinal symptoms. We were unable to demonstrate clinical or biochemical evidence of efficacy of Curcumin C3 Complex(®) in AD in this 24-week trial."[524] What does this study demonstrate, once again? It shows that most potential treatments, especially when used in the elderly with dementia, aren't effective. There are no surprises here.

D (Vitamin D)

Vitamin D refers to a group of fat-soluble secosteroids responsible for enhancing intestinal absorption of calcium, iron, magnesium, phosphate and zinc. In humans, the most important compounds in this group are vitamin D_3 (also known as cholecalciferol) and vitamin D_2 (ergocalciferol). Cholecalciferol and ergocalciferol can be ingested from the diet and from supplements. Very few foods contain vitamin D; synthesis of vitamin D (specifically cholecalciferol) in the skin is the major natural sources of the vitamin. Dermal synthesis of vitamin D from cholesterol is dependent on sun exposure (specifically UVB radiation).

Vitamin D from the diet or dermal synthesis from sunlight is biologically inactive; activation requires enzymatic conversion (hydroxylation) in the liver and kidney. Evidence indicates the synthesis of vitamin D from sun exposure is regulated by a negative feedback loop that prevents toxicity, but because of uncertainty about the cancer risk from sunlight, no recommendations are issued by the Institute of Medicine (U.S.), for the amount of sun exposure required to meet vitamin D requirements. Accordingly, the Dietary Reference Intake (DRI) for vitamin D assumes no synthesis occurs and all of a person's vitamin D is from food intake, although that will rarely occur in practice. As vitamin D is synthesized in adequate amounts by most mammals exposed to sunlight, it is not strictly a vitamin, and may be considered a hormone as its synthesis and activity occur in different locations. Vitamin D has a significant role in calcium homeostasis and metabolism. Its discovery was due to effort to find the dietary substance lacking in rickets (the childhood form of osteomalacia).

In the liver, cholecalciferol (vitamin D_3) is converted to calcidiol, which is also known as calcifediol (INN), 25-hydroxycholecalciferol (aka 25-hydroxyvitamin D_3 — abbreviated 25(OH)D_3). Ergocalciferol (vitamin D_2) is converted in the liver to 25-hydroxyergocalciferol (aka 25-hydroxyvitamin D_2 — abbreviated 25(OH)D_2). These two specific vitamin D metabolites are measured in serum to determine a person's vitamin D status. Part of the calcidiol is converted by the kidneys to calcitriol, the biologically active form of vitamin D. Calcitriol circulates as a hormone in the blood, regulating the concentration of calcium and phosphate in the bloodstream and promoting the healthy growth and remodeling of bone. Calcitriol also affects neuromuscular and immune function.

Dr. Toffanello and colleagues, publishing the results of their research in the November 5, 2014 issue of *Neurology*, tested the hypothesis that low vitamin D is associated with a higher risk of cognitive decline over a 4.4-year follow-up in 1,927 elderly subjects. Serum 25-hydroxyvitamin D (25OHD; "vitamin D") levels were measured at the baseline.

The results of our study support an independent association between low 25OHD levels and cognitive decline in elderly individuals. The authors concluded that, *"The results of our study support an independent association between low 25OHD levels and cognitive decline in elderly individuals. In cognitively intact elderly subjects, 25OHD levels below 75 nmol/L are already predictive of global cognitive dysfunction at 4.4 years."*[525]

In 2014, researchers studied the impact of treatment with vitamin D in the progression of Alzheimer's disease. They included patients with a mild stage of AD, and followed them for more than four years. Time of progression to moderate and severe AD was analyzed. The researchers noted that, "Two hundred and two patients met the inclusion criteria.

Eleven percent of the patients (n = 23) remained in the mild stage of the disease, 54 percent (n = 110) developed the moderate form in a mean time of three years while 35 percent (n = 69) developed the severe form in a mean time of 4.6 years. *Time of progression to severe stage of Alzheimer's disease was slower in patients under treatment with vitamin D compared with those without treatment (5.4 years vs. 4.4 years respectively). Treatment with vitamin D may be an independent protecting factor in the progression of Alzheimer's disease.*[526]

A separate group of researchers also studied whether or not low vitamin D concentrations are associated with an increased risk of incident all-cause dementia and Alzheimer's disease. They included 1,658 elderly ambulatory adults free from dementia, cardiovascular disease, and stroke in the study. "During a mean follow-up of 5.6 years, 171 participants developed all-cause dementia, including 102 cases of Alzheimer's disease…the risk of all-cause dementia and Alzheimer's disease markedly increased below a threshold of 50 nmol/L. *Our results confirm that vitamin D deficiency is associated with a substantially increased risk of all-cause dementia and Alzheimer disease.*"[527]

Reporting in March 2015, Dr. Annweiler and colleagues conducted research on the association between vitamin D insufficiency and abnormal brain changes. "Our objective was to investigate whether vitamin D insufficiency was associated with greater volume of white matter abnormalities (WMA) in older adults. Seventy-five Caucasian older community-dwellers (mean, 70.9; 48 percent female) received a blood test and brain MRI. The volumes of total white matter (WM) and WMA were measured. Vitamin D insufficiency was defined a priori as serum 25-hydroxyvitamin D<50 nmol/L. Participants with vitamin D insufficiency (n = 29) had a greater volume of WMA than the others, even after normalization for WM volume. Vitamin D insufficiency was associated with increased WMA volume in the studied sample of older adults. These findings may provide insight into the pathophysiology of cognitive and mobility declines in older adults with vitamin D insufficiency."[528]

E (Vitamin E)

Vitamin E refers to a group of compounds that include both tocopherols and tocotrienols. Of the many different forms of vitamin E, γ-tocopherol ("gamma"-tocopherol) is the most common in the North American diet. γ-Tocopherol can be found in corn oil, soybean oil, margarine, and dressings. α-tocopherol ("alpha"-tocopherol), the most biologically active form of vitamin E, is the second-most common form of vitamin E in the diet. This variant can be found most abundantly in wheat germ oil, sunflower, and safflower oils. As a fat-soluble antioxidant, it stops the production of reactive oxygen species formed when fat undergoes oxidation. Regular consumption of more than 1,000 mg (1,500 IU) of tocopherols per day may be expected to cause hypervitaminosis E, with an associated risk of vitamin K deficiency and consequently of bleeding problems.

The ten forms of vitamin E are divided into two groups; five are tocopherols and five are tocotrienols. They are identified by prefixes alpha- (α-), beta- (β-), gamma- (γ-), delta- (δ-), and epsilon (ε).

In 2014, researchers noted that, "Vitamin E is an important antioxidant that primarily protects cells from damage associated with oxidative stress caused by free radicals. The brain is highly susceptible to oxidative stress, which increases during aging and is considered a major contributor to neurodegeneration. High plasma vitamin E levels were repeatedly associated with better cognitive performance. Due to its antioxidant properties, the ability of vitamin E to prevent or delay cognitive decline has been tested in clinical trials in both aging population and Alzheimer's disease patients. *The difficulty in performing precise and uniform human studies is mostly responsible for the inconsistent outcomes reported in the literature. Therefore, the benefit of vitamin E as a treatment for neurodegenerative disorders is still under debate.*"[529]

According to a large literature review conducted in 2012, to assess the efficacy of vitamin E in the treatment of Alzheimer's disease and the prevention of progression of mild cognitive impairment (MCI) to dementia, "*No convincing evidence [could be found] that vitamin E is of benefit in the treatment of AD or MCI. Future trials assessing vitamin E treatment in AD should not be restricted to alpha-tocopherol [e.g., other types of vitamin E, such as gamma-tocopherol, should be included].*"[530]

Researchers conducted a literature review to comprehensively evaluate the association between dietary intakes, instead of supplements, of the most common three antioxidants (vitamin E, vitamin C, and β-carotene) and the risk of AD. Reporting their findings in the *Journal of Alzheimer's Disease*, they concluded that, "*According to the pooled relative risk (0.76 for vitamin E, 0.83 for vitamin C, and 0.88 for β-carotene), dietary intakes of the three antioxidants can lower the risk of AD, with vitamin E exhibiting the most pronounced protective effects. The findings will be of significance to the prevention and interventional treatment of AD.*"[531]

In a complex but important manner, researchers reported the following in 2014: "*Oxidative stress is a hallmark of Alzheimer's disease. We propose that rather than causing damage because of the action of free radicals[1], oxidative stress deranges signaling pathways leading to tau hyperphosphorylation, a hallmark of the disease. Indeed, incubation of neurons in culture with 5 μM beta-amyloid peptide (Aβ) causes an activation of p38 MAPK (p38) that leads to tau hyperphosphorylation. Inhibition of p38 prevents Aβ-induced tau phosphorylation. Aβ-induced effects are prevented when neurons are co-incubated with trolox (the water-soluble analog of vitamin E). We have confirmed these results in vivo, in APP/PS1 double transgenic mice of AD. We have found that APP/PS1 transgenic mice exhibit a high level of P-p38 in the hippocampus but not in cortex and this is prevented by feeding animals with a diet supplemented with vitamin E. Our results underpin the role of oxidative stress in the altered cell signaling in AD pathology and suggest that antioxidant prevention may be useful in AD therapeutics.*"[532]

---

[1]A free radical is an atom, molecule, or ion that has unpaired valence electrons; they are highly reactive with other chemicals, and can be destructive.

ALZHEIMER'S DISEASE

Dr. Mangialasche and colleagues, reporting in an 2015 issue of the *Journal of Alzheimer's Disease*, noted the following,

533

"Specific mechanisms behind the role of oxidative/nitrosative stress and mitochondrial dysfunction in Alzheimer's disease pathogenesis remain elusive. Mitochondrial aconitase (ACO2) is a Krebs cycle enzyme sensitive to free radical-mediated damage. We assessed activity and expression of ACO2 extracted from blood lymphocytes [white blood cells] of subjects with AD, mild cognitive impairment (MCI), older adults with normal cognition (OCN, age ≥65 years), and younger adults with normal cognition (YCN, age <65 years). Plasma levels and activities of antioxidants were also measured. Blood samples were collected from 28 subjects with AD, 22 with MCI, 21 OCN, and 19 YCN. ACO2 activity was evaluated in a subsample before and after in vitro exposure to free radicals. ACO2 activity was significantly lower in AD and MCI cases than controls: ACO2 median activity was 0.64 AD, 0.93 for MCI, 1.17 for OCN subjects, and 1.23 for YCN individuals. In subjects with AD and MCI, ACO2 expression was lower than OCN subjects, and *ACO2 activity correlated with vitamin E plasma levels* and Mini-Mental State Examination total score. Furthermore, free radicals exposure reduced ACO2 activity more in individuals with AD than in OCN subjects.

Our results suggest that ACO2 activity is reduced in peripheral lymphocytes of subjects with AD and MCI and correlates with antioxidant protection. Further studies are warranted to verify the role of ACO2 in AD pathogenesis and its importance as a marker of AD progression.

Another group of researchers, led by Dr. Remingon, from the University of Massachusetts Lowell, Lowell, MA, reported the results of their research in the January 1, 2015 issue of the *Journal of Alzheimer's Disease*. They noted the following, *"Increasing evidence points toward the efficacy of nutritional modifications in delaying cognitive decline and mood/behavioral difficulties in Alzheimer's disease. Nutritional supplementation with individual agents has shown varied results suggesting the need for combinatorial intervention.* We set out to determine whether nutritional intervention could positively impact cognitive performance and behavioral difficulties for individuals diagnosed with AD. A double-blind, multi-site, phase II study was conducted in which 106 individuals with AD were randomized to a nutraceutical formulation (NF; folate, alpha-tocopherol [vitamin E], B12, S-adenosyl methioinine, N-acetyl cysteine, acetyl-L-carnitine) or placebo for three or six months, followed by an open-label extension where participants received NF for 6 additional months. *The NF cohort improved versus the placebo cohort within three months.* Caregivers reported non-significant improvements in Neuropsychiatric Inventory. Both cohorts improved or maintained baseline performance during open-label extensions. Activities of Daily Living did not change for either cohort. *These findings extend phase I studies where NF maintained or improved cognitive performance and mood/behavior.* "[534]

Flavonoids and Polyphenols (Phytochemicals)

Phytochemicals are chemical compounds that occur naturally in plants (phyto means "plant" in Greek). Some are responsible for color and other organoleptic properties, such as the deep purple of blueberries and the smell of garlic. Phytochemicals may have biological significance, for example carotenoids or flavonoids, but are not established as essential nutrients.

Note, some of these compounds are discussed in this section, while others are discussed individually, in their own section. For example, quercetin, resveratrol, and green tea are discussed individually.

The definition and other characteristics of polyphenols are complicated. Please see wikipedic.org for more information. The most important food sources of phenolic compounds are commodities widely consumed in large quantities such as fruit and vegetables, green tea, black tea, red wine, coffee, chocolate, olives, and extra virgin olive oil. Herbs and spices, nuts and algae are also potentially significant for supplying certain polyphenols. Some polyphenols are specific to particular food (flavanones in citrus fruit, isoflavones in soya, phloridzin in apples); whereas others, such as quercetin, are found in all plant products such as fruit, vegetables, cereals, leguminous plants, tea, and wine.

Flavonoids (or bioflavonoids) (from the Latin word *flavus* meaning yellow, their color in nature) are a class of plant secondary metabolites. Flavonoids (specifically flavanoids such as the catechins) are the most common group of polyphenolic compounds in the human diet and are found ubiquitously in plants. Flavonols, the original bioflavonoids such as quercetin, are also found ubiquitously, but in lesser quantities. The widespread distribution of flavonoids, their variety and their relatively low toxicity compared to other active plant compounds (for instance alkaloids) mean that many animals, including humans, ingest significant quantities in their diet. Foods with a high flavonoid content include parsley, onions, blueberries and other berries, black tea, green tea and oolong tea, bananas, all citrus fruits, *Ginkgo biloba*, red wine, seabuckthorns, and dark chocolate (with a cocoa content of 70 percent or greater). Over 5000 naturally occurring flavonoids have been characterized from various plants. Further information on dietary sources of flavonoids can be obtained from the U.S. Department of Agriculture flavonoid database.

Among the most intensively studied of general human disorders possibly affected by dietary flavonoids, preliminary cardiovascular disease research has revealed the following mechanisms under investigation in patients or normal subjects:

- inhibit coagulation, thrombus formation or platelet aggregation
- reduce risk of atherosclerosis
- reduce arterial blood pressure and risk of hypertension

- reduce oxidative stress and related signaling pathways in blood vessel cells
- modify vascular inflammatory mechanisms
- improve endothelial and capillary function
- modify blood lipid levels
- regulate carbohydrate and glucose metabolism
- modify mechanisms of aging

In late 2014, one researcher noted that, "It has been suggested that altered levels/function of brain-derived neurotrophic factor (BDNF)[1] play a role in the pathophysiology of neurodegenerative diseases including Alzheimer's disease. BDNF positively contributes to neural survival and synapse maintenance...making upregulation of BDNF and/or activation of BDNF-related intracellular signaling an attractive approach to treating neurodegenerative diseases...*small natural compounds such as flavonoids successfully increase activation of the BDNF system*..."[535]

Also in late 2014, a different group of researchers noted the following, "Polyphenols are a large group of phytonutrients found in herbal beverages and foods. *They have manifold biological activities, including antioxidative, antimicrobial, and anti-inflammatory properties. Interestingly, some polyphenols bind to amyloid and substantially ameliorate amyloid diseases. Misfolding, aggregation, and accumulation of amyloid fibrils in tissues or organs leads to a group of disorders, called amyloidoses. Prominent diseases are Alzheimer's, Parkinson's, and Huntington's disease*, but there are other, less well-known diseases wherein accumulation of misfolded protein is a prominent feature. Amyloidoses are a major burden to public health. In particular, Alzheimer's disease shows a strong increase in patient numbers. Accelerated development of effective therapies for amyloidoses is a necessity.

---

[1]Brain-derived neurotrophic factor (BDNF) is a protein. BDNF acts on certain neurons of the central nervous system and the peripheral nervous system, helping to support the survival of existing neurons, and encourage the growth and differentiation of new neurons and synapses. In the brain, it is active in the hippocampus, cortex, and basal forebrain—areas vital to learning, memory, and higher thinking. BDNF itself is important for long-term memory.

A viable strategy can be the prevention or reduction of protein misfolding, thus reducing amyloid build-up by restoring the cellular aggretome. *Amyloid-binding polyphenols affect amyloid formation on various levels*, e.g. by inhibiting fibril formation or steering oligomer formation into unstructured, nontoxic pathways. Consequently, *preclinical studies demonstrate reduction of amyloid-formation by polyphenols. Intake of dietary polyphenols might be relevant to the prevention of amyloidoses. Nutraceutical strategies might be a way to reduce amyloid diseases.*"[536]

Still other researchers report that, "Polyphenolic compounds derived mainly from plant products have demonstrated neuroprotective properties in a number of experimental settings. Such protective effects have often been ascribed to antioxidant capacity, but specific augmentation of other cellular defences and direct interactions with neurotoxic proteins have also been demonstrated. With an emphasis on neurodegenerative conditions, such as Alzheimer's disease, *we highlight recent findings on the neuroprotection ascribed to bioactive polyphenols capable of directly interfering with the Alzheimer's disease hallmark toxic β-amyloid protein (Aβ), thereby inhibiting fibril and aggregate formation. This includes compounds such as the green tea polyphenol (-)-epigallocatechin-3-gallate (EGCG) and the phytoalexin resveratrol.* Targeted studies on the biomolecular interactions between dietary polyphenolics and Aβ have not only improved our understanding of the pathogenic role of β-amyloid, but also *offer fundamentally novel treatment options for Alzheimer's disease* and potentially other amyloidoses."[537]

And, Dr. Jayasena and colleagues, from the Centre for Healthy Brain Aging, School of Psychiatry, University of New South Wales, Sydney, Australia, note that, *"Alzheimer's disease is characterized by extracellular amyloid deposits, neurofibrillary tangles, synaptic loss, inflammation and extensive oxidative stress. Polyphenols, which include resveratrol, epigallocatechin gallate [EGCG] and curcumin, have gained considerable interest for their ability to reduce these hallmarks of disease and their potential to slow down cognitive decline. Although their antioxidant and free radical scavenging properties are well estab-*

lished, more recently polyphenols have been shown to produce other important effects including anti-amyloidogenic activity, cell signaling modulation, effects on telomere length and modulation of the sirtuin proteins."[538]

Drs. Williams and Spencer, from the Department of Biology and Biochemistry, University of Bath, Bath, UK reported in the journal *Free Radical Biology and Medicine*, that, "*There is increasing evidence that the consumption of flavonoid-rich foods can beneficially influence normal cognitive function. In addition, a growing number of flavonoids have been shown to inhibit the development of Alzheimer disease-like pathology and to reverse deficits in cognition in rodent models, suggestive of potential therapeutic utility in dementia.* The actions of flavonoid-rich foods (e.g., green tea, blueberry, and cocoa) seem to be mediated by the direct interactions of absorbed flavonoids and their metabolites with a number of cellular and molecular targets…Concurrently, *their effects on the vascular system may also lead to enhancements in cognitive performance through increased brain blood flow and an ability to initiate neurogenesis [nerve growth] in the hippocampus [main area for memory]. Additional mechanisms have been suggested for the ability of flavonoids to delay the initiation of and/or slow the progression of AD-like pathology and related neurodegenerative disorders,* including a potential to inhibit neuronal apoptosis [nerve cell death] triggered by neurotoxic species (e.g., oxidative stress and neuroinflammation) or disrupt amyloid β aggregation and effects on amyloid precursor protein processing through the inhibition of β-secretase (BACE-1) and/or activation of α-secretase (ADAM10). *Together, these processes act to maintain the number and quality of synaptic[1] connections in key brain regions and thus flavonoids have the potential to prevent the progression of neurodegenerative pathologies and to promote cognitive performance.*"[539]

Reporting in the August 15, 2014 issue of the journal *Neural Regeneration Research*, Dr. Subash and colleagues note that, "*Recent clinical*

---

[1] In the nervous system, a synapse is a structure that permits a neuron (or nerve cell) to pass an electrical or chemical signal to another cell (neural or otherwise).

research has demonstrated that berry fruits can prevent age-related neurodegenerative diseases and improve motor and cognitive functions. The berry fruits are also capable of modulating signaling pathways involved in inflammation, cell survival, neurotransmission and enhancing neuroplasticity[1]. *The neuroprotective effects of berry fruits on neurodegenerative diseases are related to phytochemicals such as anthocyanin, caffeic acid, catechin, quercetin, kaempferol and tannin."*[540]

Researchers report that, *"Figs are rich in fiber, copper, iron, manganese, magnesium, potassium, calcium, vitamin K, and are a good source of proanthocyanidins and quercetin which demonstrate potent antioxidant properties."* The researchers studied the effect of dietary supplementation with 4 percent figs grown in Oman on the memory, anxiety, and learning skills in an animal model of Alzheimer's disease. Without discussing the specifics of the experiment, the researchers concluded that, "Our results suggest that *dietary supplementation of figs may be useful for the improvement of cognitive and behavioral deficits in AD."*[541]

Not to be outdone, Dr. Gongadze and colleagues, from the Tbilisi State Medical University, Institute of Medical Biotechnology, Georgia, reported the following in 2014, *"Many studies have shown that biologically active components in plant-based foods, particularly phytochemicals, have important potential to modulate many processes in the development of diseases, including cancer, cardiovascular disease, diabetes, pulmonary disorders, Alzheimer's disease, and other degenerative diseases.* The aim of our study was to provide an updated understanding and analysis of various apple sorts growing in Georgia by the compounds with a particular focus on their potential role(s) in

---

[1]Neuroplasticity, also known as brain plasticity, is an umbrella term that encompasses both synaptic plasticity and non-synaptic plasticity—it refers to changes in neural pathways and synapses due to changes in behavior, environment, neural processes, thinking, emotions, as well as changes resulting from bodily injury. Neuroplasticity has replaced the formerly-held position that the brain is a physiologically static organ, and explores how - and in which ways - the brain changes throughout life.

disease risk and general human health. The Various sorts (Kekhura, Banany, Golden, Starty, Chempion, Aidaridy, Brotsky, Achabety, Sinapy, Jonagold and Antonovka) of apples were investigated. The total phenolic content and antioxidant activity were studied in peel and flesh extracts and were measured. Summarizing our data, we can conclude that, in accordance with the benefit to human health, the most prominent varieties of apples - Kekhura. It is rich with phenolic compounds, and also characterized by high scavenging activity. Also has good features Antonovka and Achabety. *It should be noted that apple peel [is] more helpful than the flesh, and therefore during consumption peeling of apples is unacceptable in terms of its usefulness.*"[542]

Reporting in the August 2014 issue of the journal *Clinical Psychopharmacology and Neuroscience*, Dr. Nakajima and colleagues noted, "When researching materials from natural resources having anti-dementia drug activity, we identified nobiletin[1], a polymethoxylated flavone from the peel of Citrus depressa. Nobiletin exhibited memory-improving effects in various animal models of dementia and exerted a wide range of beneficial effects against pathological features of AD including amyloid-β (Aβ) pathology, tau hyperphosphorylation, oxidative stress, cholinergic neurodegeneration and dysfunction of synaptic plasticity-related signaling, suggesting this natural compound could become a novel drug for the treatment and prevention of AD."[543]

Folate (Folic Acid; Vitamin B$_9$)

Folic acid or folate is a B vitamin. It is also referred to as vitamin M, vitamin B$_9$, vitamin B$_c^[$ (or folacin), pteroyl-L-glutamic acid, and pteroyl-L-glutamate. *Folate* indicates a collection of "folates" that is not chemically well-characterized. Folic acid is synthetically produced, and used in fortified foods and supplements. Folate is converted by

---

[1]Nobiletin is a chemical compound. It is an *O*-methylated flavone, a flavonoid isolated from citrus peels like in tangerine. Nobiletin was found to have anti-inflammatory and anti-tumor invasion, proliferation, and metastasis *in vitro* and in animal studies. Nobiletin was also found to potentially inhibit cartilage degradation.

humans to dihydrofolate (dihydrofolic acid), tetrahydrofolate (tetrahydrofolic acid), and other derivatives, which have various biological activities.

Folic acid is essential for numerous bodily functions. Humans cannot synthesize folates *de novo*; therefore, folic acid has to be supplied through the diet to meet their daily requirements. The human body needs folate to synthesize DNA, repair DNA, and methylate DNA as well as to act as a cofactor in certain biological reactions. It is especially important in aiding rapid cell division and growth, such as in infancy and pregnancy. Children and adults both require folate to produce healthy red blood cells and prevent anemia.

Folate and folic acid derive their names from the Latin word *folium*, which means "leaf." Folates occur naturally in many foods and, among plants, are especially plentiful in dark green leafy vegetables. A lack of dietary folates can lead to folate deficiency. A complete lack of dietary folate takes months before deficiency develops as normal individuals have about 500–20,000 µg of folate in body stores. This deficiency can result in many health problems, the most notable one being neural tube defects in developing embryos—a relatively rare birth defect affecting only 300,000 (0.002 percent) of births globally each year. Common symptoms of folate deficiency include diarrhea, macrocytic anemia with weakness or shortness of breath, nerve damage with weakness and limb numbness (peripheral neuropathy), pregnancy complications, mental confusion, forgetfulness or other cognitive deficits, mental depression, sore or swollen tongue, peptic or mouth ulcers, headaches, heart palpitations, irritability, and behavioral disorders.

Low levels of folate can also lead to homocysteine accumulation (discussed previously). In adult life, folate deficiency has been known for decades to produce a characteristic form of anaemia ("megaloblastic"). More recently *degrees of folate inadequacy, not severe enough to produce anaemia, have been found to be associated with high blood levels of the amino acid homocysteine.* Such degrees of folate inadequacy can arise because of insufficient folates in the diet or because of inefficient absorption or metabolic utilization of folates due to genetic variations.

PREVENTION

Conventional criteria for diagnosing folate deficiency may be inadequate for identifying people capable of benefiting from dietary supplementation. *High blood levels of homocysteine have been linked with the risk of arterial disease, dementia and Alzheimer's disease.* There is therefore interest in whether dietary supplements of folic acid (an artificial chemical analogue of naturally occurring folates) can improve cognitive function of people at risk of cognitive decline associated with aging or dementia, whether by affecting homocysteine metabolism or through other mechanisms. *There is a risk that if folic acid is given to people who have undiagnosed deficiency of vitamin B12 it may lead to neurological damage. Vitamin B12 deficiency produces both an anaemia identical to that of folate deficiency but also causes irreversible damage to the central and peripheral nervous systems. Folic acid will correct the anaemia of vitamin B12 deficiency and so delay diagnosis but will not prevent progression to neurological damage.*

In order to study this phenomenon, researchers conducted an extensive literature review to examine the effects of folic acid supplementation, with or without vitamin B12, on elderly healthy and demented people, in preventing cognitive impairment or retarding its progress. They found that, "There was no beneficial effect of 750 mcg of folic acid per day on measures of cognition or mood in older healthy women. *In patients with mild to moderate cognitive decline and different forms of dementia there was no benefit from folic acid on measures of cognition or mood. Folic acid plus vitamin B12 was effective in reducing the serum homocysteine concentrations.* Folic acid was well tolerated and no adverse effects were reported. More studies are needed."[544]

Dr. van der Zwaluw and colleagues, reporting the results of their research in the December 2, 2014 issue of *Neurology*, also studied the potential benefits of folic acid and vitamin B12 in an elderly population. They stated that, "We investigated the effects of 2-year folic acid and vitamin B12 supplementation on cognitive performance in elderly people with elevated homocysteine (Hcy) levels. This multicenter, double-blind, randomized, placebo-controlled trial included 2,919 elderly participants (sixty-five years and older) with Hcy levels between 12 and 50 µmol/L. Participants received daily either a tablet with 400 µg folic acid and 500 µg vitamin B12 (B-vitamin group) or a placebo tablet. Both tablets contained 15 µg vitamin D3. Mean age was 74.1 years. Hcy concentrations decreased 5.0 µmol/L in the B-vitamin group and 1.3 µmol/L in the placebo group. Cognitive domain scores did not differ over time between the two groups. *Two-year folic acid and vitamin B12 supplementation did not beneficially affect performance on four cognitive domains in elderly people with elevated Hcy levels. It may slightly slow the rate of decline of global cognition, but the reported small difference may be attributable to chance.*"[545]

But just when things seem clear (e.g., that folic acid and/or B12 are of no use), a different group of researchers did find benefit! Dr. Jerneren and colleagues, reporting in the April 15, 2015 issue of the *American Journal of Clinical Nutrition*, stated that, "Increased brain atrophy rates are common in older people with cognitive impairment, particularly in those who eventually convert to Alzheimer's disease. Plasma concentrations of omega-3 (ω-3) fatty acids ["fish oil"] and homocysteine are associated with the development of brain atrophy and dementia. *We investigated whether plasma ω-3 fatty acid concentrations* (eicosapentaenoic acid and docosahexaenoic acid) *modify the treatment effect of homocysteine-lowering B vitamins on brain atrophy rates.* This retrospective analysis included 168 elderly people (≥70 y) with mild cognitive impairment, randomly assigned either to placebo (n = 83) or to daily high-dose B vitamin supplementation (folic acid, 0.8 mg; vitamin B-6, 20 mg; vitamin B-12, 0.5 mg) (n = 85). The subjects underwent cranial magnetic resonance imaging (MRI) scans at baseline and 2 y later. The effect of the intervention was analyzed according to tertiles of baseline ω-3 fatty acid concentrations. There was a significant interaction (P = 0.024) between B vitamin treatment and plasma combined ω-3 fatty acids (eicosapentaenoic acid and docosahexaenoic acid) on brain atrophy rates. *In subjects with high baseline ω-3 fatty acids (>590 µmol/L), B vitamin treatment slowed the mean atrophy rate by 40.0 percent compared with placebo. B vitamin treatment had no significant effect on the rate of atrophy among subjects with low baseline ω-3 fatty acids (<390 µmol/L). High baseline ω-3 fatty acids were associated with a slower rate of brain atrophy in the B vitamin group but not in the placebo group.*"[546]

And finally, Drs. Shen and Ji published a review of the literature on this subject in the April 8, 2015 issue of the *Journal of Alzheimer's Disease*. They noted that, "The associations between homocysteine (Hcy), folic acid, and vitamin B12 and Alzheimer's disease have gained much interest, while remaining controversial...First, AD patients may have higher level of Hcy, and lower levels of folate and vitamin B12 in plasma than controls. Further age-subgroup analysis showed no age effect for Hcy levels in plasma between AD patients and matched controls, while the differences in folate and vitamin B12 levels further enlarged with increased age. Second, data suggests that high Hcy and low folate levels may correlate with increased risk of AD occurrence. *The comprehensive meta-analyses not only confirmed higher Hcy, lower folic acid, and vitamin B12 levels in AD patients than controls, but also implicated that high Hcy and low folic acid levels may be risk factors of AD.* Further studies are encouraged to elucidate mechanisms linking these conditions."[547]

Gelsolin

Gelsolin is a protein. Among other functions, it inhibits cell death (apoptosis) by stabilizing mitochondria. Prior to cell death, mitochondria normally lose membrane integrity and become more permeable. Gelsolin can impede the release of cytochrome C, obstructing the signal amplification that would have led to cell death.

Dr. Zhao and colleagues discussed gelsolin in the September 10, 2014 issue of the *Journal of Alzheimer's Disease*. They note that, "The presence of amyloid plaques and vascular amyloid deposits are two of the pathological features of Alzheimer's disease. Amyloid plaques and vascular deposits mainly consist of amyloid-β (Aβ), which is a metabolic product of amyloid-β protein precursor [APP] cleaved by β- and γ-secretase [two enzymes]... Intensive therapeutic efforts have been attempted in the treatment of AD targeting Aβ, including preventing Aβ generation, inhibiting Aβ aggregation, and promoting Aβ clearance...Gelsolin is suggested to be implicated in AD, based on the findings that some changes of gelsolin are correlated with disease progression rate in AD patients. *Gelsolin binds Aβ, inhibits its aggregation into fibrils, and protects cells from apoptosis induced by Aβ. More importantly, administration or overexpression of gelsolin results in significant reduction of amyloid load and decrease of Aβ level in AD transgenic mice.*"[548]

Ginkgo Biloba

Ginkgo (*Ginkgo biloba*), also known as the maidenhair tree, is a unique species of tree. The ginkgo is a living fossil, recognizably similar to fossils dating back 270 million years. Native to China, the tree is widely cultivated and was introduced early to human history. A combination of resistance to disease, insect-resistant wood and the ability to form aerial roots and sprouts makes ginkgos long-lived, with some specimens claimed to be more than 2,500 years old.

In many areas of China, it has been long cultivated, and it is common in the southern third of the country. It has also been commonly cultivated in North America for over 200 years and in Europe for close to 300, but during that time, it has never become significantly naturalized.

Ginkgo biloba special extract (EGb761) is used in most clinical trials. Potential indications include cognition and memory in Alzheimer's disease, cerebral insufficiency, intermittent claudication, and multi-infarct dementia. Dosages range from 80 to 720 mg/d for durations of two weeks to two years. Mechanisms of action include increasing cerebral blood flow, antioxidant and anti-inflammatory effects, with antiplatelet effects attributed to flavone and terpene lactones.

Possible interactions with monoamine oxidase inhibitors, alprazolam, haloperidol, warfarin, and nifedipine have been reported.

Ginkgo biloba is currently the most investigated and adopted herbal remedy for cognitive disorders and Alzheimer's disease. Nevertheless, its efficacy in the prevention and treatment of dementia still remains controversial.

PREVENTION

Research into Ginkgo biloba has been ongoing for many years, while the benefit and adverse effects of Ginkgo biloba extract EGb761 for cognitive impairment and dementia has been controversial. In the January 1, 2015 issue of the *Journal of Alzheimer's Disease*, researchers reported their review of the literature on the clinical and adverse effects of standardized Ginkgo biloba extract EGb761 for cognitive impairment and dementia. They reviewed clinical trials that included a total of 2,561 patient, mostly with a dose of 240 mg/day. There analysis showed that Ginko biloba improved activities of daily living (ADLs), cognition, and what they called neuropsychiatric symptoms (e.g., things like anxiety, irritability, and depression). They stated in conclusion, "*EGb761 at 240 mg/day is able to stabilize or to slow decline in cognition, function, behavior, and global change at 22-26 weeks in cognitive impairment and dementia, especially for patients with neuropsychiatric symptoms.*"[549]

A systematic review of the literature to evaluate the efficacy of natural medicines for the treatment of Alzheimer's disease was performed by a group of researchers in 2014. *No other "natural medicine" was found to be helpful in the prevention or treatment of AD except Ginkgo.* They noted, "Out of the literatures, twenty-one clinical reports were included in this review that satisfied the particular selection criteria. Apart from Ginkgo, other treatments we came across had minimal benefits and/or the methodological quality of the available trials was poor…*Our results suggest that Ginkgo may help established AD patients with cognitive symptoms but cannot prevent the neurodegenerative progression of the disease.*"[550]

Scientists studied whether the use of Ginkgo biloba is associated with additional cognitive and functional benefit in AD patients already in treatment with cholinesterase inhibitors (ChEIs; medications such as Aricept and Exelon). Data were from mild to moderate AD patients under ChEI treatment recruited in the Impact of Cholinergic Treatment USe (ICTUS) study. A total of 828 subjects were studied over a 12-month follow-up period. The results were mixed, but the authors concluded, "*Our findings suggest that Ginkgo biloba may provide some added cognitive benefits in AD patients already under ChEIs treatment.*

The clinical meaningfulness of such effects remains to be confirmed and clarified."[551]

In 2014, researchers from Department of Neurology, Zhongshan Hospital, Fudan University, Shanghai, China were the first to demonstate the cellular mechanisms whereby the *standard Ginkgo biloba extract EGb761 works to protect the brain from abnormal amyloid beta (Aβ) accumulation and deposition.* They concluded by stating, "Our results provide a new insight into a possible mechanism of action of EGb761. *This study provides a rational basis for the therapeutic application of EGb761 in the treatment of AD.*"[552]

There is currently on the world market a dietary supplement (Memo®) combining 750 mg of lyophilized royal jelly with standardized extracts of G. biloba 120 mg and P. ginseng 150 mg. Researchers investigated the potential benefit of this preparation, used for four weeks, on sixty-six patients with mild cognitive impairment (MCI). They concluded, "*This combined triple formula may be beneficial in treating the cognitive decline that occurs during the aging process as well as in the early phases of pathologic cognitive impairment typical of insidious-onset vascular dementia and in the early stages of Alzheimer's disease.* Larger-sized studies with longer treatment durations are needed to confirm this." [553]

In order to compare the benefits of Ginkgo biloba (120 mg daily dose) to Exelon (rivastigmine; 4.5 mg daily dose; a standard treatment for AD) in patients with Alzheimer's dementia, researchers studied 56 patients over twenty-four weeks, placing half the patients into each treatment group. They concluded, "*Our results confirm the clinical efficacy (usefulness) of rivastigmine in Alzheimer's dementia, comparing to Ginkgo biloba* [meaning that rivastigmine was superior to Ginkgo biloba in this study]."[554]

Austrian researchers studied the potential benefits of Ginkgo biloba extract EGb761 in non-institutionalized Austrian dementia patients. They studied 1,201 patients for 22-24 weeks. The researchers found that *the use of Ginkgo biloba (240 mg/day) delayed the onset of activities of daily living (ADLs) deterioration by 22.3 months compared to placebo.* This proved to be a great cost saving for the Austrian society, due to decreased requirements for home health services in the Ginkgo biloba treatment group. *In a tentative cost comparison, cholinesterase inhibitors (e.g., drugs like Aricept and Exelon) required higher expenses to achieve similar success.*[555]

A report, from the Neurobiology Laboratory for Brain Aging and Mental Health, Psychiatric University Clinics, Basel, Switzerland, notes that, "Oxidative stress and mitochondrial failure...are early stages in the development of Alzheimer's disease. *A growing volume of data confirms that Ginkgo biloba extract (GBE) reduces oxidative stress and improves mitochondrial respiration (function) and thus may be useful in preventing or slowing down the progression of AD.*" The authors also note that, *in an animal model of longevity, "Treatment with GBE-extract reduces oxidative stress and extends median lifespan compared with controls...* The flavonoids, bilobalide and some of the ginkgolides (B and J) had a high protective capacity, indicating that a combination of several compounds within standardized Gingko biloba extracts contribute disproportionately for these protective effects"[556]

Another group of researchers conducted a multi-center (e.g., different research sites and researchers), 24-week trial with 410 outpatients in order to demonstrate efficacy and safety of a 240 mg once-daily formulation of Ginkgo biloba extract EGb 761(®) in patients with mild to moderate dementia (Alzheimer's disease or vascular dementia). In their article, the researchers stated, *"In conclusion, treatment with EGb 761(®) at a once-daily dose of 240 mg was safe and resulted in a significant and clinically relevant improvement in cognition, psychopathology, functional measures and quality of life of patients and caregivers."*[557]

In 2009, in the distinguished medical journal *JAMA*, Dr. Snitz and more than sixty colleagues published the results of their research to determine whether Ginkgo biloba slows the rates of cognitive decline in older adults. They conducted the The Ginkgo Evaluation of Memory (GEM) study, a clinical trial of 3,069 community-dwelling participants aged 72 to 96 years, conducted in six academic medical centers in the United States between 2000 and 2008, with a median follow-up of 6.1 years. They summarized their (sad) results by stating, *"Compared with placebo, the use of G. biloba, 120 mg twice daily, did not result in less cognitive decline in older adults with normal cognition or with mild cognitive impairment."*[558] Perhaps starting to use a supplement at age 72 (or 92) is a little too late to expect significant benefits.

The above notwithstanding, recent research is more positive vis-à-vis the benefits of Ginko biloba (GB) in the prevention and/or treatment of Alzheimer's disease. For example, Dr. Kaur and colleagues, reporting in the June 2015 issue of the *Journal of Neuroscience Research*, reported the following, "Accumulating evidence points to roles for oxidative stress, amyloid beta (Aβ), and mitochondrial dysfunction in the pathogenesis of Alzheimer's disease...Apurinic/apyrimidinic endonuclease 1 (APE1), a multifunctional enzyme with DNA repair and reduction-oxidation activities, has been shown to enhance neuronal survival after oxidative stress...*This study presents findings from a new point of view to improve therapeutic potential for AD via the synergistic neuroprotective role played by APE1 in combination with the phytochemical GB [Gigko biloba]*."[559]

And, Dr. Bun and colleagues, reporting in the January 1, 2015 issue of the *Journal of Alzheimer's Disease*, note that, "A number of studies have examined the effect of a single supplement against Alzheimer's disease with conflicting results. Taking into account the complex and multifactorial nature of AD pathogenesis, multiple supplements may be more effective. Physical activity is another prospect against AD. An open-label intervention study was conducted to explore a potential protective effect of multiple supplements and physical activity. Participants were community-dwelling volunteers aged sixty-five or older. Among 918 cognitively normal participants included in the analyses, 171 took capsules daily for three years that contained n-3 polyunsaturated fatty acid, Ginkgo biloba leaf dry extracts, and lycopene. Two hundred and forty one participants joined the two-year exercise intervention that included a community center-based and a home-based exercise program. One-hundred and forty eight participated in both interventions. The primary outcome was AD diagnosis at follow-ups. A total of 76 participants were diagnosed with AD during follow-up periods. *Higher adherence to supplementation intervention was associated with lower AD incidence in both unadjusted and adjusted models. Exercise intervention was also associated with lower AD incidence in the unadjusted model, but not in the adjusted model. We hypothesized that the combination of supplements acted in a complementary and synergistic fashion to bring significant effects against AD occurrence."*[560]

And finally, Drs. Gauthier and Schlaefke, reported in the November 28, 2014 issue of *Clinical Interventions in Aging* their systematic review of the scientific literature to evaluate current evidence for the efficacy of Ginkgo biloba extract EGb 761(®) in dementia. They noted that, "Of 2,684 outpatients randomized to receive treatment for 22-26 weeks, 2,625 represented the full analysis sets (1,396 for EGb 761 and 1,229 for placebo). *Standardized mean differences for change in cognition, activities of daily living, and global rating significantly favored EGb 761 compared with placebo. Statistically significant superiority of EGb 761 over placebo was confirmed by responder analyses as well as for patients suffering from dementia with neuropsychiatric symptoms. Treatment-associated risks in terms of relative risks of adverse events and premature withdrawal rates did not differ noticeably between the two treatment groups. In conclusion, meta-analyses confirmed the efficacy and good tolerability of Ginkgo biloba extract EGb 761 in patients with dementia."*[561]

Ginger

Ginger (*Zingiber officinale* Roscoe) is a flowering plant in the family Zingiberaceae whose rhizome, ginger root or simply ginger, is widely used as a spice or a medicine. Other members of the family Zingiberaceae include turmeric, cardamom, and galangal.

Ginger is well known to contain a number of potentially bioactive phytochemicals having valuable medicinal properties. Although recent studies have emphasized their benefits in Alzheimer's disease, limited information is available on the possible mechanism by which it renders anti-Alzheimer activity. In order to help understand these mechanisms, researchers conducted an experiment. Without going into the complex details of their work, in 2014 the researchers noted that, "In the present study, the antioxidant activity, cholinesterase inhibition, anti-amyloidogenic potential and neuroprotective properties of dry ginger extract (GE) have been evaluated...GE expressed high antioxidant activity...Also, GE increased the cell survival against amyloid beta (Abeta) induced toxicity in primary adult rat hippocampal cell culture. Aggregation experiments showed that GE effectively prevented the formation of Abeta oligomers and dissociated the preformed oligomers. *These findings suggest that GE influences multiple therapeutic molecular targets of AD and can be considered as an effective nontoxic neutraceutical supplement for AD.*"[562]

In the June 20, 2014 issue of the journal *Biochemical and Biophysical Research Communications*, Dr. Moon and colleagues reported that, "A growing number of experimental studies suggest that 6-shogaol, a bioactive component of ginger, may play an important role as a memory-enhancing and anti-oxidant agent against neurological diseases. 6-Shogaol has also recently been shown to have anti-neuroinflammatory effects...*All these results suggest that 6-shogaol may play a role in inhibiting glial cell activation [nerve cell inflammation] and reducing memory impairment in animal models of dementia.*"[563]

Another group of researchers conducted an experiment to assess the ability of ginger root extract (GRE) to prevent behavioral dysfunction in the Alzheimer's disease rat model. The researchers concluded that, "*This experiment demonstrates that the administration of GRE reverses behavioral dysfunction and prevents AD-like symptoms in our rat model.*"[564]

Ginseng

What constitutes "ginseng" is a little confusing. Technically, Ginseng is any one of eleven species belonging to the genus *Panax* of the family

Araliaceae. Ginseng is found in North America and in eastern Asia (mostly Korea, northeast China, Bhutan, eastern Siberia), typically in cooler climates. *Panax vietnamensis*, discovered in Vietnam, is the southernmost ginseng known. Ginseng is characterized by the presence of ginsenosides. Siberian ginseng (*Eleutherococcus senticosus*) is in the same family, but not genus, as true ginseng. Like ginseng, it is considered to be an adaptogenic[1] herb. The active compounds in Siberian ginseng are eleutherosides, not ginsenosides.

Besides *P. ginseng*, many other plants are also known as or mistaken for the ginseng root. The most commonly known examples are *xiyangshen*, also known as American ginseng (*P. quinquefolius*), Japanese ginseng (*P. japonicus*), crown prince ginseng (*Pseudostellaria heterophylla*), and Siberian ginseng (*Eleutherococcus senticosus*). Although all have the name ginseng, each plant has distinctively different functions. However, true ginseng plants belong only to the *Panax* genus.

In 2010, nearly all of the world's 80,000 tons of ginseng in international commerce was produced in four countries: South Korea, China, Canada, and the United States. The product was marketed in over 35 countries. Sales exceeded $2.1 billion, of which half came from South Korea. Historically, Korea has been the largest provider, and China the largest consumer.

The root is most often available in dried form, either whole or sliced. Ginseng leaf, although not as highly prized, is sometimes also used.

---

[1]Adaptogens or adaptogenic substances, compounds, herbs or practices refer to the pharmacological concept whereby administration results in stabilization of physiological processes and promotion of homeostasis, an example being by decreased cellular sensitivity to stress. In herbal medicine the categorization of different herbs as adaptogens is very popular, often with far-reaching claims of increasing longevity, libido and well-being. Adaptogens have been claimed to treat a wide variety of medical conditions, from fatigue to cancer. However, no herbs that are considered adaptogens by the U.S. FDA have ever been conclusively shown effective in treating medical conditions, and as a result none of them are approved by the FDA to cure, treat, or prevent disease.

Folk medicine attributes various benefits to oral use of American ginseng and Asian ginseng (*P. ginseng*) roots, including roles as an aphrodisiac, stimulant, type II diabetes treatment, or cure for sexual dysfunction in men.

Ginseng may be included in small doses in energy drinks or herbal teas, such as ginseng coffee. It may be found in hair tonics and cosmetic preparations, as well, but those uses have not been shown to be clinically effective.

In 2014, researchers conducted studies in animal models of Alzheimer's diease and were able to show that, *"ginsenoside Rd, one of the main active ingredients in Panax ginseng, decreased some of the pathological changes associated with Alzheimer's disease as well as post-stroke dementia."*[565]

Chronic stress, which can induce atrophy and functional impairments in several key brain areas including the hippocampus (the main area of the brain for learning and memory), plays an important role in the generation and progression of AD. Ginsenoside Rg1 is a steroidal saponin abundantly contained in ginseng. In 2014, researchers explored the neuroprotective effects of Rg1 on chronic stress-induced learning and memory impairments in a mouse model. *Results showed that, "Rg1 "significantly protected against learning and memory impairments."*[566]

Neuroinflammatory (inflammation of nerves) responses play a crucial role in the pathogenesis of Alzheimer's disease. Ginsenoside Rg5, an abundant natural compound in Panax ginseng, has been found to be beneficial in treating Alzheimer's disease. In a recent study, *researchers demonstrated that Rg5 improved cognitive dysfunction and attenuated neuroinflammatory responses in an animal model of AD.*[567]

In yet another recent experiment using an animal model of Alzheimer's disease, researchers demonstrated that Ginseng had several protective effects through the modulation of various key enzymes and genes. The authors concluded, that, *"Panax notoginseng saponins (PNS) may be a promising agent for Alzheimer's disease."*[568]

PREVENTION

In 2008, researchers published a positive report about the use of Korean red ginseng (KRG) as an additive therapy to conventional anti-dementia medications in patients with Alzheimer's disease. The studied sixty-one patients for twelve weeks. They concluded that, *"KRG showed good efficacy for the treatment of Alzheimer's disease*; however, further studies with larger samples of patients and a longer efficacy trial should be conducted to confirm the efficacy of KRG."[569]

Also in 2008, researchers studied 97 patients in order to determine the clinical efficacy of Panax ginseng powder (4.5 g/d) for twelve weeks in the cognitive performance of AD patients. After ginseng treatment, the tests of cognitive functioning began to show improvements and continued up to twelve weeks). After discontinuing ginseng, the improved scores declined to the levels of the control group. The researchers concluded that, *"These results suggest that Panax ginseng is clinically effective in the cognitive performance of AD patients."*[570]

However, in 2009, scientists published the results of a review of all available clinical trials (e.g., the use of ginseng in human studies) in the *Journal of Alzheimer's disease*. They stated, "In conclusion, *the evidence for ginseng as a treatment of AD is scarce and inconclusive*. Further rigorous trials seem warranted."[571]

To date, animal models of Alzheimer's disease have been more convincing of ginseng's benefits than human trials. However, as noted above, more clinical trials are necessary to come to a firm conclusion. As with all substances reviewed in this book, their potential benefits in preventing AD are much greater that their use as potential treatments of Alzheimer's disease. Historically, researchers have focused on treatment rather than prevention. However, it seems that *evidence is mounting that the use of these agents, if they are to be of any help, needs to be started years before the onset of Alzheimer's disease.*

Grape Seed Extract (GSE)

Grape seed extracts are derivatives from whole grape seeds that have a great concentration of vitamin E, flavonoids, linoleic acid and phenolic procyanidins (also known as OPC or oligomeric procyanidins). The typical commercial opportunity of extracting grape seed constituents has been for chemicals known as polyphenols having antioxidant activity in vitro. A polyphenol contained in grape seeds is resveratrol (see below). Oral grape seed extract is used in capsules or tablets usually containing 50 mg or 100 mg.

Caution: In the March 1, 2015 issue of the journal *Food Chemistry*, Dr. Villani and colleagues from the New Use Agriculture and Natural Plant Products Program, Department of Plant Biology and Pathology, Rutgers University, New Brunswick, NJ issued a warning about the purity of commercially available grape seed extract products: "Fundamental concerns in quality control arise due to increasing use of grape seed extract and the complex chemical composition of GSE. Proanthocyanidin monomers and oligomers are the major bioactive compounds in GSE. *Given no standardized criteria for quality, large variation exists in the composition of commercial GSE supplements.* Twenty-one commercial GSE containing products were purchased and chemically profiled, major compounds quantitated, and compared against authenticated grape seed extract, peanut skin extract, and pine bark extract. *Nine products were adulterated, found to contain peanut skin extract. A wide degree of variability in chemical composition was detected in commercial products,* demonstrating the need for development of quality control standards for GSE."[572] So, make sure that if you decide to take GSE, it is from a reliable and trustworthy source.

It has been reported that, *"grape seed extract has biological functions including antioxidant, anti-cancer, anti-hyperglycemic (e.g., lowering blood sugar), anti-radiation, and prevention and treatment of cardiovascular diseases."*[573]

In 2014, researchers demonstrated in an animal model of diabetes that grape seed extract and vitamin E were protective against oxidative stress in the hippocampus (brain memory area). *"The protective effects of grape seed extract were more pronounced in decreasing oxidative stress and nerve cell death than those of vitamin E."*[574]

As another example of the beneficial effects of GSE, in October 2014, Dr. Kumar and colleagues, from the Department of Pharmaceutical Sciences, Skaggs School of Pharmacy and Pharmaceutical Sciences, University of Colorado Anshutz Medical Campus, Aurora, CO, documented in both animal and human cells, *"the molecular mechanisms of GSE's ability to fight colon cancer."*[575]

Reporting in the March 14, 2014 issue of the journal *Frontiers in Aging Neuroscience*, Dr. Wang and twelve collegues recently determined that a combination of *three polyphenolic preparations (grape seed extract, resveratrol, and Concord grape juice extract)*, with different polyphenolic compositions and partially redundant bioactivities, proved more effective in preventing the toxic effects of amyloid-β (Aβ) mediated nerve cell damage and cognitive impairments in a mouse model of AD. They summarized their results by stating, *"Moreover, we found greatly reduced total amyloid content in the brain following combination treatment. Our studies provided experimental evidence that application of polyphenols targeting multiple disease-mechanisms may yield a greater likelihood of therapeutic efficacy."*[576]

The research cited above underscores the fact that the brain is very complex, and that no one compound or agent is itself good enough to prevent AD. We have to take a variety of supplements, exercise, be social, and keep our minds active.

Recently, in laboratory experiments involving specific types of cells, researchers demonstrated that *one of the main ingredients of GSE, gallic acid, was able to inhibit the formation of the toxic substances associated with Alzheimer's disease.*[577]

And, in a study of the effects of GSE in an animal model of AD, *researchers reported in the journal Neurobiology of Aging profoundly positive effects.*[578]

ALZHEIMER'S DISEASE

In a review article by Drs. Pasinetti and Ho, from the Department of Neurology, Mount Sinai School of Medicine, New York, Geriatric Research, education and Clinical Center, James J. Peters veteran Affairs Medical Center, Bronx, New York, the authors state, *"Findings presented in this review article support the development of GSE as a preventative and/or therapeutic agent in Alzheimer's disease."*[579]

An interesting animal study was published in the *Journal of Alzheimer's Disease*, on "the bioavailability and brain deposition of a *grape seed polyphenolic extract (GSPE) previously found to attenuate cognitive deterioration in a mouse model of Alzheimer's disease."* They authors found that, *as opposed to a single daily dose of GSE, "Repeated daily exposure to GSPE was found to significantly increase bioavailability (of the various chemical components of GSE)."*[580]

Green (and Oolong, White, and Black) Tea

Camellia sinensis L. (tea) is the second most consumed beverage worldwide, after water. Worldwide tea consumption is growing at about 5 percent per year, with much of that growth occurring within China and India, according to the UN. Sales of tea beverages in the U.S. reached approximately $25 billion in 2014, compared to around $50 billion in coffee sales.

Tea is classified into green and white, oolong, black and red, and Pu-erh tea based on the manufacturing process: unfermented (green, yellow, and white), partially fermented (oolong), and completely fermented (black) tea.

Catechins are the main phytochemical constituents of Camellia sinensis which are known for their high antioxidant capacity. (Note: there is now a scientific journal devoted solely to phytochemicals, appropriately called *Phytomedicine*.)

Historically, the medicinal use of green tea dates back to China 4700 years ago and drinking tea continues to be regarded traditionally in Asia as a general healthful practice. Numerous scientific publications now attest to the health benefits of both black and green teas, including clinical and epidemiological studies. *Although all tea contains beneficial antioxidants, high-quality green and white teas have them in greater concentrations than black tea.*[581]

The nutritional value of tea is mostly from the tea polyphenols that are reported to possess a broad spectrum of biological activities, including anti-oxidant properties, reduction of various cancers, inhibition of inflammation, and protective effects against diabetes, hyperlipidemia and obesity. Tea polyphenols include catechins and gallic acid in green and white teas, and theaflavins and thearubigins as well as other catechin polymers in black and oolong teas.[582]

Green tea's major components are epigallocatechin gallate (EGCG), epigallocatechin (EGC), epicatechin gallate (ECG) and epicatechin (EC). Among these, EGCG is the predominant component, contributing more than 50 percent of polyphenols.[583]

There is mounting evidence that green tea possesses numerous health-promoting properties, and may potentially be beneficial to those suffering from Alzheimer's and other diseases, including cardiovascular disease and cancer. These beneficial properties are largely attributed to the high polyphenol content, particularly the catechins (including EGCG).[584]

If you don't like the taste of green tea, as some people don't, the main antioxident (EGCG) comes in pill form. It can be obtained in pharmacies, GNC, or stores like WalMart. It comes in 250 mg and smaller strength tablets. *In the greater scope of things, green tea is inexpensive and ingesting it on a regular basis is one of the very best things you can do for your heath.* Apart from helping prevent AD, it has many beneficial effects on the body. We describe a few of these benefits in order to give a sense of how wonderful green tea is, but space doesn't permit a complete discussion of them in detail.

NOTE: We strongly advise purchasing only name brand products, in order to minimize the risk of ingesting teas that may contain unhealthy

ALZHEIMER'S DISEASE

ingredients such as pesticides or heavy metals. Ingesting EGCG supplements is also a safe way to go. Dr.Schwalfenberg and colleagues from the University of Alberta, Edmonton, AB, Canada, published a disturbing report in the *Journal Toxicology* about contamination of various tea samples. Here is the summary in full:[585]

> "Increasing concern is evident about contamination of foodstuffs and natural health products. Methods: Common off-the-shelf varieties of black, green, white, and oolong teas sold in tea bags were used for analysis in this study. Toxic element testing was performed on thirty different teas by analyzing (i) tea leaves, (ii) tea steeped for 3-4 minutes, and (iii) tea steeped for 15-17 minutes. Results were compared to existing preferred endpoints. Results: All brewed teas contained lead with 73 percent of teas brewed for three minutes and 83 percent brewed for fifteen minutes having lead levels considered unsafe for consumption during pregnancy and lactation. Aluminum levels were above recommended guidelines in 20 percent of brewed teas. No mercury was found at detectable levels in any brewed tea samples. Teas contained several beneficial elements such as magnesium, calcium, potassium, and phosphorus. Of trace minerals, only manganese levels were found to be excessive in some black teas. Conclusions. *Toxic contamination by heavy metals was found in most of the teas sampled. Some tea samples are considered unsafe. There are no existing guidelines for routine testing or reporting of toxicant levels in "naturally" occurring products.* Public health warnings or industry regulation might be indicated to protect consumer safety."

For an excellent article on teas, *Do You Know What's Really In Your Tea?* By Food Babe go to: http://foodbabe.com/2013/08/21/do-you-know-whats-really-in-your-tea/ Or see (a more upbeat review) at Teaviews.com: http://www.teaviews.com/best-tea-companies/

PREVENTION

There are numerous sources of safe green tea. One such source is Lipton. Here's some of the information listed on one of their boxes of green tea, which was purchased from WalMart:

> "Pure green tea. 100 percent Natural. 40 tea bags. Based on drinking 2-3 cups per day: 150 mg tea flavonoids per serving (versus: orange juice, 58 mg; pomegranete juice, 11 mg; coffee, 0.4 mg). "Our green tea blend is selected from fresh-picked high-grown tea leaves. And we've sourced 80 percent of the tea in this package from Rainforest Alliance Certified™ tea farms…"

Below are listed some of the beneficial effects of green tea and other teas, with an emphasis on the prevention of Alzheimer's disease. There are thousands of scientific studies of tea, and those discussed below are, perforce, just a small sample.

Excessive accumulation of β-amyloid peptide (Aβ) is one of the major mechanisms responsible for neuronal (nerve cell) death in Alzheimer's disease. In 2014, a group of researchers reported that, *"Evidence is increasingly showing that epigallocatechin-3-gallate (EGCG), a flavonoid found in green tea, can partly protect cells from Aβ-mediated neurotoxicity by inhibiting Aβ aggregation."*[586]

In a recent experiment, researchers found that ascorbic acid (vitamin C) "significantly inhibited" nerve cell death in nerve cell cultures. They also studied ten flavonoids, including the main antioxidant in green tea, epigallocatechin gallate (EGCG), and reported that, *"Epicatechin, EGCG, luteolin, and myricetin showed more potent and persistent neuroprotective action than did the other compounds. These results demonstrated that oxidative stress was involved in Aβ-induced neuronal death, and antioxidative flavonoid compounds, especially epicatechin, EGCG, luteolin, and myricetin, could inhibit neuronal death. These findings suggest that these four compounds may be developed as neuroprotective agents against Alzheimer's disease."*[587]

In 2014, researchers from three different laboratories, including Astra-Zeneca-Tufts Lab for Basic and Translational Medicine, Boston, MA, showed that in a nerve cell model of Alzheimers disease, *"EGCG was able to reverse some of the characteristic damage of AD."*[588]

Cox and colleagues published a report in the July 30, 2014 issue of the journal *Neurobiology of Aging*, documenting their research. *They studied a number of flavonoid compounds in an animal model of AD, and found that "EGCG was the most potent in terms of inhibiting the pathologic process of AD.* They concluded that, *"Taken together, our results suggest that orally delivered (-)-epicatechin [EGCG] may be a potential prophylactic for Alzheimer's disease."*[589]

In another interesting study, researchers noted that, *"Polyphenols such as epigallocatechin gallate (EGCG), and resveratrol [found in red wine] have received a great deal of attention because they may contribute to the purported neuroprotective action of the regular consumption of green tea and red wine. Many studies, including those published by our group, suggest that this protective action includes their abilities to prevent the neurotoxic effects of beta-amyloid, a protein whose accumulation likely plays a pivotal role in Alzheimer's disease."* Not only did the researchers show in a cell model of Alzheimer's disease that EGCG and resveratrol were protective against the damage from beta-amyloid, *they found that these polyphenols actually increased nerve cell connections.*[590] As connections between nerve cells decrease with aging, anything that can partially reverse this process is a good thing!

Another group of researchers conducted a study to test whether daily consumption of a beverage with high antioxidant power combining extracts of green tea and apple over a period of eight months would affect inflammation in AD patients in initial phase, moderate phase and a control group. *They concluded that the antioxidant beverage, "...was more effective against inflammation in the early period of AD, and could be used as a natural complementary therapy to alleviate or improve symptoms of inflammation in early stages of AD."*[591]

In the *Journal of Nutrional Biochemistry*, Lim and colleagues reported on their experiment studying the protective effects of EGCG in an animal model of Alzheimer's disease. They found that EGCG-treated mice "exhibited significant decreases in behavioral impairment." They also discovered numerous protective effects of EGCG on a variety of critical biochemical elements. Not only that--they also found that the "treated groups showed lower levels of total cholesterol and low-density lipoprotein cholesterol [LDL; "bad cholesterol"], whereas the level of high-density lipoprotein cholesterol [HDL; "good cholesterol"] increased. *These results provide experimental evidence suggesting that EGCG can be used in the prevention of AD or treatment of AD patients.*"[592]

It is well known that tea has a variety of beneficial impacts on human health, including anti-obesity effects. It is well documented that green tea and its constituent catechins (including EGCG) suppress obesity, but the effects of other types of tea on obesity are not yet fully understood. To address this question, a recent study of oolong, black and pu-erh teas was undertaken. The researchers found that these teas also suppress the formation of fatty tissue in mice. They concluded saying, "*We found that the consumption of oolong, black or pu-erh tea for a period of one week significantly decreased visceral[1] fat without affecting body weight in male mice.*"[593] Visceral fat is known to be particularly bad for one's health, and so this is a very significant finding.

Green tea has become renowned for its many health benefits, and *researchers showed that both green and white teas were able to decrease the response to stress* in a study of eighteen students who participated in the experiment. Those students who drank white tea were also able to improve performance on an arithmetic task compared to those who

---

[1]Visceral fat is body fat that is stored within the abdominal cavity and is therefore stored around a number of important internal organs such as the liver, pancreas and intestines. Visceral fat is sometimes referred to as 'active fat' because research has shown that this type of fat plays a distinctive and potentially dangerous role affecting how our hormones function. Storing higher amounts of visceral fat is associated with increased risks of a number of health problems including type 2 diabetes.

didn't drink it, suggesting that white tea might also improve mood during and after mental stress load.[594]

Researchers from the Department of Neurology, Miller School of Medicine, University of Miami, Miami, FL *found an inverse relationship between drinking coffee or tea and various causes of death.* They studied 2,461 individuals living in Manhattan over an 11-year period. *They found that the more coffee or tea consumed, the lower the death rate. Drinking four or more cups of coffee was most beneficial in the coffee drinkers.*[595]

Oral health is associated with a variety of other health issues located far from the mouth. Inflammation of the gums, gingivitis and chronic periodontitis can be serious health problems in their own right, but may also cause serious health issues at sites distant from the mouth. A recent study investigated green tea, white tea, oolong tea, and black tea extracts with a high polyphenol content for their effects on oral hygiene. All the tea extracts inhibited the bacteria associated with gingivitis. In addition, they were shown to be highly anti-inflammatory. No marked differences in the various effects were observed among the four tea extracts. The authors concluded by saying, *"Extracts from green tea, white tea, oolong tea, and black tea show promise for controlling periodontal disease."*[596]

Hesperidin

Hesperidin is a flavanone glycoside found in citrus fruits. Its aglycone form is called hesperetin. Its name is derived from the word "hesperidium," for fruit produced by citrus trees.

In an experiment using an animal model of Alzheimer's disease, Dr. Javed and colleagues, reported in the November 6, 2014 issue of the *Journal of the Neurological Sciences*, that, "Dietary flavonoids exert chemopreventive and neuroprotective effects and comprise the most common group of plant polyphenols that provide much of the flavor and color of the vegetables and fruits. Hesperidin is a flavanone glycoside found abundantly in citrus fruits, has been reported to have antioxidant, hypolipidaemic, analgesic and anti-hypertensive activity...*The results from the present study open the possibility of using flavonoids [here, hesperidin] for potential new therapeutic strategies for sporadic dementia of Alzheimer's disease.*"[597]

In the November 2014 issue of the journal *Cellular and Molecular Neurobiology*, Dr. Wang and colleagues reported their research using an animal model of Alzheimer's to explore the effects of hesperidin against amyloid-β (Aβ)-induced cognitive dysfunction, oxidative damage and mitochondrial dysfunction in mice. They concluded by saying, "*Taken together, these findings suggest that a reduction in mitochondrial dysfunction...coupled with an increase in anti-oxidative defense, may be one of the mechanisms by which hesperidin improves cognitive function in the mouse model of AD.*"[598]

Dr. Li and colleagues, in the March 15, 2015 issue of the journal *Behavioural Brain Research*, reported on the use of hesperidin in an animal model of Alzheimer's disease. Without discussing the details of their research, they concluded that, "*Our findings suggest that hesperidin might be a potential candidate for the treatment of AD or even other neurodegenerative diseases.*"[599]

Huperzine A (Hup A; Qian Ceng Ta)

Huperzine A is a naturally occurring alkaloid compound found in the firmoss *Huperzia serrata* and in varying quantities in other *Huperzia* species. It is a reversible acetylcholinesterase inhibitor (like Aricept or Exelon) and NMDA receptor antagonist (like Namenda XR) that crosses the blood-brain barrier.

Drs. Qian and Ke, reported in the August 19, 2014 issue of the journal *Frontiers in Aging Neuroscience* that, "Huperzine A (HupA) is a natural inhibitor of acetylcholinesterase (AChE) derived from the Chinese folk medicine Huperzia serrata (Qian Ceng Ta). *It is a licensed anti-Alzheimer's disease drug in China* and is available as a nutraceutical in the U.S. A growing body of evidence has demonstrated that HupA has multifaceted pharmacological effects. *In addition to the symptomatic, cognitive-enhancing effect via inhibition of AChE, a number of recent studies have reported that this drug has "non-cholinergic" effects on AD. Most important among these is the protective effect of HupA on neurons against amyloid beta-induced oxidative injury and mitochondrial dysfunction as well as via the up-regulation of nerve growth factor and antagonizing N-methyl-d-aspartate [NMDA] receptors. The most recent discovery that HupA may reduce brain iron accumulation lends further support to the argument that HupA could serve as a potential disease-modifying agent for AD and also other neurodegenerative disorders by significantly slowing down the course of neuronal death.*[600]

In 2014, Dr. Xing and colleagues conducted an extensive literature search, referred to as a "meta-analysis" of Huperzine A (Hup A) on patients with Alzheimer's disease (AD) and vascular dementia (VD), in order to provide the basis and reference for clinical rational drug use. "The primary outcome measures assessed were mini mental state examination (MMSE) and activities of daily living scale (ADL). Eight AD trials with 733 participants and two VD trials with 92 participants that met our inclusion criteria were identified. The results showed that Hup *A could significantly improve the MMSE and ADL score of AD and VD patients, and longer durations would result in better efficacy for the patients with AD. It seemed that there was significant improvement of cognitive function measured by memory quotient (MQ) in patients with AD.* Most adverse effects in AD were generally of mild to moderate severity and transient. Compared to the patients with AD, Hup A may offer fewer side effects for participants with VD in this study. Therefore, Hup A is a well-tolerated drug that could significantly improve cognitive performance in patients with AD or VD, but we need to use it with caution in the clinical treatment."[601]

Reporting in the May 2014 issue of the journal *Neurobiology of Aging*, Dr. Huang and colleagues stated that, "In addition to acting as an acetylcholinesterase inhibitor, HupA possesses neuroprotective properties. However, the relevant mechanism is unknown. Here, we showed that the neuroprotective effect of HupA was derived from a novel action on brain iron regulation. HupA treatment reduced insoluble and soluble beta amyloid levels, ameliorated amyloid plaques formation, and hyperphosphorylated tau in the cortex and hippocampus of APPswe/PS1dE9 transgenic AD mice. Also, HupA decreased beta amyloid oligomers and amyloid precursor protein levels, and increased A Disintegrin And Metalloprotease Domain 10 (ADAM10) expression in these treated AD mice. However, these beneficial effects of HupA were largely abolished by feeding the animals with a high iron diet. In parallel, we found that HupA decreased iron content in the brain and demonstrated that HupA also has a role to reduce the expression of transferrin-receptor 1 as well as the transferrin-bound iron uptake in cultured neurons. *The findings implied that reducing iron in the brain is a novel mechanism of HupA in the treatment of Alzheimer's disease.*"[602]

Researchers conducted an extensive literature review to evaluate the beneficial and harmful effect of Huperzine A for treatment of Alzheimer's disease. They reported that, "Compared with placebo, Huperzine A showed a significant beneficial effect on the improvement of cognitive function...Activities of daily living favored Huperzine A as measured by Activities of Daily Living Scale (ADL). One trial found Huperzine A improved global clinical assessment as measured by Clinical Dementia Rating Scale (CDR). One trial demonstrated no significant change in cognitive function as measured by Alzheimer's disease Assessment Scale-Cognitive Subscale (ADAS-Cog) and activity of daily living as measured by Alzheimer's disease Cooperative Study Activities of Daily Living Inventory (ADCS-ADL) in Huperzine A group. *Huperzine A appears to have beneficial effects on improvement of cognitive function, daily living activity, and global clinical assessment in participants with Alzheimer's disease. However, the findings should be interpreted with caution due to the poor methodological quality of the included trials.*"[603]

Dr. Shao reported the results of his research in the February 15, 2015 issue of the *International Journal of Clinical and Experimental Medicine*, and noted the following:[604]

"Combined use of memantine and acetylcholinesterase inhibitors (AChEIs) has shown improved outcomes in patients with Alzheimer's disease. However, it is not clear which AChEI is the optimal for the combined treatment with memantine.

A total of 110 AD patients were randomized to receive memantine and one of the following add-on drugs: placebo, donepezil, rivastigmine, galantamine, and huperzine A for twenty-four weeks (n=22). At baseline, twelve weeks, and twenty-four weeks, the patients were evaluated using mini-mental state examination (MMSE) and Alzheimer Disease Cooperative Study-Activities of Daily Living (ADCS-ADL) scales. Adverse events were recorded to analyze the safety profile.

The MMSE scores were significantly increased and the ADL scores were significantly decreased [which is good for the ADL scale used] at twelve weeks and twenty-four weeks in all five groups compared with baseline. *At twenty-four weeks, patients treated with memantine+ huperzine A showed better MMSE and ADL scores than those treated with memantine+placebo. Huperzine A may be an optimal choice for the combined therapy with memantine in treating AD."*

Kale

Kale or borecole (*Brassica oleracea* Acephala Group) is a vegetable with green or purple leaves, in which the central leaves do not form a head. The species *Brassica oleracea* contains a wide variety of vegetables, including broccoli, cauliflower, and brussels sprouts. The cultivar group Acephala also includes spring greens and collard greens, which are similar genetically.

Kale is very high in beta carotene, vitamin K, vitamin C, and rich in calcium. Kale is a source of two carotenoids, lutein and zeaxanthin (good for eye health). Kale, as with broccoli and other brassicas, contains sulforaphane (particularly when chopped or minced), a chemical with potent anti-cancer properties.

Boiling decreases the level of sulforaphane; however, steaming, microwaving, or stir frying does not result in significant loss. *Along with other brassica vegetables, kale is also a source of indole-3-carbinol, a chemical which boosts DNA repair in cells and appears to block the growth of cancer cells.* Kale has been found to contain a group of resins known as bile acid sequestrants, which have been shown to lower cholesterol and decrease absorption of dietary fat. Steaming significantly increases these bile acid binding properties.

Although scientific research has not been conducted with kale and Alzheimer's disease, several studies of the potential benefits of kale are included because of its popularity.

One group of researchers noted the following, [605]

> "Cabbage vegetables, like Brassica group, are perceived as very valuable food products. They have a very good nutritive value, high antioxidant activity and pro-healthy potential. *Especially, kale (Brassica oleracea L. var. acephala) is characterized by good nutritional and pro-healthy properties.* The aim of this work was to assess the chemical composition and antioxidant activity of kale variety Winterbor F(1) and investigation of cooking process on selected characteristics. The chemical composition and antioxidant activity were determined in leaves of kale Winterbor F(1) variety after three subsequent years of growing. In one season, analyses were performed on raw and cooked leaves.
>
> *The investigated kale was characterized by high average contents of: β-carotene, vitamin C, alimentary fiber, and*

*ash...*The investigated kale contained polyphenolic compounds at average level of 574.9 mg of chlorogenic acid/100 g f.m., and its antioxidant activity measured as ABTS radical scavenging ability was 33.22 µM Trolox/g of fresh vegetable. It was observed a significant lowering of antioxidant compounds as a result of cooking. The losses of vitamin C were at about 89%, polyphenols at the level of 56%, in calculation on dry mass of the product. Antioxidant activity of cooked vegetable lowered and reached the level of 38 percent. There were also some losses observed in macrocomponents from 13 percent for zinc to 47 percent for sodium. The contents of harmful nitrites and nitrates in calculation on dry mass were significantly lower as a result of cooking, by 67% and 78%, respectively.

Winterbor F(1) variety of kale has a great nutritive value and high antioxidant activity. The cooking process of kale resulted in lowering of the antioxidant activity of its antioxidants especially of vitamin C, polyphenols and to the lesser extent of β-carotene what confirms that vegetable should be eaten in raw form or just undergo little processing before consumption, for example blanching."

Reporting in *The Journal of Agricultural and Food Chemistry*, researchers noted that, "*Kale is a leafy green vegetable belonging to the Brassicaceae family, a group of vegetables including cabbage, broccoli, cauliflower, and Brussels sprouts, with a high content of health-promoting phytochemicals.* The flavonoids and hydroxycinammic acids of curly kale (Brassica oleracea L. ssp. oleracea convar. acephala (DC.) Alef. var. sabellica L.), a variety of kale, were characterized and identified. Thirty-two phenolic compounds including glycosides of quercetin and kaempferol and derivatives of p-coumaric, ferulic, sinapic, and caffeic acid were tentatively identified, providing a more complete identification of phenolic compounds in curly kale than previously reported...*After acidic hydrolysis, two flavonol aglycones were identified in curly kale, quercetin* [which promotes longevity] *and*

PREVENTION

kaempferol, with total contents of 44 and 58 mg/100 g of fw, respectively."[606]

Magnesium (Mg+)

Magnesium is a chemical element with symbol Mg and atomic number 12. Magnesium is the eleventh most abundant element by mass in the human body. Its ions are essential to all cells. They interact with polyphosphate compounds such as ATP, DNA, and RNA. Hundreds of enzymes require magnesium ions to function. Magnesium compounds are used medicinally as common laxatives, antacids (e.g., milk of magnesia), and to stabilize abnormal nerve excitation or blood vessel spasm such as in eclampsia. Magnesium blood levels can easily be checked, and levels that are too high or too low can clearly be unhealthy.

A report in the journal *Advances in Nutrition* notes that:[607]

> "Magnesium has been recognized as a cofactor for >300 metabolic reactions in the body. Some of the processes in which magnesium is a cofactor include, but are not limited to, protein synthesis, cellular energy production and storage, reproduction, DNA and RNA synthesis, and stabilizing mitochondrial membranes. Magnesium also plays a critical role in nerve transmission, cardiac excitability, neuromuscular conduction, muscular contraction, vasomotor tone, blood pressure, and glucose and insulin metabolism. Because of magnesium's many functions within the body, it plays a major role in disease prevention and overall health. Low levels of magnesium have been associated with a number of chronic diseases including migraine headaches, Alzheimer's disease, cerebrovascular accident (stroke), hypertension, cardiovascular disease, and type 2 diabetes mellitus. Good food sources of magnesium include unrefined (whole) grains, spinach, nuts, legumes, and white potatoes (tubers)."

In the February 4, 2014 issue of the journal *Frontiers in Aging Neuroscience*, Dr. Cherbuin and colleagues reported that, "Higher dietary intake of potassium, calcium, and magnesium is protective against ischemic strokes while also being associated with a decreased risk of all-cause dementia. The effect of dietary iron intake on cerebral function is less clear but iron is also implicated in Alzheimer neuropathology. The aim of this study was to investigate whether dietary intake of these minerals was also associated with increased risk of mild cognitive impairment (MCI, amnestic) and other mild cognitive disorders (MCD). Associations between dietary mineral intake and risk of MCI/MCD were assessed in cognitively healthy individuals (n = 1,406, 52 percent female, mean age 62.5 years) living in the community, who were followed up over 8 years. *Higher magnesium intake was associated with a reduced risk of developing MCI/MCD. Higher intake of potassium and iron was associated with an increased risk of developing MCI/MCD.*"[608]

Dr. Li and colleagues reported in the *Journal Neuroscience* the results of their research on whether or not elevated levels of brain magnesium (Mg) can ameliorate the AD-like pathologies and cognitive deficits in a mouse model of Alzheimer's disease. They found that, "*Mg treatment reduced Aβ plaque and prevented synapse loss and memory decline in the mice. Strikingly, Mg treatment was effective even when given to the mice at the end stage of their AD-like pathological progression...Our results suggest that elevation of brain magnesium exerts substantial synaptoprotective effects in a mouse model of AD and may have therapeutic potential for treating AD in humans.*"[609]

In late 2014, another group of researchers reported the results of their research using magnesium in an animal model of Alzheimer's disease. Without going into the details of their research, they stated, "*We conclude that magnesium treatment protects cognitive function and synaptic plasticity..., which suggests a potential role for magnesium in AD therapy.*"[610]

Melatonin

Melatonin is another amazing substance that can help prevent Alzheimer's disease (and possibly other diseases as well). Melatonin is a hormone that acts as synchronizer by stabilizing bodily rhythms. Its synthesis occurs in various locations throughout the body, including the pineal gland (a small endocrine gland located in the center of the brain but outside the blood–brain barrier), skin, lymphocytes (white blood cells) and gastrointestinal (GI) tract. In addition, and a fact that most physicians are unaware of, melatonin is also produced locally in cells by most, if not all, mitochondria.[611]

When melatonin is ingested from outside the body, it is selectively taken up by mitochondria, a function not shared by [most] other antioxidants.[612] *Melatonin is a hormone that is present in the cells of almost all animals and plants.* One can only imagine that a hormone that is so ubiquitous has to have a very major role in life!

Its synthesis and secretion is controlled by light and dark conditions, whereby light decreases and darkness increases its production. Thus, melatonin is also known as the "hormone of darkness." Melatonin plays an important role in the management of depression, insomnia, epilepsy, Alzheimer's disease, diabetes, obesity, alopecia, migraine, cancer, and immune and cardiac disorders.[613]

Its secretion by the pineal gland progressively declines by age. Strong reductions of circulating melatonin are also observed in numerous disorders and diseases, including Alzheimer's disease, various other neurological and stressful conditions, pain, cardiovascular diseases, cases of cancer, endocrine and metabolic disorders, in particular diabetes type 2.[614]

There are three melatonin receptors in the brain, MT1, MT2, and MT3. Notably, a significant decrease in MT2 receptors has been observed in the hippocampus (learning and memory center) of Alzheimer's patients. *Researchers recently discovered that Depakote (valproic acid or VPA) significantly increased the number of MT2 receptors in the hip-*

pocampus in an animal experiment. This led the researchers to conclude that "a combined strategy involving VPA together with melatonin would be beneficial in neurodegenerative disorders such as Alzheimer's disease."[615]

As melatonin is produced by the body, nothing can be more "natural" than melatonin. One of its main functions is to help initiate and maintain sleep. As most of you are aware, it is an over-the-counter (OTC) supplement widely used to help treat insomnia.

It is noteworthy that there is an FDA-approved medication for insomnia, called Rozerem (ramelteon). It is chemically different than melatonin, but it works on the M1 and M2 receptors. It is available by prescription only.

Melatonin is typically used in the dose range of three to ten mg per night. It is short acting, and therefore usually doesn't leave a "hang over" when you wake up. Like everything else in life, it isn't perfect and certainly doesn't work for everyone (when it comes to insomnia).

What few people know is that melatonin is not only a natural sleep aid, it is a powerful antioxidant. And, not only is it a powerful antioxidant, it is one of the few antioxidants that works inside mitochondria, tiny cellular components that create energy for the body. *Research scientists have noted that "Melatonin is a powerful antioxidant with a particular role in the protection of nuclear and mitochondrial DNA."*[616]

This specific cellular activity by melatonin is especially important in helping to prevent Alzheimer's disease. This is because the main protein component associated with AD (Aβ peptide) can induce multiple mitochondrial dysfunctions accompanying Alzheimer's disease[617], and melatonin can help prevent this damage.

It is also important to keep in mind that melatonin has other important properties, for example it is anti-inflammatory.

So, let's review some of the scientific research supporting the use of melatonin in the prevention of Alzheimer's disease.

In 2014, researchers conducted a detailed experiment in an animal model of Alzheimer's disease, and found many benefits of melatonin. They discovered that it is neuroprotective (protecting neurons or brain cells) against several specific chemical insults. In finalizing the results of their study, they said that they, *"also determined that melatonin enhances memory function. Taken together, our data suggest that melatonin could be a promising, safe and endogenous [naturally occurring within the body] compatible antioxidant candidate for age related neurodegenerative diseases such as Alzheimer's disease."*[618]

Also in 2014, Jeong and more than a dozen colleagues found similar neuroprotective effects of melatonin in mitochondria in an experiment using human brain cells.[619] Other researchers found very significant effects on enzymes associated with AD, using both brain and non-brain cells. They noted that their findings underscored *"the preventive rather than curative nature of melatonin regarding AD treatment."*[620]

Researchers from the Department of Physics and Astronomy, McMaster University, Hamilton, Ontario, Canada discovered *"...a strongly protective effect of melatonin inhibiting the incorporation of cholesterol into beta amyloid plagues, which are characteristic of AD."*[621]

Also using an animal model of AD, researchers found that "treatment with melatonin produced marked improvement in the most studied biomarkers which was confirmed by histological investigation [e.g., tissue analysis] of the brain. In conclusion, *melatonin significantly ameliorates the neurodegeneration characteristic of AD in [an] experimental animal model due to its antioxidant, antiapoptotic, neurotrophic and anti-amyloidogenic activities."*[622]

That's a mouthful, meaning that melatonin was able to partially undo the abnormalities present in the animal model of AD, through antioxidant and non-antioxidant mechanisms.

ALZHEIMER'S DISEASE

In 2014, researchers summarized the potential usefulness of melatonin in the following way: "In recent years, research on melatonin revealed a potent activity of this hormone against oxidative and nitrosative stress-induced damage within the nervous system. Indeed, *melatonin turned out to be more effective than other naturally occurring antioxidants*, suggesting its beneficial effects in a number of diseases where oxygen radical-mediated tissue damage is involved. With specific reference to the brain, the considerable amount of evidence accumulated from studies on various neurodegeneration models and recent clinical *reports support the use of melatonin for the preventive treatment of major neurodegenerative disorders*. This review summarizes the literature on the protective effects of melatonin on Alzheimer disease, Parkinson disease, Huntington's disease and Amyotrophic Lateral Sclerosis. Additional studies are required to test the clinical efficacy of melatonin supplementation in such disorders, and to identify the specific therapeutic concentrations needed."[623]

In an animal model of Alzheimer's disease, researchers studied the protective effect of melatonin against the toxic effects of what is currently considered the main cause of AD, Amyloid-β protein (Aβ). The researchers found that when this protein was injected into the memory area of the brain, the hippocampus, learning and memory were clearly impaired. However, treatment with melatonin was able to reverse these negative effects. The researchers concluded, *"These results provide evidence for the neuroprotective action of melatonin against Aβ insults and suggest a strategy for alleviating cognition deficits of AD."*[624]

In a disturbing report (for caffeine drinkers) from the Department of Cell Biology, Microbiology, and Molecular Biology, University of South Florida, Tampa, FL, Dr. Dragicevic and colleagues report that, in animal and cellular models of Alzheimer's disease, coadministration of caffeine with melatonin blocks the beneficial effects of melatonin in mitochondria. They found *"caffeine largely blocked the large enhancement of mitochondrial function provided by melatonin... The results of this study indicate that melatonin restores mitochondrial function much more potently than caffeine in...models of Alzheimer's disease."*[625]

PREVENTION

So, although caffeine is known to improve mitochondrial function, and to be associated with a 20 percent decreased risk of AD, it impairs the positive effects of melatonin, which are much more robust and important than those of caffeine overall. The message, therefore, seems to be, decrease your caffeine intake, and increase your melatonin intake. Or, at least separate them, as in drink coffee in the morning and take melatonin at night!

In reviewing the potential benefits of melatonin in cells, animal models of Alzheimer's disease, and clinical studies in humans, researchers noted the following, "The decline in melatonin production in aged individuals has been suggested as one of the primary contributing factors for the development of age-associated neurodegenerative diseases. The efficacy of melatonin in preventing oxidative damage in either cultured neuronal (nerve) cells or in the brains of animals treated with various neurotoxic agents, *suggests that melatonin has a potential therapeutic value as a neuroprotective drug in treatment of Alzheimer's disease*, Parkinson's disease (PD), amyotrophic lateral sclerosis (ALS), Huntington's disease (HD), stroke, and brain trauma. *Therapeutic trials with melatonin indicate that it has a potential therapeutic value as a neuroprotective drug in treatment of AD, ALS, and HD.* In the case of other neurological conditions, like PD, the evidence is less compelling. Melatonin's efficacy in combating free radical damage in the brain suggests that it can be a valuable therapeutic agent in the treatment of cerebral edema following traumatic brain injury or stroke. Clinical trials employing melatonin doses in the range of 50-100 mg/day are warranted before its relative merits as a neuroprotective agent is definitively established."[626]

So, if both melatonin and exercise are beneficial in helping to prevent Alzheimer's disease, which is better? In order to answer this question, researchers studied physical exercise and melatonin in an animal model of Alzheimer's disease, with moderate to advanced phases of AD pathology. They found that, "Analysis of behavior and brain tissue at termination showed differential patterns of neuroprotection for the two treatments…Voluntary physical exercise protected against behavioral and psychological symptoms of dementia such as anxiety, a lack of exploration, and emotionality. Both treatments protected against cognitive impairment, brain oxidative stress, and a decrease in mitochondrial DNA. Interestingly, only the combined treatment of physical exercise plus melatonin was effective against the decrease of mitochondrial complexes. Therefore, *melatonin plus physical exercise may exert complementary, additive, or even synergistic (e.g., more than additive) effects against a range of disturbances present in AD.*"[627]

What about the use of melatonin in real people? A link between poor sleep quality and Alzheimer's disease has recently been suggested. Since endogenous (produced in the body) melatonin levels are already reduced at preclinical AD stages (e.g., before AD is clearly present), it is important to ask whether replenishing the missing hormone would be beneficial in AD and whether any such effects would be related to the presence of sleep disorder in patients.

In order to answer the above questions, researchers studied the effects of add-on prolonged-release melatonin (2 mg) to standard therapy (e.g. medications for AD, such as Aricept) on cognitive functioning and sleep in eighty patients diagnosed with mild to moderate AD, with and without coexisting insomnia. *Patients treated with the melatonin supplement for twenty-four weeks "had significantly better cognitive performance than those treated with placebo, particularly in those with insomnia."*[628]

In 2013, other researchers reviewed the usefulness of melatonin in the prevention and possible treatment of Alzheimer's disease, and made the following statement: "Multiple factors contribute to the etiology (cause) of AD in terms of initiation and progression. Melatonin is an endogenously (within the body) produced hormone in the brain and decreases during aging and in patients with AD. *Data from clinical trials indicate that melatonin supplementation improves sleep, ameliorates sundowning (mental confusion, typically when the sun goes down and there is less light and/or stimulation) and slows down the progression of cognitive impairment in AD patients. Melatonin efficiently protects neuronal (nerve) cells from Aβ-mediated toxicity via antioxidant and anti-amyloid properties...* The aim of this review is to stimulate interest in melatonin as *a potentially useful agent in the prevention and treatment of AD.*"[629]

Another group of researchers studied the usefulness of melatonin in mild cognitive impairment (MCI) for a second time. They had previously conducted a study using 3 to 9 mg of immediate-release melatonin for up to three years in patients with MCI. In that study, they found the treatment *"significantly improved cognitive and emotional performance and daily sleep/wake cycle in MCI patients."* In their current study, they evaluated ninety-six MCI outpatients, sixty-one of whom had received daily 3 to 24 mg of an immediate-release melatonin preparation at bedtime for fifteen to sixty months. Melatonin was given in addition to the standard medication prescribed by the attending psychiatrist. *They found that "Patients treated with melatonin exhibited significantly better [cognitive] performance. The results further support that melatonin can be a useful add-on drug for treating MCI in a clinic environment."*[630]

Researchers Angelova and Abramov, from the Department of Molecular Neuroscience, Institute of Neurology, London, U.K., reporting in the October 2014 issue of the journal *Biochemical Society Transactions*, note that, *"The pineal hormone melatonin, the glycoprotein clusterin and regulation of the membrane cholesterol can modify Aβ-induced calcium signals, ROS [reactive oxygen species] production and mitochondrial depolarization, which eventually lead to neuroprotection."*[631] And, that's a good thing!

N-acetyl cysteine (NAC)

Acetylcysteine, also known as *N*-acetylcysteine or *N*-acetyl-*L*-cysteine (NAC), is a pharmaceutical drug (such as Mucomyst) and nutritional supplement used primarily as a mucolytic agent and in the management of acetaminophen (Tylenol; Paracetamol) overdose. It is used as a cough medicine because it breaks disulfide bonds in mucus and liquefies it, making it easier to cough up. It is also this action of breaking disulfide bonds that makes it useful in thinning the abnormally thick mucus in cystic and pulmonary fibrosis patients. It is on the World Health Organization's List of Essential Medicines, a list of the most important medication needed in a basic health system.

According to the results of research published in 2014, *"N-acetyl cysteine has been shown to ameliorate cognitive deficits in Alzheimer's patients and to reduce the symptoms of blast injury in soldiers. These studies and many others in experimental models of neurodegeneration suggest that N-acetyl cysteine can protect neurons even when they are severely injured.* In the present study, we tested the hypotheses that dual hits of hydrogen peroxide and paraquat would elicit synergistic neurodegeneration and that this extreme toxicity would be prevented by N-acetyl cysteine. The findings reveal for the first time that neuronal N2a cells are much more sensitive to oxidative stress from hydrogen peroxide treatment when they have been exposed previously to the same toxin. Two hits of hydrogen peroxide also caused severe loss of glutathione. N-acetyl cysteine attenuated the loss of glutathione and reduced the near-complete loss of cells after exposure to dual hydrogen peroxide hits. *The present study supports the notion that N-acetyl cysteine can robustly protect against severe, unremitting oxidative stress in a glutathione-dependent manner."*[632]

Dr. Hsiao and colleagues, reporting on their experiment using an animal model of Alzheimer's disease, in the journal *Neurobiology of Disease,* note that, "Epidemiological study reveals that socially isolated persons have increased risk of developing Alzheimer's disease. Whether this risk arises from an oxidative stress is unclear. Here we show that *N-acetylcysteine (NAC), an anti-oxidant, is capable of preventing social isolation-induced accelerated impairment of contextual fear memory...Our results indicate that NAC is effective in mouse models of AD and has translation potential for the human disorder."*[633]

Omega 3 Fatty Acids

Omega-3 fatty acids (also called ω-3 fatty acids or *n*-3 fatty acids) are polyunsaturated fatty acids (PUFAs) with a double bond (C=C) at the third carbon atom from the end of the carbon chain. The fatty acids have two ends, the carboxylic acid (-COOH) end, which is considered the beginning of the chain, thus "alpha," and the methyl (CH$_3$) end, which is considered the "tail" of the chain, thus "omega." The way in which a fatty acid is named is determined by the location of the first double bond, counted from the methyl end, that is, the omega (ω-) or the n- end.

The three types of omega-3 fatty acids involved in human physiology are α-linolenic acid (ALA) (found in plant oils), eicosapentaenoic acid (EPA), and docosahexaenoic acid (DHA) (both commonly found in marine oils). Marine algae and phytoplankton are primary sources of omega-3 fatty acids. Common sources of plant oils containing the omega 3 ALA fatty acid include walnut, edible seeds, clary sage seed oil, algal oil, flaxseed oil, Sacha Inchi oil, *Echium* oil, and hemp oil, while sources of animal omega-3 EPA and DHA fatty acids include fish oils, egg oil, squid oils, and krill oil.

Omega-3 fatty acids are important for normal metabolism. Mammals have a limited ability to synthesize omega-3 fats when the diet includes the shorter-chain omega-3 fatty acid ALA, (eighteen carbons and three double bonds) to form the more important long-chain omega-3 fatty acids, EPA, (twenty carbons and five double bonds) and then from EPA, the most crucial, DHA, (twenty-two carbons and six double bonds) with even greater inefficiency. The ability to make the longer-chain omega-3 fatty acids from ALA may also be impaired in aging.

The 'essential' fatty acids were given their name when researchers found that they are essential to normal growth in young children and animals. The omega 3 fatty acid DHA, also known as docasohexanoic acid is found in high abundance in the human brain. It is produced by a desaturation process. However humans lack the desaturase enzyme, which acts to insert double bonds at the ω6 and ω3 position. Therefore the ω6 and ω3 polyunsaturated fatty acids cannot be synthesized and are appropriately called essential fatty acids.

ALZHEIMER'S DISEASE

Human diet has changed rapidly in recent centuries resulting in a reported increased diet of omega-6 in comparison to omega-3. The rapid evolution of human diet has presumably been too fast for humans to have adapted to resulting in biological profiles adept at utilizing omega-3 and omega-6 ratios of 1:1 and disadvantaged among modern diets. This is commonly believed to be the reason why modern diets have yielded high correlations with many inflammatory disorders.

Both omega-6 and omega-3 fatty acids are essential; i.e., humans must consume them in their diet. Omega-6 and omega-3 eighteen-carbon polyunsaturated fatty acids compete for the same metabolic enzymes, thus the omega-6:omega-3 ratio of ingested fatty acids has significant influence on the ratio and rate of production of eicosanoids, a group of hormones intimately involved in the body's inflammatory and homeostatic processes, which include the prostaglandins, leukotrienes, and thromboxanes, among others. Altering this ratio can change the body's metabolic and inflammatory state. In general, grass-fed animals accumulate more omega-3 than do grain-fed animals, which accumulate relatively more omega-6. Metabolites of omega-6 are more inflammatory (esp. arachidonic acid) than those of omega-3. This necessitates that omega-6 and omega-3 be consumed in a balanced proportion; healthy ratios of omega-6:omega-3, according to some authors, range from 1:1 to 1:4 (an individual needs more omega-3 than omega-6). Other authors believe that ratio 4:1 (when the amount of omega-6 is only four times greater than that of omega-3) is already healthy. Studies suggest the evolutionary human diet, rich in game animals, seafood, and other sources of omega-3, may have provided such a ratio.

Typical Western diets provide ratios of between 10:1 and 30:1 (i.e., dramatically higher levels of omega-6 than omega-3). The ratios of omega-6 to omega-3 fatty acids in some common vegetable oils are: canola 2:1, hemp 2–3:1, soybean 7:1, olive 3–13:1, sunflower (no omega-3), flax 1:3, cottonseed (almost no omega-3), peanut (no omega-3), grapeseed oil (almost no omega-3) and corn oil 46:1 ratio of omega-6 to omega-3.

Dr. Khorsan and colleagues completed an extensive literature review in late 2014 of the relationship between omega-3s on inflammatory biomarkers. They concluded that, *"Clinical literature on the effects of omega-3 fatty acids on inflammatory biomarkers contains mostly small sample sizes, is neutral to high quality, and report mixed effects. Larger studies examining dose and delivery are needed."*[634]

Reporting in the November 21, 2014 issue of *Neuroscience & Biobehavioral Reviews,* Dr. Ding and colleagues reviewed the literature on associations of dietary intake of long-chain omega-3 fatty acids or fish with the incidence of dementia and Alzheimer's disease. They found that, *"A higher intake of fish was associated with a 36 percent lower risk of AD. However, there was no statistical evidence for similar inverse association between long-chain omega-3 fatty acids intake and risk of dementia."*[635]

Brain health may be affected by modifiable lifestyle factors; consuming fish and antioxidative omega-3 fatty acids may reduce brain structural abnormality risk. Dr. Raji and colleagues published the results of their research on this relationship in the October 2014 issue of the *American Journal of Preventive Medicine*. To determine whether dietary fish consumption is related to brain structural integrity among cognitively normal elders, data were analyzed from 260 cognitively normal individuals. They found that, *"Weekly consumption of baked or broiled fish was positively associated with gray matter volumes in the hippocampus, precuneus, posterior cingulate, and orbital frontal cortex. These results did not change when including omega-3 fatty acid estimates in the analysis...Dietary consumption of baked or broiled fish is related to larger gray matter volumes independent of omega-3 fatty acid content. These findings suggest that a confluence of lifestyle factors influence brain health, adding to the growing body of evidence that prevention strategies for late-life brain health need to begin decades earlier."*[636]

A group of researchers, reporting in 2014, examined the consistency and strength of the impact of supplementation of omega-3 fatty acids on overall cognitive function using systematic reviews and meta-analytic methods. They concluded that, "There were differences between studies reporting outcomes for single memory function parameters. *Subgroup analysis of doses used (low versus high) indicated that subjects receiving low (<1.73 g/day) doses of omega-3 fatty acids had a significant reduction in cognitive decline rate, but there was no evidence for beneficial effects at higher doses compared with the placebo group. This study suggests that omega-3 fatty acids may be beneficial in preventing memory decline at lower doses."*[637] (Note: 1.73 g/day or grams per day is a pretty high dose, given what is typically available in retail stores. Be sure to check the bottle labels for dosing.)

Dr. Fares and colleagues, reporting in the February 2014 issue of *Current Atherosclerosis Reports*, note the following, "There has been increasing interest in the health benefits of supplemental and/or dietary omega-3 polyunsaturated fatty acids (PUFAs), particularly in their role in disease prevention. This interest escalated once their effects on cardiovascular health were observed from numerous observational studies in populations whose diet consisted mainly of fish. Research has since been undertaken on omega-3 PUFAs to investigate their health benefits in a vast array of medical conditions, including primary and secondary prevention. This article discusses the evidence and controversies concerning omega-3 PUFAs in various health conditions. *In addition to the effects on cardiovascular health, omega-3 PUFAs have been shown to prevent the development of dementia, reduce systemic inflammatory diseases, prevent prostate cancer, and possibly have a role in the treatment of depression and bipolar disorder.*"[638]

However, words of caution from Dr. Peskin from the International PEO Society, Houston, TX, who published the following in the *Journal of Lipids* in 2014:[639]

> "The medical community suffered three significant fish oil failures/setbacks in 2013. Claims that fish oil's EPA/DHA would stop the progression of heart disease were crushed when The Risk and Prevention Study Collaborative Group (Italy) released a conclusive negative finding regarding fish oil for those patients with high risk factors but no previous myocardial infarction. Fish

oil failed in all measures of CVD prevention-both primary and secondary. Another major 2013 setback occurred when fish oil's DHA was shown to significantly increase prostate cancer in men, in particular, high-grade prostate cancer, in the Selenium and Vitamin E Cancer Prevention Trial (SELECT) analysis by Brasky et al. Another monumental failure occurred in 2013 whereby fish oil's EPA/DHA failed to improve macular degeneration. In 2010, fish oil's EPA/DHA failed to help Alzheimer's victims, even those with low DHA levels. These are by no means isolated failures. The promise of fish oil and its so-called active ingredients EPA / DHA fails time and time again in clinical trials. This lipids-based physiologic review will explain precisely why there should have never been expectation for success. This review will focus on underpublicized lipid science with a focus on physiology."

The above notwithstanding, Dr. Gu and colleagues conducted a clinical study to evaluate the association between nutrient intake and plasma Aβ levels, reporting their findings in the journal *Neurology*. The widely reported associations between various nutrients and cognition may occur through many biologic pathways including those of β-amyloid (Aβ). In the study, plasma Aβ40 and Aβ42 and dietary data were obtained from 1,219 cognitively healthy elderly (age >65 years). Information on dietary intake was obtained 1.2 years, on average, before Aβ assay. The associations of plasma Aβ40 and Aβ42 levels and dietary intake of ten nutrients were examined. Nutrients examined included saturated fatty acid, monounsaturated fatty acid, ω-3 polyunsaturated fatty acid (PUFA), ω-6 PUFA, vitamin E, vitamin C, β-carotene, vitamin B(12), folate, and vitamin D. The researchers concluded that, *"Our data suggest that higher dietary intake of ω-3 PUFA is associated with lower plasma levels of Aβ42, a profile linked with reduced risk of incident Alzheimer's disease and slower cognitive decline in our cohort."*[640]

In late 2014, another group of researchers reviewed the literature to study the effect of omega-3 on cognitive decline. They concluded that, "*Studies have shown the protective role of omega-3 fatty acids in mild cognitive impairment, dementia, and the risk and progression of Alzheimer's disease in the elderly.* Further studies are needed to understand the mechanism of action of omega-3 fatty acids on cognition. Doses, composition of EPA and DHA capsules and time of supplementation should be explored."[641]

Dr. Daiello and colleagues, reported the results of their study to investigate whether the use of fish oil supplements (FOSs) is associated with concomitant reduction in cognitive decline and brain atrophy in older adults, in the June 18, 2014 issue of the journal *Alzheimer's Dementia*. They reported that, "Older adults (229 cognitively normal individuals, 397 patients with mild cognitive impairment, and 193 patients with Alzheimer's disease) were assessed with neuropsychological tests and brain magnetic resonance imaging every six months. Primary outcomes included (1) global cognitive status and (2) cerebral cortex gray matter and hippocampus and ventricular volumes. *FOS use during follow-up was associated with significantly lower mean cognitive subscale of the Alzheimer's disease Assessment Scale and higher Mini-Mental State Examination scores among those with normal cognition. Associations between FOS use and the outcomes were observed only in APOE ε4-negative participants. FOS use during the study was also associated with less atrophy in one or more brain regions of interest.*"[642] Translation: use of fish oil supplements was beneficial except in those with the APOE ε4 protein variant.

Reporting in 2014 in the *Journal of Alzheimer's Disease*, Dr. Frend-Levy and colleagues noted the following, "Oxidative stress and inflammation are two key mechanisms suggested to be involved in the pathogenesis of Alzheimer's disease. Omega-3 fatty acids (ω-3 FAs) found in fish and fish oil have several biological properties that may be beneficial in AD. However, they may also auto-oxidize and induce in vivo lipid peroxidation [which is bad].The objective of this study was to evaluate systemic oxidative stress and inflammatory biomarkers following oral supplementation of dietary ω-3 FA."[643] *The researchers concluded that oral supplementation with omega-3 fish oil did not induce inflammation in their study of forty patients with Alzheimer's disease.*

Dr. Pottala and colleagues reported the results of their research in the February 4, 2014 issue of journal *Neurology*, to test whether red blood cell (RBC) levels of marine omega-3 fatty acids measured in the Women's Health Initiative Memory Study were related to MRI brain volumes measured eight years later. The researchers reported that, "RBC eicosapentaenoic acid (EPA), docosahexaenoic acid (DHA), and MRI brain volumes were assessed in 1,111 postmenopausal women. *A higher omega-3 index was correlated with larger total normal brain volume and hippocampal volume in postmenopausal women measured eight years later. While normal aging results in overall brain atrophy, lower omega-3 index may signal increased risk of hippocampal atrophy.*"[644]

Pomegranate Extract

The pomegranate, botanical name *Punica granatum*, is a fruit-bearing deciduous shrub or small tree growing between 6–26 ft tall. The most abundant phytochemicals in pomegranate juice are polyphenols, including the hydrolyzable tannins called ellagitannins formed when ellagic acid and/or gallic acid binds with a carbohydrate to form pomegranate ellagitannins, also known as punicalagins. The red color of juice can be attributed to anthocyanins, such as delphinidin, cyanidin, and pelargonidin glycosides.

Dr. Zarfeshany and colleagues summarized the benefits of pomegranate in the March 25, 2014 issue of the journal *Advanced Biomedical Research*:[645]

> "Accumulating data clearly claimed that Punica granatum L. (pomegranate) has several health benefits. Pomegranates can help prevent or treat various disease risk factors including high blood pressure, high cholesterol, oxidative stress, hyperglycemia, and inflammatory

activities. It is demonstrated that certain components of pomegranate such as *polyphenols* have potential antioxidant, anti-inflammatory, and anticarcinogenic effects. The antioxidant potential of pomegranate juice is more than that of red wine and green tea, which is induced through ellagitannins and hydrosable tannins. Pomegranate juice can reduce macrophage oxidative stress, free radicals, and lipid peroxidation. Moreover, pomegranate fruit extract prevents cell growth and induces apoptosis [cell death], which can lead to its anticarcinogenic effects. In addition, promoter inhibition of some inflammatory markers and their production are blocked via ellagitannins."

Another group of researchers also summarized the benefits of pomegranate:[646]

"Pomegranate fruit presents strong anti-inflammatory, antioxidant, antiobesity, and antitumoral properties, thus leading to an increased popularity as a functional food and nutraceutical source since ancient times. It can be divided into three parts: seeds, peel, and juice, all of which seem to have medicinal benefits. Several studies investigate its bioactive components as a means to associate them with a specific beneficial effect and develop future products and therapeutic applications. *Many beneficial effects are related to the presence of ellagic acid, ellagitannins (including punicalagins), punicic acid and other fatty acids, flavonoids, anthocyanidins, anthocyanins, estrogenic flavonols, and flavones, which seem to be its most therapeutically beneficial components.* However, the synergistic action of the pomegranate constituents appears to be superior when compared to individual constituents. Promising results have been obtained for the treatment of certain diseases including obesity, insulin resistance, intestinal inflammation, and cancer."

PREVENTION

Other researchers report, "In recent years, the therapeutic use of non-drug substances such as herbal and medicinal foods is increasing progressively. Of these substances, Punica granatum L., which is an ancient and highly distinctive fruit, has been proposed for treatment of several different illnesses. *Ellagic acid (EA) is one of those biological molecules found in pomegranate and may have therapeutic potential in many diseases. EA has been detected not only in pomegranate but also in a wide variety of fruits and nuts such as raspberries, strawberries, walnuts, grapes and black currants, and is becoming an increasingly popular dietary supplement over recent years.* Similar to other ellagitannins (ETs), EA is quite stable under physiological conditions in the stomach. EA and ETs as active agents induce vasorelaxation, oxygen free radical scavenging, hypolipidemic, anti-inflammatory and anti-carcinogenic activities in various animal preparations."[647]

In the October 22, 2014 issue of the journal *Food & Function*, Dr. Liu and colleagues reported the following, "Advanced Glycation Endproducts (AGEs) are a heterogeneous group of molecules produced from non-enzymatic glycation. *Accumulation of AGEs in vivo plays an important role in the pathology of chronic human diseases including type-2 diabetes and Alzheimer's disease. Natural AGEs inhibitors such as the pomegranate (Punica granatum) fruit show great potential for the management of these diseases.* Herein, we investigated the anti-glycation effects of a pomegranate fruit extract (PE)...All of the samples showed anti-glycation. *Our study suggests that pomegranate may offer an attractive dietary strategy for the prevention and treatment of AGE-related diseases such as type-2 diabetes and Alzheimer's disease.*"[648]

In 2014, Dr. Ahmed and colleagues reported the results of their research in the journal *Current Alzheimer Research* on the neuroprotective effects of pomegranate juice and extracts (PE) in an animal model of Alzheimer's disease. They found that, *"PE did not improve cognitive performance of the mice, but altered levels and ratio of the Aβ42 and Aβ40 peptides which would favor a diminution in AD pathogenesis. Further analysis revealed that this reversal could be the product of the modification of γ-secretase enzyme activity, the enzyme involved in the generation of these Aβ isoforms. Our findings support a specific anti-amyloidogenic mechanism of a pomegranate extract in this aged AD animal model.*"[649]

Dr. Rojanathammanee and colleagues, from the Department of Pharmacology, Physiology, and Therapeutics, University of North Dakota, School of Medicine and Health Sciences, Grand Forks, ND, studied the anti-inflammatory effects of pomegranate in an animal model of Alzheimer's disease, publishing their findings in the *Journal of Nutrition*. Without going into the details of their research, they concluded that, "*These data indicate that dietary pomegranate produces brain anti-inflammatory effects that may attenuate AD progression.*"[650]

A separate group of researchers, publishing the results of their research of the benefits of pomegranate in an animal model of Alzheimer's disease, in the January 2015 issue of the journal *Nutrition*, concluded that, "*Our results suggest that dietary supplementation with pomegranates may slow the progression of cognitive and behavioral impairments in AD.*"[651]

Dr. Subash and colleagues, publishing the results of their research in the October 2014 issue of the *Journal of Traditional and Complementary Medicine*, noted that, "Oxidative stress may play a key role in Alzheimer's disease neuropathology. Pomegranate contains very high levels of antioxidant polyphenolic substances, as compared to other fruits and vegetables. Polyphenols have been shown to be neuroprotective in different model systems. Here, the effects of the antioxidant-rich pomegranate fruit on brain oxidative stress status were tested in the AD transgenic mouse...*The results suggest that the therapeutic potential of 4 percent pomegranate in the treatment of AD might be associated with counteracting the oxidative stress by the presence of active phytochemicals in it.*"[652]

In 2014, in another animal model of Alzheimer's disease, researchers studied the effects of citrus lemon and pomegranate juices on memory. They found that, "*These results suggest that citrus lemon and pomegranate have phytochemicals and essential nutrients which boost memory, particularly short term memory. Hence it may be concluded that flavonoids in these juices may be responsible for memory enhancing effects and a synergistic effect is observed by combinations.*"[653]

As an interesting aside, Dr. Sreekumar and colleagues reported in 2014 in the journal *BioMed Research International* on the anti-cancer properties of pomegranate. They stated, "*Earlier, we had shown its antiproliferative effect using human breast, endometrial, cervical, and ovarian cancer cell lines.*"[654]

Quercetin

Caution: The U.S. FDA has issued warning letters to emphasize that quercetin is not a defined nutrient, cannot be assigned a dietary content level and is not regulated as a drug to treat any human disease. Quercetin is contraindicated with some antibiotics; it may interact with fluoroquinolones (an antibiotic), as quercetin competitively binds to bacterial DNA gyrase. Whether this inhibits or enhances the effect of fluoroquinolones is not certain. AHFS Drug Information (2010) identifies quercetin as an inhibitor of CYP2C8 (a metabolic enzyme), and specifically names it as a drug with potential to have harmful interactions with taxol/paclitaxel. As paclitaxel is metabolized primarily by CYP2C8, its bioavailability may be increased unpredictably, potentially leading to harmful side-effects.

Quercetin is a flavonol[1] found in many fruits, vegetables, leaves and grains.

According to a group of researchers, reporting in 2014, "*Recent clinical research has demonstrated that berry fruits can prevent age-related neurodegenerative diseases and improve motor and cognitive functions. The berry fruits are also capable of modulating signaling pathways involved in inflammation, cell survival, neurotransmission and enhancing neuroplasticity. The neuroprotective effects of berry fruits on*

---

[1]Flavonols are a class of flavonoids.

neurodegenerative diseases are related to phytochemicals such as anthocyanin, caffeic acid, catechin, quercetin, kaempferol and tannin."[655]

Dr. Sabogal-Guaqueta and colleagues published the results of their research on the neuroprotective effects of quercetin in an animal model of Alzheimer's disease, in the February 7, 2015 issue of the journal *Neuropharmacology*. Without discussing the actual experiment, they concluded that, "Our data show that quercetin decreases extracellular β-amyloidosis, tauopathy, astrogliosis and microgliosis in the hippocampus and the amygdala. These results were supported by a significant reduction in the paired helical filament (PHF), β-amyloid (βA) 1-40 and βA 1-42 levels and a decrease in BACE1-mediated cleavage of APP (into CTFβ). *Additionally, quercetin induced improved performance on learning and spatial memory tasks and greater risk assessment behavior based on the elevated plus maze test. Together, these findings suggest that quercetin reverses histological hallmarks of AD and protects cognitive and emotional function in aged 3xTg-AD mice.*"[656] (And that's a good thing!)

In 2014, a separate group of researchers studied the effects of quercetin in a different animal model of Alzheimer's disease. In short, they found quercetin to be very beneficial in this model, concluding that, "*The polyphenol quercetin, by specifically activating macroautophagy and proteasomal degradation pathways, proved able to prevent Aβ(1-42) aggregation and paralysis.*"[657] (And that's another good thing!)

The most commonly used, FDA-approved, medication for the treatment of Alzheimer's disease, and as discussed previously, is Aricept (donepezil), which works as an acetylcholine-esterase (AchE) inhibitor. According to one group of researchers, "Quercetin is a plant flavonoid compound which can act as AchE inhibitor and it may be a better alternative to current AchE inhibitors in terms of effectiveness with no or fewer side effects." These researchers performed numerous computer simulation experiments comparing Aricept (and similar agents) and quercetin, concluding that, *"This in silico[1] [QSAR] study has conclusively predicted the superiority of the natural compound quercetin over the conventional drugs as AchE inhibitors* and it sets the need for further in-vitro study of this compound in the future."[658]

The beneficial effects of dietary polyphenols on health are due not only to their antioxidant properties but also to their antibacterial, anti-inflammatory and/or anti-tumoral activities. It has recently been proposed that protection of mitochondrial function (which is altered in several diseases such as Alzheimer's, Parkinson's, obesity and diabetes) by these compounds, may be important in explaining the beneficial effects of polyphenols on health. Researchers conducted a cell experiment "to evaluate the protective effects of dietary polyphenols quercetin, rutin, resveratrol (from red wine and red grapes, and peanuts) and epigallocatechin gallate (EGCG; green tea) against the alterations of mitochondrial function induced by indomethacin (INDO) in intestinal epithelial Caco-2 cells...Quercetin, resveratrol and rutin protected Caco-2 cells against INDO-induced mitochondrial dysfunction, while no protection was observed with epigallocatechin gallate. *Quercetin was the most efficient in protecting against mitochondrial dysfunction; this could be due to its ability to enter cells and accumulate in mitochondria [as do CoQ10 and melatonin].* Additionally its structural similarity with rotenone could favor its binding to the ubiquinone site of complex I, protecting it from inhibitors such as INDO or rotenone. *These findings suggest a possible new protective role for dietary polyphenols for mitochondria, complementary of their antioxidant property. This new role might expand the preventive and/or therapeutic use of PPs [polyphenols] in conditions involving mitochondrial dysfunction and associated with increased oxidative stress at the cellular or tissue levels [such as Alzheimer's disease].*"[659]

Dr. Simonyi and colleagues, from the MU Center for Botanical Interaction Studies, University of Missouri, Columbia, MO, reported the results of their research in the March 2, 2015 issue of the journal *Life*

---

[1] *In silico* is an expression used to mean "performed on computer or via computer simulation."

Science. They reported that, "Elderberry (Sambucus spp.) is one of the oldest medicinal plants noted for its cardiovascular, anti-inflammatory, and immune-stimulatory properties. In this study, we investigated the anti-inflammatory and anti-oxidant effects of the American elderberry (Sambucus nigra subsp. canadensis) pomace as well as some of the anthocyanins (cyanidin chloride and cyanidin 3-O-glucoside) and flavonols (quercetin and rutin) in bv-2 mouse microglial cells. Reactive oxygen species (ROS) and nitric oxide (NO) production (indicating oxidative stress and inflammatory response) were measured. These results demonstrated differences in oxidative and inflammatory effects of elderberry extracts depending on solvents used. *Results further identified quercetin as the most active component in suppressing oxidative stress and inflammatory responses on microglial [a type of nerve cell] cells.*"[660]

Resveratrol

Resveratrol is a polyphenol that plays a potentially important role in many disorders and has been studied in different diseases. The research on this chemical started through the "French paradox," which describes improved cardiovascular outcomes despite a high-fat diet in French people. Since then, resveratrol has been broadly studied and shown to have antioxidant, anti-inflammatory, anti-proliferative, and anti-angiogenic effects, with those on oxidative stress possibly being most important and underlying some of the others, but many signaling pathways are among the molecular targets of resveratrol. In concert they may be beneficial in many disorders, particularly in diseases where oxidative stress plays an important role.[661]

Food sources of resveratrol include the skin of grapes, blueberries, raspberries, and mulberries. In grapes, resveratrol is found primarily in the skin. The levels of resveratrol found in food varies greatly. Red wine contains between 0.2 and 5.8 mg/l, depending on the grape variety, while white wine has much less, because red wine is fermented with the skins, allowing the wine to extract the resveratrol, whereas white wine is fermented after the skin has been removed. The composition of wine is different from that of grapes since the extraction of resveratrols from grapes depends on the duration of the skin contact.

Low-to-moderate red wine consumption has been shown to reduce age-related neurological disorders including macular degeneration, stroke, and cognitive deficits with or without dementia. Resveratrol has been considered as one of the key ingredients responsible for the preventive action of red wine since it displays a neuroprotective action in various models of toxicity.[662]

While red wine is a good source of resveratrol (in general: Cabernet Sauvignon > Merlot > Chianti), one can only drink so much wine. The recommended limits for drinking all forms of alcohol are two drinks per day for males and one drink per day for females. This clearly limits the amount of resveratrol one can ingest….far better to take a supplement to get an adequate amount. Such preparations are available as OTC (over-the-counter) supplements in a variety of stores, such as pharmacies, health food stores such as GNC, and big-box stores, such as Walmart, Target, SAMS Club, COSTCO, and so forth, generally from 100 mg to 250 mg per pill.

One promising source of resveratrol is peanuts, especially sprouted peanuts where the content rivals that in grapes. According to a scientific review published in 2014, "Peanuts are important dietary food source of resveratrol with potent antioxidant properties implicated in reducing risk of cancer, cardiovascular and Alzheimer's disease, and delaying aging."[663]

The fruit of the mulberry (esp. the skin) is a source, and is sold as a nutritional supplement.

Cocoa powder, baking chocolate, and dark chocolate also have low levels of resveratrol in normal consumption quantities (0.35 to 1.85 mg/kg).

As with green tea, melatonin, and curcumin, resveratrol has many, many beneficial effects on the body. It is considered to have a number

ALZHEIMER'S DISEASE

of beneficial effects, including anticancer, anti-athrogenic [artery plaque forming], anti-oxidative, anti-inflammatory, anti-microbial and estrogenic activity.

We will touch on some of these diverse positive effects, but our main focus will be on resveratrol's protective effect on the brain. (While there is some overlap in the focus of the articles reviewed, specific research on resveratrol's effects on longevity will be reviewed in the special section, Longevity.)

Dr. Poulsen and colleagues summarized the scientific literature on resveratrol in the July 2013 issue of the *Annals of the New York Academy of Science*. They summarized their findings by stating, "In the search for novel preventive and therapeutic modalities in the management of metabolic diseases and obesity, resveratrol has attracted great attention over the past decades. Preclinical trials [non-human studies] suggest that resveratrol mimics the metabolic effects of calorie restriction (CR)...In experimental animals, this potential translates into prevention or improvement of glucose metabolism, anti-inflammation, cancer, and nonalcoholic fatty liver disease. Moreover, and in accordance with CR, supplementation with resveratrol promotes longevity in several primitive species and protects against diet-induced metabolic abnormalities in rodents. Despite the substantial preclinical evidence, human clinical data are very scarce, and even though the compound is widely distributed as an over-the-counter human nutritional supplement, its therapeutic rationale has not been well characterized."[664] This tepid conclusion belies much of the powerful data supporting its beneficial effects, which are discussed below.

The following article summary uses a bit of scientific jargon, but it is important to the overall understanding of the importance of resveratrol:[665]

> "From the Department of Genetics, Harvard Medical School, Boston, MA, Drs. Hubbard and Sinclair reported in March 2014 that, "Recent studies in mice have identified single molecules that can delay multiple dis-

eases of aging and extend lifespan. In theory, such molecules could prevent dozens of diseases simultaneously, potentially extending healthy years of life. In this review, we discuss recent advances, controversies, opportunities, and challenges surrounding the development of *SIRT1 activators* [like resveratrol], molecules with the potential to delay aging and age-related diseases. Sirtuins [including SIRT1] comprise a family of NAD^+-dependent deacylases [enzymes] that are central to the body's response to diet and exercise. New studies indicate that both natural and synthetic sirtuin activating compounds (STACs) work via a common allosteric mechanism to stimulate sirtuin activity, thereby conferring broad health benefits in rodents, primates, and possibly humans. *The fact that two-thirds of people in the USA who consume multiple dietary supplements consume resveratrol, a SIRT1 activator*, underscores the importance of understanding the biochemical mechanism, physiological effects, and safety of STACs."

Presented here as an example of the potential beneficial and diverse effects of resveratrol, Dr. Aguirre and colleagues reported in the November 14, 2014 issue of the journal *Molecules* that, "Resveratrol has been recently reported as preventing obesity." They reviewed the scientific literature concerning this topic and, without explaining all of their findings, they concluded, "...consequently the associated energy dissipation, can contribute to explaining the body-fat lowering effect of resveratrol."[666]

What about resveratrol's effects on Alzheimer's disease? Dr. Pasinettie and colleagues, from the Department of Neurology, Friedman Brain Institute, Icahn School of Medicine at Mount Sinai, New York, NY, reported the following in October 2014:[667]

> "There is mounting evidence that dietary polyphenols, including resveratrol, may beneficially influence Alzheimer's disease (AD). Based on this consideration, sev-

eral studies reported in the last few years were designed to validate sensitive and reliable translational tools to mechanistically characterize brain bioavailable polyphenols as disease-modifying agents to help prevent the onset of AD dementia and other neurodegenerative disorders. *Several research groups worldwide with expertise in AD, plant biology, nutritional sciences, and botanical sciences have reported very high quality studies that ultimately provided the necessary information showing that polyphenols [such as resveratrol] and their metabolites, which come from several dietary sources, including grapes, cocoa etc., are capable of preventing AD. The ultimate goal of these studies was to provide novel strategies to prevent the disease even before the onset of clinical symptoms. The studies discussed in this review article provide support that the information gathered in the last few years of research will have a major impact on AD prevention by providing vital knowledge on the protective roles of polyphenols, including resveratrol."*

Professor Ghobeh and colleagues, from the Institute of Biochemistry and Biophysics, University of Tehran, Tehran, Iran, reported in the November 2014 issue of the journal *Biopolymers*, that, *"resveratrol was able to destabilize some of the plaque formations characteristic of Alzheimer's disease,* in an animal model."[668]

Recently, researchers found that resveratrol was also helpful in an animal model of vascular dementia, which has a different type of pathology than Alzheimer's dementia. They stated that, *"resveratrol improved learning and memory ability...These results confirmed that the neuroprotective effects of resveratrol on vascular dementia were associated with its anti-oxidant properties."*[669]

Researchers reported that, "Polyphenols such as epigallocatechin gallate (EGCG) [found in green tea] and resveratrol [found in red wine] have received a great deal of attention because they may contribute to the purported neuroprotective action of the regular consumption of green tea and red wine. Many studies, including those published by our group, suggest that this protective action includes their abilities to prevent the neurotoxic effects of beta-amyloid, a protein whose accumulation likely plays a pivotal role in Alzheimer's disease." The researchers went on to discuss their current research on the protective effects of EGCG and resveratrol in preventing the death of nerve cells challenged with a specific toxic agent.[670]

Two separate research groups from China, using different animal models of Alzheimer's disease, *demonstrated the protective effects of resveratrol against the characteristic pathologic lesions of AD.*[671,672]

Inflammatory molecules have been implicated in the pathogenesis of neurodegenerative diseases such as Parkinson's disease, Alzheimer's disease, and multiple sclerosis. Researchers studied the anti-inflammatory effects of resveratrol and concluded that, *"Collectively, these studies suggest that resveratrol may be an effective therapeutic agent in neurodegenerative diseases initiated or maintained by inflammatory processes."*[673]

Nerve cell branching is required for proper nerve cell or neuronal connectivity. SIRT1[1] has been associated with aging and longevity, which in neurons is linked to neuronal differentiation and neuroprotection. Using cultured memory nerve cells from animals, the role of SIRT1 in nerve cell development was evaluated. Neurons with higher levels of SIRT1 showed increased nerve cell branching. The researchers reported that, *"The effect of SIRT1 was mimicked by treatment with resveratrol, a well-known activator of SIRT1, indicating that the effect of resveratrol was specifically mediated by SIRT1."* The researchers also found that memory nerve cells treated with resveratrol were protected from nerve cell damage induced by Aβeta proteins.[674]

---

[1]SIRT1 is one of a group of proteins. Sirtuins have been implicated in influencing a wide range of cellular processes like aging, cell death, inflammation and stress resistance, as well as energy efficiency and alertness during low-calorie situations. Sirtuins can also control circadian clocks and mitochondrial biogenesis.

ALZHEIMER'S DISEASE

Dr. Scuderi and colleagues, reporting in 2014 in the *Frontiers of Pharmacology*, noted that in an animal model of Alzheimer's disease, resveratrol, which is a SIRT1 activator, "was able to reduce astrocyte[1] activation as well as the production of pro-inflammatory mediators. These data disclose novel findings about the therapeutic potential of SIRT modulators, and suggest novel strategies for AD treatment."[675]

Dr.Pasinetti and colleagues, from the Department of Neurology, Friedman Brain Institute, Icahn School of Medicine at Mount Sinai, New York, NY, reported in the June 2015 issue of *Biochimica et Biophysica Acta*, "There is mounting evidence that dietary polyphenols, including resveratrol, may beneficially influence Alzheimer's disease...Several research groups worldwide with expertise in AD, plant biology, nutritional sciences, and botanical sciences have reported very high quality studies that ultimately provided the necessary information showing that polyphenols and their metabolites, which come from several dietary sources, including grapes, cocoa etc., are capable of preventing AD. The ultimate goal of these studies was to provide novel strategies to prevent the disease even before the onset of clinical symptoms. The studies discussed in this review article provide support that the information gathered in the last few years of research will have a major impact on AD prevention by providing vital knowledge on the protective roles of polyphenols, including resveratrol."[676]

Dr. Bastianetto, from the Douglas Mental Health University Institute, McGill University, Montreal, Canada, and colleagues, reported on the many benefits of resveratrol in the June 2015 issue of the journal *Biochimica et Biophysica Acta*:[677]

---

[1]Astrocytes also known collectively as astroglia, are characteristic star-shaped glial cells in the brain and spinal cord. They are the most abundant cells of the human brain. They perform many functions, including biochemical support of endothelial cells that form the blood–brain barrier, provision of nutrients to the nervous tissue, maintenance of extracellular ion balance, and a role in the repair and scarring process of the brain and spinal cord following traumatic injuries.

"Low-to-moderate red wine consumption appeared to reduce age-related neurological disorders including macular degeneration, stroke, and cognitive deficits with or without dementia. Resveratrol has been considered as one of the key ingredients responsible for the preventive action of red wine since the stilbene displays a neuroprotective action in various models of toxicity. *Besides its well documented free radical scavenging and anti-inflammatory properties, resveratrol has been shown to increase the clearance of beta-amyloid, a key feature of Alzheimer's disease, and to modulate intracellular effectors associated with oxidative stress (e.g. heme oxygenase), neuronal energy homeostasis (e.g. AMP kinase), program cell death (i.e. AIF) and longevity (i.e. sirtuins).*"

Rhodiola Rosea

Rhodiola rosea (commonly golden root, rose root, roseroot, western roseroot, Aaron's rod, Arctic root, king's crown, *lignum rhodium*, orpin rose) is a perennial flowering plant in the family Crassulaceae. It grows in cold regions of the world, including much of the Arctic, the mountains of Central Asia, scattered in eastern North America from Baffin Island to the mountains of North Carolina, and mountainous parts of Europe, such as the Alps, Pyrenees, and Carpathian Mountains, Scandinavia, Iceland, Great Britain and Ireland. It grows on sea cliffs and on mountains at altitudes up to 2280 meters.

According to wikipedia.com: Some studies have found support for it having antidepressant effects. It is not approved by the U.S. Food and Drug Administration (FDA) to cure, treat, or prevent any disease. In fact, the FDA has forcibly removed some products containing *R. rosea* from the market due to disputed claims that it treats cancer, anxiety, influenza, the common cold, bacterial infections, and migraines. *R. rosea* may be effective for improving mood and alleviating depression.

Pilot studies on human subjects showed it improves physical and mental performance, and may reduce fatigue.

In Russia and Scandinavia, *R. rosea* has been used for centuries to cope with the cold Siberian climate and stressful life. Such effects were provided with evidence in laboratory models of stress using the nematode *C. elegans*, and in rats in which *Rhodiola* effectively prevented stress-induced changes in appetite, physical activity, weight gain and the estrus cycle.

The plant has been used in traditional Chinese medicine, where it is called *hóng jǐng tiān* (红景天). The medicine can be used to prevent altitude sickness.

Dr. Jacob and colleagues, reported the results of their research on the protective effects of Rhodiola rosea in an animal model of oxidative stress, in the journal *Annals of Neurosciences*.

The researchers note that, "Aging and age-related neurodegenerative changes including Parkinson's disease [and Alzheimer's disease] are characterized by an important role of reactive oxygen species. It is characterized by signs of major oxidative stress and mitochondrial damage in the pars compacta of substantia nigra. Present study was designed to investigate whether Rhodiola rosea extract would prevent MPTP [a neurotoxin] induced neurotoxicity in Male wistar rats...MPTP induced rats showed behavioral alterations in elevated plus maze testing... Histological evidence revealed that MPTP treated rats shown pathological changes like cellular inflammation and vascular degeneration in brain tissue. The oxidative stress and related biochemical alteration by MPTP were attenuated by Rhodiola rosea treatment."[678]

We have included the details of the following research so that the reader can get a sense of how complicated and detailed most the research reported in this book is. Publishing the results of their research in the journal *Behavioural Brain Research*, Dr. Zhang and colleagues note that,

PREVENTION

"Beta amyloid (Aβ)-induced oxidative stress and chronic inflammation in the brain are considered to be responsible for the pathogenesis of Alzheimer's disease. *Salidroside, the major active ingredient of Rhodiola crenulata, has been previously shown to have antioxidant and neuroprotective properties* in vitro [in the laboratory]. The present study aimed to investigate the protective effects of salidroside on Aβ-induced cognitive impairment in vivo [in animals and humans]. Rats received intrahippocampal Aβ1-40 injection were treated with salidroside (25, 50 and 75 mg/kg p.o.) once daily for twenty-one days. Learning and memory performance were assessed in the Morris water maze (days 17-21). After behavioral testing, the rats were sacrificed and hippocampi were removed for biochemical assays (reactive oxygen species (ROS), superoxide dismutase (SOD), glutathione peroxidase (GPx), malondialdehyde (MDA), acetylcholinesterase (AChE), acetylcholine (ACh)) and molecular biological analysis (Cu/Zn-SOD, Mn-SOD, GPx, nicotinamide adenine dinucleotide phosphate (NADPH) oxidase, nuclear factor κB (NF-κB), inhibitor of κB-alpha (IκBα), cyclooxygenase-2 (COX-2), inducible nitric oxide synthase (iNOS), receptor for advanced glycation end products (RAGE)). Our results confirmed that Aβ1-40 peptide caused learning and memory deficits in rats. Further analysis demonstrated that the NADPH oxidase-mediated oxidative stress was increased in Aβ1-40-injected rats. Furthermore, NF-κB was demonstrated to be activated in Aβ1-40-injected rats, and the COX-2, iNOS and RAGE expression were also induced by Aβ1-40. *However, salidroside (50 and 75 mg/kg p.o.) reversed all the former alterations. Thus, the study indicates that salidroside may have a protective effect against AD via modulating oxidative stress and inflammatory mediators.*"[679]

Rhodiola also has other interesting properties, as discussed below.

In 2014, Drs. Yan and Choi reported in the *Journal of Pharmacological Sciences* that, "Salidroside is a biologically active ingredient of Rhodiola rosea, which has several interesting biological properties, including anti-oxidant and anti-inflammatory; however, its anti-allergic effects are poorly understood. The objective of this study is to determine whether salidroside attenuates the inflammatory response in an asthma model." Without going into the technical aspects of their research, the authors concluded, "*Our data support the utility of salidroside as a potential medicine for the treatment of asthma.*"[680]

Dr. Song and colleagues reported the results of their research studying the anti-inflammatory effects of Rhodiola rosea in a cellular model of inflammation in the *Journal of Medicinal Food*. Without going into all of the details of their research, which is quite technical, but for those readers who are interested in some of the science behind the researcher's findings, we include the following, "The aim of this study was to evaluate the effect of salidroside on lipopolysaccharide (LPS)-induced nitric oxide (NO) and prostaglandin E_2 (PGE_2) production in RAW 264.7 macrophages and related anti-inflammatory mechanism...The data showed salidroside inhibited LPS-induced NO and PGE_2 production and reduced iNOS and COX-2 protein expression in RAW 264.7 macrophages...In addition, we further investigated signal transduction mechanisms and found that the activation of NF-κB was suppressed by salidroside in a dose-dependent manner. These results suggest that salidroside suppresses NO and PGE_2 production by inhibiting iNOS and COX-2 protein expression, level of $[Ca^{2+}](i)$, and activation of NF-κB signal transduction pathway." [681] Summarizing, we can say that Rhodiola suppresses nitric oxide (NO) and prostaglandin E_2 (PGE_2) production (both associated with inflammation), and is a COX-2 inhibitor[1].

---

[1]COX-2 selective inhibitor is a form of non-steroidal anti-inflammatory drug (NSAID) that directly targets cyclooxygenase-2, COX-2, an enzyme responsible for inflammation and pain. Targeting selectivity for COX-2 reduces the risk of peptic ulceration, and is the main feature of celecoxib, rofecoxib and other members of this

Another interesting research study shows that, like many supplements, rhodiola has numerous different and beneficial properties. In the September 2014 issue of the journal *Pharmacology Biochemistry & Behavior*, Dr. Yang and colleagues reported the results of their research using Rhodiola in an animal model of depression. They found that, "Chronic treatment with SA could remarkably reduce TNF-α and IL-1β levels in hippocampus. Western blot showed that SA could markedly increase glucocorticoid receptor (GR) and brain-derived neurotrophic factor (BDNF) expression in the hippocampus. Besides, SA could also attenuate corticotropin-releasing hormone (CRH) expression in hypothalamus, as well as reducing significantly the levels of serum corticosterone. In conclusion, this study demonstrated that OBX rats treated with SA could significantly improve the depressive-like behaviors. *The antidepressant mechanisms of SA might be associated with its anti-inflammatory effects* and the regulation of HPA axis activity. Reversal of abnormalities of GR may be partly responsible for those effects. *These findings suggested that SA might become a beneficial agent to prevent and treat the depression.*"[682]

Saffron (Crocus sativus L.)

For those that want to use a "natural" treatment for Alzheimer's disease as opposed to medications, here is a recent report demonstrating that Saffron, extracted from a plant, is as effective in the management of moderate to severe AD as is Namenda (memantine; 20 mg/day). Using a typical research protocol, sixty-eight patients with moderate to severe AD were treated with either Namenda or Saffron for twelve months. *Both treatment groups showed similar outcomes, slowing cognitive decline*, and the frequency of adverse events was not significantly different between the two groups as well.[683]

---

drug class. After several COX-2 inhibiting drugs were approved for marketing, data from clinical trials revealed that COX-2 inhibitors caused a significant increase in heart attacks and strokes, with some drugs in the class having worse risks than others. Rofecoxib (commonly known as Vioxx) was taken off the market in 2004 because of these concerns and celecoxib and traditional NSAIDs received boxed warnings on their labels.

Selenium

Selenium is a chemical element with symbol Se and atomic number 34. Selenium salts are toxic in large amounts, but trace amounts are necessary for cellular function in many organisms, including all animals, and is an ingredient in many multi-vitamins and other dietary supplements, including infant formula. Selenium is a component of the antioxidant enzymes glutathione peroxidase and thioredoxin reductase (which indirectly reduce certain oxidized molecules in animals and some plants). It is also found in three deiodinase enzymes, which convert one thyroid hormone to another.

Dietary selenium comes from nuts, cereals, meat, mushrooms, fish, and eggs. Brazil nuts are the richest ordinary dietary source (though this is soil-dependent, since the Brazil nut does not require high levels of the element for its own needs). In descending order of concentration, high levels are also found in kidney, tuna, crab, and lobster.

Selenium as a dietary supplement is available in many forms, including multi-vitamins. In 2013 the U.S. Food and Drug Administration (FDA) proposed the requirement of minimum and maximum levels of selenium in infant formula.

Dr. Cardoso and colleagues, reporting in the October 2014 issue of the *Journal of Trace Elements in Medicine and Biology*, described the results of their study on the relationship between selenium (Se) and cognitive decline. "Studies show that decreased antioxidant system is related to cognitive decline. Thus we aimed to measure selenium (Se) status in Alzheimer's disease (AD) and mild cognitive impairment (MCI) in the elderly and compared them with a control group (CG). Twenty-seven AD, seventeen MCI and twenty-eight control elderly were evaluated. Se concentration was determined in plasma and erythrocyte [red blood cells]...*The AD group exhibited the lowest plasma [blood] Se level when compared to the MCI and CG groups. It is observed that erythrocyte Se decreases as cognition function does...Our findings suggest that the deficiency of Se may contribute to cognitive decline among aging people.*"[684]

In a 2014 article reviewing the importance of selenium in brain disorders, the authors noted that, *"Selenoproteins are important for normal brain function, and decreased function of selenoproteins can lead to impaired cognitive function and neurological disorders...Selenium deficiency is associated with cognitive decline, and selenoproteins may be helpful in preventing neurodegeneration in Alzheimer's disease."*[685]

In 2014, Dr. Song and colleagues, from the College of Life Sciences, Shenzhen University, Shenzhen, China, reported in the *Journal of Alzheimer's Disease* that, "Disruption of the intracellular balance between free radicals and the antioxidant system is a prominent and early feature in the neuropathology of Alzheimer's disease. Selenium, a vital trace element with known antioxidant potential, has been reported to provide neuroprotection through resisting oxidative damage but its therapeutic effect on AD remains to be investigated. The objective of our study was to investigate the potential of selenomethionine (Se-Met), an organic form of selenium, in the treatment of cognitive dysfunction and neuropathology [in an animal model of AD]...*Thus Se-Met improves cognitive deficit in a murine*[1] *model of AD, which is associated with reduction in tau expression and hyperphosphorylation, amelioration of inflammation, and restoration of synaptic proteins and antioxidants. This study provides a novel therapeutic approach for the prevention of AD.*"[686]

Souvenaid®

Dr. Ritchie and colleagues, from the Department of Medicine, Imperial College, London, UK, published the following in the March 2014 issue of the *Journal of Nutrition, Health & Aging*:[687]

> "Synaptic loss correlates closely with cognitive deficits in Alzheimer's disease and represents a new target for intervention. Souvenaid® is the first medical nutrition product to be designed to support synapse formation and function in early Alzheimer's disease, and has under-

---

[1]Murine: of or relating to a murid genus (*Mus*) or its subfamily (Murinae) which includes the common household rats and mice.

gone an extensive, 12-year development programme. The relatively large amount of clinical data available for Souvenaid® is unusual for a medical nutrition product. Souvenaid® contains omega-3 polyunsaturated fatty acids (docosahexaenoic acid and eicosapentaenoic acid), uridine (as uridine monophosphate) and choline which are nutritional precursors required for synaptic membrane phospholipid synthesis, together with phospholipids and other cofactors [vitamins E, C, B12, and B6, folic acid, and selenium]. Souvenaid® has demonstrated cognitive benefits in patients with mild Alzheimer's disease but not in patients with mild-to-moderate Alzheimer's disease. Two randomized, double-blind, controlled trials (duration twelve and twenty-four weeks) in patients with mild Alzheimer's disease untreated with acetylcholinesterase inhibitors and/or memantine have demonstrated that Souvenaid® is well tolerated and improves episodic memory performance.

The daily intake of Souvenaid® has not been associated with any harmful effects or interactions with medications and none are anticipated. The ongoing, 24-month, European Union-funded LipiDiDiet trial in subjects with prodromal Alzheimer's disease is evaluating the potential benefits of Souvenaid® on memory and in slowing progression to Alzheimer's dementia. If Souvenaid® induces synaptogenesis and improved synaptic function, it may provide benefits in other clinical conditions characterised by neurodegeneration. A number of trials are ongoing and planned to evaluate the potential wider benefits of Souvenaid®."

Dr. de Waal and colleagues published the results of their research on Souvenaid® in the January 27, 2014 issue of *PLOS ONE*[1]. The authors

---

[1] *PLOS ONE* (originally *PLoS ONE*) is a peer-reviewed, open access, scientific journal published by the Public Library of Science (PLOS) since 2006.

noted that, "Synaptic loss is a major hallmark of Alzheimer's disease. Disturbed organization of large-scale functional brain networks in AD might reflect synaptic loss and disrupted neuronal communication. The medical food Souvenaid®, containing the specific nutrient combination Fortasyn Connect, is designed to enhance synapse formation and function and has been shown to improve memory performance in patients with mild AD in two randomised controlled trials." They studied 179 drug-nieve mild AD patients who participated in the Souvenir II study, for twenty-four weeks. They concluded that, *"The current results suggest that Souvenaid preserves the organization of brain networks in patients with mild AD within twenty-four weeks, hypothetically counteracting the progressive network disruption over time in AD*. The results strengthen the hypothesis that Souvenaid® affects synaptic integrity and function."[688]

However, Dr. Shah and colleagues, publishing the results of their research on Souvenaid® in the November 26, 2013 issue of the journal *Alzheimer's Research & Therapy*, found no advantage of the complex. The researchers wanted to better understand whether or not Souvenaid® slows cognitive decline in treated persons with mild-to-moderate Alzheimer's disease. They reported that, "In a 24-week, double-masked clinical trial at forty-eight clinical centers, 527 participants [52 percent women, mean age 76.7 years, and mean Mini-Mental State Examination score 19.5] taking AD medications [such as Aricept, Exelon or Namenda] were randomized 1:1 to daily, 125-mL, oral intake of the active product (Souvenaid®) or an iso-caloric control. The primary outcome of cognition was assessed by the 11-item Alzheimer's disease Assessment Scale-Cognitive Subscale (ADAS-cog). *Cognitive performance as assessed by ADAS-cog showed decline over time in both control and active study groups, with no significant difference between study groups. Add-on intake of Souvenaid® during twenty-four weeks did not slow cognitive decline in persons treated for mild-to-moderate AD*."[689]

St John's Wort

Hypericum perforatum, known as Perforate St John's-wort, Common Saint John's wort and St John's wort, is a flowering plant of the genus *Hypericum* and a medicinal herb with antidepressant activity and potent anti-inflammatory properties as an arachidonate 5-lipoxygenase inhibitor and COX-1 inhibitor.

Some studies have supported the use of St John's wort preparations as a treatment for depression in humans. In contrast, the National Center for Complementary and Integrative Medicine of the United States' National Institutes of Health warn that St. John's wort is not a proven treatment for depression. [This, once again, flies in the face of reality—see the following paragraph.]

In the November 2014 issue of the journal *Archives of Medical Research*, Dr. Pahnke and colleagues noted the following:[690]

> "In elderly subjects, depression and dementia often coincide but the actual reason is currently unknown. Does a causal link exist or is it just a reactive effect of the knowledge of suffering from dementia? The ABC transporter superfamily may represent a causal link between these mental disorders. *Since the transporters ABCB1 and ABCC1 have been discovered as major β-amyloid-exporting molecules at the blood-brain barrier and ABCC1 was found to be directly activated by St. John's wort (SJW), depression and dementia certainly share an important pathophysiologic link. It was recognized that herbal anti-depressant formulations made from SJW are at least as effective for the treatment of unipolar depression in old age as classical pharmacotherapy [antidepressants like Prozac, Zoloft, Paxil, etc.], while having fewer side effects (Cochrane reports[1], 2008).* SJW is

---

[1]The Cochrane Collaboration is an independent, non-profit, non-governmental organization consisting of a group of more than 31,000 volunteers in more than 120 countries. The collaboration was formed to organize medical research information in a

PREVENTION

known to activate various metabolizing and transport systems in the body, with cytochrome P450 enzymes [metabolic enzymes] and ABC transporters being most important.

Does the treatment of depression in elderly subjects using pharmacological compounds or phytomedical extracts target a mechanism that also accounts for peptide storage in Alzheimer's disease and perhaps other proteopathies of the brain? *In this review we summarize recent data that point to a common mechanism and present the first promising causal treatment results of demented elderly subjects with distinct SJW extracts. Insufficient trans-barrier clearance may indeed present a common problem in all the proteopathies of the brain where toxic peptides are deposited in a location-specific manner. Thus, activation of efflux molecules holds promise for future treatment of this large group of devastating disorders."*

And, the experimental use of an extract of St. John's wort, in an animal model of Alzheimer's disease, also supports the benefits of SJW in helping to reverse some of the pathology associated with AD. Dr. Hofrichter and colleagues, reported the following in the December 2013 issue of journal *Current Alzheimer Research*:[691]

"Soluble β-amyloid peptides (Aβ) and small Aβ oligomers[1] represent the most toxic peptide moieties recognized in brains affected by Alzheimer's disease. *Here we*

---

systematic way to facilitate the choices that health professionals, patients, policy makers and others face in health interventions according to the principles of evidence-based medicine. The group conducts systematic reviews of randomized controlled trials of health-care interventions, which it publishes in The Cochrane Library.
[1]In chemistry, an oligomer is a molecular complex that consists of a few monomer units, in contrast to a polymer, where the number of monomers is, in principle, not limited. Dimers, trimers, and tetramers are, for instance, oligomers composed of two, three and four monomers, respectively.

provide the first evidence that specific St. John's wort (SJW) extracts both attenuate Aβ-induced histopathology and alleviate memory impairments in APP-transgenic mice. Importantly, these effects are attained independently of hyperforin. *Specifically, two extracts characterized by low hyperforin content (i) significantly decrease intracerebral Aβ42 levels, (ii) decrease the number and size of amyloid plaques, (iii) rescue neocortical neurons, (iv) restore cognition to normal levels, and (iv) activate microglia in vitro and in vivo. Mechanistically, we reveal that the reduction of soluble Aβ42 species is the consequence of a highly increased export activity in the bloodbrain barrier ABCC1transporter, which was found to play a fundamental role in Aβ excretion into the bloodstream.* These data (i) support the significant beneficial potential of SJW extracts on AD proteopathy, and (ii) demonstrate for the first time that hyperforin concentration does not necessarily correlate with their therapeutic effects. *Hence, by activating ABC transporters, specific extracts of SJW may be used to treat AD and other diseases involving peptide accumulation and cognition impairment. We propose that the anti-depressant and anti-dementia effects of these hyperforin-reduced phytoextracts could be combined for treatment of the elderly,* with a concomitant reduction in deleterious hyperforin-related side effects."

Similarly, Dr. Brenn and colleagues, reporting in the January 2014 issue of the journal *Brain Pathology*, noted that:[692]

"The adenosine triphosphate-binding cassette transport protein P-glycoprotein (ABCB1) *is involved in the export of beta-amyloid from the brain into the blood, and there is evidence that age-associated deficits in cerebral P-glycoprotein content may be involved in Alzheimer's disease pathogenesis. P-glycoprotein function and expression can be pharmacologically induced by a variety of compounds including extracts of Hypericum perforatum (St. John's Wort).* To clarify the effect of St. John's Wort on the accumulation of beta-amyloid and P-glycoprotein expression in the brain, St. John's Wort extract was fed to mice. *Mice receiving St. John's Wort extract showed (i) significant reductions of parenchymal beta-amyloid 1-40 and 1-42 accumulation; and (ii) moderate, but statistically significant increases in cerebrovascular P-glycoprotein expression. Thus, the induction of cerebrovascular P-glycoprotein may be a novel therapeutic strategy to protect the brain from beta-amyloid accumulation, and thereby impede the progression of Alzheimer's disease."*

Walnuts

A walnut is the nut of any tree of the genus *Juglans* (Family Juglandaceae), particularly the Persian or English walnut, *Juglans regia*. Walnuts are a nutrient-dense food: 100 grams of walnuts contain 15.2 grams of protein, 65.2 grams of fat, and 6.7 grams of dietary fiber. The protein in walnuts provides many essential amino acids.

While English walnuts are the most common, their nutrient density and profile are significantly different from those of black walnuts. For example, the Omega-3 fatty acid content of English walnuts is approximately 4.5 times that of black walnuts.

Unlike most nuts that are high in monounsaturated fatty acids, walnut oil is composed largely of polyunsaturated fatty acids (47.2 percent), particularly alpha-linolenic acid (9.1 percent) and linoleic acid (38.1 percent).

Dr. Hicyilmaz and colleagues published the results of their experiment, in the December 18, 2014 issue of the journal *Nutritional Neuroscience*, studying the effects of walnuts in an animal model of Alzheimer's disease. Without discussing the specifics of their work, they concluded by stating, *"We suggested that walnut supplementation may have protective effects against the decline of cognitive functions by regulating NMDAR [N-methyl d-aspartate receptors] and lipid peroxidation levels in the hippocampus. The study provides evidence that selected dietary factors (polyunsaturated fatty acids, melatonin, vitamin E, and flavonoids) within walnut may help to trigger hippocampal neuronal signal transduction for the formation of learning and memory."*[693]

As an interesting aside, Dr.Mohammadifard and colleagues published a report, in the October 14, 2014 issue of the *European Journal of Nutrition*, on the association between nut intake and obesity. They studied 9,660 randomly chosen adults aged ≥19 years whose nutritional behaviors included regular intake of walnuts, almonds, pistachios, hazelnuts and sunflower seeds. They compared the rate of obesity based on nut consumption and found, *"...a significant association between high nut consumption and lower prevalence of overweight or general obesity as well as abdominal obesity in women, but not men. Frequent nuts and seeds consumption, particularly ≥1 time/day, had an inverse association with all classes of obesity among women."*[694]

Drs. Jackson and Hu, from the Department of Nutrition, Harvard School of Public Health, Boston, MA, reported significant health benefits from eating nuts, in the June 2014 issue of the *American Journal of Clinical Nutrition*:[695]

> "There is some concern that the high-fat, energy-dense content of nuts may promote weight gain. Nuts, however, are rich in protein and dietary fiber, which are associated with increased satiety. They also contain high amounts of vitamins, minerals, antioxidants, and phytoesterols that may confer health benefits for cardiovascular disease and type 2 diabetes delay and prevention. Therefore, it is important to determine the association between nut consumption and long-term weight change and disease risk to reach scientific consensus and to make evidence-based public health rec-

ommendations. Several cross-sectional analyses have shown an inverse association between higher nut consumption and lower body weight. In addition, several independent prospective studies found that increasing nut consumption was associated with lower weight gain over relatively long periods of time. *Moreover, high consumption of nuts (especially walnuts) has been associated with lower diabetes risk. Therefore, regular consumption (approximately one handful daily) of nuts over the long term, as a replacement to less healthful foods, can be incorporated as a component of a healthy diet for the prevention of obesity and type 2 diabetes."*

As another interesting aside, but without discussing the details of their experiment on the effects of walnuts on human cancer cells, Dr. Le and colleagues, reporting in 2014 in the Journal of *Nutrition and Cancer*, note that, "Walnuts contain many bioactive components that may slow cancer growth."[696]

And, another group of researchers note that, *"Our results suggest that a diet rich in ET-containing [polyphenols, mainly ellagitannins (ETs)] foods, such as walnuts, could contribute to the prevention of prostate cancer."*[697]

From the Department of Biochemistry and Microbiology, Marshall University School of Medicine, Huntington, WV, Dr. Hardman, reporting in the April 2014 issue of the Journal of Nutrition, noted that:[698]

> *"Cancer may not be completely the result of novel or inherited genetic mutations but may in fact be a largely preventable disease. Researchers have identified biochemicals, including n-3 (ω-3) fatty acids, tocopherols [vitamin E], β-sitosterol, and pedunculagin, that are found in walnuts and that have cancer-prevention properties.*

Mouse studies in which walnuts were added to the diet have shown the following compared with the control diet: (1) the walnut-containing diet inhibited the growth rate of human breast cancers implanted in nude mice by ~80 percent; (2) the walnut-containing diet reduced the number of mammary gland tumors by ~60 percent in a transgenic mouse model; (3) the reduction in mammary gland tumors was greater with whole walnuts than with a diet containing the same amount of n-3 fatty acids, supporting the idea that multiple components in walnuts additively or synergistically contribute to cancer suppression; and (4) walnuts slowed the growth of prostate, colon, and renal cancers by antiproliferative and antiangiogenic mechanisms. Cell studies have aided in the identification of the active components in walnuts and of their mechanisms of action. This review summarizes these studies and presents the notion that *walnuts may be included as a cancer-preventive choice in a healthy diet."*

From the laboratory of Dr. Fisher and colleagues, as reported in the August 25, 2014 issue of the journal, *Nutritional Neuroscience*, "The shift in equilibrium toward excess reactive oxygen or nitrogen species production from innate antioxidant defenses in the brain is a critical factor in the declining neural function and cognitive deficit accompanying age. *Previous studies from our laboratory have reported that walnuts, rich in polyphenols, antioxidants, and omega fatty acids such as alpha-linolenic acid and linoleic acid, improve the age-associated declines in cognition and neural function in rats...These results suggest antioxidant and anti-inflammatory protection or enhancement of membrane-associated functions in brain cells by walnut serum metabolites."*[699]

Dr. Muthaiyah and colleagues examined the effects of walnuts in an animal model of Alzheimer's disease, reporting their findings in 2014 in the *Journal of Alzheimer's Disease*. They noted, "*Previous in vitro studies have shown that walnut extract can inhibit amyloid-β (Aβ) fibrillization, can solubilize its fibrils, and has a protective effect against Aβ-induced oxidative stress and cellular death.* In this study, we analyzed the effect of dietary supplementation with walnuts on learning skills, memory, anxiety, locomotor activity, and motor coordination in a mouse model of Alzheimer's disease...*These findings suggest that dietary supplementation with walnuts may have a beneficial effect in reducing the risk, delaying the onset, or slowing the progression of, or preventing AD.*"[700]

Dr. Poulose and colleagues, from the USDA-Agricultural Research Services, Human Nutrition Research Center on Aging, Tufts University, Boston, MA, noted in the April 2014 issue of the *Journal of Nutrition* the following:[701]

"Because of the combination of population growth and population aging, increases in the incidence of chronic neurodegenerative disorders [especially Alzheimer's disease] have become a societal concern, both in terms of decreased quality of life and increased financial burden. Clinical manifestation of many of these disorders takes years, with the initiation of mild cognitive symptoms leading to behavioral problems, dementia and loss of motor functions, the need for assisted living, and eventual death. Lifestyle factors greatly affect the progression of cognitive decline, with high-risk behaviors including unhealthy diet, lack of exercise, smoking, and exposure to environmental toxins leading to enhanced oxidative stress and inflammation.

Although there exists an urgent need to develop effective treatments for age-related cognitive decline and neurodegenerative disease [like Alzheimer's disease], prevention strategies have been underdeveloped. Primary prevention in many of these neurodegenerative diseases could be achieved earlier in life by consuming a healthy diet, rich in antioxidant and anti-inflammatory phyto-

> *chemicals, which offers one of the most effective and least expensive ways to address the crisis.*
>
> *English walnuts (Juglans regia L.) are rich in numerous phytochemicals, including high amounts of polyunsaturated fatty acids, and offer potential benefits to brain health. Polyphenolic compounds found in walnuts not only reduce the oxidant and inflammatory load on brain cells but also improve interneuronal signaling, increase neurogenesis, and enhance sequestration of insoluble toxic protein aggregates."*

A different group of researchers from the USDA-Agricultural Research Service, Jean Mayer Human Nutrition Research Center on Aging at Tufts University, Boston, MA, led by Dr. Joseph, reported the following in 2014 in the *Journal of Nutrition*:[702]

> *"Numerous studies have indicated that individuals consuming a diet containing high amounts of fruits and vegetables exhibit fewer age-related diseases such as Alzheimer's disease. Research from our laboratory has suggested that dietary supplementation with fruit or vegetable extracts high in antioxidants (e.g. blueberries, strawberries, walnuts, and Concord grape juice) can decrease the enhanced vulnerability to oxidative stress that occurs in aging and these reductions are expressed as improvements in behavior. Additional mechanisms involved in the beneficial effects of fruits and vegetables include enhancement of neuronal communication via increases in neuronal signaling and decreases in stress signals induced by oxidative/inflammatory stressors (e.g. nuclear factor kappaB). Moreover, collaborative findings indicate that blueberry or Concord grape juice supplementation in humans with mild cognitive impairment increased verbal memory performance, thus translating our animal findings to humans. Taken together, these results suggest that a greater intake of high-antioxidant*

foods such as berries, Concord grapes, and walnuts may increase "health span" and enhance cognitive and motor function in aging."

And rounding out some of the health benefits of walnuts, Dr. Kris-Etherton, from the Department of Nutritional Sciences, Pennsylvania State University, University Park, PA, reported in 2014 on the benefits of walnuts vis-à-vis the heart and cardiovascular system. According to Dr. Kris-Etherton:[703]

> "Given the pressing need to reduce cardiovascular disease (CVD) morbidity and mortality, there has been a focus on optimizing dietary patterns to reduce the many contributing risk factors. Over the past two decades, many studies have been conducted that have evaluated the effects of walnut consumption on CVD risk factors. *Walnuts have been shown to decrease low density lipoprotein cholesterol (by ~9-16 percent) and blood pressure (diastolic blood pressure by ~2-3 mm Hg), 2 major risk factors for CVD. In addition, walnuts improve endothelial function, decrease both oxidative stress and some markers of inflammation, and increase cholesterol efflux. The effect of walnuts on multiple CVD targets over relatively short periods of time supports recommendations for their inclusion in a heart-healthy diet."*

And finally, and also in 2014, Dr. Hosseini and colleagues studied the effects of walnuts on patients with type II diabetes. After reviewing the results of their experiment, they said, *"In conclusion, treatment of type II diabetic patients with 100mg Juglans regia leaf [walnut] extract two times a day for three months improves lipid profile and glycemic control without any tangible adverse effects."*[704]

Zinc

Zinc is a chemical element with symbol Zn and atomic number 30. It is an essential mineral. Zinc deficiency affects about two billion people in the developing world and is associated with numerous diseases. In children it causes growth retardation, delayed sexual maturation, infection susceptibility, and diarrhea. Enzymes with a zinc atom in the reactive center are widespread in biochemistry. However, consumption of excess zinc can cause ataxia, lethargy and copper deficiency.

Zinc is found in between 100 to 300 specific enzymes. It is the second most abundant transition metal in organisms after iron and it is the only metal which appears in all enzyme classes. There are 2-4 grams of zinc distributed throughout the human body. Most zinc is in the brain, muscle, bones, kidney, and liver, with the highest concentrations in the prostate and parts of the eye. Semen is particularly rich in zinc, which is a key factor in prostate gland function and reproductive organ growth.

In humans, zinc plays ubiquitous biological roles. It interacts with a wide range of organic molecules, and has roles in the metabolism of RNA and DNA, signal transduction, and gene expression. It also regulates apoptosis (cell death). A 2006 study estimated that about 10 percent of human proteins (2,800) potentially bind zinc, in addition to hundreds which transport and traffic zinc.

In the brain, zinc is stored in specific synaptic vesicles by glutamatergic neurons and can modulate brain excitability. It plays a key role in synaptic plasticity and so in learning. However, it has been called "the brain's dark horse," because it also can be a neurotoxin, suggesting zinc homeostasis plays a critical role in normal functioning of the brain and central nervous system.

Dr. Flinn and colleagues, reporting in the October 22, 2014 issue of the journal *Frontiers in Aging Neuroscience*, conducted an experiment to study the effects of zinc in an animal model of Alzheimer's disease. Without discussing the details of the experiment here, the researchers

PREVENTION

concluded that, *"These data suggest that increased dietary Zn can significantly impair spatial memory...These findings are particularly relevant because increased intake of dietary supplements, such as Zn, are common in the elderly, a population already at risk for AD."*[705] The researchers found that this risk was significantly higher in the animals who carried the ApoE ε4 gene.

Another group of researchers, also reporting in 2014, noted that, "The precise regulation of zinc homeostasis is essential for central nervous system and for the whole organism. Zinc plays a significant role in the brain development and in the proper brain function at every stage of life... Zinc imbalance can result not only from insufficient dietary intake, but also from impaired activity of zinc transport proteins and zinc dependent regulation of metabolic pathways. *It is known that some neurodegenerative processes are connected with zinc dyshomeostasis and it may influence the state of Alzheimer's disease, depression and aging-connected loss of cognitive function.* The exact role of zinc and zinc-binding proteins in CNS pathogenesis processes is being placed under intensive investigation. *The appropriate zinc supplementation in brain diseases may help in the prevention as well as in the proper treatment of several brain dysfunctions."*[706] [Unfortunately the "appropriate" amount is unclear.]

Another group of researchers, using an animal model of Alzheimer's disease, noted the following, "Dysregulation of metal homeostasis has been perceived as one of the key factors in the progression of neurodegeneration. *Aluminium (Al) has been considered as a major risk factor, which is linked to several neurodegenerative diseases, especially Alzheimer's disease*, whereas zinc (Zn) has been reported as a vital dietary element, which regulates a number of physiological processes in the central nervous system. The present study was conducted to explore the protective potential of zinc, if any, in ameliorating neurotoxicity induced by aluminium. Without discussing the specifics of their experiment here, the researchers concluded, *"Therefore, zinc has the potential to alleviate aluminium-induced neurodegeneration."*[707]

In summary, one can say that zinc is very important in cellular function. However, how much we should be getting is far from clear. Sticking with the recommended daily dietary guidelines is probably the best idea.

Other Prevention Programs

Introduction

The Alzheimer's Association is one of the largest nonprofit funders of AD and dementia research in the world. During the 2014 fiscal year, the association made investments totaling nearly $14 million to 88 scientific investigations. Included in this funding is this latest round of research grants, which supports 42 projects across the United States, Canada, Italy, France, the United Kingdom, and Australia.

For example, a Finnish study reported at the Alzheimer's Association International Conference in July 2014 gave strong evidence that lifestyle intervention targeting a variety of risk factors simultaneously can be beneficial in overall healthy aging and preventing cognitive decline. The study enrolled 1,260 adults aged 60 to 77 years.

As reported by *Medscape Medical News* at that time, *"An intervention that included nutritional guidance, physical exercise, cognitive training, social activities, and management of cardiac risk factors resulted in better overall cognitive performance on a comprehensive neuropsychological test battery vs regular health advice. The advantage for this approach was seen on each of the individual cognitive domains tested as well, including memory, executive function, and psychomotor speed."*[708]

Anti-Stress

Physiological or biological stress is an organism's response to a stressor such as an environmental condition or a stimulus. Stress is a body's method of reacting to a challenge. According to the stressful event, the body's way to respond to stress is by sympathetic nervous system activation which results in the fight-or-flight response. Because the body cannot retain this state for long periods of time, the parasympathetic system returns the body's physiological conditions to normal (homeostasis). In humans, stress typically describes a negative condition or a positive condition that can have an impact on a person's mental and physical well-being.

Stress has a significant effect on memory formation and learning. In response to stressful situations, the brain releases hormones and neurotransmitters (ex. glucocorticoids and catecholamines) which affect memory encoding[1] processes in the hippocampus[2]. Behavioral research on animals shows that chronic stress produces adrenal hormones which impact the hippocampal structure in the brains of rats. An experimental study by German cognitive psychologists L. Schwabe and O. Wolf demonstrates how learning under stress also decreases memory recall in humans. In this study, forty-eight healthy female and male university students participated in either a stress test or a control group. Those randomly assigned to the stress test group had a hand immersed in ice cold water (the reputable SECPT or 'Socially Evaluated Cold Pressor Test') for up to three minutes, while being monitored and videotaped. Both the stress and control groups were then presented with thirty-two words to memorize. Twenty-four hours later, both groups were tested to see how many words they could remember (free recall) as well as how many they could recognize from a larger list of words (recognition performance). The results showed a clear impairment of memory performance in the stress test group, who recalled 30 percent fewer words

---

[1]Memory has the ability to encode, store and recall information. Memories give an organism the capability to learn and adapt from previous experiences as well as build relationships. Encoding allows the perceived item of use or interest to be converted into a construct that can be stored within the brain and recalled later from short term or long term memory.

[2]The hippocampus is a major component of the brains of humans and other vertebrates. Humans and other mammals have two hippocampi, one in each side of the brain. It belongs to the limbic system and plays important roles in the consolidation of information from short-term memory to long-term memory and spatial navigation.

than the control group. The researchers suggest that *stress experienced during learning distracts people by diverting their attention during the memory encoding process.*

Dr. Justice, from the Institute of Molecular Medicine, Program in Neuroscience, and Huffington Center on Aging and Department of Human and Molecular Genetics, Baylor College of Medicine, Houston, Texas, and colleagues, reported in the Feburary 11, 2015 issue of the *Journal of Neuroscience* that, "*Recent studies have found that those who suffer from posttraumatic stress disorder (PTSD) are more likely to experience dementia as they age, most often Alzheimer's disease.* These findings suggest that the symptoms of PTSD might have an exacerbating effect on AD progression. AD and PTSD might also share common susceptibility factors such that those who experience trauma-induced disease were already more likely to succumb to dementia with age."[709]

In 2014, Dr. Machado and colleagues reviewed the scientific literature on the relationship between chronic stress and Alzheimer's disease. Without discussing the details of their analysis here, they concluded that, "*All these data support the idea that chronic stress could be considered a risk factor for AD.*"[710]

Suffice it to say, avoiding or decreasing chronic stress probably lowers the risk of Alzheimer's disease.

Dental Care

As previously discussed, poor dental care and periodontitis is associated with a higher risk of Alzheimer's disease. As such, it is common sense that maintaining optimal dental and gingival health will help minimize the risk of Alzheimer's disease.

Pets

In the October 2014 issue of the *Journal of Behavioral Medicine*, Drs. Polheber and Matchock reported the results of their experiment in which they examined the effects of social support on salivary cortisol (a stress hormone) and heart rate (HR). "Forty-eight participants were randomly assigned to three different conditions (human friend, novel dog, or control)...For participants paired with a dog, overall cortisol levels were attenuated throughout the experimental procedure, and HR was attenuated during the Trier Social Stress Test... *"These results suggest that short-term exposure to a novel dog in an unfamiliar setting can be beneficial."*[711]

Religion

Midlife habits may be important for the later development of Alzheimer's disease. To further evaluate this relationship, with regard to religious practices, researchers conducted a door-to-door survey. Praying was assessed by the number of monthly praying hours at midlife. Seven hundred seventy-eight individuals [normal controls (n=448), AD (n=92) and MCI (n=238)] were included in the study. The researchers found that, "A higher proportion of cognitively normal individuals engaged in prayer at midlife [(87 percent) versus MCI (71 percent) or AD (69 percent)]. Since 94 percent of males engaged in prayer, the effect on cognitive decline could not be assessed in men. Among women, stepwise logistic regression adjusted for age and education, showed that prayer was significantly associated with reduced risk of MCI but not AD. *Among individuals endorsing prayer activity, the amount of prayer was not associated with MCI or AD in either gender. Praying at midlife is associated with lower risk of mild cognitive impairment in women.*"[712]

Dr. Norton and colleagues, from the Department of Family Consumer and Human Development, Utah State University, Logan, Utah, as well as thirty-three collaborators from Cache County, reported the results of their study in the March 2012 issue of the *Journal of the American Geriatrics Society*. They wanted to identify distinct behavioral patterns of diet, exercise, social interaction, church attendance, alcohol consumption, and smoking and to examine their association with subsequent dementia risk. They included 2,491 participants without dementia (51 percent male, average age 73.0 ± 5,7; average education 13.7 ± 4.1 years) who initially reported no problems in activities of daily living and no stroke or head injury within the past five years. "Six dichotomized lifestyle behaviors were examined (diet: high ≥ median on the Dietary Approaches to Stop Hypertension scale; exercise: ≥5 h/wk of light activity and at least occasional moderate to vigorous activity; church attendance: attending church services at least weekly; social Interaction: spending time with family and friends at least twice weekly; alcohol: currently drinking alcoholic beverages ≥ 2 times/wk; non-smoker: no current use or fewer than 100 cigarettes ever)...Follow-up averaged 6.3 ± 5.3 years, during which 278 cases of incident dementia (200 Alzheimer's disease) were diagnosed. Four distinct lifestyle classes were identified. Unhealthy-religious (UH-R; 11.5 percent), unhealthy-nonreligious (UH-NR; 10.5 percent), healthy-moderately religious (H-MR; 38.5 percent), and healthy-very religious (H-VR; 39.5 percent). *UH-NR, H-MR, and H-VR had significantly lower dementia risk than UH-R*. Results were comparable for AD, except that UH-NR was less definitive. Functionally independent older adults appear to cluster into subpopulations with distinct patterns of lifestyle behaviors with different levels of risk for subsequent dementia and AD."[713]

Sleep

Making memories occurs through a three step process, which can be enhanced by sleep. The three steps are as follows: 1) acquisition, which is the process of storage and retrieval of new information in memory; 2) consolidation, and 3) recall. Sleep does not affect acquisition or recall while one is awake. Therefore, sleep has the greatest effect on memory consolidation. During sleep, the neural connections in the brain are strengthened. This enhances the brain's abilities to stabilize and retain memories. There have been several studies which show that sleep improves the retention of memory, as memories are enhanced through active consolidation. When you are sleeping, the hippocampus replays the events of the day for the neocortex. The neocortex then reviews and processes memories, which moves them into long term memory. When you do not get enough sleep it makes it more difficult to learn, as these neural connections are not as strong, resulting in a lower retention rate of memories. Sleep deprivation makes it harder to focus, resulting in inefficient learning. One of the primary functions of sleep is thought to be the improvement of the consolidation of information, as several studies have demonstrated that memory depends on getting sufficient sleep between training and test.

Dr. Liguori, from the Neurophysiopathology Unit, Sleep Medicine Centre, Department of Systems Medicine, University of Rome Tor Vergata, Rome, Italy, and colleagues, reported the results of their research on sleep in the December 1, 2014 issue of the Journal *JAMA Neurology*.

According to the researchers, "*Nocturnal sleep disruption develops in Alzheimer disease owing to the derangement of the sleep-wake cycle regulation pathways*. Orexin[1] contributes to the regulation of the sleep-wake cycle by increasing arousal levels and maintaining wakefulness." The researchers studied forty-eight individuals, "To study cerebrospinal fluid (CSF) levels of orexin in patients with AD, to evaluate the relationship of orexin cerebrospinal fluid levels with the degree of dementia and the cerebrospinal fluid AD biomarkers (tau proteins and β-amyloid 1-42), and to analyze potentially related sleep architecture changes measured by polysomnography...*Our results demonstrate that, in AD, increased cerebrospinal fluid orexin levels are related to a parallel sleep deterioration, which appears to be associated with cognitive decline*. Therefore, *the orexinergic system seems to be dysregulated in AD, and its output and function appear to be overexpressed along the progression of the neurodegenerative process*. This overexpression may result from an imbalance of the neurotransmitter networks regulating the wake-sleep cycle toward the orexinergic system promoting wakefulness."[714]

---

[1]Orexin, also called hypocretin, is a neurotransmitter that regulates arousal, wakefulness, and appetite. The most common form of narcolepsy, in which the sufferer briefly loses muscle tone (cataplexy), is caused by a lack of orexin in the brain due to destruction of the cells that produce it.

As an interesting aside, according to an article published December 22, 2014:[715]

> "Planning to read in bed tonight? It may be better to read an actual book instead of an e-book reader. A small study has found that reading light-emitting electronic devices before bedtime is a recipe for poor sleep.
>
> Researchers randomly assigned twelve healthy young adults to one of two activities: reading a light-emitting e-book in a dimly lit room for about four hours before bedtime on five consecutive evenings, or reading a printed book for the same amount of time. All participants did both tasks.
>
> The researchers took blood samples to measure melatonin levels, and electronically tracked how long it took to fall asleep and how much time was spent in each sleep stage. The study, done at Brigham and Women's Hospital in Boston, is online in the Proceedings of the National Academy of Sciences.
>
> *Compared with a printed book, a light-emitting e-book decreased sleepiness, reduced REM sleep (often called dream sleep), and substantially suppressed the normal bedtime rise of melatonin, the hormone that regulates the sleep and wake cycle. The e-book users took longer to fall asleep and felt sleepier in the morning.*"

Social Relations

In December 2014, researchers reported the findings of their study of elderly patients (n = 2,300, with a mean age of 82.45 years), where they examined the relationship between social support, physical activity, depression, and Alzheimer's disease. The researchers found that, "Higher depressive symptoms and lower cognitive and physical activity were associated with an increased risk of subsequent all-cause dementia and Alzheimer's dementia. While neither social engagement nor the general social support scale was associated with subsequent dementia, a higher level of social integration was associated with a lower dementia risk. In combined models, the results for activity variables remained similar, but the strength of the association between depressive symptoms and the subsequent risk of dementia decreased, and the association with social integration disappeared. Depressive symptoms increased and activity variables decreased the risk of subsequent dementia; however, activity variables, namely cognitive and physical activity, partly mediated the effect of depressive symptoms on the subsequent risk of all-cause dementia and AD. *In many cases, social support was not associated with a risk of subsequent dementia.*"[716]

Researchers followed 2,089 individuals for up to fifteen years in order to study the association between several social network variables and quality of relationships with the risk of dementia and Alzheimer's disease. During the study, 461 individuals developed dementia (373 Alzheimer's disease cases). The researchers found that, *"Participants who felt satisfied with their relations had a 23 percent reduced dementia risk. Participants who reported that they received more support than they gave over their lifetime had a 55 percent and 53 percent reduced risk for dementia and Alzheimer's disease, respectively. The only variables associated with subsequent dementia or Alzheimer's disease were those reflecting the quality of relationships."*[717]

CHAPER TEN:
LONGEVITY

Introduction

NOTE: Many of the supplements, vitamins, medications, and other lifestyle factors (such as exercise) previously discussed help improve health and extend life, by their very nature. This chapter goes even further in discussing specific research on extending life.

Life expectancy at birth in the United States was at an all-time high of 78.8 years in 2012, with much of the improvement attributed to reductions in death rates from major causes of death, such as heart disease, cancer, stroke, and chronic lower respiratory tract diseases, according to a report released in October 2014 from the Centers for Disease Control and Prevention (CDC).[718]

Life expectancy was higher for women (81.2 years) than for men (76.4 years).

Few scientific topics are as compelling as the field of aging, and when it comes to brain aging, few research areas are better funded. For example, although heart disease is America's No. 1 killer, that field will receive an estimated $1.2 billion in federal research funding. The field of aging alone will receive $2.5 billion, more than twice that amount. Perhaps as part of our survival instinct, many are seeking a scientific fountain of youth.

Life expectancies at birth have increased for males and females in the more developed economies across the 20th century. The 21st century is expected to see this development continue with life expectancies moving toward 100 years.[719]

LONGEVITY

Once a backwater in medical sciences, aging research has emerged and now threatens to take the forefront. This dramatic change of stature is driven from three major events. First and foremost, the world is rapidly getting old. Never before have we lived in a demographic environment like today, and the trends will continue such that 20 percent of the global population of 9 billion will be over the age of sixty by 2050. A second major driver on the rise is the dramatic progress that aging research has made using invertebrate models such as worms, flies, and yeast. Genetic approaches using these organisms have led to hundreds of aging genes and, perhaps surprisingly, strong evidence of evolutionary conservation among longevity pathways between disparate species, including mammals. Current studies suggest that this conservation may extend to humans. Finally, *"...small molecules such as rapamycin and resveratrol have been identified that slow aging in model organisms, although only rapamycin to date impacts longevity in mice. The potential now exists to delay human aging, whether it is through known classes of small molecules or a plethora of emerging ones."*[720]

Aging and longevity are unquestioningly complex. Several thoughts and mechanisms of aging, such as pathways involved in oxidative stress, lipid and glucose metabolism, inflammation, DNA damage and repair, growth hormone axis and insulin-like growth factor (GH/IGF), and environmental exposure have been proposed. *To date, the most promising leads for longevity are caloric restriction, particularly target of rapamycin (TOR), sirtuins, hexarelin and hormetic responses.*[721]

The following is from an article published February 2014, entitled, How Silicon Valley is trying to cure aging:[722]

> "Death has always been considered one of life's only real certainties, but now some of the world's top scientists are challenging the assumption. Scientists believe that aging is simply a medical problem for which a solution can be found
>
> Humanity has long been in search of the mythical Fountain of Youth, from Alexander the Great to knights of

the Crusades. But now Silicon Valley scientists believe they are on the cusp of discovering the cause of aging, which will help them achieve the unthinkable: find a cure.

Earlier this year, doctor and investor Joon Yun launched the Palo Alto Longevity Prize, offering $1 million (£650,000) to anyone who could "hack the code of life" and come up with a way to keep us young.

"It's always been said that there's two certainties in life: death and taxation, but death isn't looking so certain anymore," says Stuart Kim, one of fifty world-class advisers on the prize board and a professor in Developmental Biology and Genetics at Stanford University. He believes aging is simply a medical problem for which a solution can be found. The prize will be awarded to the first team to unlock what many believe to be the secret to aging: homeostatic capacity, or the ability of the body's systems to stabilize in response to stressors.

Scientists could effectively slow down the body's clock and enable us to remain middle aged for fifty years or more, meaning we can feel fifty when we are really eighty. The future could see us not just living longer, but staying healthier for longer.

The first half of the prize will be awarded next year to the team that can restore the homeostatic capacity of an aging adult mammal to that of a young one, thereby reversing the effects of aging. The second half to the team that can then extend the lifespan of their chosen mammal by 50 percent of published norms. So far fifteen teams have entered, including a handful from Stanford University as well as from further afield at the genetics department at George Washington University in D.C. and the Albert Einstein College of Medicine, New York.

But they face even fiercer competition outside the prize. Google recently unveiled its own $1.2 billion research centre Calico, or the California Life Company, aiming to achieve the tech giant's boldest ambition yet – extend the human lifespan.

While their work, which is led by Arthur Levinson, former CEO of biotech firm Genentech, is shrouded in secrecy, *they are said to be focusing on developing drugs for age-related neurodegenerative disorders [like Alzheimer's disease].*

Meanwhile, Craig Venter, the geneticist who sequenced the first human genome, has set up his own company, Human Longevity Inc., alongside stem cell pioneer Robert Hariri. They plan to sequence one million human genomes, including those of several supercentenarians, in order to build the world's largest database of human genetic variation. By looking at the DNA, they hope to discover a common feature among those living longer.

Dr. de Grey, a British gerontologist at the SENS Foundation in Silicon Valley, has dedicated his life's work to solving the perennial problem of death. He believes it should be treated as a disease and can be postponed indefinitely.

The idea of reverse-engineering aging is not a new one. The American Academy of Anti-Aging Medicine was set up in 1992, but only recently has the idea gained traction in mainstream medicine.

Life-extending technology has become a booming industry in Silicon Valley. Google X and Proteus Digital Health are among a dozen or so companies working on "ingestible tech" that they hope will go some way toward keeping us alive and healthy for longer. Google's pill, which is filled with tiny iron-oxide nanoparticles that enter the bloodstream, is able to identify cancer tumor cells, which give off early biochemical signals when they contract the disease. Proteus, having already gained FDA approval, is now in talks with Britain's National Health Service about the possible use of its sensor pill, which sends biological information it retrieves from the body to a smartphone.

At the same time, the XPrize Foundation, a charity that runs technology competitions, is working on developing a hand-held all-in-one diagnostic device. With one drop of blood, the "tricorder" will be able to accurately detect conditions such as diabetes and tuberculosis as well as measuring blood pressure and temperature – all from the comfort of your home. Grant Campany, director of the XPrize, told The Sunday Telegraph: "It will all but eradicate the need to see a doctor for check-ups. The device will help people take their health back into their own hands."

The Longevity Prize's Dr Kim, who has spent the last ten years looking into the causes of aging, believes we cannot afford not to come up with a solution. *"We shouldn't just be thinking of how to treat diseases like cancer [and Alzheimer's disease], we should be looking at how to prevent* them by figuring out why old people are much more likely to get them," he says. "If you could take 80-year-olds and make them biologically more like 60-year-olds, that's a 15-fold decrease in the rate of cancer right there."

Definition of Aging

Aging is the process of becoming older. It represents the accumulation of changes in a person over time. In humans, aging refers to a multidimensional process of physical, psychological, and social change. Reaction time, for example, may slow with age, while knowledge of world events and wisdom may expand. Aging is an important part of all human societies reflecting the biological changes that occur, but also reflecting cultural and societal conventions. Aging is among the largest known risk factors for most human diseases.

According to a recent article, "Biological aging means a time-dependent accumulation of changes to which a living organism is being exposed during its lifetime. Biological aging normally concurs with chronological aging, the time frame of which is set by an upper limit, the lifespan (in humans approximately 120 years). New findings in experimental biogerontology are challenging both the dogma of irreversibility of biological aging and the preset species-specific limitations of life."[723]

According to Dr. Rattan, from the Laboratory of Cellular Aging, Department of Molecular Biology and Genetics, Aarhus University, Denmark, reporting in the June 1, 2014 issue of *Aging and Disease*, "Although aging is the common cause of all age-related diseases, aging in itself cannot be considered a disease…*Age-induced health problems, for which there are no other clear-cut causative agents, may be better tackled by focusing on health mechanisms and their maintenance, rather than only disease management and treatment. Continuing the disease-oriented research and treatment approaches, as opposed to health-oriented and preventive strategies, are economically, socially and psychologically unsustainable.*"[724]

What is successful aging? Dr. Marin and colleagues discussed the answer to this question in the May 18, 2014 issue of the journal *Gerontologist*. They stated, "Everyone wants to age successfully; however, *the definition and criteria of successful aging remain vague for laypersons, researchers, and policymakers in spite of decades of research on the topic*…Additional views on successful aging emphasize subjective versus objective perceptions of successful aging and relate successful aging to studies on healthy and exceptional longevity. Additional theoretical work is needed to better understand successful aging, including the way it can encompass disability and death and dying. The extent of rapid social and technological change influencing views on successful aging also deserves more consideration."[725]

Dr. de Cabo, from the Translational Gerontology Branch, National Institute on Aging, National Institutes of Health, Baltimore, Maryland, and colleagues, reported in the June 19, 2014 issue of the journal *Cell*, *"Recent evidence is shaping a picture where low caloric regimes and exercise may improve healthy senescence, and several pharmacological strategies have been suggested to counteract aging. Surprisingly, the most effective interventions proposed to date converge on only a few cellular processes, in particular nutrient signaling, mitochondrial efficiency, proteostasis[1], and autophagy[2]."*[726]

In September 2014, Dr. Allison and twenty-four colleagues, as part of a coordinated effort to expand research activity at the interface of aging and energetics, reported that, "A team of investigators at the University of Alabama at Birmingham systematically assayed and catalogued the top research priorities identified in leading publications in that domain, believing the result would be useful to the scientific community at large…Ten research categories were identified from the forty papers. These included: (1) *Calorie restriction (CR) longevity response, (2) role of mTOR (mechanistic target of Rapamycin) and related factors in*

---

[1]Proteostasis, a portmanteau of the words protein and homeostasis, is the concept that there are competing and integrated biological pathways within cells that control the biogenesis, folding, trafficking and degradation of proteins present within and outside the cell. The concept of proteostasis maintenance is central to understanding the cause of diseases associated with excessive protein misfolding and degradation leading to loss-of-function phenotypes, as well as aggregation-associated degenerative disorders. Therefore, adapting proteostasis should enable the restoration of proteostasis once its loss leads to pathology. Cellular proteostasis is key to ensuring successful development, healthy aging, resistance to environmental stresses, and to minimize homeostasis perturbations by pathogens such as viruses.
[2]Autophagy (or autophagocytosis) is the basic catabolic mechanism that involves cell degradation of unnecessary or dysfunctional cellular components through the actions of lysosomes. The breakdown of cellular components promotes cellular survival during starvation by maintaining cellular energy levels. Autophagy allows the degradation and recycling of cellular components.

lifespan extension, (3) nutrient effects beyond energy (especially resveratrol, omega-3 fatty acids, and selected amino acids), 4) autophagy and increased longevity and health, (5) aging-associated predictors of chronic disease, (6) use and effects of mesenchymal stem cells (MSCs), (7) telomeres relative to aging and energetics, (8) accretion and effects of body fat, (9) the aging heart, and (10) mitochondria, reactive oxygen species, and cellular energetics."[727]

Dr. Darzynkiewicz and colleagues, from the Brander Cancer Research Institute and Department of Pathology, New York Medical College, Valhalla, New York, published the results of their review in the May 2014 issue of *Cytometry Part A*, on the mechanisms of aging. This is a very technical article and the details won't be presented here. The authors did note, among other findings, that, "Outlined are critical sites along these pathways, including autophagy, as targets for potential antiaging (gero-suppressive) and/or chemopreventive agents… to monitor activation along these pathways in response to the reported antiaging drugs rapamycin, metformin, berberine, resveratrol, vitamin D3, 2-deoxyglucose, and acetylsalicylic acid [Aspirin]. Specifically, effectiveness of these agents to attenuate the level of constitutive mTOR signaling was tested…"[728]

Definition of Longevity

The word "longevity" is sometimes used as a synonym for "life expectancy" in demography - however, the term "longevity" is sometimes meant to refer only to especially long-lived members of a population, whereas "life expectancy" is always defined statistically as the average number of years remaining at a given age. For example, a population's life expectancy at birth is the same as the average age at death for all people born in the same year (in the case of cohorts). *Longevity is best thought of as a term for general audiences meaning 'typical length of life'* and specific statistical definitions should be clarified when necessary.

Well known things that limit longevity, such as war, smoking, excessive drinking, use of illicit drugs, poverty, lack of healthcare, and so forth are self evident and won't be discussed here. Some less well known factors that impact longevity, such as early life experiences, will be discussed, but the focus of this section will be on things that adults can do to improve their chances of living longer.

There are many books and a great deal of scientific research devoted to this topic. We focus on current research (and will, of course, be updating this with each new edition of this book). This is an extremely exciting area. Regardless of this fact, there seems to be a very large gap between basic scientific research and common knowledge, let alone translating scientific discoveries into daily practice. Change is difficult for most of us, and the fact is no different in this area.

Theories of Aging

By way of introduction, Dr. Longo and colleagues, from the Davis School of Gerontology and Department of Biological Sciences, Longevity Institute, University of Southern California, Los Angeles, CA, published their consensus findings from a conference on aging, held in Italy, in the April 22, 2015 issue of the journal *Aging Cell*:[729]

> "The workshop entitled 'Interventions to Slow Aging in Humans: Are We Ready?' was held to bring together leading experts in the biology and genetics of aging and obtain a consensus related to the discovery and development of safe interventions to slow aging and increase healthy lifespan in humans.
>
> *There was consensus that there is sufficient evidence that aging interventions will delay and prevent disease onset for many chronic conditions of adult and old age.*
>
> Essential pathways have been identified, and behavioral, dietary, and pharmacologic approaches have emerged. Although many gene targets and drugs were discussed

and there was not complete consensus about all interventions, the participants selected a subset of the most promising strategies that could be tested in humans for their effects on healthspan. These were: (i) dietary interventions mimicking chronic dietary restriction (periodic fasting mimicking diets, protein restriction, etc.); (ii) drugs that inhibit the growth hormone/IGF-I axis; (iii) drugs that inhibit the mTOR-S6K pathway; or (iv) drugs that activate AMPK or specific sirtuins. These choices were based in part on consistent evidence for the pro-longevity effects and ability of these interventions to prevent or delay multiple age-related diseases and improve healthspan in simple model organisms and rodents and their potential to be safe and effective in extending human healthspan. The authors of this manuscript were speakers and discussants invited to the workshop."

Caloric Restriction

Caloric restriction (CR) or dietary restriction (DR), is a dietary regimen that is based on low calorie intake. "Low" can be defined relative to the subject's previous intake before intentionally restricting calories, or relative to an average person of similar body type. Calorie restriction without malnutrition has been shown to work in a variety of species, among them yeast, fish, rodents and dogs to decelerate the biological aging process, resulting in longer maintenance of youthful health and an increase in both median and maximum lifespan. The life-extending effect of calorie restriction is not universal. Wild mice, for instance, do not live longer when on a calorie restricted diet.

According to Dr. Selman, from the Institute of Biodiversity, Animal Health and Comparative Medicine, College of Medicine, Veterinary and Life Sciences, University of Glasgow, UK, reporting in the May 2014 issue of the journal *Proceedings of The Nutrition Society* stated, "Dietary restriction (DR) has been shown to extend both median and maximum lifespan in a range of animals, although recent findings suggest that these effects are not universally enjoyed across all animals. In particular, the lifespan effect following DR in mice is highly strain-specific and there is little current evidence that DR induces a positive effect on all-cause mortality in non-human primates. However, *the positive effects of DR on health appear to be highly conserved across the vast majority of species, including human subjects. Despite these effects on health, it is highly unlikely that DR will become a realistic or popular life choice for most human subjects given the level of restraint required. Consequently significant research is focusing on identifying compounds that will bestow the benefits of DR without the obligation to adhere to stringent reductions in daily food intake. Several such compounds, including rapamycin, metformin and resveratrol, have been identified as potential DR mimetics[1]*."[730]

In 2014, another group of researchers noted the following, "Calorie restriction (CR) with adequate nutrition is the only non-genetic, and the most consistent non-pharmacological intervention that extends lifespan in model organisms from yeast to mammals, and protects against the deterioration of biological functions, delaying or reducing the risk of many age-related diseases. However, most people would not comply with such a rigorous dietary program; research is thus increasingly aimed at determining the feasibility and efficacy of natural and/or pharmacological CR mimetic molecules/ treatments without lowering food intake, particularly in mid- to late-life periods. *Likely candidates act on the same signaling pathways as CR, and include resveratrol and other polyphenols, rapamycin, 2-deoxy-D-glucose and other glycolytic inhibitors, insulin pathway and AMP-activated protein kinase activators, autophagy stimulators, alpha-lipoic acid, and other antioxidants.*"[731]

Dr. Martin and colleagues, reporting in the journal *Current Medicinal Chemistry*, state the following:[732]

> "The pronounced effects of the epigenetic diet (ED) [previously discussed] and caloric restriction (CR) have

---

[1]Mimetic: Of or relating to an imitation; imitative.

on epigenetic gene regulation have been documented in many pre-clinical and clinical studies. *Understanding epigenetics is of high importance because of the concept that external factors such as nutrition and diet may possess the ability to alter gene expression without modifying the DNA sequence. The ED introduces bioactive medicinal chemistry compounds such as sulforaphane[1] (SFN), curcumin (CCM), epigallocatechin gallate (EGCG) and resveratrol (RSV) that are thought to aid in extending the human lifespan.* CR, although similar to ED in the target of longevity, mildly reduces the total daily calorie intake while concurrently providing all beneficial nutrients. Both CR and ED may act as epigenetic modifiers to slow the aging process through histone modification, DNA methylation, and by modulating microRNA expression. *CR and ED have been proposed as two important mechanisms that modulate and potentially slow the progression of age-related diseases such as cardiovascular disease (CVD), cancer, obesity, Alzheimer's and osteoporosis to name a few."*

Dr. Wang, in the October 2014 issue of *Diabetes & Metabolism Journal*, commented on the life-extending mechanism of caloric restriction, stating, "Although it has been known for more than 80 years that calorie restriction increases lifespan, a mechanistic understanding of this phenomenon remains elusive. Yeast silent information regulator 2 (Sir2), the founding member of the sirtuin family of protein deacetylases [enzymes], and its mammalian homologue Sir2-like protein 1 (SIRT1), have been suggested to promote survival and longevity of organisms. *SIRT1 exerts protective effects against a number of age-associated disorders. Caloric restriction increases both Sir2 and SIRT1 activity.*"[733]

---

[1]Sulforaphane is a molecule within the isothiocyanate group of organosulfur compounds. It is obtained from cruciferous vegetables such as broccoli, Brussels sprouts or cabbages..

Dr. Mirzaei and colleagues, from the Longevity Institute and Davis School of Gerontology, University of Southern California, Los Angeles, CA, commented in the November 2014 issue of the journal *Trends in Endocrinology & Metabolism*, *"Many of the effects of dietary restriction (DR) on longevity and health span in model organisms have been linked to reduced protein and amino acid (AA) intake and the stimulation of specific nutrient signaling pathways. Studies in yeast have shown that addition of serine, threonine, and valine in media promotes cellular sensitization and aging by activating different but connected pathways. Protein or essential AA restriction extends both lifespan and healthspan in rodent models. In humans, protein restriction (PR) has been associated with reduced cancer, diabetes, and overall mortality. Thus, interventions aimed at lowering the intake of proteins or specific AAs can be beneficial and have the potential to be widely adopted and effective in optimizing healthspan."* [734]

In 2014, one researcher discusses the conflicting data about weight and longevity, stating, "Normal BMI [body mass index] ranges from 18.5 to 24.9; many epidemiological studies show an inverse relationship between mortality and BMI inside the normal BMI range. Other studies show that the lowest mortality in the entire range of BMI is obtained in the overweight range (25-29.9). Reconciling the extension of life span in laboratory animals by experimental CR with the BMI-mortality curve of human epidemiology is not trivial. In fact, one interpretation is that the CR data are identifying a known: *"excess fat is deleterious for health;"* although a second interpretation may be that: *"additional leanness from a normal body weight may add health and life span, delaying the process of aging."*[735]

Another group of researchers note the following:[736]

> "During aging there is an increasing imbalance of energy intake and expenditure resulting in obesity, frailty, and metabolic disorders. For decades, research has shown that caloric restriction (CR) and exercise can postpone detrimental aspects of aging. These two interventions invoke a similar physiological signature involving pathways asso-

ciated with stress responses and mitochondrial homeostasis. Nonetheless, *CR is able to delay aging processes that result in an increase of both mean and maximum lifespan, whereas exercise primarily increases healthspan.* Due to the strict dietary regime necessary to achieve the beneficial effects of CR, most studies to date have focused on rodents and non-human primates. As a consequence, *there is vast interest in the development of compounds such as resveratrol, metformin and rapamycin that would activate the same metabolic- and stress-response pathways induced by these interventions without actually restricting caloric intake."*

Exercise

Dr. Avin and colleagues, from the Department of Physical Medicine and Rehabilitation, University of Pittsburgh Pittsburgh, PA, USA; Division of Geriatric Medicine, Department of Medicine, University of Pittsburgh PA, USA, reported in the June 17, 2014 issue of the journal *Frontiers in Physiology* that:[737]

"Klotho is a powerful longevity protein that has been linked to the prevention of muscle atrophy, osteopenia, and cardiovascular disease. Similar anti-aging effects have also been ascribed to exercise and physical activity... Our pilot clinical findings performed in young and aged individuals suggest that *circulating Klotho levels are upregulated in response to an acute exercise bout, but that the response may be dependent on fitness level. A similar upregulation of circulating Klotho is also observed in response to an acute exercise in young and old mice,* suggesting that this may be a good model for mechanistically probing the role of physical activity on Klotho expression...It is hoped that this review will stimulate further consideration of the relationship between skeletal muscle activity and Klotho expression,

potentially leading to important insights into *the well-documented systemic anti-aging effects of exercise.*"

In another very interesting and important article, Dr. Zhang and colleagues, reported in the April 22, 2015 issue of the *International Journal of Sports Medicine*:[738]

> "*Physical fitness has been reported to decrease the risk of lifestyle-related diseases. The present study evaluated genome-wide methylation under the hypothesis that interval walking training (IWT) imparted beneficial effects on health, particularly by epigenetically ameliorating susceptibility to inflammation…we found the NFκB2 [nuclear factor kappa beta] gene to have increased methylation in multiple regions of its promoter sequence following participation in an exercise regimen…The increase in NFκB2 gene promoter methylation by IWT indicates that this regimen may suppress pro-inflammatory cytokines[1]. Thus, these results provide an additional line of evidence that IWT is advantageous in promoting health from an epigenetic perspective by ameliorating susceptibility to inflammation.*"

Free Radical Theory of Aging

In a very interesting, long, and comprehensive analysis of the free radical theory of aging, Dr. Sadowska-Bartosz and colleagues, in 2014 reviewed the effects of numerous antioxidants. It is a free article well worth reading. The authors note, "If aging is due to or contributed by free radical reactions, as postulated by the free radical theory of aging,

---

[1] *Cytokines* are a broad and loose category of small proteins that are important in cell signaling. They are released by cells and affect the behavior of other cells, and sometimes the releasing cell itself. Cytokines include chemokines, interferons, interleukins, lymphokines, tumor necrosis factor but generally not hormones or growth factors (despite some terminologic overlap). Cytokines are produced by a broad range of cells, including immune cells like macrophages, B lymphocytes, T lymphocytes and mast cells, as well as endothelial cells, fibroblasts, and various stromal cells.

lifespan of organisms should be extended by administration of exogenous antioxidants. *This paper reviews data on model organisms concerning the effects of exogenous antioxidants (antioxidant vitamins, lipoic acid, coenzyme Q, melatonin, resveratrol, curcumin, other polyphenols, and synthetic antioxidants including antioxidant nanoparticles) on the lifespan of model organisms.* Mechanisms of effects of antioxidants, often due to indirect antioxidant action or to action not related to the antioxidant properties of the compounds administered, are discussed. The legitimacy of antioxidant supplementation in humans is considered."[739]

Dr. Strong and colleagues report that, "The National Institute on Aging Interventions Testing Program (ITP) was established to evaluate agents that are hypothesized to increase life span and/or health span in genetically heterogeneous mice. It is the goal of the ITP to publish all results, negative or positive. We report here on the results of lifelong treatment of mice, beginning at four months of age, with each of five agents, that is, green tea extract (GTE), curcumin, oxaloacetic acid, medium-chain triglyceride oil, and resveratrol, on the life span of genetically heterogeneous mice. Each agent was administered beginning at four months of age. *None of these five agents had a statistically significant effect on life span of male or female mice, by log-rank test, at the concentrations tested, although a secondary analysis suggested that GTE might diminish the risk of midlife deaths in females only.*"[740]

Genetics

A group of researchers, led by Dr. Garagnani, reported in 2014 in the journal *BioMed Research International*, that the genetics of human longevity consists of the nuclear genome (nDNA), mitochondrial DNA (mtDNA), and gut microbiota (GM). They stated that, "we have to add another level of complexity represented by the microbiota, that is, the whole set of bacteria present in the different parts of our body with their whole set of genes. In particular, *several studies investigated the role of gut microbiota (GM) modifications in aging and longevity and an age-related GM signature was found*. In this view, *human beings*

ALZHEIMER'S DISEASE

must be considered as "metaorganism" and a more holistic approach is necessary to grasp the complex dynamics of the interaction between the environment and nDNA-mtDNA-GM of the host during aging."[741]

In a complicated but very interesting and important study of longevity, Dr. Jylhava and colleagues, reporting in the September 11, 2014 issue of *BMC Medical Genomics*, stated the following:[742]

> "Prediction models for old-age mortality have generally relied upon conventional markers such as plasma-based factors and biophysiological characteristics. However, it is unknown whether the existing markers are able to provide the most relevant information in terms of old-age survival or whether predictions could be improved through the integration of whole-genome expression profiles. We assessed the predictive abilities of survival models containing only conventional markers, only gene expression data or both types of data together in a Vitality 90+ study cohort consisting of n = 151 nonagenarians. The all-cause death rate was 32.5 percent (49 of 151 individuals), and the median follow-up time was 2.55 years...
>
> The multivariate Cox regression model was used to adjust for the conventional mortality prediction markers, i.e., the body mass index, frailty index and cell-free DNA level, *revealing that 331 transcripts[1] were independently associated with survival. The final mortality-predicting transcriptomic signature derived from the Ridge regression model was mapped to a network that identified nuclear factor kappa beta (NF-κB) as a central node. Together with the loss of physiological reserves, the transcriptomic predictors centered around NF-κB underscored the role of immunoinflammatory*

---

[1] A transcription unit is a linear sequence of DNA that extends from a transcription start site to a transcription stop site.

signaling, the control of the DNA damage response and cell cycle, and mitochondrial functions as the key determinants of old-age mortality."

Immunological Theory of Aging

In 2014, in the journal *Interdisciplinary Topics in Gerontology and Geriatrics*, Dr. Fulop and colleagues, from the Research Center on Aging, University of Sherbrooke, Sherbrooke, Que., Canada, note the following:[743]

> "Aging is a complex phenomenon the cause of which is not fully understood, despite the plethora of theories proposed to explain it. As we age, changes in essentially all physiological functions, including immunity, are apparent. Immune responses decrease with aging, contributing to the increased incidence of different chronic diseases with an inflammatory component (sometimes referred to as 'inflamm-aging'). It is clear from many studies that human longevity may be influenced by these changes in the immune system, but how they proceed is not clearly determined…*Many data in humans support the notion that age-associated immune dysfunction may at least in part explain the aging process. Explanatory power may be enhanced by combination with other theories such as the free radical theory."*

And, from Drs. Bravo-San Pedro and Senovilla, reporting in the journal *Aging* (Albany NY):[744]

> "During the past two decades, several interventions have been shown to increase the healthy lifespan of model organisms as evolutionarily distant from each other as yeast, worms, flies and mammals. These anti-aging maneuvers include (but are not limited to) cycles of caloric restriction, physical exercise as well as the administra-

tion of multiple, chemically unrelated agents, such as resveratrol, spermidine and various rapamycin-like compounds collectively known as rapalogs. Most, if not all, lifespan-extending agents promote macroautophagy (hereafter referred to as autophagy[1]), an evolutionarily old mechanism that contributes to the maintenance of intracellular homeostasis and plays a critical role in the adaptive response of cells to stress.

In line with this notion, *the activation of autophagy appears to mediate significant anti-aging effects in several organisms*, including mice. *Here, we focus on rapalogs to discuss the possibility that part of the beneficial activity of lifespan-extending agents stems from their ability to exert immunostimulatory effects. Accumulating evidence indicates indeed that the immune system can recognize and eliminate not only cells that are prone to undergo malignant transformation, but also senescent cells, thus playing a significant role in the control of organismal aging. In addition, it has recently become clear that rapamycin and other rapalogs, which for a long time have been viewed (and used in the clinic) as pure immunosuppressants, can mediate robust immunostimulatory functions, at least in some circumstances."*

Klotho

Dr. Dubal, from the Gladstone Institute of Neurological Disease, San Francisco, California, and the Department of Neurology, University of California, San Francisco, California, and colleagues, reported the fol-

---

[1] Autophagy is the basic catabolic mechanism that involves cell degradation of unnecessary or dysfunctional cellular components through the actions of lysosomes. The breakdown of cellular components promotes cellular survival during starvation by maintaining cellular energy levels. Autophagy allows the degradation and recycling of cellular components.

lowing in the February 11, 2015 issue of *The Journal of Neuroscience*:[745]

> "Aging is the principal demographic risk factor for Alzheimer's disease, the most common neurodegenerative disorder. *Klotho is a key modulator of the aging process and, when overexpressed, extends mammalian lifespan, increases synaptic plasticity, and enhances cognition.* Whether klotho can counteract deficits related to neurodegenerative diseases, such as AD, is unknown. Here we show that elevating klotho expression decreases premature mortality and network dysfunction in human amyloid precursor protein (hAPP) transgenic mice, which simulate key aspects of AD. Increasing klotho levels prevented depletion of NMDA receptor (NMDAR) subunits in the hippocampus and enhanced spatial learning and memory in hAPP mice. Klotho elevation in hAPP mice increased the abundance of the GluN2B subunit of NMDAR in postsynaptic densities and NMDAR-dependent long-term potentiation, which is critical for learning and memory. *Thus, increasing wild-type klotho levels or activities improves synaptic and cognitive functions, and may be of therapeutic benefit in AD and other cognitive disorders.*"

Mitochondrial Theory of Aging

A new perspective on the mitochondrial theory of aging is provided by Dr. Shokolenko and colleagues, from the Inna N Shokolenko, Biomedical Sciences Department, Patt Capps Covey College of Allied Health Professions, University of South Alabama, Mobile, AL, in the November 20, 2014 issue of the *World Journal of Experimental Medicine*:[746]

> "The mitochondrial theory of aging, a mainstream theory of aging which once included accumulation of mitochondrial DNA (mtDNA) damage by reactive oxygen

species (ROS)[1] as its cornerstone, has been increasingly losing ground and is undergoing extensive revision due to its inability to explain a growing body of emerging data. Concurrently, the notion of the central role for mtDNA in the aging process is being met with increased skepticism. Our progress in understanding the processes of mtDNA maintenance, repair, damage, and degradation in response to damage has largely refuted the view of mtDNA as being particularly susceptible to ROS-mediated mutagenesis due to its lack of "protective" histones and reduced complement of available DNA repair pathways.

Recent research on mitochondrial ROS production has led to the appreciation that mitochondria, even in vitro, produce much less ROS than previously thought, automatically leading to a decreased expectation of physiologically achievable levels of mtDNA damage. New evidence suggests that both experimentally induced oxidative stress and radiation therapy result in very low levels of mtDNA mutagenesis. Recent advances provide evidence against the existence of the "vicious" cycle of mtDNA damage and ROS production. *Meta-studies reveal no longevity benefit of increased antioxidant defenses. Simultaneously, exciting new observations from both comparative biology and experimental systems indicate that increased ROS production and oxidative damage to cellular macromolecules, including mtDNA, can be associated with extended longevity. A novel paradigm suggests that increased ROS production in aging may be the result of adaptive signaling rather than a*

---

[1]Reactive oxygen species (ROS) are chemically reactive molecules containing oxygen. Examples include oxygen ions and peroxides. ROS are formed as a natural by-product of the normal metabolism of oxygen and have important roles in cell signaling and homeostasis. However, during times of environmental stress (e.g., UV or heat exposure), ROS levels can increase dramatically. This may result in significant damage to cell structures. Cumulatively, this is known as oxidative stress.

detrimental byproduct of normal [cellular] respiration that drives aging."

In another interesting analysis, Drs. Hill and Van Remmen, from the Free Radical Biology and Aging Research Program, Oklahoma Medical Research Foundation, Oklahoma City, OK, report in the July 27, 2014 issue of the journal *Redox Biology*, that, "…the role of mitochondrial stress signaling in longevity has been expansively studied. *Current and exciting studies provide evidence that mitochondria can also signal among tissues to up-regulate cytoprotective activities to promote healthy aging. Alternatively, mitochondria release signals to modulate innate immunity and systemic inflammatory responses and could consequently promote inflammation during aging.*"[747]

In the March 2015 issue of the journal, *Nature Cell Biology*, Drs. Riera and Dillin, from the Department of Molecular and Cell Biology, University of California, Berkeley, note that, "A hallmark of aging is dysfunction in nutrient signaling pathways that regulate glucose homeostasis, negatively affecting whole-body energy metabolism and ultimately increasing the organism's susceptibility to disease. *Maintenance of insulin sensitivity depends on functional mitochondrial networks, but is compromised by alterations in mitochondrial energy metabolism during aging.*"[748]

Sirtuins

Dr. Giblin, from the Department of Human Genetics, University of Michigan, Ann Arbor, MI, and colleagues briefly commented on sirtuins[1] in the July 2014 issue of the journal *Trends in Genetics*, noting that, "The first link between sirtuins and longevity was made fifteen years ago in yeast. These initial studies sparked efforts by many laboratories working in diverse model organisms to elucidate the relations

---

[1]Sirtuin are a class of enzymatic proteins. Sirtuins have been implicated in influencing a wide range of cellular processes like aging, transcription, apoptosis, inflammation and stress resistance, as well as energy efficiency and alertness during low-calorie situations. Sirtuins can also control circadian clocks and mitochondrial biogenesis.

between sirtuins, lifespan, and age-associated dysfunction. We focus primarily on mammalian sirtuins SIRT1, SIRT3, and SIRT6, the three sirtuins for which the most relevant data are available. *Strikingly, a large body of evidence now indicates that these and other mammalian sirtuins suppress a variety of age-related pathologies and promote healthspan. Moreover, increased expression of SIRT1 or SIRT6 extends mouse lifespan. Overall, these data point to important roles for sirtuins in promoting mammalian health, and perhaps in modulating the aging process.*"[749]

Drs. Sinclair and Guarente, from the Glenn Laboratories for the Biological Mechanisms of Aging, Department of Genetics, Harvard Medical School, Boston, Massachusetts, noted the following in 2014 in the journal *Annual Review of Pharmacology and Toxicology*, "The *mammalian sirtuins (SIRT1-7) play central roles in cell survival, inflammation, energy metabolism, and aging. Members of this family of enzymes are considered promising pharmaceutical targets for the treatment of age-related diseases including cancer, type 2 diabetes, inflammatory disorders, and Alzheimer's disease. SIRT1-activating compounds (STACs), which have been identified from a variety of chemical classes, provide health benefits in animal disease models...Compared with polyphenols such as resveratrol, the synthetic STACs show greater potency, solubility, and target selectivity.* Although considerable progress has been made regarding SIRT1 activation, key questions remain, including how the molecular contacts facilitate SIRT1 activation, whether other sirtuin family members will be amenable to activation, and whether STACs will ultimately prove safe and efficacious in humans."[750]

Dr. Chen and colleagues reported in 2015 that, "Sirtuins [sirtuin (SIRT)1-SIRT7] mediate the longevity-promoting effects of calorie restriction in yeast, worms, flies, and mice. Additionally, *SIRT3 is the only SIRT analog whose increased expression has been shown to be associated with longevity in humans. The polyphenol resveratrol (RSV) is the first compound discovered able to mimic calorie restriction by stimulating SIRTs.*"[751]

Telomere Length

Telomere length has been found to be associated with longevity. According to Dr. Rizvi and colleauges, reporting in the January 22, 2015 issue of the journal *Current Aging Science*:[752]

> "Telomeres are gene sequences present at chromosomal ends and are responsible for maintaining genome integrity. Telomere length is maximum at birth and decreases progressively with advancing age and thus is considered as a biomarker of chronological aging. *This age associated decrease in the length of telomere is linked to various ageing associated diseases like diabetes, hypertension, Alzheimer's disease, cancer etc. and their associated complications. Telomere length is a result of combined effect of oxidative stress, inflammation and repeated cell replication on it, and thus forming an association between telomere length and chronological aging and related diseases. Thus, decrease in telomere length was found to be important in determining both the variations in longevity and age-related diseases in an individual.*"

Dr. Ornish and colleagues from the Department of Medicine, University of California San Francisco, San Francisco, CA, USA; Preventive Medicine Research Institute, Sausalito, CA, noted that, "Telomere shortness in human beings is a prognostic marker of aging, disease, and premature morbidity." The researchers studied a group of men for five years. "Men in the intervention group followed a programme of comprehensive lifestyle changes (diet, activity, stress management, and social support), and the men in the control group underwent active surveillance alone. We took blood samples at five years and compared relative telomere length and telomerase enzymatic activity at baseline, and assessed their relation to the degree of lifestyle changes…*Our comprehensive lifestyle intervention was associated with increases in relative telomere length after five years of follow-up*, compared with controls, in this small pilot study. Larger randomized controlled trials are warranted to confirm this finding."[753]

In the March 5, 2015 issue of *Peer J*, Dr. Wang, from the Tropical Medicine Institute, Guangzhou University of Chinese Medicine, Guangzhou, China, and colleagues reported the following:[754]

> "Calorie restriction is known to extend lifespan among organisms by a mechanism underlying nitric oxide-driven mitochondrial biogenesis. We report here that *nitric oxide generators including artemisinin[1], sodium nitroprusside[2], and L-arginine[3] mimic calorie restriction* and resemble hydrogen peroxide to initiate the nitric oxide signaling cascades and elicit the global antioxidative responses in mice. The large quantities of antioxidant enzymes are correlated with the low levels of reactive oxygen species, which allow the down-regulation of tu-

---

[1]Artemisinin, also known as Qinghaosu (Chinese: 青蒿素), and its derivatives are a group of drugs that possess the most rapid action of all current drugs against Plasmodium falciparum malaria. The medicinal value of this plant has been known to the Chinese for at least 2,000 years.

[2]Sodium nitroprusside is an inorganic compound. This compound is used as a drug. In this role it is abbreviated SNP, and it has trade names like Nitropress. It acts as a drug by releasing nitric oxide; it belongs to the class of NO-releasing drugs as a result. This drug is used as a vasodilator to reduce blood pressure.

[3]*L-arginine:* In mammals, arginine is classified as a semi-essential or conditionally essential amino acid, depending on the developmental stage and health status of the individual. Preterm infants are unable to synthesize or create arginine internally, making the amino acid nutritionally essential for them. Most healthy people do not need to supplement with arginine because their body produces sufficient amounts. Arginine is found in a wide variety of foods, including: Animal sources: dairy products (e.g., cottage cheese, ricotta, milk, yogurt, whey protein drinks), beef, pork (e.g., bacon, ham), gelatin, poultry (e.g. chicken and turkey light meat), wild game (e.g. pheasant, quail), seafood (e.g., halibut, lobster, salmon, shrimp, snails, tuna); Plant sources: wheat germ and flour, lupins, buckwheat, granola, oatmeal, peanuts, nuts (coconut, pecans, cashews, walnuts, almonds, Brazil nuts, hazelnuts, peanuts), seeds (pumpkin, sesame, sunflower), chickpeas, cooked soybeans, *Phalaris canariensis* (canaryseed or alpiste).

mor suppressors and accessory DNA repair partners, *eventually leading to the compromise of telomere shortening.* Accompanying with the up-regulation of signal transducers and respiratory chain signatures, mitochondrial biogenesis occurs with the elevation of adenosine triphosphate levels upon exposure of mouse skeletal muscles to the mimetics of calorie restriction. *In conclusion, calorie restriction-triggered nitric oxide provides antioxidative protection and alleviates telomere attrition via mitochondrial biogenesis, thereby maintaining chromosomal stability and integrity, which are the hallmarks of longevity."*

Reporting in the December 2, 2014 issue of the *British Medical Journal*, Dr. Crous-Bou, from the Channing Division of Network Medicine, Department of Medicine, Brigham and Women's Hospital and Harvard Medical School, Boston, MA 02115, USA Department of Epidemiology, Program in Genetic Epidemiology and Statistical Genetics, Harvard School of Public Health, Boston, MA, and colleagues conducted a study to examine whether adherence to the Mediterranean diet was associated with longer telomere length, a biomarker of aging. They examined the results of blood tests from 4,676 disease-free women, a subset of women within the Nurses' Health Study. They found that, *"In this large study, greater adherence to the Mediterranean diet was associated with longer telomeres. These results further support the benefits of adherence to the Mediterranean diet for promoting health and longevity."*[755]

Things That Predict Longevity

Introduction

Numerous things can predict longevity. For example, Dr. Tencza and colleagues, from the University of Pennsylvania, reported in the July 2014 issue of the journal *Demographic Research* that, "Factors including smoking, drinking, substance abuse, obesity, and health care have all been shown to affect health and longevity." The authors conducted research wherein, "The analysis calculates age-standardized death rates by cause of death from 2000-2009 for white men and women separately. Only premature deaths between ages 20-64 are included...*Smoking and obesity, substance abuse, and rural/urban residence are the three factors that make the largest contributions to state-level mortality variation among males. The same factors are at work for women but are less vividly revealed.*"[756]

Reporting in the 2014 *Living to 100* monograph, researchers reported the following:[757]

> "Knowledge of strong predictors of mortality and longevity is very important for actuarial science and practice. Earlier studies found that parental characteristics as well as early-life conditions and midlife environment play a significant role in survival to advanced ages. However, little is known about the simultaneous effects of these three factors on longevity. This ongoing study attempts to fill this gap by comparing centenarians born in the United States in 1890-91 with peers born in the same years who died at age sixty-five. The records for centenarians and controls were taken from computerized family histories, which were then linked to 1900 and 1930 U.S. censuses. As a result of this linkage procedure, 765 records of confirmed centenarians and 783 records of controls were obtained.
>
> Analysis found that parental longevity and some midlife characteristics proved to be significant predictors of longevity while the role of childhood conditions was less important. More centenarians were born in the second half of the year compared to controls, suggesting early origins of longevity. We found the existence of both general and gender-specific predictors of human longevity.

General predictors common for men and women are paternal and maternal longevity.

Gender-specific predictors of male longevity are the farmer occupation at age forty, Northeastern region of birth in the United States and birth in the second half of year.

A gender-specific predictor of female longevity is surprisingly the availability of radio in the household according to the 1930 U.S. census.

Given the importance of familial longevity as an independent predictor of survival to advanced ages, we conducted a comparative study of biological and non-biological relatives of centenarians using a larger sample of 1,945 validated U.S. centenarians born in 1880-95. We found that male gender of centenarian has significant positive effect on survival of adult male relatives (brothers and fathers) but not female blood relatives. Life span of centenarian siblings-in-law is lower compared to life span of centenarian siblings and does not depend on centenarian gender. Wives of male centenarians (who share lifestyle and living conditions) have a significantly better survival compared to wives of centenarians' brothers. This finding demonstrates an important role of shared familial environment and lifestyle in human longevity. The results of this study suggest that familial background, early-life conditions and midlife characteristics play an important role in longevity."

Biomarkers & Genetics

Drs. Shadyab and LaCroix published an overview of genetic influences in longevity in the November 5, 2014 issue of the journal *Aeging Research Reviews*. They stated that:[758]

> "Besides maintaining healthy lifestyle behaviors, positive aging outcomes may also be heritable, with estimates ranging from 20 percent to 35 percent [implying that approximately 70 percent of longevity is NOT based on genetics]. Recent studies not only confirm the association of APOE with longevity in different populations, but also implicate several other pathways that may influence longevity including nitric oxide production, inflammation, immunity, and DNA damage response and repair. Recent evidence also suggests that mitochondrial DNA may play an important role in attaining longevity. Despite these implicated pathways, longevity may be a polygenic trait influenced by a complex interplay of multiple genes."

Serum dehydroepiandrosterone-sulfate (DHEAS), the most abundant adrenal steroid hormone, may predict aging status and longevity in humans. To examine this possible relationship, researchers "...investigated correlations of serum DHEAS with age or conventional health indices (body mass index, blood pressure, and twelve serum/blood tests) and associations of serum DHEAS with lifestyle factors (smoking, drinking, exercise, sleep) in 384 healthy men aged 30-49 years, randomly selected from voluntary attendees at a checkup." The researchers found that, *"Serum DHEAS had an inverse and stronger correlation with age than with any conventional health indices used here. Serum DHEAS rose in parallel with increased smoking and alcohol intake, but had no significant relationships with exercise or sleep. Serum DHEAS reflects age better than health status evaluated by conventional health indices, and may increase with cigarette smoking and alcohol drinking in middle-aged healthy men."*[759]

One exciting new biomarker vis-à-vis longevity is DNA methylation. According to an article published January 30, 2015:[760]

> "*A biological clock in people's DNA could tell scientists how long they will live.* Researchers have found that chemical changes in DNA can help us understand peo-

ple's "biological age" — a measure of how old their body is that seems to be able to predict when people are going to die. Scientists found that people whose biological age showed them as older than their real age were more likely to die sooner. That still held true, even accounting for other factors like smoking and heart disease.

Four independent studies tracked 5,000 people for up to fourteen years. Researchers measured each of their biological ages, and then compared it over time. Scientists found that the link between biological age and the chance of death held up.

The study's principal investigator, Professor Ian Deary, from the University of Edinburgh's Centre for Cognitive Ageing and Cognitive Epidemiology, said: *"This new research increases our understanding of longevity and healthy ageing. It is exciting as it has identified a novel indicator of ageing, which improves the prediction of lifespan over and above the contribution of factors such as smoking, diabetes and cardiovascular disease."*

Scientists measured people's biological age by looking at a chemical modification that happens to DNA, known as methylation. *It plays an important role in biological processes, and can turn genes on and off."*

In November 2014, researchers completed a literature review to determine the association of the apolipoprotein E (ApoE) gene with exceptional longevity (EL, i.e. reaching 100+years). The researchers identified possible unequal distribution of alleles/genotypes in the common variants ε2, ε3 and ε4 among centenarians and younger population. The association of ApoE with EL was analyzed in a total of 2,776 centenarians (cases) and 11,941 younger controls. The researchers noted that, "The main result for all ethnic groups combined was that the likelihood of reaching EL was negatively associated with ε4-allele carriage and with ε4/ε4, ε3/ε4 and ε2/ε4 genotypes. *In contrast, the ε2/ε3 genotype was positively associated with EL. When compared with ε3-allele, the ε2-allele was not associated with increased odds of EL). The present meta-analysis confirms that, besides its previously documented influence on Alzheimer's and cardiovascular disease risk, the ApoE gene is associated with the likelihood of reaching EL.*[761]

Early-Life Nutrition

According to one researcher, reporting in 2014, *"Available data from both experimental and epidemiological studies suggest that inadequate diet in early life can permanently change the structure and function of specific organs or homoeostatic pathways, thereby 'programming' the individual's health status and longevity. Sufficient evidence has accumulated showing significant impact of epigenetic regulation mechanisms in nutritional programming phenomenon. The essential role of early-life diet in the development of aging-related chronic diseases is well established and described in many scientific publications."*[762]

Exercise, Activity & Fitness Levels

According to an article published in March 2015:[763]

> *"Cardiologists at Johns Hopkins University School of Medicine have devised a formula that estimates an individual's risk of dying based on their ability to exercise on a treadmill.*
>
> *In a new study published in the journal Mayo Clinic Proceedings, researchers analyzed data from 58,000 heart stress tests and created an algorithm to gauge mortality risk over a decade based solely on treadmill exercise performance. While exercise-based risk scoring systems for short-term mortality exist, they are only used for patients with established heart disease or overt*

signs of cardiovascular trouble. *This new algorithm, the FIT Treadmill Score, is applicable to anyone.*

"The notion that being in good physical shape portends lower death risk is by no means new, but we wanted to quantify that risk precisely by age, gender and fitness level, and do so with an elegantly simple equation that requires no additional fancy testing beyond the standard stress test," lead investigator Dr. Haitham Ahmed, a cardiology fellow at the Johns Hopkins University School of Medicine, said in a news release.

The FIT Treadmill Score factors in age, gender, peak heart rate reached during intense exercise and the ability to tolerate physical exertion. The last factor is measured by metabolic equivalents (METs), a gauge of how much energy the body expends during exercise. More vigorous activity requires higher energy output (higher METs), better exercise tolerance and higher fitness level, according to the news release. For example, slow walking equals two METs, but running is eight METs.

One benefit of the test is that it's easy to calculate and costs nothing beyond the cost of the treadmill test itself, researchers said.

"We hope the score will become a mainstay in cardiologists' and primary clinicians' offices as a meaningful way to illustrate risk among those who undergo cardiac stress testing and propel people with poor results to become more physically active, senior study author Dr. Michael Blaha, director of clinical research at the Johns Hopkins Ciccarone Center for the Prevention of Heart Disease, said in the news release.

According to researchers, the new data shows that varying degrees of fitness among those with "normal" exercise stress test results reveal telling clues about cardiac and respiratory fitness— and therefore overall death risk over time.

Researchers analyzed data on 58,020 people, ages 18 to 96, who underwent standard exercise stress tests between 1991 and 2009 in Detroit, Michigan. They then tracked how many participants within each fitness level died from any cause over the next decade.

Among people of the same age and gender, fitness level as measured by METs and peak heart rate reached during exercise were the greatest indicators of death risk. Additionally, fitness level was the single most powerful predictor of death and survival, even after accounting for important variables such as diabetes and family history of premature death.

An example of their analysis found that a 45-year-old woman with a fitness score in the bottom fifth percentile is estimated to have a 38 percent risk of dying over the next decade, compared to a 2 percent risk for a 45-year-old woman with a top fitness score. "We hope that illustrating risk that way could become a catalyst for patients to increase exercise and improve cardiovascular fitness," Blaha said."

The following is an article published in the *American Journal of Clinical Exercise* and later online by CBS Atlanta on January 15, 2015:[764]

"Study: Lack Of Exercise Causes Twice As Many Deaths As Obesity

Researchers out of the University of Cambridge in Britain found that *as little as a 20-minute daily walk can help prevent heart attacks.*

"Just a small amount of physical activity each day could have substantial health benefits for people who are physically inactive," Ulf Ekelund, a professor at the University of Cambridge said in a statement obtained by *The Oregonian*. "Physical activity has many proven health benefits and should be an important part of our daily lives."

Over 334,000 men and women participated in the study. Researchers followed the participants for over twelve years. Researchers measured each participant's height, weight, and waist. They also asked each participant how much physical activity they had in their daily lives. Over the course of the study, 21,438 participants died.

Researchers analyzed the cause of death and found that the greatest reduction in risk of an early demise was found in people who were moderately active as compared to those who were not active at all. The researchers also found that a 20-minute walk can help reduce the risk of a premature death by up to 30 percent.

According to the Centers for Disease Control and Prevention (CDC), there has been a dramatic increase in obesity in the United States over the last twenty years and rates remain high. More than one-third of U.S. adults and approximately 17 percent of children and adolescents have obesity."

Unfortunately, according to Dr. Aviroop and colleagues, who published the results of their research in 2015 in the journal *Annals of Internal Medicine*, exercising is not enough! They conducted a literature review to quantify the association between sedentary time and hospitalizations, all-cause mortality, cardiovascular disease, diabetes, and cancer in adults independent of physical activity. They found positive associations between all the variables studied and sedentary time. "The degree of risk with sedentary time and outcomes was generally more pronounced at lower levels of physical activity than at higher levels...*Prolonged sedentary time was independently associated with deleterious health outcomes regardless of physical activity.*"[765]

Dr. Garatachea and colleagues published the results of their literature review of the mortality of elite athletes in the September 2014 issue of the journal *Mayo Clinic Proceedings*. Six studies provided data on cardiovascular disease (CVD) and five on cancer (in a total of 35,920 and 12,119 athletes, respectively). The researchers concluded that, "*The evidence available indicates that top-level athletes live longer than the general population and have a lower risk of two major causes of mortality, namely, CVD and cancer.*"[766]

An article, titled Short spurts of vigorous exercise helps prevent early death, says study, published in April 2015, noted the following:[767]

> "*Scientists found that those who engaged in some kind of vigorous exercise such as jogging lived longer on average than those who exercised gently. Short spurts of vigorous exercise that get you out of breath are better than longer bouts of gentle exercise when it comes to preventing an early death, according to a study of middle-aged men and women.*
>
> Scientists followed more than 200,000 people for six years and found that those who engaged in some kind of vigorous exercise such as jogging or aerobics lived longer on average than those who exercised gently. The researchers believe the effect was statistically significant, lowering the risk of premature death by between 9 and 13 per cent compared to those who undertook moderate exercise only, such as gentle swimming or household chores. *The findings contradict the basic assumption of current health advice which is that two minutes of moderate exercise is roughly equivalent in terms of health benefits to one minute of vigorous exercise*, said the researchers.

"Current World Health Organization guidelines, adopted in the UK, are that adults should exercise with moderate activity for 150 minutes per week or 75 minutes if the activities are vigorous," said Melody Ding of the University of Sydney, a co-author of the study. "The guidelines leave individuals to choose their level of exercise intensity, or a combination of levels, with two minutes of moderate exercise considered the equivalent of one minute of vigorous activity," Dr Ding said. "It might not be the simple two-for-one swap that is the basis of current guidelines. Our research indicates that encouraging vigorous activities may help to avoid preventable deaths at an earlier age," she said.

The study, published in *JAMA Internal Medicine*, found that the health benefits of vigorous exercise were true for middle-aged men as well as women, and extended to people with weight problems and pre-existing cardiovascular disease. "Our research indicates that even small amounts of vigorous activity could help reduce your risk of early death," said Klaus Gerbel of James Cook University in Cairns, Queensland, the lead author of the study.

"The benefits of vigorous activity applied to men and women of all ages, and were independent of the total time spent being active. The results indicate that whether or not you are obese, and whether or not you have heart disease or diabetes, if you can manage some vigorous activity it could offer significant benefits for longevity," Dr Gerbel said.

The participants in the study were classified into three groups. Those said that up to 30 per cent of their activity was vigorous had a mortality rate 9 per cent lower than those with no vigorous exercise, while those who reported more than 30 per cent vigorous activity had a 13 per cent reduction in mortality.

Dr Gerbel warned, however, that people who do not exercise regularly should talk to their doctor first before considering an exercise regime of vigorous activity that could seriously raise their heartbeat or get them out of breath. "For those with medical conditions, for older people in general and for those who have never done any vigorous exercise before, it's always important to talk to a doctor first," Dr Gerbel said.

"Previous studies indicate that interval training with short bursts of vigorous effort, is often manageable for older people, including those who are overweight or obese," he said."

So, how much jogging is the "right" amount? Dr. Schnohr and colleagues studied this issue and reported their findings in the February 10, 2015 issue of *The Journal of the American College of Cardiology*. According to the authors:[768]

> "People who are physically active have at least a 30 percent lower risk of death during follow-up compared with those who are inactive. However, the ideal dose of exercise for improving longevity is uncertain. The aim of this study was to investigate the association between jogging and long-term, all-cause mortality by focusing specifically on the effects of pace, quantity, and frequency of jogging.
>
> As part of the Copenhagen City Heart Study, 1,098 healthy joggers and 3,950 healthy nonjoggers have been prospectively followed up since 2001. Compared with sedentary nonjoggers, *1 to 2.4 h of jogging per week was associated with the lowest mortality. The optimal frequency of jogging was two to three times per week.* The

optimal pace was slow or average. The joggers were divided into light, moderate, and strenuous joggers. The lowest HR for mortality was found in light, followed by moderate and strenuous joggers.

The findings suggest a U-shaped association between all-cause mortality and dose of jogging as calibrated by pace, quantity, and frequency of jogging. *Light and moderate joggers have lower mortality than sedentary nonjoggers, whereas strenuous joggers have a mortality rate not statistically different from that of the sedentary group."*

Facial Scans

According to an article published in March 2015, titled Face scans show how fast a person is aging:[769]

> *"Every face tells a story, and that story apparently includes hints of how quickly a person is aging,* a new study contends. *Facial features have proven even more reliable than blood tests in spotting those for whom time is taking a heavier toll,* a Chinese research team reports in the March 31 [2015] issue of the journal *Cell Research*. A computerized 3-D facial imaging process uncovered a number of "tells" that show if a person is aging more rapidly, including a widening mouth, bulging nose, sagging upper lip, shrinking gums and drooping eye corners, the researchers said.
>
> "This suggests not only that youth is 'skin deep,' but also that health is 'written' on the face," the study authors concluded, *suggesting that facial scanning could more accurately assess a person's general health than a routine physical exam.*

ALZHEIMER'S DISEASE

This sort of facial imaging is part of a cutting-edge technology aimed at estimating life expectancy and assessing health risk factors simply by taking a scan of your face, said Jay Olshansky, a professor at the University of Illinois at Chicago's School of Public Health and a board member of the American Federation for Aging Research.

"A lot of your risk factor for disease shows up in your face," Olshansky said. *"You can identify the precise places on the face where these risk factors show up."*

In fact, Olshansky predicts that insurance companies eventually could turn to such technology to improve underwriting of life insurance, predicting a person's future health with a simple face scan rather than a complex panel of blood tests.

"All of that blood chemistry, all of the money spent on it, is mostly a waste of money and time," he said. *"You can get at these risks a much simpler way through a combination of facial analytics and asking the right questions."* In the new study, researchers at the Chinese Academy of Sciences collected 3-D facial images of 332 people of Chinese descent between the ages of seventeen and seventy-seven. Based on this data, the researchers constructed a model for predicting age, generating a map of the aging human face that recognized certain patterns of aging based on specific facial features.

They found that up to age forty, people of the same chronological age could differ by up to six years in facial age. Those older than forty showed even wider variation in facial age.

"In aging science, we know people who look young for their age are aging more slowly," Olshansky said. "They look younger because they probably are younger. One year of clock time is matched by something less than one year of biological time. It's real. We can see it." The researchers compared the results of their facial scans to routine blood tests they took from the participants, and found that age estimates based on facial features were more accurate than blood screenings for cholesterol, uric acid or the blood protein albumin.

The findings track with what doctors already know about how age can affect a person's face, said Dr. Anne Taylor, chairwoman of the American Society of Plastic Surgeons' Public Education Committee. "Our lips are shrinking, and the distance between the nose and the mouth increases as we age," Taylor said. "And there's a reason for the saying, 'Long in the tooth.' Your gums are shrinking as you age, so more of your teeth are showing."

Olshansky added that facial features also reveal evidence of behaviors that can affect your health. Smokers tend to develop wrinkles around the mouth, caused by constant pursing of the lips to suck on a cigarette, he said. Drinkers develop a "W.C. Fields" nose, red and bulbous at the tip."

Fiber

According to an article published January 12, 2015:[770]

> *"People who ate the most fiber were less likely to die of any cause during a recent study of nearly one million people.* The finding might be explained by fiber's potential to lower the risk of chronic diseases including heart

disease, stroke, diabetes and several types of cancer, researchers say.

Individuals should be encouraged to increase their dietary fiber intake "to potentially decrease the risk of premature death," Yang Yang, of the Shanghai Cancer Institute in China, and colleagues write in the *American Journal of Epidemiology*. They pooled data from seventeen previous studies that tracked 982,411 men and women, mostly in Europe and the U.S., and recorded about 67,000 deaths.

Yang's team divided participants into five groups based on their daily fiber intake. Those in the top fifth, who ate the greatest amount of fiber daily, were 16 percent less likely to die than those in the bottom fifth, who consumed the least amount of fiber. In addition, eight studies showed a 10 percent drop in risk for any cause of death with each 10-gram per day increase in fiber intake.

The U.S. Department of Agriculture recommends that adults consume fourteen grams of fiber in every 1,000 calories they take in, the authors point out. That translates to approximately 25 grams a day for women and 38 grams daily for men.

"On average, intakes of dietary fiber in the U.S. and other economically developed countries are much lower than recommended goals – in the U.S., about half of what is advised," said Victoria Burley, a nutrition researcher at the University of Leeds in the UK, who was not involved in the study.

These study results are "very much in line with earlier published meta-analyses of the relationship between dietary fiber and risk of major chronic diseases such as cardiovascular disease, and cancers," Burley told Reuters Health in an email.

She said *the benefits of consuming fiber-rich foods have been known for decades, including lowering of blood cholesterol, blood pressure, blood glucose and insulin, and possibly reducing inflammation.* High-fiber foods may also make people feel full sooner, and for longer, which helps curb overeating and weight gain, she added. "Some or all of these factors may underlie the reduction in mortality observed here."

It's not difficult to consume an extra ten grams of fiber per day, Burley said. "This can come from two servings of whole grain foods, such as breakfast cereal and two servings of fruit or vegetables, for example."

Little is known about the best sources of fiber for reducing disease risk - whether the best sources are fruit and vegetables, legumes or grains, Burley pointed out. "Although there is increasing evidence that cereal grains may offer the best risk reductions for colorectal and cardiovascular disease," she said.

Friend-rated Personality Traits

According to Dr. Jackson, from the Department of Psychology, Washington University in St. Louis, and colleagues, who reported the results of their research in the January 12, 2015 issue of *Psychological Science,* "*Self-rated personality traits predict mortality risk.*" To study whether or not one's friends can perceive personality characteristics that predict one's mortality risk, the researchers reviewed data from a 75-year longitudinal study (the Kelly/Connolly Longitudinal Study on Personality and Aging). According to the researchers, "In that study, 600 participants were observed beginning in 1935 through 1938, when they were in their mid-20s, and continuing through 2013. *Male partici-*

pants seen by their friends as more conscientious and open lived longer, whereas friend-rated emotional stability and agreeableness were protective for women. Friends' ratings were better predictors of longevity than were self-reports of personality, in part because friends' ratings could be aggregated to provide a more reliable assessment. Our findings demonstrate the utility of observers' reports in the study of health and provide insights concerning the pathways by which personality traits influence health."[771]

Handshake Strength

Who could have known that the expression, "Get a grip," held such meaning. According to an article published online May 14, 2015, "A firm handshake could indicate robust health, a new study suggests." The research, published in the medical journal, *The Lancet*, found:[772]

> "The vigor of a person's hand-grip could predict the risk of heart attacks and strokes, and was a stronger predictor of death than checking systolic blood pressure. Experts said a grip test could be a simple, low-cost way to predict the risk of heart attacks and strokes.
>
> The international study, involving almost 140,000 adults in seventeen countries found weak grip strength is linked with shorter survival and a greater risk of having a heart attack or stroke. It also found that grip strength is a stronger predictor of death than systolic blood pressure.
>
> Reduced muscular strength, which can be measured by grip strength, has been consistently linked with early death, disability, and illness. But there has been limited research on whether grip strength could be used to indicate heart health. The new study followed 139,691 adults aged between thirty-five and seventy living in seventeen countries from The Prospective Urban-Rural

Epidemiology (PURE) study for an average of four years. Grip strength was assessed using a handgrip dynamometer. It is measured as the force exerted when a subject squeezes an object as hard as possible with their hands.

The findings show that every five kilos (approximately ten pounds) decline in grip strength was associated with a 16 per cent increased risk of death from any cause; a 17 per cent greater risk of cardiovascular death; a 17 per cent higher risk of non-cardiovascular mortality; and more modest increases in the risk of having a heart attack (seven per cent) or a stroke (nine per cent).

Overall, grip strength was a stronger predictor of all-cause deaths, including deaths from heart disease, than systolic blood pressure, which is normally seen as a "robust causal factor" for death, the study showed. The associations persisted even after taking into account differences in other factors that can affect mortality or heart disease such as age, education level, employment status, physical activity level, and tobacco and alcohol use.

A low grip strength was linked with higher death rates in people who suffer a heart attack or stroke and non-cardiovascular diseases, for example cancer, suggesting muscle strength can predict the risk of death in people who develop a major illness. Lead author Dr. Darryl Leong, of McMaster University in Canada, said: "Grip strength could be an easy and inexpensive test to assess an individual's risk of death and cardiovascular disease. Further research is needed to establish whether efforts to improve muscle strength are likely to reduce an individual's risk of death and cardiovascular disease."

"Healthy" Diet

"You are what you eat."[1] According to Dr. Jankovic and colleagues, who published the results of their research in the November 15, 2014 issue of the *American Journal of Epidemiology*, "The World Health Organization (WHO) has formulated guidelines for a healthy diet to prevent chronic diseases and postpone death worldwide. Our objective was to investigate the association between the WHO guidelines, measured using the Healthy Diet Indicator (HDI), and all-cause mortality in elderly men and women from Europe and the United States. We analyzed data from 396,391 participants (42 percent women) in eleven prospective cohort studies who were sixty years of age or older at enrollment (in 1988-2005)...During 4,497,957 person-years of follow-up, 84,978 deaths occurred...*These estimates translate to an increased life expectancy of two years at the age of sixty years. Greater adherence to the WHO guidelines is associated with greater longevity in elderly men and women in Europe and the United States.*"[773]

Heart Rate

According to Dr. Gent and colleagues, from the Institute for Pathophysiology, West German Heart and Vascular Center, University School of

---

[1] You are what you eat. In the 1920s and 30s, the nutritionist Victor Lindlahr, who was a strong believer in the idea that food controls health, developed the Catabolic Diet. That view gained some adherents at the time and the earliest known printed example is from an advert for beef in a 1923 edition of the *Bridgeport Telegraph*, for 'United Meet [sic] Markets': "Ninety per cent of the diseases known to man are caused by cheap foodstuffs. You are what you eat." In 1942, Lindlahr published *You Are What You Eat: how to win and keep health with diet*. That seems to be the vehicle that took the phrase into the public consciousness. Lindlahr is likely to have also used the term in his radio talks in the late 1930s (now lost unfortunately), which would also have reached a large audience. The phrase got a new lease of life in the 1960s hippy era. The food of choice of the champions of this notion was macrobiotic wholefood and the phrase was adopted by them as a slogan for healthy eating. The belief in the diet in some quarters was so strong that when Adelle Davis, a leading spokesperson for the organic food movement, contracted the cancer that later killed her, she attributed the illness to the junk food she had eaten at college.

Medicine, Essen, Germany, reporting in the March 2015 issue of the journal *Basic Research in Cardiology*, "*Heart rate correlates inversely with life span across all species, including humans. In patients with cardiovascular disease, higher heart rate is associated with increased mortality, and such patients benefit from pharmacological heart rate reduction*...We studied the effects of a life-long pharmacological heart rate reduction on longevity in mice. We hypothesized, that the total number of cardiac cycles is constant, and that a 15 percent heart rate reduction might translate into a 15 percent increase in life span...Ivabradine reduced heart rate by 14 percent throughout life, and median life span was increased by 6.2 percent...*Life span was not increased to the same extent as heart rate was reduced, but nevertheless significantly prolonged by 6.2 percent.*"[774]

Dr. Bohm and colleagues published the results of their literature review, on the association between resting heart rate and longevity, in the October 15, 2014 issue of the *American Journal of Medicine*. The authors noted that, "*Resting heart rate is central to cardiac output and is influenced by changes occurring in numerous diseases. It predicts longevity and cardiovascular diseases and current evidence suggests that it is also an important marker of outcome in cardiovascular disease including heart failure.* Beta blockers[1] improve outcomes in heart failure; however, they have effects outside reducing heart rate. Ivabradine[2]

---

[1] Beta blockers are a class of drugs that are particularly used for the management of cardiac arrhythmias, protecting the heart from a second heart attack (myocardial infarction) after a first heart attack (secondary prevention), and, in certain cases, hypertension. Beta blockers block the action of endogenous catecholamines epinephrine (adrenaline) and norepinephrine (noradrenaline) -in particular on adrenergic beta receptors, of the sympathetic nervous system, which mediates the fight-or-flight response. Some block all activation of β-adrenergic receptors and others are selective.

[2] Ivabradine is a novel medication used for the symptomatic management of stable angina pectoris (heart-related chest pain). It is marketed by Servier under the trade names Procoralan (worldwide), Coralan (in Hong Kong, Singapore, Australia and some other countries), Corlentor (in Armenia, Spain, Italy and Romania) and Coraxan (in Russia and Serbia). It is also marketed in India under the brand names Ivabid and Bradia. Ivabradine acts by reducing the heart rate via specific inhibition of the funny channel, a mechanism different from beta blockers and calcium channel blockers, two commonly prescribed antianginal drugs. Ivabradine is a cardiotonic agent.

has demonstrated efficacy in reducing rehospitalizations and mortality in heart failure and in improving exercise tolerance and reducing angina attacks in patients with coronary artery disease, while selective heart rate reduction may also prove to be beneficial in therapeutic areas outside those where ivabradine has already demonstrated clinical efficacy."[775]

Isolation

According to an article published March 16, 2015, being alone is as bad as smoking or excessive drinking: "More Americans are choosing to live alone than ever before. And while it's healthy to have "down time" by yourself, one study says too much alone time may shorten your life. Researchers at Brigham Young University studied 3 million people. *They found people who said they were lonely, felt socially isolated or lived alone, had a 30 percent increased likelihood of death. The study says loneliness and isolation are as damaging as obesity. The impact of loneliness has also been likened to smoking fifteen cigarettes a day or excessive drinking. So partner up.*"[776]

Matthew Effect

One of the things that *may* predict long life is old age itself. Some studies have shown, for example, that if you are eighty years old, you stand a better chance of reaching ninety years of age than if you are sixty years old. This is an example of the Matthew Effect, as explained in 2014 by Dr. Pere, from the Faculty of Natural Sciences and Mathematics, University of Maribor, Maribor, Slovenia:[777]

> "The Matthew effect describes the phenomenon that in societies, the rich tend to get richer and the potent even more powerful. It is closely related to the concept of preferential attachment in network science, where the more connected nodes are destined to acquire many more links in the future than the auxiliary nodes. Cumulative advantage and success-breeds-success also both

describe the fact that advantage tends to beget further advantage. The concept is behind the many power laws and scaling behavior in empirical data, and it is at the heart of self-organization across social and natural sciences. Here, we review the methodology for measuring preferential attachment in empirical data, as well as the observations of the Matthew effect in patterns of scientific collaboration, socio-technical and biological networks, the propagation of citations, the emergence of scientific progress and impact, career longevity, the evolution of common English words and phrases, as well as in education and brain development."

However, recent discoveries cast doubt on this phenomenon vis-à-vis longevity. Dr. Gavrilov and colleagues, from the Center on Aging, NORC at the University of Chicago, Chicago, Ill, published the following in the December 20, 2014 issue of the journal *Gerontology*:[778]

"Biodemography is a promising scientific approach based on using demographic data and methods for getting insights into biological mechanisms of observed processes. *Recently, new important developments have happened in biodemographic studies of aging and longevity that call into question conventional aging theories and open up novel research directions. Recent studies found that the exponential increase of the mortality risk with age (the famous Gompertz law) continues even at extreme old ages in humans, rats, and mice, thus challenging traditional views about old-age mortality deceleration, mortality leveling-off, and late-life mortality plateaus.* This new finding represents a challenge to many aging theories, including the evolutionary theory that explains senescence by a declining force of natural selection with age.

Innovative ideas are needed to explain why exactly the same exponential pattern of mortality growth is observed not only at reproductive ages, but also at very-old postreproductive ages (up to 106 years), long after the force of natural selection becomes negligible (when there is no room for its further decline). Another important recent development is the discovery of long-term 'memory' for early-life experiences in longevity determination. *Siblings born to young mothers have significantly higher chances to live up to 100 years*, and this new finding, confirmed by two independent research groups, calls for its explanation. As recent studies found, even *the place and season of birth matter for human longevity*. Beneficial longevity effects of young maternal age are observed only when children of the same parents are compared, while the maternal age effect often could not be detected in across-families studies, presumably being masked by between-family variation. It was also found that *male gender of centenarian has a significant positive effect on the survival of adult male biological relatives (brothers and fathers) but not of female relatives*. Finally, large gender differences are found in longevity determinants for males and females, suggesting a higher importance of occupation history for male centenarians as well as a higher importance of home environment history for female centenarians."

Mediterranean diet

Dr. Crous-Bou from the Channing Division of Network Medicine, Department of Medicine, Brigham and Women's Hospital and Harvard Medical School, Boston, MA, and the Department of Epidemiology, Program in Genetic Epidemiology and Statistical Genetics, Harvard School of Public Health, Boston, MA, and colleagues, published the results of their research examining whether or not adherence to the Mediterranean diet was associated with longer telomere length, a biomarker of aging in the December 2, 2014 issue of the *British Medical Journal*. To do so, they studied 4,676 disease-free women from the

Nurses' Health Study. They found that, *"In this large study, greater adherence to the Mediterranean diet was associated with longer telomeres. These results further support the benefits of adherence to the Mediterranean diet for promoting health and longevity."*[779]

Milk Consumption

According to an article published October 29, 2014:[780]

> "Drinking lots of milk could be bad for your health, a new study reports. Previous research has shown that the calcium in milk can help strengthen bones and prevent osteoporosis. These benefits to bone health have led U.S. health officials to recommend milk as part of a healthy diet. *But this new study found that drinking large amounts of milk did not protect men or women from bone fractures, and was linked to an overall higher risk of death during the study period.* However, the researchers said the results should be viewed with caution.
>
> *Women who drank three glasses of milk or more every day had a nearly doubled risk of death and cardiovascular disease, and a 44 percent increased risk of cancer compared to women who drank less than one glass per day, the researchers found.*
>
> *Men's overall risk of death increased about 10 percent when they drank three or more glasses of milk daily*, said the study, published online Oct. 28 in *BMJ* [*British Medical Journal*].
>
> "The study findings have, for myself, been strong enough to cut down on my milk consumption," said lead author Karl Michaelsson, a professor in the department of surgical sciences at Uppsala University in Sweden. Still, the findings only suggest an association and not a direct link, said Mary Schooling, a professor at the City

ALZHEIMER'S DISEASE

University of New York School of Public Health, who wrote an editorial accompanying the study.

The study involved more than 61,000 women and 45,000 men in Sweden who previously filled out dietary questionnaires for other research projects, the women in the late 1980s and the men in 1997. All were over thirty-nine years of age. Researchers compared their reported milk-drinking habits to health data kept by Swedish officials, to see whether milk consumption could be linked to risk of death or health problems.

The investigators found that a large amount of milk in a daily diet did appear to be linked to an increased risk of death in both men and women during the study period. In addition, excessive milk drinking appeared to actually increase a woman's risk of broken bones, compared with women who drank little milk. The risk of any bone fracture increased 16 percent in women who drank three or more glasses daily, and the risk of a broken hip increased 60 percent, the findings indicated.

Lots of milk did not appear to either protect against or promote broken bones in men. Michaelsson and colleagues said *the increased risk of death they observed could be explained by the high levels of sugars contained in milk, specifically lactose and galactose. Galactose has been shown to prematurely age mice in the laboratory, Michaelsson said, noting that the milk sugar promotes inflammation.*

By contrast, a high intake of fermented milk products with low lactose content -- such as yogurt and cheese -- was associated with reduced rates of death and fracture, particularly in women, the researchers reported.

While interesting, these findings are too preliminary to warrant a change in nutritional guidelines, said Isabel Maples, a registered dietitian in Haymarket, Va., and spokesperson for the Academy of Nutrition and Dietetics. About 55 percent of older adults -- 44 million Americans -- either have osteoporosis or are at high risk for brittle bones, Maples said. She added that the U.S. Dietary Guidelines recommend three servings of dairy per day, not just for bone health, but also to reduce the risk of heart disease, type 2 diabetes and high blood pressure. "They don't base the guidelines on fads. They don't base it on trends. They don't base it on what has been the traditional advice. They look at the scientific evidence," she said."

Nut Consumption

Increased nut consumption has been associated with a reduced risk of major chronic diseases, including cardiovascular disease and type 2 diabetes mellitus. In order to study the relationship between nut consumption and mortality risk, researchers studied nut consumption and subsequent total and cause-specific mortality among 76,464 women in the Nurses' Health Study (1980-2010) and 42,498 men in the Health Professionals Follow-up Study (1986-2010). Participants with a history of cancer, heart disease, or stroke were excluded. Nut consumption was assessed at baseline and updated every two to four years. The researchers found that, "During 3,038,853 person-years of follow-up, 16,200 women and 11,229 men died. *Nut consumption was inversely associated with total mortality among both women and men, after adjustment for other known or suspected risk factors. Significant inverse associations were also observed between nut consumption and deaths due to cancer, heart disease, and respiratory disease.*"[781]

Oral Health

Dr. Kaufman and colleagues, from the Section of Geriatrics, Department of Medicine, Boston Medical Center, Boston, Massachusetts; Department of General Dentistry, Boston University, Henry M. Goldman School of Dental Medicine, Boston, Massachuset, published the results of their research, on the relationship between oral health and longevity, in the June 2014 issue of the *Journal of the American Geriatrics Society*. They "studied seventy-three centenarians, 467 offspring, and 251 offspring generation-reference cohort subjects from the NECS. The edentulous rate [e.g., those with no teeth] of centenarians (36.5 percent) was lower than that of their birth cohort (46 percent) when they were aged sixty-five to seventy-four in 1971 to 1974 (according to National Center of Health Statistics). Adjusting for confounding factors, the reference cohort was more likely to be edentulous, less likely to have all or more than half of their own teeth, and less likely to report excellent or very good oral health than the centenarian offspring. *Centenarians and their offspring have better oral health than their respective birth cohorts. Oral health may prove to be a helpful marker for systemic health and healthy aging.*"[782]

Purpose in life

According to Dr. Hill and colleagues, who reported the results of their analysis in May 2014, "Having a purpose in life has been cited consistently as an indicator of healthy aging for several reasons, including its potential for reducing mortality risk. In the current study, we sought to extend previous findings by examining whether purpose in life promotes longevity across the adult years, using data from the longitudinal Midlife in the United States (MIDUS) sample. Proportional-hazards models demonstrated that purposeful individuals lived longer than their counterparts did during the fourteen years after the baseline assessment, even when controlling for other markers of psychological and affective well-being. *Moreover, these longevity benefits did not appear to be conditional on the participants' age, how long they lived during the follow-up period, or whether they had retired from the workforce. In other words, having a purpose in life appears to widely buffer against mortality risk across the adult years."* [783]

Another study finds that having a sense of meaning and purpose in your life might do more than just give you focus -- it might help you live longer, too:[784]

> "The study, involving more than 9,000 British people averaging sixty-five years of age, found that those who professed to feeling worthwhile and having a sense of purpose in life were less likely to die during the more than eight years the researchers tracked them.
>
> Over the study period, 9 percent of people with the highest levels of this type of well-being died, compared with 29 percent of those with the lowest levels, according to the report in the Nov. 7 [2014] issue of *The Lancet*.
>
> The study comes on the heels of similar research published Monday in the *Proceedings of the National Academy of Sciences*. In that study, a team led by Eric Kim of the University of Michigan found that older adults with a strong sense of purpose in life may be particularly likely to get health screenings such as colonoscopies and mammograms.
>
> The new British study was led by Andrew Steptoe, director of the Institute of Epidemiology and Health Care at University College London. His team found that, after taking other factors into account, *people with the highest levels of "purpose in life" were 30 percent less likely to die during the study period, living an average of two years longer than those with the lowest levels."*

ALZHEIMER'S DISEASE

RDW (Red Blood Cell Distribution Width)

Dr. Darzynkiewicz and colleagues, from the Brander Cancer Research Institute and Department of Pathology, New York Medical College, Valhalla, New York, reported their analysis of antiaging molecules in the May 2014 issue of the journal *Cytometry Part A*. This is a complex article, but very informative vis-à-vis aging and longevity. Presented below are a few critical snipits of the article:[785]

> "This review presents the evidence in support of the IGF-1/mTOR/S6K1 signaling as the primary factor contributing to aging and cellular senescence. Reviewed are also specific interactions between mTOR/S6K1 and ROS-DNA damage signaling pathways. Outlined are critical sites along these pathways, including autophagy, as targets for potential antiaging (gero-suppressive) and/or chemopreventive agents...to monitor activation along these pathways in response to the reported antiaging drugs rapamycin, metformin, berberine, resveratrol, vitamin D3, 2-deoxyglucose, and acetylsalicylic acid [Aspirin]. Specifically, effectiveness of these agents to attenuate the level of constitutive mTOR signaling was tested by cytometry and confirmed by Western blotting through measuring phosphorylation of the mTOR-downstream targets including ribosomal protein S6. The ratiometric analysis of phosphorylated to total protein along the mTOR pathway offers a useful parameter reporting the effects of gero-suppressive agents... Discussed is cytometric analysis of cell size and heterogeneity of size as a potential biomarker used to assess gero-suppressive agents and longevity...
>
> Downstream of these signals, the kinase activity of mTOR (raptor) is directly suppressed by its specific inhibitor, rapamycin. The evidence that rapamycin has gero-suppressive properties is so persuasive that it prompted some authors to advise its instant implementa-

tion as a human antiaging drug/supplement extending the lifespan, preventing the age-associated diseases and reducing costs of health care. Indirect inhibition of mTOR is achieved through activation of AMPK. Metformin and berberine are among its activators that have been shown to have gero-suppressive properties. Both these drugs are effective to treat diabetes type 2. Their mechanism of AMPK activation involves inhibition of electron transport chain in mitochondria that leads to a decline in content of ATP, an increase of AMP/ATP ratio and thus provides the trigger activating AMPK. There is ample evidence of the gero-suppressive properties of metformin. Particularly convincing are results of recent experiments showing extended longevity and health-span of mice fed with this drug. Similar as in the case of rapamycin, with its long-term clinical usage and already well-known pharmacokinetics and toxicity profile, the use of metformin as an antiaging drug has been recently postulated...

Berberine, a naturally occurring alkaloid with a long history of medicinal use in both Ayurvedic and old Chinese medicine, was also shown to have antiaging properties and found to be effective in treatment of several age associated diseases [including Alzheimer's disease]. We have recently reported that both metformin and berberine suppress mTOR signaling...

Of particular interest in the area of aging/longevity and flow cytometry are tantalizing observations, overlooked in the literature pertaining to cytometry, that the red blood cell distribution width (RDW) is a remarkably strong predictor of longevity, including all causes of death, for adults aged forty-five years and older. The RDW is a measure of heterogeneity of size of erythrocytes [red blood cells], expressed as coefficient of variation (CV) of the mean value of the erythrocyte Coulter volume, routinely reported in a standard complete blood count, and increased in certain types of anemia. However, this predictor remains strongly associated with mortality even after excluding all types of red cell blood diseases or other conditions that can affect red blood cells, e.g., such as vitamin B12 deficiency. Incredibly, the persons with the bottom quintile of the CV (<12.60%) at age ≥65 have over 60% longer survival after twelve years compared to persons with the top quintile (>14.05%).

It is tempting to speculate that IGFs/mTOR signaling is one of the factors, if not the key factor, that plays a role in the observed correlation between the RDW and mortality. In support of this contention are the data that IGF-1 can enhance erythropoiesis by activation of erythropoietin and also can affect the final stages of erythroid maturation. The IGFs/mTOR signaling dramatically affects the cell size as shown in the case of 32D-derived myeloid cells which were 50% smaller after having deleted IGF-1 receptor. It is possible therefore that persistent activation of erythropoiesis through IGF-1/mTOR signaling leads to heterogeneity of erythrocyte sizes because of their higher turnover rate. Further support to this contention provide recent findings by Kozlitina and Garcia on the association between telomere length, size of erythrocytes, and RDW, which show that persons having short telomeres have increased fraction of larger red cells and most importantly, increased heterogeneity of their sizes revealed by RDW. However, while there is an association between the level of IGF-1 in serum and telomere length it is unclear whether there are mechanistic bases for this association. *Given the above, the easily measured RDW may be a useful biomarker of the constitutive level of IGF-1 signaling, the critical factor accountable for longevity."*

Dr. Yoon and colleagues, reporting in the May 11, 2015 issue of *Plos One*, note that:[786]

> "Red blood cell distribution width (RDW) is a robust marker of adverse clinical outcomes in various populations. The purpose of this study was to determine the prognostic importance of a change in RDW in end-stage renal disease (ESRD) patients. Three hundred twenty-six dialysis patients were analyzed. Temporal changes in RDW during twelve months after dialysis initiation were assessed. The associations between rising RDW and mortality and cardiovascular (CV) events were investigated. During a median follow-up of 2.7 years, seventy-five deaths (24.0 percent) and sixty non-fatal CV events (18.4 percent) occurred. After categorizing patients according to baseline RDW, the event-free survival rate was lowest in patients with a baseline RDW >14.9 percent and increased RDW, and highest in patients with a baseline RDW ≤14.9 percent and decreased RDW. In multivariate analysis, *rising RDW was independently associated with the composite of end-points, whereas the baseline RDW was not. This study shows that a progressive rise in RDW independently predicted mortality and CV events in ESRD patients. Rising RDW could be an additive predictor for adverse CV outcomes for ESRD patients.*"

Dr. Marinez-Velilla and colleagues, reported the results of their research on the significance of changing RDW values, in the 2015 issue of *The Journal of Nutrition, Health and Aging*. They note that:[787]

> "Most of the studies that evaluate the association between red blood cell distribution width (RDW) and mortality assess it on a single occasion instead of doing so through serial measurements. Very few studies have investigated repeated measurements of RDW and its prognostic value, and most of them are focused on patients

with cardiovascular diseases. RDW is a dynamic value so we aimed at determining the prognostic value of sequential RDW assessment in the last years of life in patients enrolled in a Department of Geriatrics. Patients were consecutively recruited for the study at admission in a tertiary hospital and then followed up for at least five years. A total of fifty-five patients with repeated RDW assessments during all the five years before their death were selected from the total cohort of 122 patients.

We found a strong correlation between progressive rise in RDW and mortality risk, especially during the last year of life. There was a gradual significant increase in the RDW values along the last five years of life, with means growing up from 14.8 to 16.37. In our group of geriatric patients, *RDW is a dynamic variable that is modified during the last five years of life, irrespective of their age, and especially during the last year."*

And finally, Dr. Horne, from the Intermountain Heart Institute, Intermountain Medical Center, Salt Lake City, UT, and colleagues, reported in the March 7, 2015 issue of the *European Journal Of Clinical Investigation* the following: [788]

> "The red cell distribution width (RDW) predicts mortality among many populations. RDW is calculated as the standard deviation (SD) of the red blood cell (RBC) volume divided by mean corpuscular volume (MCV). Because higher MCV also predicts mortality, we hypothesized that the RDW numerator (one SD of RBC volume or 1SD-RDW) predicts mortality more strongly than the RDW.
>
> Adult subjects hospitalized during a contemporary clinical era (10/2005-1/2014, N = 135,963) and a historical era (1/1999-9/2005, N = 119,530) were studied. The RDW was obtained from the complete blood count

(CBC), while 1SD-RDW was calculated (RDW multiplied by MCV and divided by 100).

1SD-RDW was a superior predictor of mortality compared to RDW. This superiority remained after adjustment for age, sex, basic metabolic profile components and other CBC factors excluding MCV. Findings were similar for the 1999-2005 cohort.

The 1SD-RDW predicted mortality more strongly than RDW, suggesting that 1SD-RDW is superior to RDW as an individual risk predictor. Further, these results indicate that the dispersion of RBC volume and its mean are independent risk markers. Further research is required to understand the clinical value and mechanistic basis of these associations."

Real vs. Perceived Age

According to an article published on December 15, 2014:[789]

"How old do you feel? Think carefully — the answer might help predict how much longer you'll live. That's according to British research posing that question to about 6,500 adults. *Those who felt younger than their real age lived the longest over the following eight years.*

The average real age of those questioned was about sixty-six years. *Most adults felt at least three years younger than their real age. Those who felt younger had the least chances of dying over about eight years after the age question was asked. Adults who felt older than their actual age had the greatest chances of dying in that period.*

The researchers analyzed data from a study in England on aging that included information on deaths during a follow-up period that ended in February 2013; deaths totaled 1,030. About 14 percent of the young-feeling adults died during the follow-up, versus 19 percent of those who felt their actual age and 25 percent of those who felt older.

Feeling older was a predictor of death even when the researchers accounted for things that could affect death rates, including illnesses, wealth, education, smoking, alcohol intake and physical activity. *Older-feeling adults were about 40 percent more likely to die than younger-feeling adults."*

Sleep

In 2014, researchers studied the sleep patterns and biochemical profiles of oldest old individuals (N = 10, age 85-105 years old) and compare them to young adults (N = 15, age 20-30 years old) and older adults (N = 13, age 60-70 years old). The researchers found that, "The oldest old individuals showed lower sleep efficiency and REM sleep when compared to the older adults...*Oldest old individuals maintained strictly regular sleep-wake schedules and also presented higher HDL-cholesterol and lower triglyceride levels than older adults*...Taken together with the favorable lipid profile, these results contribute with evidence to the importance of sleep and lipid metabolism regulation in the maintenance of longevity in humans."[790]

Researchers from the Department of Psychology, University of California and the Department of Psychology, University of Pennsylvania, reported the results of their research in late 2014, on whether or not childhood sleep duration is associated with lifelong mortality risk. Without discussing the specifics of their research, they found that, "Male children with shorter or longer sleep durations than expected for their age were at increased risk of death at any given age in adulthood. The findings suggest that sleep may be a core biobehavioral trait, with implications for new models of sleep and health throughout the entire life span."[791]

Sun Activity When Born

According to an article published January 7, 2015, the sun may determine lifespan at birth:[792]

> "Paris (AFP) - Could the Sun be your lucky -- or unlucky -- star? In an unusual study published Wednesday, Norwegian scientists said people *born during periods of solar calm may live longer, as much as five years on average, than those who enter the world when the Sun is feisty.*
>
> The team overlaid demographic data of Norwegians born between 1676 and 1878 with observations of the Sun.
>
> The lifespan of those born in periods of solar maximum – interludes marked by powerful flares and geomagnetic storms – was "5.2 years shorter" on average than those born during a solar minimum, they found. "Solar activity at birth decreased the probability of survival to adulthood," thus truncating average lifespan, according to the paper published in the journal Proceedings of the Royal Society B. There was a stronger effect on girls than boys, it said.
>
> The Sun has cycles that last eleven years, give or take, from one period of greatest activity or solar maximum, to the next. Solar maxima are marked by an increase in sunspots, solar flares and coronal mass ejections that can disrupt radio communications and electrical power on Earth, damage satellites and disturb navigational equipment.

Solar activity is also linked to levels of ultraviolet radiation-- an environmental stressor known to affect survival and reproductive performance, possibly by causing cell and DNA damage, according to the study authors.

The team, from the Norwegian University of Science and Technologybased their study on demographic data from church records of some 8,600 individuals from two different mid-Norwegian populations, one poor and one wealthy. This was matched to maps of historical solar cycles. On top of lifespan, being born in a solar maximum period also "significantly reduced" fertility for women born into the poor category, but not for wealthier women or for men, said the authors. *"We show for the first time that not only infant survival and thus lifespan but also fertility is statistically associated with solar activity at birth,"* they wrote.

It was not clear whether the same would necessarily hold true for people born in the modern era. One explanation could be ultraviolet-induced degradation of the B vitamin folate, a shortage of which before birth has been linked to higher rates of illness and death, the team theorized. "Our findings suggest that maternal exposure to solar activity during gestation can affect the fitness of female children," the authors wrote.

"The effect of socio-economic status on the relationship between solar activity and fertility suggests that high-status pregnant women were better able to avoid the adverse effects of high solar activity" – possibly by staying out of the Sun or because a healthier diet curbed the harm. The team did not have data about how early or late into a solar maximum event the children were born -- a limitation of the study.

"This study is the first to emphasise the importance of UVR (ultraviolet radiation) in early life," the authors said. "UVR is a global stressor with potential ecological impacts and the future levels of UVR are expected to increase due to climate change and variation in atmospheric ozone."

Volatile Organic Compounds (VOCs)

According to research published in late 2014, exhaled breath volatile organic compounds (VOCs) have been suggested as a new biomarker to detect and monitor physiological processes. The researchers reported that, "In the present study we investigated, in real time, the breath properties and VOC exhaled content in healthy centenarians [individuals 100 years of age or older] as compared with non-centenarian seniors and young healthy subjects. We found distinctly different breath pattern and distribution profiles of VOCs in the centenarians. Thus, the VOCs measurement allowed to discriminate the differences between the agegroups. *We propose a VOCs fingerprint as a biomarker underlying the physiological mechanisms of aging and longevity.*"[793]

Medications

Antidepressants

Dr. Tsiouris and colleagues, who published the results of their research in the July 2014 issue of the *Journal of Clinical Psychiatry*, investigated the effects of antidepressants on longevity, age at dementia onset, and survival after onset among adults with Down syndrome. To do so, they reviewed the charts of 357 adults with Down syndrome (mean age at first visit = 46.3 years); 155 patients were diagnosed with depressive disorders, and 78 of whom received antidepressants for over 90 days. Of 160 patients who developed dementia, the estimated mean age at onset was 52.8 years. Longevity and age at estimated onset among those receiving and not receiving antidepressants were compared. The researchers reported that, "The mean age at dementia onset among those receiving antidepressants before onset was 53.75 years versus 52.44 years among others. Mean age at death or at end of study for those receiving antidepressants was 54.71 years; among others, it was 52.60 years...*The findings in this retrospective study revealed that antidepressant use was associated with delayed dementia onset and increased longevity in adults with Down syndrome.*"[794]

Angiotensin II Blockade

Dr. de Cavanagh, from the School of Biomedical Sciences, Austral University-Arterial Hypertension Center, Austral University Hospital, Buenos Aires, Argentina, note that, "Caloric restriction (CR), rapamycin-mediated mTOR inhibition and renin angiotensin system blockade (RAS-bl) increase survival and retard aging across species. Prolonged mTORC1 activation may lead to age-related disease progression; thus, rapamycin-mediated mTOR inhibition and CR may extend lifespan and retard aging through mTORC1 interference...Here we review how mTOR-inhibition extends lifespan, Klotho functions as an aging-suppressor, sirtuins mediate longevity, Vitamin-D loss may contribute to age-related disease, and how they relate to mitochondrial function. Also, we discuss how RAS-bl downregulates mTOR, upregulates Klotho, sirtuin and VitaminD-receptor expression, suggesting that at least some of RAS-bl benefits in aging are mediated through the modulation of mTOR, klotho and sirtuin expression and Vitamin-D signaling, paralleling CR actions in age retardation. Concluding, the available evidence endorses the idea that RAS-bl is among the interventions that may turn out to provide relief to the spreading issue of age-associated chronic disease."[795]

NSAIDS (Non-steroidal Anti-inflamatory Drugs)

According to an article published in late 2014, cheap painkillers can slow aging and fight disease:[796]

"Researchers have found that regular doses of ibuprofen can increase life expectancy. Regular doses of ibuprofen could allow people to live up to twelve years longer. In tests, the drug appears to hold back the aging process as well as helping fight disease. *Ibuprofen, which is used every day at home by people to treat inflammation, pain and fever, may be the key to developing a long sought after anti-aging drug.*

Dr Brian Kennedy, president and chief executive of the Buck Institute for Research on Aging in California, said: *"There is a lot to be excited about. The research shows that ibuprofen impacts a process not yet implicated in aging, giving us a new way to study and understand the aging process.*

Ibuprofen is a relatively safe drug, found in most people's medicine cabinets. *There is every reason to believe there are other existing treatments that can impact health span and we need to be studying them."* Lead researcher Professor Michael Polymenis of Texas A&M University agreed. He said: *"It should be possible to find other drugs like ibuprofen with even better ability to extend lifespan, with the aim of adding healthy years of life in people."*

In laboratory tests, ibuprofen was found to extend the lives of worms and flies by the equivalent of about twelve years in human terms. The creatures not only lived longer, they appeared to maintain their fitness and health as they got older. Despite the huge evolutionary gap between worms and people, the researchers believe they have found a new aspect to aging that could have major implications for humans.

It should be possible to find other drugs like ibuprofen with even better ability to extend lifespan. Professor

ALZHEIMER'S DISEASE

Polymenis said: "We are not sure why this works but it is worth exploring further. This study was a proof of principle, to show that common, relatively safe drugs in humans can extend the lifespan of very diverse organisms."

Ibuprofen is a non-steroidal anti-inflammatory drug, sold under its own name and under a variety of brand names such as Nurofen, Advil and Motrin. The World Health Organization includes the drug on its list of "essential medications." Although considered relatively safe, high doses can have harmful side effects.

In the new research, scientists exposed three test organisms – baker's yeast, the lab worm Caenorhabditis elegans and the fruit fly – to ibuprofen. The doses used were broadly the equivalent of those taken by humans. The treatment added about 15 per cent to the lives of the different species, which in human terms amounts to an extra dozen or so years of life. It was also considered to be healthy living time. Both the treated flies and worms appeared healthier in old age than those left untreated, the scientists reported in the online journal *Public Library of Science Genetics*.

Dr Kennedy said the study opens the door for a new exploration of anti-aging medicines. He added: "Our institute is interested in finding out why people get sick when they get old. "We think that by understanding those processes, we can intervene and find ways to extend human health span, keeping people healthier longer and slowing down aging. "That's our ultimate goal."

Earlier this year, researchers at Newcastle University found that the cheap anti-inflammatory drug could also help fight a host of chronic diseases such as Type 2 diabetes, arthritis and dementia.

They discovered that chronic inflammation may accelerate aging and trigger disease by stopping the body's cells regenerating. Once a patient suffers inflammation from one disease, it increases the risk of them developing other conditions.

The drug should be taken with or after food because it can damage the stomach lining. The NHS advises that anyone with questions over the use of ibuprofen should speak to their GP [general practitioner]."

Rapamycin

Rapamycin, also called sirolimus, is a drug characterized primarily by its ability to suppress the immune system, which led to its use in the prevention of transplant rejection.

In 2014, Dr. Ehnigerand and colleagues noted that, "The Federal Drug Administration (FDA)-approved compound rapamycin was the first pharmacological agent shown to extend maximal lifespan in both genders in a mammalian species. A major question then is whether the drug slows mammalian aging or if it has isolated effects on longevity by suppressing cancers, the main cause of death in many mouse strains...*Currently available evidence seems to best fit a model, wherein rapamycin extends lifespan by suppressing cancers. In addition the drug has symptomatic effects on some aging traits, such as age-related cognitive impairments.*"[797]

Dr. Richarfson and colleagues discussed the benefits of rapamycin in the December 3, 2014 issue of *Experimental Gerontology*. "The discovery that rapamycin increases lifespan in mice and restores/delays many aging phenotypes has led to the speculation that rapamycin has 'anti-aging' properties...*Rapamycin has been shown to prevent (and possibly restore in some cases) the deficit in memory observed in the mouse model of Alzheimer's disease as well as reduce Aβ and tau aggregation, restore cerebral blood flow and vascularization, and reduce microglia activation. All of these parameters are widely recognized as symptoms central to the development of AD. Furthermore, rapamycin has also been shown to improve memory and reduce anxiety and depression in several other mouse models that show cognitive deficits as well as in 'normal' mice.*"[798]

Senolytic Drugs

Dr. Zhu and thirty-two colleagues published the results of their research in the March 9, 2015 issue of *Aging Cell*, where they described the rationale for identification and validation of a new class of drugs termed senolytics, which selectively kill senescent (aging) cells. They found that, "Drugs targeting these [certain] factors selectively killed senescent cells. Dasatinib[1] eliminated senescent [aging] human fat cell progenitors [cells that turn into fat cells], while quercetin[2] was more effective against senescent human endothelial [blood vessel] cells... In vivo [here, in animal models], this combination reduced senescent cell burden in chronologically aged, radiation-exposed mice. *In old mice, cardiac function and carotid vascular reactivity were improved five days after a single dose. Following irradiation of one limb in mice, a single dose led to improved exercise capacity for at least seven months following drug treatment. Periodic drug administration extended healthspan in mice, delaying age-related symptoms and pathology, osteoporosis and loss of intervertebral disc proteoglycans. These results demonstrate the feasibility of selectively ablating [killing] senescent cells and the efficacy of senolytics for alleviating symptoms of frailty and extending healthspan.*"[799]

Metformin

Dr. Hans and colleagues, published the results of their research of the impacts of aspirin and metformin in an animal of longevity, in April

---

[1]Sprycel® (dasatinib) is a prescription medicine used to treat adults who have certain types of leukemia.
[2]Quercetin is a flavonol found in many fruits, vegetables, leaves and grains. It is commercially available as a supplement. (See wikipedia.org for more information.)

2015. They reported that, "We examined the impacts of aspirin and metformin on the life history of the cricket Acheta domesticus (growth rate, maturation time, mature body size, survivorship, and maximal longevity). Both drugs significantly increased survivorship and maximal life span. Maximal longevity was 136 days for controls, 188 days (138 % of controls) for metformin, and 194 days (143 % of controls) for aspirin. Metformin and aspirin in combination extended longevity to a lesser degree (163 days, 120 % of controls). Increases in general survivorship were even more pronounced, with low-dose aspirin yielding mean longevity 234 % of controls (i.e., health span)…Unlike the reigning dietary restriction paradigm, low aspirin conformed to a paradigm of "eat more, live longer." In contrast, metformin-treated females were only ~67 % of the mass of controls. Our results suggest that hormetic[1] agents like metformin may derive significant trade-offs with life extension, whereas health and longevity benefits may be obtained with less cost by agents like aspirin that regulate geroprotective pathways."[800]

Dr. Wang and colleagues, who published the results of their research in 2014 in the *Journal of Endocinology, Diabetes*, studied whether or not the protective effect of metformin against death is modified by frailty status in older adults with type 2 diabetes. The researchers reported that, "…of 2,415 veterans, 307 (12.7%) were metformin users, 2,108 (87.3%) were sulfonylurea users, the mean age was 73.7, the mean study period was 5.6 years, the mean HbA1c at baseline was 6.7, 23% had diabetes for ≥10 years, and 43.6% (N=1,048) died during the study period. Our study suggests that metformin could potentially promote longevity via preventing frailty in older adults with type 2 diabetes."[801]

Dr. De Haes and colleagues, publishing the results of their research in the June 17, 2014 issue of the *Proceedings of the National Academy of*

---

[1]Hormesis is the term for generally favorable biological responses to low exposures to toxins and other stressors. A pollutant or toxin showing hormesis thus has the opposite effect in small doses as in large doses. Hormetics is the term proposed for the study and science of hormesis. In toxicology, hormesis is a dose response phenomenon characterized by a low dose stimulation, high dose inhibition, resulting in either a J-shaped or an inverted U-shaped dose response.

Sciences of the United States of America, noted that,"The antiglycemic drug metformin, widely prescribed as first-line treatment of type II diabetes mellitus, has lifespan-extending properties...We show that metformin extends lifespan through the process of mitohormesis[1] and propose a signaling cascade in which metformin-induced production of reactive oxygen species increases overall life expectancy. We further address an important issue in aging research, wherein so far, the key molecular link that translates the reactive oxygen species signal into a prolongevity cue remained elusive. We show that this beneficial signal of the mitohormetic pathway is propagated by the peroxiredoxin PRDX-2. Because of its evolutionary conservation, peroxiredoxin signaling might underlie a general principle of prolongevity signaling."[802]

Supplements & Vitamins

Introduction

According to Dr. Uysal and colleagues, "Slowing aging is a widely shared goal. Plant-derived polyphenols, which are found in commonly consumed food plants such as tea, cocoa, blueberry and grape, have been proposed to have many health benefits, including slowing aging. In-vivo studies have demonstrated the lifespan-extending ability of six polyphenol-containing plants. These include five widely consumed foods (tea, blueberry, cocoa, apple, and pomegranate) and a flower commonly used as a folk medicine (betony). These and multiple other plant polyphenols have been shown to have beneficial effects on aging-associated changes across a variety of organisms from worm and fly to

---

[1]Mitohormesis: ROS (reactive oxygen species) may perform an essential and potentially lifespan-promoting role as redox signaling molecules which transduce signals from the mitochondrial compartment to other compartments of the cell. Increased formation of ROS within the mitochondria may cause an adaptive reaction which produces increased stress resistance and a long-term reduction of oxidative stress. This kind of reverse effect of the response to ROS stress has been named mitochondrial hormesis or mitohormesis and is hypothesized to be responsible for the respective lifespan-extending and health-promoting capabilities of glucose restriction and physical exercise.

rodent and human."[803] See also, berberine, immediately above, in the "Metformin" section. Vitamin D and resveratrol has also shown antiaging properties, as discussed below.

In an article published October 22, 2014 in the journal *Aging Cell*, titled, "Effects Of Vitamins And Minerals On Aging," Dr. Lee and colleagues, from the Department of Life Sciences, Pohang University of Science and Technology, Pohang, Gyeongbuk, South Korea, discussed their review based on many literature citations:[804]

> "Although vitamins and minerals are not generally considered energy sources, these essential nutrients act as cofactors for diverse biological processes, such as mitochondrial energy metabolism and hormonal signaling. Humans cannot synthesize minerals or most vitamins; therefore, these must be supplied through dietary consumption. Deficiencies of essential vitamins and minerals can impair biological functions and promote the development of various diseases. Many studies indicate that vitamins and minerals also influence organismal lifespan...
>
> Studies have shown that dietary vitamins increase lifespan in various organisms primarily by functioning as antioxidants. For example, vitamin E/tocopherol intake significantly increases the lifespan of rotifers, nematodes, and fruit flies. Vitamin E also increases the replicative lifespan of cultured adrenocortical cells and protects these cells from DNA-strand breaks in peroxide-treated conditions. Vitamin P/hesperidin increases the lifespan of yeast by reducing ROS. Supplementation of vitamin C/ascorbic acid, a well-known antioxidant, increases the lifespan of the bean beetle *Callosobruchus maculatus*. Although vitamin C feeding does not change the lifespan of *D. melanogaster*, vitamin C content declines with age in flies, suggesting that decreased vitamin C may be an indicator of aging. Furthermore, diets

that include vitamin C rescue the short lifespan of *wrn-1* (Werner helicase 1) mutant *C. elegans* by reducing the high levels of ROS and increasing the low levels of ATP in these mutant animals. Many members of the vitamin B family also lengthen the lifespan of flies, Zucker fatty rats, and *C. elegans*. For example, supplementation with vitamin B3 (nicotinic acid and nicotinamide) lengthens the lifespan of *C. elegans* through SIR-2.1, a worm homolog of SIRT1. These studies confirm the public belief that vitamins are generally beneficial for health, mostly because they moderate levels of ROS…

Although vitamins are generally considered to have beneficial effects on health, there is increasing evidence that vitamins also reduce lifespan. The antioxidant functions of vitamin C/ascorbic acid decrease the long lifespan conferred by mildly increased ROS in *C. elegans*. Feeding vitamin C and/or E shortens lifespan in the phlebotomine sand flies *Lutzomyia longipalpis* and in wild-derived voles. In addition, vitamin C feeding reduces the enhanced mitochondrial functions caused by exercise in rats. This is associated with reduced expression of PGC-1, nuclear respiratory factor 1 (NRF-1), and mitochondrial transcription factor A (mTFA), which are key transcription factors required for mitochondrial biogenesis. Consistently, vitamin C and E supplementation decreases oxidative stress but inhibits the beneficial effects of physical exercise on enhanced insulin sensitivity in humans. Vitamin E intake causes hypertension in patients with type 2 diabetes. Moreover, a mega-dose of vitamins and minerals mildly increases human mortality. A meta-analysis of 385 publications indicates that overall levels of antioxidant supplementation positively correlate with mortality. In the case of multiple sclerosis, supplementation with vitamin A for six months increases the level of C-reactive protein (CRP), which is indicative of the level of inflammation.

Because moderate levels of ROS are beneficial for health and longevity, antioxidant vitamins may interfere with the beneficial roles of ROS. In addition to these antioxidant vitamins, vitamin B9/folate displays a negative correlation with longevity in certain conditions, as reduced dietary vitamin B9 extends lifespan in *C. elegans*. Supplementation with nicotinamide, which is one form of vitamin B3, shortens the lifespan of budding yeast by decreasing the deacetylase activity of Sir2. Overall, these studies indicate that the conventional view that vitamins promote health benefits and delay aging should be modified or applied with caution…

How can we explain these differential effects of vitamin supplementation on lifespan? One plausible interpretation is hormesis, which is defined as beneficial effects of low doses of substances that are toxic at higher doses. Thus, hormetic effects of vitamins predict that high doses of vitamins have negative effects on the health and aging, while low doses are beneficial for health. In the same context, although the amount of vitamins that are required for the proper functions of our body is relatively small, deficiency of vitamins causes diseases. The triage theory may help explain the effects of vitamin deficiency on health. According to this theory, when a micronutrient is insufficient, nature prioritizes biological functions essential for short-term survival by the expense of nonessential functions. This leads to long-term consequences that may cause age-related diseases. In any case, these possibilities are consistent with the fact that adequate amounts of vitamins are crucial for the management of health.

In comparison with vitamins, the effects of dietary minerals on aging are not as well known. Examples of the beneficial effects of minerals are rare. One example is a study showing that dietary intake of selenium (Se), an antioxidant mineral, significantly reduces DNA breakage and extends the replicative lifespan of cultured adrenocortical cells. However, supplementation with high doses of minerals generally decreases organismal lifespan. Supplementation with various doses of selenium (Se), iron (Fe), manganese (Mn), copper (Cu), or zinc (Zn) leads to reduced lifespan in *D. melanogaster* and *C. elegans*. Overexpression of metal-responsive transcription factor, MTF-1, rescues the reduced lifespan of flies induced after supplementation with high, millimolar doses of metals. Thus, excessive amounts of dietary minerals are generally harmful to organisms."

According to an article by Dr. McCarty, published in April 2014:[805]

"AMP-activated kinase (AMPK) [an enzyme] is activated when the cellular (AMP+ADP)/ATP ratio rises; it therefore serves as a detector of cellular "fuel deficiency." AMPK activation is suspected to mediate some of the health-protective effects of long-term calorie restriction. Several drugs and nutraceuticals which slightly and safely impede the efficiency of mitochondrial ATP generation-most notably metformin and berberine-can be employed as clinical AMPK activators and, hence, may have potential as calorie restriction mimetics for extending health span.

Indeed, current evidence indicates that AMPK activators may reduce risk for atherosclerosis, heart attack, and stroke; help to prevent ventricular hypertrophy and manage congestive failure; ameliorate metabolic syndrome, reduce risk for type 2 diabetes, and aid glycemic control in diabetics; reduce risk for weight gain; decrease risk for a number of common cancers while improving prognosis in cancer therapy; decrease risk for dementia and possibly other neurodegenerative disorders; help to preserve the proper structure of bone and cartilage; and possibly aid in the prevention and control of autoimmunity.

While metformin and berberine appear to have the greatest utility as clinical AMPK activators-as reflected by their efficacy in diabetes management-regular ingestion of vinegar, as well as moderate alcohol consumption, may also achieve a modest degree of health-protective AMPK activation. The activation of AMPK achievable with any of these measures may be potentiated by clinical doses of the drug salicylate [Aspirin], which can bind to AMPK and activate it allosterically."

So, metformin, berberine, moderate alcohol consumption, and vinegar can help prevent disease and extend life. Furthermore, Aspirin can potentiate the positive effects of all of these.

Alpinia Zerumbet

Alpinia zerumbet, commonly known as shell ginger, is a perennial species of ginger native to East Asia. They can grow up to eight to ten feet tall and bear colorful funnel-shaped flowers. They are grown as ornamentals and their leaves are used in cuisine and traditional medicine. They are also sometimes known as the pink porcelain lily, variegated ginger or butterfly ginger.

The plant's long leaf blades are still used for wrapping zongzi. In Okinawa, Japan, *A. zerumbet* is known in the local dialect as *sannin*, or in Japanese as *getto*. Its leaves are sold as herbal tea and are also used to flavor noodles and wrap mochi rice cakes. Its tea has hypotensive, diuretic and antiulcerogenic properties. Decoction of leaves has been used during bathing to alleviate fevers. The leaves and rhizomes have been proven effective against HIV-1 integrase and neuraminidase enzymes, and has also shown anti-diabetic effect through inhibitions of formation of advanced glycation end products. The antioxidant activities of different parts of *Alpinia zerumbet* have been reported.

According to one group of researchers, "The beneficial effects of the phytochemical compounds in fruits and vegetables have been extrapolated mainly from in vitro studies or short-term dietary supplementation studies. Recent approaches using animal models of Caenorhabditis elegans are becoming quite popular, and in this regard the effects of Alpinia zerumbet leaf extract (ALP) on C. elegans lifespan were investigated under both normal and stress conditions. ALP significantly increased, mean lifespan by 22.6 percent, better than the positive control, resveratrol. Furthermore, both under thermal and oxidative stressed conditions, ALP increased the survival rate significantly better than quercetin...These results suggest that phytochemical compounds in A. zerumbet have beneficial effects on the lifespan of C. elegans, and that they can be used as a source of dietary supplements for aging and age-related diseases."[806]

Apart from its antiaging property, Dr. Bevilaqua and colleagues, reported the results of their research on Alpinia zerumbet in the April 17, 2015 issue of the journal *Pharmaceutical Biology*, noted that, "The traditional uses of Alpinia zerumbet (Pers.) B.L.Burtt & R.m.SM (Zingiberaceae), popularly known as colonia or pacová, suggest that the species has antihypertensive, diuretic, and sedative properties...Moreover, Alpinia zerumbet presented antioxidant and anxiolytic-like effects in mice...These results [showing antidepressant properties] indicated that Alpinia zerumbet most likely acts through the dopaminergic and/or noradrenergic system but not through the serotoninergic or glutamatergic systems. This study reinforces the idea that the available biodiversity in Brazil can serve as a basis for innovation in the development of new drugs."[807]

And, concerning the protective effects against cardiovascular diseases of Alpinia zerumbet, Dr. Chen, from the Department of Pharmacology of Materia Medica, Guiyang Medical University, Guiyang, Guizhou, China; and the The Key Lab of Optimal Utilization of Natural Medicine Resources, Guiyang Medical University, Guiyang, Guizhou, China, and colleagues, reported the results of their research in 2014 in the journal Evidence-Based Complementary and Alternative Medicine. They noted that, "Alpinia zerumbet is a miao folk medicinal plant widely used in the Guizhou Province of southwest China that contains several bioactive constituents and possesses protective effects against cardiovascular diseases."[808]

Drs. Tu and Tawata, reporting in the October 15, 2014 issue of the journal *Molecules*, note that, "Obesity and its related disorders have become leading metabolic diseases. In the present study, we used 3T3-L1 adipocytes [fat cells] to investigate the anti-obesity activity of hispidin and two related compounds that were isolated from Alpinia zerumbet (alpinia) rhizomes[1]. The results showed that hispidin, dihydro-5,6-dehydrokawain (DDK), and 5,6-dehydrokawain (DK) have promising anti-obesity properties...These results highlight the potential for developing hispidin and its derivatives [from Alpinia zerumbet] as anti-obesity compounds."[809]

D (Vitamin D)

A large scientific review of the literature on the relationship between vitamin D levels and death rates, by Dr. Schottker and colleagues, was published in the June 17, 2014 issue of the *British Medical Journal*. They included 26,018 men and women aged fifty to seventy-nine years from the general population in Europe and the United States, comparing vitamin D concentrations and all-cause, cardiovascular, and cancer mortality. They found that:[810]

> "25(OH)D concentrations varied strongly by season (higher in summer), country (higher in U.S. and northern Europe) and sex (higher in men), but no consistent trend with age was observed. During follow-up, 6,695 study participants died, among whom 2,624 died of cardiovascular diseases and 2,227 died of cancer. For each cohort [group] and analysis, 25(OH)D quintiles were defined with cohort and subgroup specific cut-off values.

---

[1]In botany, a rhizome is a modified subterranean stem of a plant that is usually found underground, often sending out roots and shoots from its nodes. Rhizomes are also called creeping rootstalks and rootstocks.

Comparing bottom versus top quintiles[1] resulted in a pooled risk ratio[2] of 1.57 for all-cause mortality [e.g., highest death rate in those with the lowest vitamin D levels]. Risk ratios for cardiovascular mortality were similar in magnitude to that for all-cause mortality in subjects both with and without a history of cardiovascular disease at baseline. With respect to cancer mortality, an association was only observed among subjects with a history of cancer (risk ratio, 1.70 [e.g., highest death rate in those with a history of cancer and low vitamin D blood levels]). No strong age, sex, season, or country specific differences were detected. Despite levels of 25(OH)D strongly varying with country, sex, and season, the association between 25(OH)D level and all-cause and cause-specific mortality was remarkably consistent."

Extra Virgin Olive Oil

Dr. Vasto and colleagues, reporting in 2014 in the journal *Gerontology*, note the following:[811]

"Traditional Mediterranean diet (MedDiet) is a common dietary pattern characterizing a lifestyle and culture proven to contribute to better health and quality of life in Mediterranean countries. By analyzing the diet of centenarians from the Sicani Mountains and eating habits of inhabitants of Palermo, it is reported that a close adherence to MedDiet is observed in the countryside, whereas in big towns this adherence is not so close. This has an effect on the rates of mortality at old age (and reciprocally longevity) that are lower in the countryside than in big towns. Concerning the health effects of the diet, the

---

[1] In statistics, a quantile is where the sample or population is divided into fifths.
[2] Risk ratio (or relative risk) of 1.0 means no risk, with higher values indicating increased risk, and lower values indicating lower risk.

low content of animal protein and the low glycemic index of the Sicilian MedDiet might directly modulate the insulin/IGF-1 and the mTOR pathways, known to be involved in aging and longevity. In particular, the reduction of animal protein intake may significantly reduce serum IGF-1 concentrations and inhibit mTOR activity with a down-regulation of the signal that leads to the activation of FOXO3A and, consequently, to the transcription of homeostatic genes that favor longevity. The down-regulation of both IGF-1 and mTORC1 also induces an anti-inflammatory effect. In addition to the effects on sensing pathways, many single components of MedDiet are known to have positive effects on health, reducing inflammation, optimizing cholesterol and other important risk factors of age-related diseases. However, a key role is played by polyphenols represented in high amount in the Sicilian MedDiet (in particular in extra virgin olive oil) that can work as hormetins that provide an environmental chemical signature regulating stress resistance pathways such as nuclear factor erythroid 2-related factor 2."

Dr. Menendez and colleagues, from the Metabolism and Cancer Group, Translational Research Laboratory, Catalan Institute of Oncology, Girona, Spain, report the results of their analysis of the beneficial effects of extra virgin olive oil on health in the journal *Cell Cycle*. Without delving into most of their analysis, which is very technical, we just note the following, "Aging can be viewed as a quasi-programmed phenomenon driven by the over activation of the nutrient-sensing mTOR gerogene. mTOR-driven aging can be triggered or accelerated by a decline or loss of responsiveness to activation of the energy-sensing protein AMPK, a critical gerosuppressor of mTOR. The occurrence of age-related diseases, therefore, reflects the synergistic interaction between our evolutionary path to sedentarism, which chronically increases a number of mTOR activating gero-promoters (e.g., food, growth factors, cytokines [inflammatory signaling proteins] and insulin) and the "defective design" of central metabolic integrators such as mTOR and

AMPK...nature of complex polyphenols naturally present in extra virgin olive oil (EVOO), a pivotal component of the Mediterranean style diet that has been repeatedly associated with a reduction in age-related morbid conditions and longer life expectancy...EVOO secoiridoids, which provide an effective defense against plant attack by herbivores and pathogens, are bona fide xenohormetins that are able to activate the gerosuppressor AMPK and trigger numerous resveratrol-like anti-aging transcriptomic signatures. As such, EVOO secoiridoids constitute a new family of plant-produced gerosuppressant agents that molecularly "repair" the aimless (and harmful) AMPK/mTOR-driven quasi-program that leads to aging and aging-related diseases, including cancer."[812] And that's a good thing! So, include more extra virgin olive oil in your diet.

Garlic

Dr. Huang and colleagues reported the results of their research on the effects of garlic on longevity in the April 2, 2015 issue of *The Journal of Nutritional Biochemistry*. They note that:[813]

> "The beneficial effects of garlic (Allium sativum) consumption in treating human diseases have been reported worldwide over a long period of human history. The strong antioxidant effect of garlic extract (GE) has also recently been claimed to prevent cancer, thrombus formation, cardiovascular disease and some age-related maladies. Using Caenorhabditis elegans[1] as a model organism, aqueous GE was herein shown to increase the

---

[1]*Caenorhabditis elegans* is a free-living (not parasitic), transparent nematode (roundworm), about 1 mm in length, that lives in temperate soil environments. In 1963, Sydney Brenner proposed research into *C. elegans* primarily in the area of neuronal development. In 1974, he began research into the molecular and developmental biology of *C. elegans*, which has since been extensively used as a model organism. *C. elegans* was the first multicellular organism to have its whole genome sequenced, and as of 2012, the only organism to have its connectome (neuronal "wiring diagram") completed.

expression of longevity-related FOXO transcription factor daf-16 and extend lifespan by 20%. To investigate the garlic components functionally involved in longevity, an integrated metabolo-proteomics approach was employed to identify metabolites and protein components associated with treatment of aqueous GE. Among potential lifespan-promoting substances, mannose-binding lectin and N-acetylcysteine were found to increase daf-16 expression. Our study points to the fact that the lifespan-promoting effect of aqueous GE may entail the DAF-16-mediated signaling pathway."

Resveratrol

Resveratrol has emerged in recent years as a compound conferring strong protection against metabolic, cardiovascular and other age-related complications, including neurodegeneration (such as Alzheimer's disease) and cancer. This has generated the notion that resveratrol treatment acts as a calorie-restriction mimetic, based on the many overlapping health benefits observed upon both interventions in diverse organisms, including yeast, worms, flies and rodents.[814] These organisms are the ones most often used in studies of longevity.

Caloric restriction (CR) can extend the average and maximum life span and delay the onset of age-associated changes in many organisms. CR elicits coordinated and adaptive stress responses at the cellular and whole-organism level. The overall effect of these adaptive stress responses is an increased resistance to subsequent stress, thus delaying age-related changes and promoting longevity. According to a recent report, "In humans, CR could delay many diseases associated with aging including cancer, diabetes, atherosclerosis, cardiovascular disease, and neurodegenerative diseases [such as Alzheimer's disease]. As an alternative to CR, several CR mimetics have been tested on animals and humans. At present, the most promising alternatives to the use of CR in humans seem to be exercise, alone or in combination with reduced calorie intake, *and the use of plant-derived polyphenol resveratrol as a food supplement.*"[815]

In 2015, other researchers noted that, "A number of small molecules with the ability to extend the lifespan of multiple organisms have recently been discovered. *Resveratrol, amongst the most prominent of these*, has gained widespread attention due to its ability to extend the lifespan of yeast, worms, and flies, and its ability to protect against age-related diseases such as cancer, Alzheimer's, and diabetes in mammals."[816]

Dr. Giacosa and his group, in September 2014, summed up the benefits of moderate wine drinking as follows:[817]

> "The Copenhagen Prospective Population Studies demonstrated in the year 2000 that wine intake may have a beneficial effect on all-cause mortality that is additive to that of alcohol. Wine contains various poliphenolic substances which may be beneficial for health and in particular flavonols (such as myricetin and quercetin), catechin and epicatechin, proanthocyanidins, anthocyanins, various phenolic acids and the stilbene resveratrol. *In particular, resveratrol seems to play a positive effect on longevity because it increases the expression level of Sirt1* [an enzyme, discussed below], *besides its antioxidant, anti-inflammatory and anticarcinogenic properties*. Moderate wine drinking is part of the Mediterranean diet, together with abundant and variable plant foods, high consumption of cereals, olive oil as the main fat and a low intake of meat. This healthy diet pattern involves a "Mediterranean way of drinking," that is a regular, moderate wine consumption mainly with food [up to two glasses a day for men and one glass for women is the maximum recommended amount]. Moderate wine drinking increases longevity, reduces the risk of cardiovascular diseases and does not appreciably influence the overall risk of cancer."

Sirtuins are a family of enzymes highly conserved in evolution, meaning they are present in many different species, and involved in mechanisms known to promote healthy aging and longevity. One sirtuin, *SIRT1*, is now known to promote longevity and to provide neuroprotection against cognitive aging and Alzheimer's disease pathology.[818]

Researchers demonstrated, in an animal model of aging, that resveratrol has many positive effects on health and "significantly extends the life span." They showed that the mechanism for these effects was through activation of the enzyme SIRT1.[819]

Recently, Dr. Das and his group showed that resveratrol's positive effects work though SIRT1 and other enzymes, and that this "paves the way to an anti-aging environment."[820]

Researchers studied the beneficial effects of resveratrol in an animal model of Alzheimer's disease and aging, and found that, "Resveratrol increases metabolic rate, insulin sensitivity, mitochondrial biogenesis [the creation of mitochondria] and physical endurance, and reduces fat accumulation in mice. In addition, resveratrol may be a powerful agent to prevent age-associated neurodegeneration and to improve cognitive deficits in Alzheimer's disease...We found that resveratrol supplements increased mean life expectancy and maximal life span. It also reduces cognitive impairment and has a neuroprotective role, decreasing the amyloid burden and reducing tau hyperphosphorylation [two characteristic lesions in AD]."[821]

As previously noted, not all studies (with any medical subject) are positive. Dr. Semba and colleagues, in the July 2014 issue of the journal *JAMA*, published negative findings of a study to determine whether resveratrol levels achieved with diet are associated with inflammation, cancer, cardiovascular disease, and mortality in humans. Over nine years of follow up, the researchers studied 7,832 men and women sixty-five years or older, in two villages in the Chianti area in Italy. They concluded that, "Resveratrol levels achieved with a Western diet did not have a substantial influence on health status and mortality risk of the population in this study."[822]

Also in 2014, researchers reported on experiments using animal models of aging, focusing on caloric restriction and supplementation with resveratrol. Importantly, they discovered a high rate of genetic variability in response to these two interventions. They concluded, "Thus, this experiment suggests that careful re-examination of resveratrol effects using diverse genotypes is required."[823] They implied that individual animals respond to caloric restriction and/or supplementation with resveratrol differently, and that this needs to be considered in the overall understanding of the effects of caloric restriction and/or supplementation with resveratrol.

Dr. Marchal and colleagues summarized the current situation, as of July 2013, with resveratrol in the *Annals of The New York Academy of Sciences*:[824]

> "Through its antioxidant, anticarcinogenic, and anti-inflammatory properties, resveratrol has become a candidate for drug development in the context of aging studies. Scientific evidence has highlighted its potential as a therapeutic agent for cardiovascular diseases and some cancers but also as an antiaging molecule. Resveratrol is thought to mimic the beneficial effects of chronic and moderate calorie restriction. Nevertheless, no study has demonstrated the prolongation of life span in healthy non-obese mammal models...In our opinion, more studies should be performed to assess the effects of a chronic dietary intake of resveratrol in long-lived species close to humans, such as non-human primates. This will certainly generate more evidence about the ability of resveratrol to achieve the physiological benefits that have been observed in small mammal laboratory models and feature the eventual unwanted secondary effects that may occur under high levels of resveratrol."

A similar review was reported in October 2013 by Lam and others, in the journal *Experimental Gerontology*. The authors stated:[825]

> "Calorie restriction extends lifespan and confers metabolic benefits similar to the effect of lifestyle interventions. Poor compliance to long-term dietary restriction, however, hinders the success of this approach. Evidence is now persuasive for a role of resveratrol supplementation [a polyphenol in red grapes] as potential alternative to calorie restriction. ...Resveratrol activates SIRT1 and the associated improvement in energy utilization and insulin sensitivity closely resembles the benefits of calorie restriction. Current data largely support resveratrol as a potential calorie restriction mimetic to improve metabolic and probably functional health. Future studies which characterize the bioavailability and efficacy of resveratrol supplementation are critical to provide evidence for its long-term health benefits."

An interesting experiment in honey bees was conducted in 2012 to determine the effects of resveratrol on longevity. The researchers found that, "...two resveratrol treatments [using different concentrations of resveratrol] lengthened average lifespan in wild-type honey bees by 38 percent and 33 percent, respectively. Both resveratrol treatments also lengthened maximum and median lifespan...Honey bees that were not fed resveratrol exhibited greater responsiveness to sugar, while those supplemented with resveratrol were less responsive to sugar. We also discovered that individuals fed a high dose of resveratrol-compared to controls-ingested fewer quantities of food under ad libitum [chosen by the animal] feeding conditions."[826]

And finally (for now!) two reports, the first one from 2012, the more negative, and the second report, from 2014, the more positive:

> [2012] "Resveratrol has shown evidence of decreasing cancer incidence, heart disease, metabolic syndrome and neural degeneration in animal studies. However, the ef-

fects on longevity are mixed. We aimed to quantify the current knowledge of life extension from resveratrol. We used meta-analytic techniques to assess the effect resveratrol has on survival, using data from nineteen published papers, including six species: yeast, nematodes, mice, fruit flies, Mexican fruit flies and turquoise killifish. Overall, our results indicate that resveratrol acts as a life-extending agent. The effect is most potent in yeast and nematodes, with diminished reliability in most higher-order species. Turquoise killifish were especially sensitive to life-extending effects of resveratrol but showed much variation. Much of the considerable heterogeneity in our analysis was owing to unexplained variation between studies. In summary, we can report that few species conclusively show life extension in response to resveratrol. As such, we question the practice of the substance being marketed as a life-extending health supplement for humans."[827]

[2014] "Wine is a traditional beverage that has been associated with both healthy and harmful effects. Conceptions like the so-called "French paradox" or the beneficial impact of the Mediterranean diet suggest benefit. Wine has a complex composition, which is affected by whether it is red or white or by other variables, like the variety of grapes or others. Alcohol and phenolic compounds have been attributed a participation in the benefits ascribed to wine. The case of alcohol has been extensively studied, but the key question is whether wine offers additional benefits. Resveratrol, a non-flavonoid compound, and quercetin, a flavonol, have received particular attention. There is much experimental work confirming a beneficial balance for both substances, particularly resveratrol, in various organs and systems. The pharmacological dosages used in many of those experiments have shed doubt, however, on the clinical translation of those findings. Clinical studies are limited by their observational nature as well as for the difficulties to abstract the benefits of wine from other confounders. Notwithstanding the doubts, there is reasonable unanimity in beneficial effects of moderate wine consumption in cardiovascular disease, diabetes, osteoporosis, maybe neurological diseases, and longevity. Observations are less enthusiastic in what refers to cancer. While considering these limitations, clinicians may spread the message that the balance of moderate wine consumption seems beneficial."[828]

Pomegranite Juice

Dr. Balasubramani and colleagues published the results of their research of the benefits of pomegranate juice in an animal model of longevity, in the December 16, 2014 issue of the journal *Frontiers in Public Health*. They noted that:[829]

"Rasayana is a dedicated branch of Ayurveda (an Indian medicine) that deals with methods to increase vitality and delay aging through the use of diet, herbal supplements, and other lifestyle practices. The life-span and health-span enhancing actions of the fruits of pomegranate (Punica granatum L.), a well-known Rasayana, were tested on Drosophila melanogaster (fruit fly) model. Supplementation of standard corn meal with 10 percent (v/v) pomegranate juice (PJ) extended the life-span of male and female flies by 18 and 8 percent, respectively. When male and female flies were mixed and reared together, there was 19 percent increase in the longevity of PJ fed flies, the median survival days MSD was 24.8. MSD for control and resveratrol (RV) groups was at 20.8 and 23.1 days, respectively. PJ thus outperformed both control and RV groups in the life-span and health-span parameters tested. This study provides the scope to explore the potential of PJ as a nutraceutical to improve health span and lifespan in human beings."

In an article published in the April-June 2015 issue of *Pharmacognosy Magazine*, Dr. Kihicgun and colleagues reported the results of their research using pomegranate in an animal model of longevity:[830]

"The aim of this study was to identify the possible longevity, fertility and growth promoting properties of different ethanolic extract concentrations of pomegranate in Caenorhabditis elegans, which is increasingly popular and has proven to be a very useful experimental model organism for aging studies as well as for testing antioxidants and other compounds for effects on longevity. In this study, five experimental groups (20, 10, 5, 2.5 and 1.25 mg pomegranate extract/mL and one control group) were used to determine the most effective dose of pomegranate in terms of longevity, fertility and growth parameters. It was seen that, pomegranate extracts up to the concentration of 5 mg/mL, had the potential to promote longevity, formation of new generations, fertility of new generations and growth properties of C. elegans although higher concentrations significantly reduced these parameters. These findings indicated that pomegranate could be used as a supplement to enhance longevity, fertility and growth rate for the other living organisms and human beings, but the dose should be carefully adjusted to avoid adverse effects."

Summary of Steps To Take

What steps to take is, at once, both simple and complicated. We have outlined the basic steps that we believe most people should take. More sophisticated steps have to be individually tailored. Be sure to go to our website, http://FIVESTARBRAIN.COM to sign up for periodic emails with breaking news and cutting-edge research on Alzheimer's disease and longevity, as well as times and dates of free teleseminars, webinars, and seminars.

Basic Steps To Take:

1. Exercise: This is the foundation of a healthy, long life, and preventing Alzheimer's disease. Exercise a minimum of twice weekly. Three to five times is better, but don't overdo it. You don't need a gym membership to accomplish this goal. START SLOW AND CHECK WITH YOUR HEALTH PROVIDER BEFORE YOU EMBARK ON ANY STRENUOUS EXERCISE.

   Once you are "medically cleared," work up to the point that you are consistently getting out of breath during each exercise period.

   Get your resting heart rate down, below 60 beats per minute (bpm).

   Note: Even significantly handicapped people can often do a lot more exercise than they are currently doing. Here, you should think like the military: "Yes, sir; No, sir; No excuse, sir!" No excuses!

   Biking, swimming, and many other activities are absolutely great. You can actually work up a sweat playing ping pong. For numerous reasons, a sport like racquetball might be the ideal activity. Remember, you don't have to be great at it, or even good at it; you just have to do it!

2. Minimize your sitting -- no matter how much you exercise. Stand up; walk around. Increase your speed of walking. Decrease your sit-down time.

3. Maintain good oral health -- brush, floss, and use mouthwash twice daily. See your dentist regularly.

4. Get restful sleep. Use good sleep hygiene. Sleep between 7-9 hours per night. If you are not getting good sleep, or are always tired during the day, you may have obstructive sleep apnea, which can only be diagnosed by a sleep study; speak with your healthcare provider.

5. Be mentally active.

6. Socialize.

7. If you are monolingual, become bilingual!

8. Think young.

9. Have a purpose in life.

10. Don't overuse your GPS!

11. Gradually switch to the Mediteranian Diet, or a similar healthy diet. (We are developing our own diet that will optimize the concepts outlined in this book.) Be sure to include:

    a. Extra virgin olive oil.
    b. Walnuts and other nuts (one handful per day).
    c. Berries: blueberries; strawberries; raspberries; blackberries; other berries.
    d. Fish (especially salmon, sardines, and mackerel; once or twice per week; not fried).
    e. Minimize dairy products.
    f. Minimize red meat.
    g. Eat fruits and vegetables (but minimal carrots).
    h. Drink pomegranate juice.

12. Maintain healthy weight. Most of us need to lose weight. This requires...not exercise, but eating less! Watch what you eat and eat

LONGEVITY

less! Do not eat to relieve stress…exercise or do yoga or meditate or engage in mindfulness! Do not eat to relieve boredom…don't be bored!

13. Aspirin – ask your healthcare provider if it is okay for you to take a baby (81 mg) Aspirin (ASA). Do not take without your provider giving you the go-ahead, as this can cause gastrointestinal (GI) bleeding or other serious (or even fatal) side effects.

14. Gradually start adding supplements to your diet, one at a time, in order to ensure that you can tolerate any particular supplement. The amounts are not written in stone, but are general recommendations. Here are some you can start with, listed in alphabetical order:

   a. Ashwagandha – 470 mg per day
   b. B12 – 100 to 1000 micrograms per day.
   c. Berberine – 500 mg per day.
   d. CoQ10 – 100 mg per day.
   e. Green tea –drink some regularly; take a supplement of 500 mg per day.
   f. Melatonin – 3-10 mg per night (take this whether or not you have insomnia).
   g. Omega-3 fish oil (or similar) – 300 mg (of the actual omega-3 oil) per day.
   h. Quercetin – 500 mg per day.
   i. Resveratrol – minimum 100 mg per day; better 250 mg (even twice daily). It's hard to get too much!
   j. Rhodiola – 340 mg per day
   k. Turmeric – 1000 mg per day.
   l. Vitamin D – 2000 units per day.

Basic Things to Avoid:

1. If you smoke, stop.
2. Minimize carrot intake.

3. Do not take supplemental folate unless you are pregnant, or a female who may become pregnant in the near future.
4. Do not take more than the recommended daily amount (RDA) of vitamin E (absolute maximum is 400 i.u. per day).
5. Consume minimal red meat.
6. Limit alcohol (maximum is: two drinks per day for men; one drink per day for women).
7. Limit the use of anticholinergic medications (e.g., Benadryl – which is diphenhydramine or other sleep agents (use melatonin); Elavil – which is amitriptyline. See the text for a more complete list of anticholinergic medications.
8. Don't purchase "junk food," and limit your intake.
9. Avoid refined sugar.
10. Limit soft drinks (regular or diet).
11. Limit intake of processed foods.

Conclusion

In conclusion, we all want to live a long time, be healthy, and not suffer with Alzheimer's disease. While the number of people living in the United States with Alzheimer's disease is rapidly increasing, we don't want to be among them. Fortunately, we are on the cusp of being able to easily, rapidly, and cheaply diagnose this type of dementia. Even more exciting is the fact that there are *now* preventative measures that we can take that, for most of us, can limit or stop its development. It is vital to understand that, at the present time, treatment of Alzheimer's disease is unsatisfactory. Prevention is the key. Given that the disease begins decades prior to the onset of its clinical presentation, early intervention is critical.

Wearing a seatbelt does not guarantee that you won't get into an accident, or, if you are in an accident, that you won't be seriously injured or even killed. Wearing a seatbelt does, however, shift the odds most definitely in your favor. Does stopping smoking guarantee that you won't get lung cancer? Of course not. However, doing so dramatically shifts the odds in your favor. Taking some of the steps outlined in his book does not guarantee longevity or that you will be free of Alzheimer's disease. However, taking some of these steps discussed here will definitely shift the odds of having a healthier and longer life in your favor. Statistically, you will be light years ahead.

We wish you and yours the very best—a long, healthy, and happy life.

RESOURCES

1. Alzheimer's Association (alz.org). This is, of course, the main web site for Alzheimer's disease and is loaded with lots of information.

2. For a list of the 20 best blogs in 2015 for Alzheimer's disease, go to: http://www.healthline.com/health-slideshow/best-alzheimers-dementia-blogs#1.

   One of my favorites is the Azheimer's Reading Room, run by Bob DeMarco. The goal of the Alzheimer's Reading Room is to Educate and Empower Alzheimer's caregivers, their families, and the entire Alzheimer's community; www.alzheimersreadingroom.com.

3. Fivestarbrain.com – follow for current updates about Alzheimer's disease, longevity, and wellness, operated by the author. To contact the author, just use the contact form on the website.

4. The Stadter Center: A 70-bed psychiatric hospital, which includes a 20-bed geriatric unit. Located in Grand Forks, ND. For information about the Stadter Center, go to: www.stadtercenter.com. This is owned and operated by Dr. Thomas Peterson:

   Dr. Thomas Peterson, MD, is a founding partner, president and medical director of the Stadter Center. Dr. Peterson received his Medical Doctorate at the University of North Dakota School of Medicine in Grand Forks, North Dakota. His specialty is General Psychiatry and he completed his Psychiatry Resident Program in 1994 at the University of North Dakota School of Medicine. After founding the Center of Psychiatric Care, a private outpatient mental health clinic, he in conjunction with others, founded the Stadter Center, a private inpatient mental health hospital, which opened in May of 2000. Dr. Peterson is the hospital's president and medical director, and works closely with the hospital's administrative work team. A member of the American Psychiatric Association, he received his Board Certification in Psychiatry in 1996. A true entrepreneur, Dr. Peterson is involved in the development of other medical projects to enhance the medical park upon which the Stadter Center currently resides.

5. The Center for Psychiatric Care. Affiliated with the Stadter Center, and located in the same complex, The Center provides outpatient psychiatric services, including evaluations for dementia. Information about The Center can be found at: http://www.centerforpsychiatriccare.com/. Call for an appointment for a comprehensive evaluation for dementia by the author. Telephone: (701) 772-2500.

GLOSSARY

AD. This is the abbreviation used for Alzheimer's disease in the text.

ADLs. This is the abbreviation for activities of daily living, a term used in healthcare to refer to daily self-care activities. ADLs are defined as "the things we normally do...such as feeding ourselves, bathing, dressing, grooming, work, homemaking, and leisure."

ADAPTOGENIC or ADAPTOGENS. These are substances, compounds, herbs whose

administration results in stabilization of physiological processes and promotion of homeostasis, an example being by decreased cellular sensitivity to stress.

AFFECTIVE. In psychology and psychiatry this refers to emotionality; for example, being happy or sad. It can also refer to the look on someone's face.

AGNOSIA. This is the inability to process sensory information; a failure to recognize.

ALLELE. One of a number of alternative forms of the same gene or same genetic locus.

AMYLOID. Amyloids are insoluble fibrous protein aggregates sharing specific structural traits. They arise from at least eighteen inappropriately folded versions of proteins and polypeptides present naturally in the body. These misfolded structures alter their proper configuration such that they erroneously interact with one another or other cell components, forming insoluble fibrils. They have been associated with the pathology of more than twenty serious human diseases in that abnormal accumulation of amyloid fibrils in organs may lead to amyloidosis, and may play a role in various neurodegenerative disorders.

AMYLOID B-PEPTIDE (AB). The amyloid-β peptide protein fragment that aggregates into clumps called "plaques" in the brains of Alzheimer's disease patients.

AMINO ACIDs. Biologically important organic compounds composed of amine (-NH$_2$) and carboxylic acid (-COOH) functional groups, along with a side-chain specific to each amino acid. The key elements of an amino acid are carbon, hydrogen, oxygen, and nitrogen, though other elements are found in the side-chains of certain amino acids. About 500 amino acids are known and can be classified in many ways.

ANIMAL MODELS (OF ALZHEIMER'S DISEASE). Mice, which are genetically modified in a variety of ways, are most commonly used to study Alzheimer's disease.

ANIMAL MODELS (OF LONGEVITY). Fruit flies, specific worms, mice, and a large variety of other species are used to study longevity.

ANTICHOLINERGIC. An anticholinergic agent is a substance that blocks the neurotransmitter acetylcholine in the central and the peripheral nervous system. Anticholinergics inhibit parasympathetic nerve impulses by selectively blocking the binding of the neurotransmitter acetylcholine to its receptor in nerve cells. The nerve fibers of the parasympathetic system are responsible for the involuntary movement of smooth muscles present in the gastrointestinal tract, urinary tract, lungs, etc. Anticholinergic side effects from a medication might include dry mouth, constipation, blurry vision, confusion, difficulty urinating, memory impairment, and fast heart rate.

ANTIOXIDANT. An antioxidant is a molecule that inhibits the oxidation of other molecules. Oxidation is a chemical reaction involving the loss of electrons or an increase in oxidation state. Oxidation reactions can produce free radicals. In turn, these radicals can start chain reactions. When the chain reaction occurs in a cell, it can cause damage or death to the cell. Antioxidants terminate these chain reactions by removing free radical intermediates, and inhibit other oxidation reactions.

ANTIPSYCHOTIC. Antipsychotics (also known as neuroleptics or major tranquilizers) are a class of psychiatric medication primarily used to manage psychosis (including delusions, hallucinations, or disordered thought), in particular in schizophrenia and bipolar disorder, and are increasingly being used in the management of non-psychotic disorders, such as agitation associated with dementia or delirium.

APOE4 (APOLIPOPROTEIN E4) ALLELE. Apolipoprotein E (ApoE) is a class of apolipoproteins. In the central nervous system, ApoE is mainly produced by astrocytes (specific nerve cells), and transports cholesterol to neurons via ApoE receptors. ApoE has three major types (called "alleles"): ApoE2, ApoE3, and ApoE4. Although these allelic forms differ from each other by only one or two amino acids, these differences alter apoE structure and function. E4 has a frequency of approximately 14 percent. E4 has been implicated in atherosclerosis, Alzheimer's disease, impaired cognitive function, reduced hippocampal volume, HIV, faster disease progression in multiple sclerosis, unfavorable outcome after traumatic brain injury, ischemic cerebrovascular disease, sleep apnea, accelerated telomere shortening and reduced neurite outgrowth.

APP (AMYLOID PRECURSOR PROTEIN). The membrane protein present in many tissues and concentrated in the synapses of neurons. Its primary function is not known, though it has been implicated as a regulator of synapse formation, neural plasticity and iron export. APP is best known as the precursor molecule whose cleavage generates beta amyloid or amyloid B peptide (Aβ). a 37 to 49 amino acid peptide whose amyloid fibrillar form is the primary component of amyloid plaques found in the brains of Alzheimer's disease patients.

APRAXIA. A motor disorder caused by damage to the brain, in which someone has difficulty with the motor planning to perform tasks or movements when asked, provided that the request or command is understood and he/she is willing to perform the task.

ASTROCYTES. A type of nerve cell. These are also known collectively as astroglia, are characteristic star-shaped glial cells in the brain and spinal cord. They are the most abundant cells of the human brain. They perform many functions, including biochemical support of endothelial cells that form the blood–brain barrier, provision of nutrients to the nervous tissue, maintenance of extracellular ion balance, and a role in the repair and scarring process of the brain and spinal cord following traumatic injuries.

ATROPHY. The partial or complete wasting away of a part of the body. In Alzheimer's disease, this means shrinkage of the brain.

AUTOPHAGY (OR AUTOPHAGOCYTOSIS). The basic mechanism that involves cell degradation of unnecessary or dysfunctional cellular components.

B-AMYLOID (AB) PEPTIDE – BETA AMYLOID. See "AMYLOID B-PEPTIDE (AB)" above.

BBB (BLOOD-BRAIN BARRIER). The blood–brain barrier (BBB) is a highly selective permeability barrier that separates the circulating blood from the brain extracellular fluid (BECF) in the central nervous system (CNS). The blood–brain barrier is formed by capillary endothelial cells, which are connected by tight junctions. The blood–brain barrier allows the passage of water, some gases, and lipid soluble molecules by passive diffusion, as well as the selective transport of molecules such as glucose and amino acids that are crucial to neural function.

BIMS (Brief Interview for Mental Status). This is similar to the MMSE, but is used primarily for elderly patients in nursing homes as part of the Minimum Data Set 3.0 (MDS 3.0), which is part of the Centers for Medicare and Medicaid Services (CMS) requirements. It is used as a performance-based cognitive screener that can be easily completed by nursing home staff. The range of scores is 0-15, with 15 being the best possible scores. The cutoff for normal is 12. Below this is considered abnormal, and indicates possible early dementia.

BIOMARKERS. A biomarker, or biological marker, generally refers to a measurable indicator of some biological state or condition. Biomarkers are often measured and evaluated to examine normal biological processes, pathogenic processes, or pharmacologic responses to a therapeutic intervention. Many things, including routine blood tests, are biomarkers.

BIOAVAILABILITY. The proportion of a drug or other substance that enters the circulation when introduced into the body and so is able to have an active effect.

BODY MASS INDEX (BMI). This is a measure of relative size based on the mass and height of an individual. The BMI for a person is defined as their body mass divided by the square of their height—with the value universally being given in units of kg/m^2. So if the weight is in kilograms and the height in meters, the result is immediate, if pounds and inches are used, a conversion factor of 703 $(kg/m^2)/(lb/in^2)$ must be applied.

BRAIN-DERIVED NEUROTROPHIC FACTOR (BDNF). BDNF is a protein and a member of the neurotrophin family of growth factors, which are related to Nerve Growth Factor. Neurotrophic factors are found in the brain and the periphery. BDNF acts on certain neurons (nerve cells) of the central nervous system and the peripheral nervous system, helping to support the survival of existing neurons, and encourage the growth and differentiation of new neurons and synapses. In the brain, it is active in the hippocampus, cortex, and basal forebrain—areas vital to learning, memory, and higher thinking.

CAPGRAS DELUSION (OR CAPGRAS SYNDROME). A disorder in which a person has a delusion that a friend, spouse, parent, or other close family member (or pet) has been replaced by an identical-looking impostor.

CARDIOVASCULAR. Of or relating to the heart and blood vessels.

CARDIOVASCULAR RISK FACTORS. Traditional risk factors include such things as high blood pressure (hypertension), smoking, obesity, age, lack of physical activity, high cholesterol (hyperlipidemia). However, there are now many other risk factors that also have to be considered. For a full discussion, see: http://emedicine.medscape.com/article/164163-overview.

CIRCADIAN. For biological processes, recurring naturally on a twenty-four-hour cycle, even in the absence of light fluctuations. Referred to as a "circadian rhythm."

CORONARY ARTERY DISEASE (CAD). Also known as atherosclerotic heart disease (ASHD), coronary heart disease (CHD), or ischemic heart disease (IHD), is the most common type of heart disease and cause of heart attacks. The disease is caused by plaque building up along the inner walls of the arteries of the heart, which narrows the lumen (opening) of arteries and reduces blood flow to the heart.

CEREBRAL CORTEX. The furrowed outer layer of gray matter in the cerebrum of the brain, associated with the higher brain functions, as voluntary movement, coordination of sensory information, learning and memory, and the expression of individuality.

CHOLESTEROL. A sterol that occurs in all animal tissues, especially in the brain, spinal cord, and adipose tissue, functioning chiefly as a protective agent in the skin and myelin sheaths of nerve cells, a detoxifier in the bloodstream, and as a precursor of many steroids: deposits of cholesterol form in certain pathological conditions, as gallstones and atherosclerotic plaques.

COGNITION (AND COGNITIVE). The act or process of knowing or thinking; perception.

CONTROL SUBJECTS. In a clinical trial, the group that does not receive the new treatment being studied. This group is compared to the group that receives the new treatment, to see if the new treatment works.

CORTEX. The outer region of an organ or structure, as the outer portion of the brain.

CORTICAL GRAY MATTER. The gray nervous tissue found in the cortex of the cerebrum and cerebellum. It is predominantly composed of neuron cell bodies and unmyelinated axons.

CT (COMPUTED TOMOGRAPHY) SCAN. The abbreviated term for computed or computerized axial tomography. The test may involve injecting a radioactive contrast into the body. Computers are used to scan for radiation and create cross-sectional images of internal organs. This is the most common type of "brain scan."

CYTOKINES. Are a broad and loose category of small proteins that are important in cell signaling. They are released by cells and affect the behavior of other cells. Cytokines include chemokines, interferons, interleukins, lymphokines, and tumor necrosis factor. They act through receptors, and are especially important in the immune system. They are important in health and disease, specifically in host responses to infection, immune responses, inflammation, trauma, sepsis, cancer, and reproduction.

DELUSIONS. A delusion is an unshakable belief in something untrue. These irrational beliefs defy normal reasoning, and remain firm even when overwhelming proof is presented to dispute them. Delusions are often accompanied by hallucinations and/or feelings of paranoia, which act to strengthen confidence in the delusion. Delusions are distinct from culturally or religiously based beliefs that may be seen as untrue by outsiders.

DEMENTIA. A loss of mental ability severe enough to interfere with normal activities of daily living, lasting more than six months, not present since birth, and not associated with a loss or alteration of consciousness. Dementia is a group of symptoms caused by gradual death of brain cells. The loss of cognitive abilities that occurs with dementia leads to impairments in memory, reasoning, planning, and behavior. While the overwhelming number of people with dementia are elderly, dementia is not an inevitable part of aging; instead, dementia is caused by specific brain diseases. Alzheimer's disease is the most common cause, followed by vascular or multi-infarct dementia.

DNA (DEOXYRIBONUCLEIC ACID). Double helix molecule containing nucleotide bases adenine (A), guanine (G), cytosine (C), and thymine (T). It carries the cell's genetic information and hereditary characteristics via its nucleotides and their sequence and is capable of self-replication and RNA synthesis.

DOPAMINE. A monoamine neurotransmitter formed in the brain and essential to the normal functioning of the central nervous system. A reduction in its concentration within the brain is associated with Parkinson's disease. It is the main neurotransmitter associated with pleasure. Too much dopamine is associated with psychosis and schizophrenia.

EFFICACY. In the context of evidence-based medicine, the capacity of a drug or therapy to positively influence the course or duration of a disease at the dose tested in the patient population for which it is designed and has been tested.

ELECTRON MICROSCOPY. The electron microscope is a type of microscope that uses a beam of electrons to create an image of the specimen. It is capable of much higher magnifications and has a greater resolving power than a light microscope, allowing it to see much smaller objects in finer detail.

ENDOGENOUS. Growing or originating from within an organism.

ENDOTHELIAL. The endothelium is the thin layer of simple squamous cells that lines the interior surface of blood vessels and lymphatic vessels, forming an interface between circulating blood or lymph in the lumen and the rest of the vessel wall.

EPIDEMIOLOGY. Epidemiology is the science that studies the patterns, causes, and effects of health and disease conditions in defined populations. It is the cornerstone of public health, and informs policy decisions and evidence-based practice by identifying risk factors for disease and targets for preventive healthcare.

EPIGENETIC. Epigenetics is the study of cellular and physiological trait variations that are *not* caused by changes in the DNA sequence; epigenetics describes the study of dynamic alterations in the transcriptional potential of a cell. These alterations may or may not be heritable, although the use of the term epigenetic to describe processes that are not heritable is controversial.

EXECUTIVE FUNCTION. An umbrella term for the management (regulation, control) of cognitive processes, including working memory, reasoning, task flexibility, and problem solving, as well as planning and execution.

ETIOLOGY. The cause, set of causes, or manner of causation of a disease or condition.

FDA (FOOD and DRUG ADMINISTRATION). A United States Federal agency responsible for monitoring trading and safety standards in the food and drug industries. Any new medication must be approved by the FDA before it can be marketed for use in the United States.

FLAVONOIDS. Any of a group of oxygen-containing aromatic antioxidant compounds that includes many common pigments (as the anthocyanins and flavones).

FOLATE (FOLIC ACID). Folic acid or folate is a B vitamin. It is also referred to as vitamin B_9. Food supplement manufacturers often use the term *folate* for something different than "pure" folic acid. *Folate* indicates a collection of "folates" that is not chemically well-characterized. Folic acid is synthetically produced, and used in fortified foods and supplements.

FREE RADICAL. Free radicals play an important role in a number of biological processes. Many of these are necessary for life, such as the killing of bacteria by white blood cells. However, because of their reactivity, these same free radicals can participate in unwanted side reactions resulting in cell damage. Excessive amounts of these free radicals can lead to cell injury and death, which may contribute to many diseases such as cancer, stroke, myocardial infarction, diabetes, neurodegenerative disorders (e.g., Alzheimer's disease, Parkinson's disease, and so forth), and other diseases.

GENETIC. In biology, the science of genes, heredity, and the variation of organisms.

GERIATRICS. Geriatrics or geriatric medicine is a specialty that focuses on health care of elderly people. It aims to promote health by preventing and treating diseases and disabilities in older adults. There is no set age at which patients may be under the care of a geriatrician or geriatric physician, a physician who specializes in the care of elderly people. Rather, this decision is determined by the individual patient's needs, and the availability of a specialist.

Geriatrics, the care of aged people, differs from gerontology which is the study of the aging process itself.

GLUCOSE. A sugar that is made during photosynthesis in plants from water and carbon dioxide, using energy from sunlight. Glucose is a primary source of energy for the brain, so its availability influences psychological processes. When glucose is low, psychological processes requiring mental effort (e.g., self-control, effortful decision-making) are impaired.

GREY (GRAY) MATTER. A major component of the central nervous system, consisting of neuronal cell bodies, neuropil (dendrites and myelinated as well as unmyelinated axons), glial cells (astroglia and oligodendrocytes), synapses, and capillaries. Grey matter is distinguished from white matter, in that grey matter contains numerous cell bodies and relatively few myelinated axons, while white matter is composed chiefly of long-range myelinated axon tracts and contains relatively very few cell bodies.

HALLUCINATIONS. A perception in the absence of external stimulus that has qualities of real perception. Hallucinations are vivid, substantial, and located in external objective space. Hallucinations can occur in any sensory modality, with the primary modalities being visual, auditory (sound), olfactory (smell), gustatory (taste), and tactile (touch).

HDL (HIGH-DENSITY LIPOPROTEINS). One of the five major groups of lipoproteins. HDL are sometimes referred to as "good cholesterol" because they can transport fat molecules (including cholesterol, triglycerides, etc.) out of artery walls, and thus help prevent, even regress atherosclerosis over weeks, years, decades, thereby helping prevent cardiovascular disease, stroke(s) and other vascular disease complications body wide.

HEAVY METALS. There is no widely agreed criteria-based definition of a heavy metal. Numerous metals can be toxic at high levels. Three very toxic heavy metals, that are tested for in a blood test referred to as a "heavy metal screen," are lead, arsenic, and mercury.

HEMOSTASIS. The arrest of bleeding by the physiological properties of vasoconstriction and coagulation.

HIPPOCAMPUS. A major component of the brains of humans and other vertebrates. Humans and other mammals have two hippocampi, one in each side of the brain. The hippocampus belongs to the limbic system and plays important roles in the consolidation of information from short-term memory to long-term memory and spatial navigation. The hippocampus is located under the cerebral cortex.

HOMOCYSTEINE. A naturally occurring amino acid found in blood plasma. High levels of homocysteine in the blood are believed to increase the chance of heart disease, stroke, Alzheimer's disease, and osteoporosis.

HYPERCHOLESTEROLEMIA. Hypercholesterolemia (also sometimes referred to as dyslipidemia or hyperlipidemia) is the presence of high levels of cholesterol in the blood.

HYPERGLYCEMIA. Condition characterized by excessively high levels of glucose in the blood, and occurs when the body does not have enough insulin or cannot use the insulin it does have to turn glucose into energy. Hyperglycemia is often indicative of diabetes that is out of control.

HYPERTENSION (NTH). Hypertension is high blood pressure. Blood pressure is the force of blood pushing against the walls of arteries as it flows through them. Arteries are the blood vessels that carry oxygenated blood from the heart to the body's tissues. As blood flows through arteries it pushes against the inside of the artery walls. The more pressure the blood exerts on the artery walls, the higher the blood pressure will be.

Blood pressure is highest when the heart beats to push blood out into the arteries. When the heart relaxes to fill with blood again, the pressure is at its lowest point. Blood pressure when the heart beats is called systolic pressure. Blood pressure when the heart is at rest is called diastolic pressure. When blood pressure is measured, the systolic pressure is stated first and the diastolic pressure second. Blood pressure is measured in millimeters of mercury (mm Hg). For example, if a person's systolic pressure is 120 and diastolic pressure is 80, it is written as 120/80 mm Hg. A normal reading is now considered to be less than 120 over less than 80.

Hypertension is a major health problem, especially because it has no symptoms. Many people have hypertension without knowing it. In the United States, about 50 million people age six and older have high blood pressure. Hypertension is more common in men than women and in people over the age of sixty-five than in younger persons. More than half of all Americans over the age of sixty-five have hypertension. It also is more common in African-Americans than in white Americans.

Hypertension is serious because people with the condition have a higher risk for heart disease and other medical problems than people with normal blood pressure. Serious complications can be avoided by getting regular blood pressure checks and treating hypertension as soon as it is diagnosed.

INCIDENCE. The rate at which a certain event occurs, as the number of new cases of a specific disease occurring during a certain period in a population at risk.

INSULIN RESISTANCE. Insulin resistance is a condition in which cells fail to respond to the normal actions of the hormone insulin. The body (pancreas) produces insulin, but the cells in the body become resistant to insulin and are unable to use it as effectively, leading to elevated blood sugar (hyperglycemia). Beta cells in the pancreas subsequently increase their production of insulin, further contributing to elevated insulin levels (hyperinsulinemia).

INTRACELLULAR. Occurring or situated within a cell or cells.

IN VITRO. Studies that are performed with cells or biological molecules studied outside their normal biological context; for example proteins are examined in solution, or cells in artificial culture medium. Colloquially called "test tube experiments." these studies in biology and its sub-disciplines are traditionally done in test-tubes, flasks, petri dishes, and so forth. In contrast, *in vivo* studies are those conducted in animals including humans, and whole plants.

IN VIVO. Occurring or carried out in a living organism.

KETONE BODIES. Three water-soluble molecules that are produced by the liver from fatty acids during periods of low food intake (fasting) or carbohydrate restriction for cells of the body to use as energy instead of glucose.

LDL (LOW-DENSITY LIPOPROTEINS). One of the five major groups of lipoproteins. LDL particles are sometimes referred to as "bad cholesterol" because they can transport their content of fat molecules into artery walls, attract macrophages (shite blood cells), and thus drive atherosclerosis.

LEPTIN. The "satiety hormone," is a hormone made by fat cells, which regulates the amount of fat stored in the body. It does this by adjusting both the sensation of hunger, and adjusting energy expenditures. Hunger is inhibited (satiety) when the amount of fat stored reaches a certain level. Leptin is then secreted and circulates through the body, eventually activating leptin receptors in the hypothalamus.

LIPID. A group of naturally occurring molecules that include fats, waxes, sterols, fat-soluble vitamins (such as vitamins A, D, E, and K), monoglycerides, diglycerides, triglycerides, phospholipids, and others. The main biological functions of lipids include storing energy, signaling, and acting as structural components of cell membranes. Although the term *lipid* is sometimes used as a synonym for fats, fats are a subgroup of lipids called triglycerides. Lipids also encompass molecules such as fatty acids and their derivatives (including tri-, di-, monoglycerides, and phospholipids), as well as other sterol-containing metabolites such as cholesterol.

MCI (MILD COGNITIVE IMPAIRMENT). A brain function syndrome involving the onset and evolution of cognitive impairments beyond those expected based on the age and education of the individual, but which are not significant enough to interfere with their daily activities. It may occur as a transitional stage between normal aging and dementia. Although MCI can present with a variety of symptoms, when memory loss is the predominant symptom it is termed "amnestic MCI" and is frequently seen as a prodromal stage of Alzheimer's disease. Studies suggest that these individuals tend to progress to probable Alzheimer's disease at a rate of approximately 10 to 15 percent per year.

MELATONIN. A substance found in essentially all animals, plants, fungi and bacteria. In animals, melatonin is involved in the entrainment (synchronization) of the circadian rhythms of physiological functions including sleep timing, blood pressure regulation, seasonal reproduction and many others. Many of melatonin's biological effects in animals are produced through activation of melatonin receptors, while others are due to its role as a pervasive and powerful antioxidant, with a particular role in the protection of nuclear and mitochondrial DNA.

THE METABOLIC EQUIVALENT OF TASK (MET). Also referred to as simply metabolic equivalent, it is a physiological measure expressing the energy cost of physical activities and is defined as the ratio of metabolic rate (and therefore the rate of energy consumption) during a specific physical activity to a reference metabolic rate. 1 MET is also defined as 58.2 W/m^2 (18.4 $Btu/h·ft^2$), which is equal to the rate of energy produced per unit surface area of an average person seated at rest.

META-ANALYSIS. In statistics, meta-analysis comprises statistical methods for contrasting and combining results from different studies in the hope of identifying patterns among study results, sources of disagreement among those results, or other interesting relationships that may come to light in the context of multiple studies. Meta-analysis can be thought of as "conducting research about previous research."

MITOCHONDRION (PLURAL = MITOCHONDRIA). A membrane-bound organelle found in most cells. Mitochondria range from 0.5 to 1.0 μm in diameter. These structures are sometimes described as "the powerhouse of the cell" because they generate most of the cell's supply of adenosine triphosphate (ATP), used as a source of chemical energy. In addition to supplying cellular energy, mitochondria are involved in other tasks such as signaling, cellular differentiation, cell death, as well as maintaining the control of the cell cycle and cell growth.

MMSE (MINI MENTAL STATUS EXAM). A sensitive, valid and reliable 30-point questionnaire that is used extensively in clinical and research settings to measure cognitive impairment. It is commonly used to screen for dementia. It is also used to estimate the severity and progression of cognitive impairment and to follow the course of cognitive changes in an individual over time; thus making it an effective way to document an individual's response to treatment.

MORBIDITY. A diseased state, disability, or poor health due to any cause. The term may be used to refer to the existence of any form of disease, or to the degree that the health condition affects the patient. Comorbidity is the simultaneous presence of two or more medical conditions, such as schizophrenia and substance abuse. In epidemiology and actuarial science, the term "morbidity rate" can refer to either the incidence rate, or the prevalence of a disease or medical condition. This measure of sickness is contrasted with the mortality rate of a condition, which is the proportion of people dying during a given time interval.

MORPHOLOGY. In biology, the study of the form or shape of an organism or part thereof.

MORTALITY. The state of being mortal, or susceptible to death; the opposite of immortality. Mortality rate is a measure of the number of deaths in a given population.

MRI (MAGNETIC RESONANCE IMAGING). A medical imaging technique used in radiology to investigate the anatomy and physiology of the body in both health and disease. MRI scanners use magnetic fields and radio waves to form images of the body. The technique is widely used in hospitals for medical diagnosis, staging of disease and for follow-up without exposure to ionizing radiation (which is used with CAT or CT scans, for example).

mTOR. The mechanistic target of rapamycin, also known as mammalian target of rapamycin, is a protein kinase (enzyme) that regulates cell growth, cell proliferation, cell motility, cell survival, protein synthesis, transcription, and longevity.

MYELIN. A dielectric (electrically insulating) material that forms a layer, the myelin sheath, usually around only the axon of a neuron (nerve cell). It is essential for the proper functioning of the nervous system. It is an outgrowth of a type of glial cell. The production of the myelin sheath is called myelination.

MYOPATHY. A muscular disease in which the muscle fibers do not function for any one of many reasons, resulting in muscular weakness. This meaning implies that the primary defect is within the muscle, as opposed to the nerves ("neuropathies" or "neurogenic" disorders) or elsewhere (e.g., the brain). Muscle cramps, stiffness, and spasm can also be associated with myopathy.

N. The number of individuals in an experimental study.

NEURODEGENERATIVE. The umbrella term for the progressive loss of structure or function of neurons (nerve cells), including death of neurons. Many neurodegenerative diseases including ALS, Parkinson's, Alzheimer's, and Huntington's occur as a result of neurodegenerative processes.

NEUROGENESIS. Neurogenesis (birth of neurons) is the process by which neurons are generated from the neural stem cells and progenitor cells. Neurogenesis is most active during pre-natal development, and is responsible for populating the growing brain with neurons. Neurogenesis has been shown to occur in two parts of the brains of adult mammals: the hippocampus and the subventricular zone.

NEUROINFLAMMATION. inflammation of the nervous tissue. It may be initiated in response to a variety of cues, including infection, traumatic brain injury, toxic metabolites, or autoimmunity. In the central nervous system, including the brain and spinal cord, microglia are the resident innate immune cells that are activated in response to these cues.

NEURON. Also known as a neuron or nerve cell is an electrically excitable cell that processes and transmits information through electrical and chemical signals. These signals between neurons occur via synapses, specialized connections with other cells. Neurons can connect to each other to form neural networks. Neurons are the core components of the nervous system, which includes the brain, spinal cord–which together comprise the central nervous system (CNS)–and the ganglia of the peripheral nervous system.

NEUROPATHOLOGY. The study of disease of nervous system tissue, usually in the form of either small surgical biopsies or whole autopsies. Neuropathology is a subspecialty of anatomic pathology, neurology, and neurosurgery. It should not be confused with neuro*pathy*, which refers to disorders of the nerves (usually in the peripheral nervous system).

NEUROPSYCHIATRY. A branch of medicine that deals with mental disorders attributable to diseases of the nervous system. It preceded the current disciplines of psychiatry and neurology, which had common training. However, psychiatry and neurology subsequently split apart and are typically practiced separately. Nevertheless, neuropsychiatry has become a growing subspecialty of psychiatry and it is also closely related to the fields of neuropsychology and behavioral neurology, which is a subspecialty of neurology that addresses clinical problems of cognition and/or behavior caused by brain injury or brain disease of different etiologies.

NEUROTOXICITY. Neurotoxicity occurs when exposure to natural or artificial toxic substances, which are called neurotoxins, alters the normal activity of the nervous system in such a way as to cause damage to nervous tissue. This can eventually disrupt or even kill neurons, key cells that transmit and process signals in the brain and other parts of the nervous system. Neurotoxicity can result from exposure to substances used in chemotherapy, radiation treatment, drug therapies, certain drug abuse, and organ transplants, as well as exposure to heavy metals, certain foods and food additives, pesticides, industrial and/or cleaning solvents, cosmetics, and some naturally occurring substances. Symptoms may appear immediately after exposure or be delayed. They may include limb weakness or numbness, loss of memory, vision, and/or intellect, uncontrollable obsessive and/or compulsive behaviors, delusions, headache, cognitive and behavioral problems and sexual dysfunction.

NEUROTROPHIC FACTORS. A family of proteins that are responsible for the growth and survival of developing neurons (nerve cells) and the maintenance of mature neurons. Recent research has shown that neurotrophic factors promote the initial growth and development of neurons in the central nervous system and peripheral nervous system and that they are capable of regrowing damaged neurons in test tubes and animal models. Neurotrophic factors are often released by the target tissue in order to guide the growth of developing axons.

NEUROTRANSMITTER. Neurotransmitters are endogenous (produced within the body) chemicals that transmit signals across a synapse from one neuron (nerve cell) to another "target" neuron. Neurotransmitters are released from synaptic vesicles in synapses into the synaptic cleft, where they are received by receptors on other synapses. Many neurotransmitters are synthesized from plentiful and simple precursors such as amino acids, which are readily available from the diet and only require a small number of biosynthetic steps to convert them. Neurotransmitters play a major role in shaping everyday life and functions. Their exact numbers are unknown but more than 100 chemical messengers have been identified. Some examples include dopamine, serotonin, norepinephrine, and glutamate.

NOREPINEPHRINE. A catecholamine with multiple roles including those as a hormone and a neurotransmitter. It is the hormone and neurotransmitter most responsible for vigilant concentration in contrast to the chemically similar hormone, dopamine, which is most responsible for cognitive alertness.

OBSERVATIONAL STUDY. In epidemiology and statistics, an observational study draws inferences about the possible effect of a treatment on subjects, where the assignment of subjects into a treated group versus a control group is outside the control of the investigator. This is in contrast with experiments, such as randomized controlled trials, where each subject is randomly assigned to a treated group or a control group.

OXYGEN "FREE" RADICALS. A radical (often, but unnecessarily called a free radical) is an atom or group of atoms that have one or more unpaired electrons. Radicals can have positive, negative or neutral charge. They are formed as necessary intermediates in a variety of normal biochemical reactions, but when generated in excess or not appropriately controlled, radicals can wreak havoc on a broad range of macromolecules. A prominent feature of radicals is that they have extremely high chemical reactivity, which explains not only their normal biological activities, but how they inflict damage on cells. There are many types of radicals, but those of most concern in biological systems are derived from oxygen, and known collectively as *reactive oxygen species*. Oxygen has two unpaired electrons in separate orbitals in its outer shell. This electronic structure makes oxygen especially susceptible to radical formation. Free radicals play an important role in a number of biological processes. Many of these are necessary for life, such as the intracellular killing of bacteria. Researchers have also implicated free radicals in certain cell signaling processes known as redox signaling. The two most important oxygen-centered radicals are superoxide and hydroxyl radical. They derive from molecular oxygen under reducing conditions. However, because of their reactivity, these same radicals can participate in unwanted side reactions resulting in cell damage. Excessive amounts of these radicals can lead to cell injury and death, which may contribute to many diseases such as Alzheimer's disease, cancer, stroke, myocardial infarction, diabetes and other major disorders.

OXIDATIVE STRESS. Oxidative stress reflects an imbalance between the systemic manifestation of reactive oxygen species and a biological system's ability to readily detoxify the reactive intermediates or to repair the resulting damage. Disturbances in the normal redox state of cells can cause toxic effects through the production of peroxides and free radicals that damage all components of the cell, including proteins, lipids, and DNA. Oxidative stress from oxidative metabolism causes base damage, as well as strand breaks in DNA. Some reactive oxidative species act as cellular messengers in redox signaling. Thus, oxidative stress can cause disruptions in normal mechanisms of cellular signaling. In humans, oxidative stress is thought to be involved in the development of cancer, Parkinson's disease, Alzheimer's disease, atherosclerosis, heart failure, myocardial infarction, fragile X syndrome, Sickle Cell Disease, lichen planus, vitiligo, autism, infection, and chronic fatigue syndrome. However, reactive oxygen species can be beneficial, as they are used by the immune system as a way to attack and kill pathogens. Short-term oxidative stress may also be important in prevention of aging by induction of a process named mitohormesis.

PARKINSON'S DISEASE. Also known as paralysis agitans; a degenerative disorder of the central nervous system mainly affecting the motor system. The motor symptoms of Parkinson's disease result from the death of dopamine-generating cells in the substantia nigra, a region of the midbrain. The cause of this cell death is poorly understood. Early in the course of the disease, the most obvious symptoms are movement-related; these include shaking, rigidity, slowness of movement and difficulty with walking and gait. Later, thinking and behavioral problems may arise, with dementia commonly occurring in the advanced stages of the disease, whereas depression is the most common psychiatric symptom. Other symptoms include sensory, sleep and emotional problems. Parkinson's disease is more common in older people, with most cases occurring after the age of 50; when it is seen in young adults, it is called young onset PD (YOPD).

PATHOGENESIS. The pathogenesis of a disease is the biological mechanism (or mechanisms) that lead to the diseased state. The term can also describe the origin and development of the disease, and whether it is acute, chronic, or recurrent. The pathogenic mechanisms of a disease (or condition) are set in motion by underlying etiological causes, which if controlled would allow the disease to be prevented.

PATHOLOGY. A significant component of the causal study of disease and a major field in modern medicine and diagnosis. Also, pathological features considered collectively; the typical behavior of a disease.

PCP (PRIMARY CARE PROVIDER). A health care practitioner who sees people that have common medical problems. This person is usually a doctor, but may be a physician assistant or a nurse practitioner.

PEPTIDE. A compound consisting of two or more amino acids linked in a chain. Typically, peptides are distinguished from proteins by their shorter length, although the cut-off number of amino acids for defining a peptide and protein can be arbitrary.

PHARMACOKINETICS. Pharmacodynamics is often summarized as the study of what a drug does to the body, whereas pharmacokinetics is the study of what the body does to a drug.

PET (POSITRON EMISSION TOMOGRAPHY) SCAN. A nuclear medicine, functional imaging technique that produces a three-dimensional image of functional processes in the body. The system detects pairs of gamma rays emitted indirectly by a positron-emitting radionuclide (tracer), which is introduced into the body on a biologically active molecule. Three-dimensional images of tracer concentration within the body are then constructed by computer analysis.

PHYTOCHEMICAL. Chemical compounds that occur naturally in plants. Some are responsible for color and other organoleptic properties, such as the deep purple of blueberries and the smell of garlic. Phytochemicals may have biological significance, for example carotenoids or flavonoids, but are not established as essential nutrients. There may be as many as 4,000 different phytochemicals.

PLACEBO. A placebo (Latin *placēbō*, "I shall please;" from *placeō*, "I please") is a simulated or otherwise medically ineffectual treatment for a disease or other medical condition intended to deceive the recipient. Sometimes patients given a placebo treatment will have a perceived or actual improvement in a medical condition, a phenomenon commonly called the placebo effect or placebo response. The placebo effect consists of several different effects woven together, and the methods of placebo administration may be as important as the administration itself. In medical research, placebos are given as control treatments and depend on the use of measured suggestion. Common placebos include inert tablets, vehicle infusions, sham surgery, and other procedures based on false information.

POLYPHENOLS. A structural class of mainly natural, but also synthetic or semisynthetic, organic chemicals characterized by the presence of large multiples of phenol structural units. The number and characteristics of these phenol structures underlie the unique physical, chemical, and biological (metabolic, toxic, therapeutic, etc.) properties of particular members of the class. Many polyphenolic extracts, for example from grape skin, grape seeds, olive pulp and maritime pine bark are sold as ingredients in functional foods, dietary supplements and cosmetics without any legal health claims. Some of them have self-affirmed GRAS status in the U.S. There are no recommended Dietary Reference Intake levels established for polyphenols.

PREVALENCE. The proportion of a population who have (or had) a specific characteristic in a given time period – in medicine, typically an illness, a condition, or a risk factor such as depression or smoking.

PROGNOSIS. A medical term for predicting the likely outcome of one's current standing. A complete prognosis includes the expected duration, the function, and a description of the course of the disease, such as progressive decline, intermittent crisis, or sudden, unpredictable crisis.

PROPHYLACTIC. A medicine or course of action used to prevent disease.

PROTEIN. Any of a class of nitrogenous organic compounds that consist of large molecules composed of one or more long chains of amino acids and are an essential part of all living organisms, especially as structural components of body tissues such as muscle, hair, collagen, and so forth, and as enzymes and antibodies.

PSEUDOBULBAR AFFECT (PBA). Refers to a neurologic disorder characterized by involuntary crying or uncontrollable episodes of crying and/or laughing, or other emotional displays. PBA occurs secondary to a neurologic disease or brain injury.

PSYCHOTROPIC MEDICATIONS. Any medication capable of affecting the mind, emotions, or behavior.

RANDOMIZED CONTROLLED TRIAL (RCT). A study design that randomly assigns participants into an experimental group or a control group. As the study is conducted, the only expected difference between the control and experimental groups in a randomized controlled trial (RCT) is the outcome variable being studied.

RDA (RECOMMENDED DAILY ALLOWANCE). The amount of a nutriment (as a vitamin or mineral) that is recommended for daily consumption by the Food and Nutrition Board of the National Academy of Sciences—abbreviation RDA.

RED MEAT. In traditional culinary terminology, this is meat which is red when raw and not white when cooked. Red meat also includes the meat of most adult mammals. The meat from mammals such as cows, sheep, veal calves, lamb, pigs, horses is invariably considered red, while chicken and rabbit meat is invariably considered white.

RNA. ribonucleic acid, a nucleic acid present in all living cells. Its principal role is to act as a messenger carrying instructions from DNA for controlling the synthesis of proteins, although in some viruses RNA rather than DNA carries the genetic information.

SENILE PLAQUES. Extracellular deposits of amyloid beta in the grey matter of the brain. Degenerative neural (nerve cell) structures and an abundance of microglia and astrocytes (specific nerve cell types) can be associated with senile plaque deposits. These deposits can also be a by-product of senescence (aging). However, large numbers of senile plaques and neurofibrillary tangles are characteristic features of Alzheimer's disease. In Alzheimer's disease they are primarily composed of amyloid beta peptides. These polypeptides tend to aggregate and are believed to be neurotoxic.

SEROTONIN. A monoamine neurotransmitter. Biochemically derived from tryptophan, serotonin is primarily found in the gastrointestinal tract (GI tract), blood platelets, and the central nervous system (CNS) of animals, including humans. Approximately 90 percent of the human body's total serotonin is located in the GI tract, where it is used to regulate intestinal movements. The remainder is synthesized in serotonergic neurons of the CNS, where it has various functions. These include the regulation of mood, appetite, and sleep. Serotonin also has some cognitive functions, including memory and learning. Modulation of serotonin at synapses is thought to be a major action of several classes of pharmacological antidepressants.

SIRTUIN MODULATORS. Are a group of proteins (including SIRT1 through SIRT7). Sirtuins have been implicated in influencing a wide range of cellular processes like aging, cell death, inflammation and stress resistance, as well as energy efficiency and alertness during low-calorie situations. Sirtuins can also control circadian clocks and mitochondrial biogenesis.

SSRIs (SELECTIVE SEROTONIN REUPTAKE INHIBITORs). A class of compounds typically used as antidepressants in the treatment of major depressive disorder and anxiety disorders.

SSRIs are believed to increase the extracellular level of the neurotransmitter serotonin by inhibiting its reuptake into the presynaptic cell, increasing the level of serotonin in the synaptic cleft available to bind to the postsynaptic receptor. They have varying degrees of selectivity for the other monoamine transporters, with pure SSRIs having only weak affinity for the norepinephrine and dopamine transporter. SSRIs are the most widely prescribed antidepressants in many countries.

STEM CELLS. Are undifferentiated biological cells that can differentiate into specialized cells and can divide to produce more stem cells.

SUBCORTICAL. Relating to or denoting the region of the brain below the cortex. (The cortex is the outer layer of the cerebrum (the *cerebral cortex*), composed of folded gray matter and playing an important role in consciousness.)

SUNDOWNING. A psychological phenomenon associated with increased confusion and restlessness in patients with some form of dementia. Most commonly associated with Alzheimer's disease, but also found in those with mixed dementia, the term "sundowning" was coined due to the timing of the patient's confusion. For patients with sundowning syndrome, a multitude of behavioral problems begin to occur in the evening or while the sun is setting. Sundowning seems to occur more frequently during the middle stages of Alzheimer's disease and mixed dementia. Patients are generally able to understand that this behavioral pattern is abnormal. Sundowning seems to subside with the progression of a patient's dementia. Research shows that 20–45 percent of Alzheimer's patients will experience some sort of sundowning confusion.

SYNAPSE. In the nervous system, a synapse is a structure that permits a neuron (or nerve cell) to pass an electrical or chemical signal to another cell (neural or otherwise).

SYNERGISTIC. More than additive. When synergistic parts work together, they accomplish more than they could alone. Synergetic is often used to describe the effect of drugs working together — where one drug increases the other's effectiveness.

TRIGLYCERIDE. An ester formed from glycerol and three fatty acid groups. Triglycerides are the main constituents of natural fats and oils, and high concentrations in the blood indicate an elevated risk of stroke.

VASCULAR RISK FACTORS. Traditional risk factors include such things as high blood pressure (hypertension), smoking, obesity, age, lack of physical activity, and high cholesterol (hyperlipidemia). However, there are now many other risk factors that also have to be considered. For a full discussion, see: http://emedicine.medscape.com/article/164163-overview.

VISCERAL. Referring to the viscera, the internal organs of the body, specifically those within the chest (as the heart or lungs) or abdomen (as the liver, pancreas or intestines).

WHITE MATTER. The part of the brain that contains myelinated nerve fibers. The white matter is white because it is the color of myelin, the insulation that covers nerve fibers.

INDEX

"Atypical" Antipsychotic Medications, 186
"Healty" Diet, 496
"Mood Stabilizers", 186
A (Vitamin A), 317
Abilify (aripiprazole), 186
Acetyl-L-carnitine, 319
Alcohol Consumption, 38
Alpha-lipoic Acid, 320
Alpinia Zerumbet, 527
Aluminum, 51
Alzheimer's Disease, 10
Amyloid hypothesis, 81
Amyloid precursor protein (APP), 95
Anabolic Steroids, 38
Angiotensin II Blockade, 516
Anti-Alzheimer's Diet, 269
Antibodies and Immunotherapy, 207
Antidepressants, 189, 221, 515
Anti-diabetic Medications, 238
Antihistamines (and anticholinergics), 39
Anti-hypertensive Agents, 248
Anti-inflammatory Medications, 244
Anti-Stress, 444
APOE4, 81
Arginine, 79
Aricept (donepezil), 178
Arsenic, 49
Ascorbic Acid (Vitamin C), 321
Ashwagandha, 322
Ativan (lorazepam), 192
Autophagy, 214
B Vitamins, 326
B12 (Vitamin B12), 328
Basic Blood Tests, 123
Benzodiazepine Use, 41
Benzodiazepines, 192
Berberine, 334
BIMS (Brief Interview for Mental Status), 111
Binswanger's Disease, 103
Biomarkers & Genetics, 479
Black Pepper, 336
Blessed Dementia Rating Scale (BDRS), 111
blood-brain barrier, 172
Body mass index (BMI), 282
brain-derived neurotrophic factor (BDNF), 15
Brain-derived neurotrophic factor (BDNF), 129
CADASIL, 102
Caloric Restriction, 461
Cancer, 42
Carotenoids (Including Lycopene, Lutein and Zeaxanthin), 336

Cause(s) and Pathology, 78
Celexa (citalopram), 189, 222
Cerebral Spinal Fluid (CSF), 142
CFI (Cognitive Function Instrument), 112
Chia, 340
Chinese Herbal Preparations, 342
Cholinergic hypothesis, 80
Cholinergic Medications, 174
Circadian, 204
Clinical Dementia Rating (CDR), 112
Clinical Evaluation, 117
Clock Drawing Test, 113
Coconut, 344
Coenzyme Q_{10} (CoQ10), 346
Coffee, 345
Cognex (tacrine), 177
Cognitive Training & Mindfulness, 198
Cognitive Training/Activity, 273
Combination Treatments, 185
Complete Blood Count (CBC), 124
Complete Metabolic Panel (CMP), 124
CoQ10 Blood Levels, 134
C-reactive protein (CRP), 127
Creutzfeldt–Jakob disease, 104
Cromolyn Sodium, 248
CT (Computed Tomography) Scan, 149
Curcumin (Turmeric), 349
Cytokines, 86

D (Vitamin D), 351, 529
Definition of Aging, 456
Definition of Longevity, 459
Delirium, 98
Dementia Severity Rating Scale, 114
Dental Care, 446
Depression, 98
Depression Screening, 118
Diabetes, 42, 89
Diabetes mellitus (DM), 238
Diabetic Medications, 211
Diagnosis, 13, 107
Diets, 255
Differential Diagnosis of Alzheimer's disease, 96
E (Vitamin E), 354
Early Onset Alzheimer Disease (EOAD), 36
Early-Life Nutrition, 482
Educational Level, 43
EEG (Electroencephalogram), 158
EGCG, 381
Electromagnetic Fields, 43
Epigenetic Diet, 265
Epigenetic Therapies, 211
Epigenetics, 212
Estrogens, 252
Event Related Potential P3, 171
executive function, 35
Exelon (rivastigmine), 179
Exercise, 465
Exercise, Activity & Fitness Levels, 482
Experimental Treatments, 206
Extra Virgin Olive Oil, 530

Eye Movements, 169
Facial Scans, 489
Female Gender, 45
Fetzima (levomilnacipran), 226
Fiber, 491
Fish Diet, 268
Flavinoids and Polyphenols (Phytochemicals), 357
Folate (Folic Acid; Vitamin B_9), 363
Free Radical Theory of Aging, 466
Free radicals, 307
Friend-rated Personality Traits, 493
Frontotemporal Lobar Degeneration, 96
Gait & Balance Assessment, 165
Garlic, 532
Gelsolin, 367
Genetic Testing, 138
Genetics, 80, 467
Geodon (ziprazadone), 186
Ginger, 373
Ginkgo Biloba, 368
Ginseng, 374
Glaucoma, 45
Glutamate, 253
Gout, 48
Grape Seed Extract, 378
Green (and Oolong, White, and Black) Tea, 380
Handshake Strength, 494
Healthy Lifestyle, 271
Heart Rate, 496
Heavy Metal Exposure, 48

Height, 53
Hemoglobin A_1C (HgbA_1C), 125
Herpes simplex virus (HSV), 52
Hesperidin, 386
High Fat Diet, 53
Higher Education, 275
hippocampus, 8
Homeostasis, 94
Homocysteine, 83, 127
Huperzine A, 387
hypercholesterolemia, 53
Hyperketonemia, 212
Immunological Theory of Aging, 469
Inbreeding, 54
Infections, 54
Inflammation, 84
Instrumental Activities of Daily Living, 114
Insulin Receptor Substrate-1 (IRS-1, 133
insulin resistance, 90
Invega (palperidone), 186
Isolation, 498
Kale, 390
Keppra (levetiracetam), 227
Ketogenic Diet, 268
Klonopin (clonazepam), 192
Klotho, 470
Lack of Purpose in Life, 56
Latuda (lurasidone), 186
Learning a Language, 276
Leptin, 92
Lewy Body Disease, 97
Lexapro (escitalopram), 191

Life Space, 165, 272
Lifespan with Alzheimer's Disease, 32
Lipid Profile or Panel (Cholesterol), 125
Lithium, 227
Loneliness, 57
Longevity, 452
Low Testosterone, 57
Magnesium (Mg+), 393
Magnetoencephalographic Imaging (MEGI), 157
Matthew Effect, 498
Meat Diet, 257
Meditation, 277
Mediterranean and DASH Diets, 259
Mediterranean diet, 500
Melatonin, 395
Memory, 6
Mental Activities, 273
Mental Issues, 58
Mercury, 50
Meta-analysis, 200
Metformin, 242, 520
Methylmalonic Acid, 129
Mild Cognitive Impairment, MCI, 25
Milk Consumption, 501
Mindfulness, 279
Mitochondrial dysfunction, 88
Mitochondrial Theory of Aging, 471
MMSE (Mini-Mental State Exam), 115
MRI (Magnetic Resonance Imaging), 150
mTOR, 280
N-acetyl cysteine, 401
Namenda XR (memantine), 182
Namzaric (donepezil + memantine), 185
Nanosolution, 213
Nanotubes, 214
Neuroimaging (Brain Scans), 148
Neuropathology, 17
Neuropsychological Testing, 116
Neurosurgical Treatments, 201
NMDA (*N*-Methyl-D-aspartate), 182
normal pressure hydrocephalus (NPH),, 104
NSAIDs, 244
NSAIDS, 516
NT-proBNP, 135
Nut Consumption, 503
Obesity, 59
Omega 3 Fatty Acids, 402
Oral Health, 504
Osteoporosis, 61
Other Prevention Programs, 444
Other Types of Dementia (DSM-V), 96
Paleo Diet, 263
Paper-and-Pencil Testing, 110
Parkinson's Disease, 98
Patient Health Questionnaire (PHQ-9), 123
Paxil (paroxetine), 190
Periodontitis, 62
Pesticides, 64

Pets, 446
Physical Activity, 280
Physical Activity Trackers, 291
Platelet Proteins, 134
Pollution, 66
Pomegranate Extract, 409
Pomegranite Juice, 539
Positron Emission Tomography (PET) Scan, 154
Predicting Alzheimer's Disease, 33
Prevention, 218
Primary Progressive Aphasia, 101
Progressive Supranuclear Palsy (PSP), 104
Protriptyline, 227
Prozac (fluoxetine), 192, 224
Pulse Wave Velocity (PWV), 168
Purpose in life, 504
Quercetin, 413
Rapamycin, 519
RDW, 506
Reactive oxygen species (ROS), 310
Real vs. Perceived Age, 511
Relatives With Alzheimer's, 67
Religion, 447
Reminiscence Therapy, 205
Reminyl (galantamine), 180
Resveratrol, 416, 533
Retinal Assessment, 169
Rhodiola Rosea, 423
Risperdal (risperidone), 186
Saffron, 427
Saphris (asenapine), 186

SATNAV or GPS, 45
Selenium, 428
Senolytic Drugs, 520
Seroquel (quetiapine), 187
Sirtuins, 473
Sleep, 448, 512
Sleep Apnea, 68
Sleep Issues, 68
Sleep Study, 163
Smell Test, 160
Smoking, 70
Social Interaction, 202
Social Relations, 450
Souvenaid®, 429
SSRIs, 189, 221
St John's Wart, 432
Statins (HMG-CoA Reductase Inhibitors), 233
Stem Cells, 214
Stress, 71
Subjective memory impairment (SMI), 23
Summary, 541
Sun Activity When Born, 513
Sundowing, 30
Supplements & Vitamins, 522
Supplements, Antioxidants, and Micronutrients, 294
Support Groups, 202
Tailored Lighting Intervention, 204
Tau hypothesis, 82
TDP-43 (A Protein), 83
Telomer Length, 475
Tests Related to Abeta Amyloid and Tau Proteins, 135

The Geriatric Depression Scale, 122
Theories of Aging, 460
Things That Predict Longevity, 477
Thyroid Tests, 129
Tooth Loss, 72
Transcranial LED therapy, 204
Transcranial Stimulation, 205
Transcranial Ultrasound, 170
transient ischemic attack (TIA), 102
Traumatic Brain Injury (TBI), 72
Treatment, 172
Turmeric, 349
Ultrasound, 215
Use of Proton Pump Inhibitors, 73
Vaccines, 216
Vascular and Cholesterol Risk, 73
Vascular Disease, 97
VDRL, 129
Viagra (sildenafil), 254
Virtual Reality, 163
Visceral fat, 385
Visual-spatial construction, 91
Volatile Organic Compounds (VOCs), 169, 515
Walnuts, 435
white matter hyperintensities (WMHs), 59
Whole-food Diet, 267
Xanax (alprazolam), 192
Zinc, 442
Zoloft (sertraline), 190
Zoloft (Sertraline), 225

REFERENCES

[1] Take Action to Promote Brain Health: IOM Report. Megan Brooks, April 14, 2015. http://www.medscape.com/viewarticle/843108.

[2] Recollection and familiarity in aging individuals with mild cognitive impairment and Alzheimer's disease: a literature review. Schoemaker D^1, Gauthier S, Pruessner JC. Neuropsychol Rev. 2014 Sep;24(3):313-31.

[3] Is magnetite a universal memory molecule? Størmer FC. Med Hypotheses. 2014 Nov;83(5):549-51.

[4] RAND Corp., news release, Mary Elizabeth Dallas; HealthDay; Oct. 28, 2014. http://www.nlm.nih.gov/medlineplus/news/fullstory_149204.html [The citation will not be available after January, 2015.]

[5] CDC National Health Report: Leading Causes of Morbidity and Mortality and Associated Behavioral Risk and Protective Factors-United States, 2005-2013. Johnson NB, Hayes LD, Brown K, Hoo EC, Ethier KA. MMWR Surveill Summ. 2014 Oct 31;63:3-27.

[6] Memory Lapses May Signal Stroke Risk: Study. Robert Preidt. December 11, 2014 http://www.nlm.nih.gov/medlineplus/news/fullstory_149918.html (*this news item will not be available after 03/11/2015).

[7] Characteristics of residents living in residential care communities, by community bed size: United States, 2012. Caffrey C, Harris-Kojetin L, Rome V, Sengupta M. NCHS Data Brief. 2014 Nov;(171):1-8.

[8] Expanding efforts to address Alzheimer's disease: The Healthy Brain Initiative. Anderson LA, Egge R. Alzheimers Dement. 2014 Oct;10(5 Suppl):S453-6.

[9] Prediction of dementia by subjective memory impairment: effects of severity and temporal association with cognitive impairment. Jessen F, Wiese B, Bachmann C, Eifflaender-Gorfer S, Haller F, Kölsch H, Luck T, Mösch E, van den Bussche H, Wagner M, Wollny A, Zimmermann T, Pentzek M, Riedel-Heller SG, Romberg HP, Weyerer S, Kaduszkiewicz H, Maier W, Bickel H; German Study on Aging, Cogni-

tion and Dementia in Primary Care Patients Study Group (Collaborators 22). Arch Gen Psychiatry. 2010 Apr;67(4):414-22.

[10] Cortical Thinning in Individuals with Subjective Memory Impairment. Meiberth D, Scheef L, Wolfsgruber S, Boecker H, Block W, Träber F, Erk S, Heneka MT, Jacobi H, Spottke A, Walter H, Wagner M, Hu X, Jessen FJ Alzheimers Dis. 2014 Dec 2.

[11] Self-rated and informant-rated everyday function in comparison to objective markers of Alzheimer's disease. Rueda AD, Lau KM, Saito N, Harvey D, Risacher SL, Aisen PS, Petersen RC, Saykin AJ, Tomaszewski Farias S; Alzheimer's disease Neuroimaging Initiative. Alzheimers Dement. 2014 Nov 15. pii: S1552-5260(14)02823-4.

[12] Self-reported memory complaints: implications from a longitudinal cohort with autopsies. Kryscio RJ, Abner EL, Cooper GE, Fardo DW, Jicha GA, Nelson PT, Smith CD, Van Eldik LJ, Wan L, Schmitt FA. Neurology. 2014 Oct 7;83(15):1359-65.

[13] Follow-up study of olfactory deficits, cognitive functions, and volume loss of medial temporal lobe structures in patients with mild cognitive impairment. Lojkowska W, Sawicka B, Gugala M, Sienkiewicz-Jarosz H, Bochynska A, Scinska A, Korkosz A, Lojek E, Ryglewicz D. Curr Alzheimer Res. 2011 Sep;8(6):689-98.

[14] Subjective Memory Complaint Only Relates to Verbal Episodic Memory Performance in Mild Cognitive Impairment. Gifford KA, Liu D, Damon SM, Chapman WG, Romano RR, Samuels LR, Lu Z, Jefferson AL. J Alzheimers Dis. 2014 Oct 3.

[15] Subjective cognitive complaints contribute to misdiagnosis of mild cognitive impairment. Edmonds EC, Delano-Wood L, Galasko DR, Salmon DP, Bondi MW; Alzheimer's disease Neuroimaging Initiative. Collaborators (431). J Int Neuropsychol Soc. 2014 Sep;20(8):836-47.

[16] Motoric cognitive risk syndrome: Multicenter incidence study. Verghese J, Ayers E, Barzilai N, Bennett DA, Buchman AS, Holtzer R, Katz MJ, Lipton RB, Wang C. Neurology. 2014 Oct 31.

[17] Mild physical impairment predicts future diagnosis of dementia of the Alzheimer'stype. Wilkins CH, Roe CM, Morris JC, Galvin JE. J Am Geriatr Soc. 2013 Jul;61(7):1055-9.

[18] Association of muscle strength with the risk of Alzheimer disease and the rate of cognitive decline in community-dwelling older persons. Boyle PA, Buchman AS, Wilson RS, Leurgans SE, Bennett DA. Arch Neurol. 2009 Nov;66(11):1339-44.

[19] Motor phenotype of decline in cognitive performance among community-dwellers without dementia: population-based study and meta-analysis. Beauchet O, Allali G, Montero-Odasso M, Sejdić E, Fantino B, Annweiler C. PLoS One. 2014 Jun 9;9(6):e99318.

[20] Association between acute care and critical illness hospitalization and cognitive function in older adults. Ehlenbach WJ, Hough CL, Crane PK, Haneuse SJ, Carson SS, Curtis JR, Larson EB. JAMA. 2010 Feb 24;303(8):763-70.

[21] Natural history of cognitive decline in the old old. Howieson DB, Camicioli R, Quinn J, Silbert LC, Care B, Moore MM, Dame A, Sexton G, Kaye JA. Neurology. 2003 May 13;60(9):1489-94.

[22] Sundown syndrome in persons with dementia: an update. Khachiyants N, Trinkle D, Son SJ, Kim KY. Psychiatry Investig. 2011 Dec;8(4):275-87.

[23] Disruptive behavior as a predictor in Alzheimer disease. Scarmeas N, Brandt J, Blacker D, Albert M, Hadjigeorgiou G, Dubois B, Devanand D, Honig L, Stern Y. Arch Neurol. 2007 Dec;64(12):1755-61.

[24] Delusions and hallucinations are associated with worse outcome in Alzheimer disease. Scarmeas N, Brandt J, Albert M, Hadjigeorgiou G, Papadimitriou A, Dubois B, Sarazin M, Devanand D, Honig L, Marder K, Bell K, Wegesin D, Blacker D, Stern Y. Arch Neurol. 2005 Oct;62(10):1601-8.

[25] The natural history of dementia. Kua EH, Ho E, Tan HH, Tsoi C, Thng C, Mahendran R. Psychogeriatrics. 2014 Sep;14(3):196-201.

[26] Independent predictors of cognitive decline in healthy elderly persons. Marquis S, Moore MM, Howieson DB, Sexton G, Payami H, Kaye JA, Camicioli R. Arch Neurol. 2002 Apr;59(4):601-6.

[27] Memory impairment on free and cued selective reminding predicts dementia. Grober E[1], Lipton RB, Hall C, Crystal H. Neurology. 2000 Feb 22;54(4):827-32.

[28] The course of cognitive impairment in preclinical Alzheimer disease: three- and 6-year follow-up of a population-based sample. Small BJ[1], Fratiglioni L, Viitanen M, Winblad B, Bäckman L. Arch Neurol. 2000 Jun;57(6):839-44.

[29] A-78Cognitively Normal Older Adults with Preclinical Alzheimer's disease Demonstrate Slower Processing Speed on Everyday Financial Tasks. Triebel K, Martin R, Christianson T, Swenson-Dravis D, Pankratz V, Petersen R, Marson D. Arch Clin Neuropsychol. 2014 Sep;29(6):531-2.

[30] A-76 Associations between Brain Atrophy and Financial Capacity in Prodromal and Clinical AD. Kerr D, Bartel T, McLaren D, Marson D. Arch Clin Neuropsychol. 2014 Sep;29(6):531.

[31] A-75 Financial Decline in Patients with Mild Cognitive Impairment: A Six-year Longitudinal Study. Martin R, Triebel K, Falola M, Cutter G, Kerr D, Marson D. Arch Clin Neuropsychol. 2014 Sep;29(6):530-1.

[32] An updated Alzheimer's disease progression model: incorporating non-linearity, beta regression, and a third-level random effect in NONMEM. Conrado DJ[1], Denney WS, Chen D, Ito K. J Pharmacokinet Pharmacodyn. 2014 Dec;41(6):581-98.

[33] Brain pathology contributes to simultaneous change in physical frailty and cognition in old age. Buchman AS[1], Yu L[2], Wilson RS[3], Boyle PA[3], Schneider JA[4], Bennett DA[2]. J Gerontol A Biol Sci Med Sci. 2014 Dec;69(12):1536-44.

[34] Clinical, genetic, and neuroimaging features of early onset Alzheimer disease: the challenges of diagnosis and treatment. Alberici A, Benussi A, Premi E, Borroni B, Padovani A. Curr Alzheimer Res. 2014;11(10):909-17.

[35] Low concentrations of ethanol protect against synaptotoxicity induced by Aβ in hippocampal neurons. Muñoz G, Urrutia JC, Burgos CF, Silva V, Aguilar F, Sama M, Yeh HH, Opazo C, Aguayo LG. Neurobiol Aging. 2014 Oct 17. pii: S0197-4580(14)00674-5.

[36] 17β-trenbolone, an anabolic-androgenic steroid as well as an environmental hormone, contributes to neurodegeneration. Ma F, Liu D. Toxicol Appl Pharmacol. 2014 Nov 25. pii: S0041-008X(14)00422-0.

[37] Cumulative Use of Strong Anticholinergics and Incident Dementia: A Prospective Cohort Study. Gray SL, Anderson ML, Dublin S, Hanlon JT, Hubbard R, Walker R, Yu O, Crane PK, Larson EB. JAMA Intern Med. 2015 Jan 26.

[38] Adult asthma increases dementia risk: a nationwide cohort study. Peng YH, Wu BR, Su CH, Liao WC, Muo CH, Hsia TC, Kao CH. J Epidemiol Community Health. 2015 Feb;69(2):123-8.

[39] Link between Alzheimer's disease and benzodiazepines suspected. No author listed. Nurs Older People. 2014 Nov 28;26(10):13.

[40] Association of cancer history with Alzheimer's disease onset and structural brain changes. Nudelman KN[1], Risacher SL[2], West JD[2], McDonald BC[3], Gao S[4], Saykin AJ[5]; Alzheimer's disease Neuroimaging Initiative. Front Physiol. 2014 Oct 31;5:423.

[41] Diabetes and Cognition. Mayeda ER[1], Whitmer RA[2], Yaffe K[3]. Clin Geriatr Med. 2015 Feb;31(1):101-115.

[42] Low amyloid-β deposition correlates with high education in cognitively normal older adults: a pilot study. Yasuno F, Kazui H, Morita N, Kajimoto K, Ihara M, Taguchi A, Yamamoto A, Matsuoka K, Kosaka J, Kudo T, Iida H, Kishimoto T. Int J Geriatr Psychiatry. 2014 Nov 26.

[43] Neuronal cellular responses to extremely low frequency electromagnetic field exposure: implications regarding oxidative stress and neurodegeneration. Reale M, Kamal MA, Patruno A, Costantini E, D'Angelo C, Pesce M, Greig NH. PLoS One. 2014 Aug 15;9(8):e104973.

[44] Neurodegenerative disease and magnetic field exposure in UK electricity supply workers. Sorahan T, Mohammed N. Occup Med (Lond). 2014 Sep;64(6):454-60.

[45] Short-term effects of extremely low frequency electromagnetic fields exposure on Alzheimer's disease in rats. Zhang Y, Liu X, Zhang J, Li N. Int J Radiat Biol. 2014 Nov 14:1-7.

[46] Glaucoma, Alzheimer's disease, and Parkinson's disease: an 8-year population-based follow-up study. Lin IC[1], Wang YH[2], Wang TJ[3], Wang IJ[4], Shen YD[1], Chi NF[5], Chien LN[6]. PLoS One. 2014 Oct 2;9(9):e108938.

[47] Is your satnav harming your brain? Scientists warn over-use of modern technology may be linked to memory loss and depression in later life. John Naish. Daily Mail. March 2, 2015.

[48] Relation between Uric Acid and Alzheimer's disease in Elderly Jordanians. Al-Khateeb E[1], Althaher A[1], Al-Khateeb M[2], Al-Musawi H[3], Azzouqah O[3], Al-Shweiki S[3], Shafagoj Y[1]. J Alzheimers Dis. 2014 Oct 31.

[49] Exposure to As-, Cd-, and Pb-Mixture Induces Aβ, Amyloidogenic APP Processing and Cognitive Impairments via Oxidative Stress-Dependent Neuroinflammation in Young Rats. Ashok A[1], Rai NK[1], Tripathi S[2], Bandyopadhyay S[3]. Toxicol Sci. 2014 Oct 6.

[50] Heavy metals and neurodegenerative diseases: an observational study. Giacoppo S[1], Galuppo M, Calabrò RS, D'Aleo G, Marra A, Sessa E, Bua DG, Potortì AG, Dugo G, Bramanti P, Mazzon E. Biol Trace Elem Res. 2014 Nov;161(2):151-60.

[51] The Effects of Arsenic Exposure on Neurological and Cognitive Dysfunction in Human and Rodent Studies: A Review. Tyler CR, Allan AM. Curr Environ Health Rep. 2014 Mar 21;1:132-147.

[52] Does inorganic mercury play a role in Alzheimer's disease? A systematic review and an integrated molecular mechanism. Mutter J[1], Curth A, Naumann J, Deth R, Walach H. J Alzheimers Dis. 2010;22(2):357-74.

[53] Metal concentrations in plasma and cerebrospinal fluid in patients with Alzheimer's disease. Gerhardsson L[1], Lundh T, Minthon L, Londos E. Dement Geriatr Cogn Disord. 2008;25(6):508-15.

[54] Increase in mercury in Pacific yellowfin tuna. Drevnick, P. E., Lamborg, C. H. and Horgan, M. J. Environmental Toxicology and Chemistry. Feb 2015.

[55] Systematic review of potential health risks posed by pharmaceutical, occupational and consumer exposures to metallic and nanoscale aluminum, aluminum oxides, aluminum hydroxide and its soluble salts. Willhite CC[1], Karyakina NA, Yokel RA, Yenugadhati N, Wisniewski TM, Arnold IM, Momoli F, Krewski D. Crit Rev Toxicol. 2014 Oct;44 Suppl 4:1-80.

[57] Herpes simplex virus type 1 and Alzheimer's disease: increasing evidence for a major role of the virus. Itzhaki RF. Front Aging Neurosci. 2014 Aug 11;6:202.

[58] Herpes simplex infection and the risk of Alzheimer's disease-A nested case-control study. Lövheim H, Gilthorpe J, Johansson A, Eriksson S, Hallmans G, Elgh F. Alzheimers Dement. 2014 Oct 7. pii: S1552-5260(14)02770-8.

[59] Height in relation to dementia death: individual participant meta-analysis of 18 UK prospective cohort studies. Tom C. Russ, Mika Kivimäki, John M. Starr, Emmanuel Stamatakis, G. David Batty. http://bjp.rcpsych.org/content/205/5/348.abstract.

[60] Prenatal high fat diet alters the cerebrovasculature and clearance of β-amyloid in adult offspring. Hawkes CA[1], Gentleman SM, Nicoll JA, Carare RO. J Pathol. 2014 Oct 24.

[61] Inbreeding among Caribbean Hispanics from the Dominican Republic and its effects on risk of Alzheimer disease. Vardarajan BN, Schaid DJ, Reitz C, Lantigua R,

Medrano M, Jiménez-Velázquez IZ, Lee JH, Ghani M, Rogaeva E, St George-Hyslop P, Mayeux RP. Genet Med. 2014 Nov 13.

[62] Link between chronic bacterial inflammation and Alzheimer disease. Bibi F, Yasir M, Sohrab SS, Azhar EI, Al-Qahtani MH, Abuzenadah AM, Kamal MA, Naseer MI[1]. CNS Neurol Disord Drug Targets. 2014;13(7):1140-7.

[63] The role of viruses in neurodegenerative and neurobehavioral diseases. Karim S, Mirza Z, Kamal MA, Abuzenadah AM, Azhar EI, Al-Qahtani MH, Damanhouri GA, Ahmad F, Gan SH, Sohrab SS[1]. CNS Neurol Disord Drug Targets. 2014;13(7):1213-23.

[64] Cytomegalovirus Infection and Risk of Alzheimer Disease in Older Black and White Individuals. Barnes LL[1], Capuano AW[2], Aiello AE[3], Turner AD[4], Yolken RH[5], Torrey EF[5], Bennett DA[2]. J Infect Dis. 2014 Aug 8.

[65] Helicobacter pylori Filtrate Induces Alzheimer-Like Tau Hyperphosphorylation by Activating Glycogen Synthase Kinase-3β. Xiu-Lian W[1], Ji Z[2], Yang Y[3], Yan X[3], Zhi-Hua Z[4], Mei Q[3], Xiong Y[3], Xu-Ying S[3], Qing-Zhang T[3], Rong L[3], Jian-Zhi W[3]. J Alzheimers Dis. 2014 Jul 30.

[66] Helicobacter pylori infection and dementia: can actual data reinforce the hypothesis of a causal association? Adriani A[1], Fagoonee S, De Angelis C, Altruda F, Pellicano R. Panminerva Med. 2014 Sep;56(3):195-9.

[67] Effect of a purpose in life on risk of incident Alzheimer disease and mild cognitive impairment in community-dwelling older persons. Boyle PA, Buchman AS, Barnes LL, Bennett DA. Arch Gen Psychiatry. 2010 Mar;67(3):304-10.

[68] Relationship between loneliness, psychiatric disorders and physical health ? A review on the psychological aspects of loneliness. Mushtaq R, Shoib S, Shah T, Mushtaq S. J Clin Diagn Res. 2014 Sep;8(9):WE01-4.

[69]Diet-induced obesity and low testosterone increase neuroinflammation and impair neural function. Jayaraman A, Lent-Schochet D, Pike CJ[1]. J Neuroinflammation. 2014 Sep 16;11:162.

[70] Midlife personality and risk of Alzheimer disease and distress: A 38-year follow-up. Johansson L[1], Guo X[2], Duberstein PR[2], Hällström T[2], Waern M[2], Ostling S[2], Skoog I[2]. Neurology. 2014 Oct 21;83(17):1538-44.

[71] Relationships between Personality Traits, Medial Temporal Lobe Atrophy, and White Matter Lesion in Subjects Suffering from Mild Cognitive Impairment. Duron

E[1], Vidal JS[1], Bounatiro S[2], Ben Ahmed S[2], Seux ML[1], Rigaud AS[1], Hanon O[1], Viollet C[2], Epelbaum J[2], Martel G[2]. Front Aging Neurosci. 2014 Jul 29;6:195.

[72] Severe psychiatric disorders in mid-life and risk of dementia in late- life (age 65-84 years): a population based case-control study. Zilkens RR, Bruce DG, Duke J, Spilsbury K, Semmens JB[1]. Curr Alzheimer Res. 2014;11(7):681-93.

[73] Body mass index in dementia. García-Ptacek S[1], Faxén-Irving G[2], Cermáková P[3], Eriksdotter M[4], Religa D[5]. Eur J Clin Nutr. 2014 Nov;68(11):1204-1209.

[74] Adipokines: a link between obesity and dementia? Kiliaan AJ[1], Arnoldussen IA[1], Gustafson DR[2]. Lancet Neurol. 2014 Sep;13(9):913-23.

[75] Obesity-induced cerebral hypoperfusion derived from endothelial dysfunction: one of the risk factors for Alzheimer's disease. Toda N, Ayajiki K, Okamura T[1]. Curr Alzheimer Res. 2014;11(8):733-44.

[76] Effects of diet-induced obesity and voluntary exercise in a tauopathy mouse model: implications of persistent hyperleptinemia and enhanced astrocytic leptin receptor expression. Koga S[1], Kojima A[2], Ishikawa C[3], Kuwabara S[1], Arai K[4], Yoshiyama Y[5]. Neurobiol Dis. 2014 Nov;71:180-92.

[77] Body mass index and mild cognitive impairment-to-dementia progression in 24 months: a prospective study. Sobów T[1], Fendler W[2], Magierski R[3]. Eur J Clin Nutr. 2014 Nov;68(11):1216-1219.

[78] Bone loss and osteoporosis are associated with conversion from mild cognitive impairment to Alzheimer's disease. Zhou R, Zhou H, Rui L, Xu J[1]. Curr Alzheimer Res. 2014;11(7):706-13.

[79] Connection between periodontitis and Alzheimer's disease: possible roles of microglia and leptomeningeal cells. Wu Z[1], Nakanishi H. J Pharmacol Sci. 2014;126(1):8-13.

[80] Periodontal health condition in patients with Alzheimer's disease. Martande SS[1], Pradeep AR[2], Singh SP[3], Kumari M[4], Suke DK[3], Raju AP[5], Naik SB[6], Singh P[7], Guruprasad CN[3], Chatterji A[8]. Am J Alzheimers Dis Other Demen. 2014 Sep;29(6):498-502.

[81] Periodontal disease associates with higher brain amyloid load in normal elderly. Kamer AR[1], Pirraglia E[2], Tsui W[2], Rusinek H[3], Vallabhajosula S[4], Mosconi L[2], Yi L[2], McHugh P[2], Craig RG[5], Svetcov S[6], Linker R[6], Shi C[6], Glodzik L[2], Williams S[2], Cor-

by P[7], Saxena D[8], de Leon MJ[2]. Neurobiol Aging. 2014 Nov 5. pii: S0197-4580(14)00704-0.

[82] Neuroactive insecticides: targets, selectivity, resistance, and secondary effects. Casida JE, Durkin KA. Annu Rev Entomol. 2013;58:99-117.

[83] Elevated Serum Pesticide Levels and Risk for Alzheimer Disease. Jason R. Richardson, PhD[1,2]; Ananya Roy, ScD[2]; Stuart L. Shalat, ScD[1,2]; Richard T. von Stein, PhD[2]; Muhammad M. Hossain, PhD[1,2]; Brian Buckley, PhD[2]; Marla Gearing, PhD[4]; Allan I. Levey, MD, PhD[3]; Dwight C. German, PhD.[5] JAMA Neurol. 2014;71(3):284-290.

[84] Ozone, Particulate Matter, and Newly Diagnosed Alzheimer's disease: A Population-Based Cohort Study in Taiwan. Jung CR[1], Lin YT[1], Hwang BF[2]. J Alzheimers Dis. 2014 Oct 13.

[85] Air pollution and your brain: what do you need to know right now. Calderón-Garcidueñas L[1], Calderón-Garcidueñas A[2], Torres-Jardón R[3], Avila-Ramírez J[4], Kulesza RJ[5], Angiulli AD[6]. Prim Health Care Res Dev. 2014 Sep 26:1-17.

[86] Brain atrophy rates in first degree relatives at risk for Alzheimer's. Lampert EJ[1], Roy Choudhury K[2], Hostage CA[2], Rathakrishnan B[1], Weiner M[3], Petrella JR[2], Doraiswamy PM[4]; Alzheimer's disease Neuroimaging Initiative. Neuroimage Clin. 2014 Sep 4;6:340-6.

[87] Can sleep apnea cause Alzheimer's disease? Pan W, Kastin AJ. Neurosci Biobehav Rev. 2014 Oct 30;47C:656-669.

[88] Impact of sleep on the risk of cognitive decline and dementia. Spira AP, Chen-Edinboro LP, Wu MN, Yaffe K.
Curr Opin Psychiatry. 2014 Nov;27(6):478-83.

[89] Self-reported sleep disturbance is associated with Alzheimer's disease risk in men. Benedict C, Byberg L, Cedernaes J, Hogenkamp PS, Giedratis V, Kilander L, Lind L, Lannfelt L, Schiöth HB. Alzheimers Dement. 2014 Oct 27. pii: S1552-5260(14)02819-2.

[90] Long sleep duration in elders without dementia increases risk of dementia mortality (NEDICES). Benito-León J, Louis ED, Villarejo-Galende A, Romero JP, Bermejo-Pareja F. Neurology. 2014 Oct 21;83(17):1530-7.

[91] Sleep facilitates clearance of metabolites from the brain: glymphatic function in aging and neurodegenerative diseases. Mendelsohn AR, Larrick JW. Rejuvenation Res. 2013 Dec;16(6):518-23.

[92] Association of smoking and alcohol drinking with dementia risk among elderly men in China. Zhou S, Zhou R, Zhong T, Li R, Tan J, Zhou H[1]. Curr Alzheimer Res. 2014;11(9):899-907.

[93] Chronic stress as a risk factor for Alzheimer's disease. Machado A, Herrera AJ, de Pablos RM, Espinosa-Oliva AM, Sarmiento M, Ayala A, Venero JL, Santiago M, Villarán RF, Delgado-Cortés MJ, Argüelles S, Cano J. Rev Neurosci. 2014;25(6):785-804.

[94] Psychological distress and risk of peripheral vascular disease, abdominal aortic aneurysm, and heart failure: pooling of sixteen cohort studies. Batty GD[1], Russ TC[2], Stamatakis E[3], Kivimäki M[3]. Atherosclerosis. 2014 Oct;236(2):385-8.

[95] Chronic Stress Decreases Basal Levels of Memory-Related Signaling Molecules in Area CA1 of At-Risk (Subclinical) Model of Alzheimer's disease. Alkadhi KA[1], Tran TT. Mol Neurobiol. 2014 Aug 12.

[96] Association between Tooth Loss and the Development of Mild Memory Impairment in the Elderly: The Fujiwara-kyo Study. Okamoto N[1], Morikawa M[2], Tomioka K[1], Yanagi M[3], Amano N[3], Kurumatani N[1]. J Alzheimers Dis. 2014 Oct 31.

[97] A-26Self-Reported Head Injury and Earlier Age of Diagnosis of Mild Cognitive Impairment. LoBue C, Lacritz L, Hart J Jr, Kyle W, Cullum M. Arch Clin Neuropsychol. 2014 Sep;29(6):512.

[98] Risk of dementia in elderly patients with the use of proton pump inhibitors. Haenisch B[1], von Holt K, Wiese B, Prokein J, Lange C, Ernst A, Brettschneider C, König HH, Werle J, Weyerer S, Luppa M, Riedel-Heller SG, Fuchs A, Pentzek M, Weeg D, Bickel H, Broich K, Jessen F, Maier W, Scherer M. Eur Arch Psychiatry Clin Neurosci. 2014 Oct 24.

[99] Adverse Vascular Risk is Related to Cognitive Decline in Older Adults. Jefferson AL[1], Hohman TJ[1], Liu D[2], Haj-Hassan S[1], Gifford KA[1], Benson EM[1], Skinner JS[3], Lu Z[2], Sparling J[4], Sumner EC[1], Bell S[5], Ruberg FL[6]. J Alzheimers Dis. 2014 Dec 2.

[100] Hypertension drives parenchymal β-amyloid accumulation in the brain parenchyma. Bueche CZ[1], Hawkes C[2], Garz C[3], Vielhaber S[1], Attems J[4], Knight RT[5], Reymann K[6], Heinze HJ[1], Carare RO[2], Schreiber S[1]. Ann Clin Transl Neurol. 2014 Feb;1(2):124-9.

[101] Hypertension Accelerates the Progression of Alzheimer-Like Pathology in a Mouse Model of the Disease. Cifuentes D[1], Poittevin M[1], Dere E[1], Broquères-You D[1], Bonnin P[1], Benessiano J[1], Pocard M[1], Mariani J[1], Kubis N[1], Merkulova-Rainon T[1], Lévy BI[2]. Hypertension. 2014 Oct 20.

[102] Effect of hypertension on the resting-state functional connectivity in patients with Alzheimer's disease (AD). Son SJ[1], Kim J[2], Lee E[3], Park JY[3], Namkoong K[3], Hong CH[1], Ku J[4], Kim E[5], Oh BH[3]. Arch Gerontol Geriatr. 2015 Jan-Feb;60(1):210-6.

[103] Coronary heart disease and cortical thickness, gray matter and white matter lesion volumes on MRI. Vuorinen M[1], Damangir S[2], Niskanen E[3], Miralbell J[4], Rusanen M[1], Spulber G[2], Soininen H[1], Kivipelto M[5], Solomon A[5]. PLoS One. 2014 Oct 10;9(10):e109250.

[104] Atherosclerotic calcification is related to a higher risk of dementia and cognitive decline. Bos D[1], Vernooij MW[1], de Bruijn RF[2], Koudstaal PJ[3], Hofman A[4], Franco OH[4], van der Lugt A[5], Ikram MA[6]. Alzheimers Dement. 2014 Aug 20. pii: S1552-5260(14)02493-5.

[105] HDL and cognition in neurodegenerative disorders. Hottman DA[1], Chernick D[2], Cheng S[1], Wang Z[1], Li L[3]. Neurobiol Dis. 2014 Dec;72PA:22-36.

[106] A neurodegenerative vascular burden index and the impact on cognition. Heinzel S[1], Liepelt-Scarfone I[2], Roeben B[1], Nasi-Kordhishti I[1], Suenkel U[1], Wurster I[1], Brockmann K[1], Fritsche A[3], Niebler R[4], Metzger FG[4], Eschweiler GW[4], Fallgatter AJ[5], Maetzler W[1], Berg D[2]. Front Aging Neurosci. 2014 Jul 9;6:161.

[107] Interactive effects of vascular risk burden and advanced age on cerebral blood flow. Bangen KJ[1], Nation DA[2], Clark LR[3], Harmell AL[3], Wierenga CE[4], Dev SI[3], Delano-Wood L[4], Zlatar ZZ[5], Salmon DP[6], Liu TT[7], Bondi MW[1]. Front Aging Neurosci. 2014 Jul 7;6:159.

[108] Key network approach reveals new insight into Alzheimer's disease. Schluesener JK, Zhu X, Schluesener HJ, Wang GW, Ao P. IET Syst Biol. 2014 Aug;8(4):169-75.

[109] Arginine deprivation and immune suppression in a mouse model of Alzheimer's disease. Kan MJ[1], Lee JE[2], Wilson JG[2], Everhart AL[2], Brown CM[3], Hoofnagle AN[4], Jansen M[2], Vitek MP[2], Gunn MD[5], Colton CA[6].
J Neurosci. 2015 Apr 15;35(15):5969-82.

[110] Amyloid β-peptide and Alzheimer's disease. Allsop D, Mayes J. Essays Biochem. 2014;56:99-110.

[111] Water influx into cerebrospinal fluid is significantly reduced in senile plaque bearing transgenic mice, supporting beta-amyloid clearance hypothesis of Alzheimer's disease. Igarashi H, Suzuki Y, Kwee IL, Nakada T. Neurol Res. 2014 Dec;36(12):1094-8.

[112] Spreading of amyloid-β peptides via neuritic cell-to-cell transfer is dependent on insufficient cellular clearance. Domert J, Rao SB, Agholme L, Brorsson AC, Marcusson J, Hallbeck M, Nath S. Neurobiol Dis. 2014 May;65:82-92.

[113] Inconsistencies and controversies surrounding the amyloid hypothesis of Alzheimer's disease. Morris GP, Clark IA, Vissel B. Acta Neuropathol Commun. 2014 Sep 18;2:135.

[114] Moving beyond anti-amyloid therapy for the prevention and treatment of Alzheimer's disease. Castello MA, Jeppson JD, Soriano S. BMC Neurol. 2014 Sep 2;14:169.

[115] Tau pathology induces intraneuronal cholesterol accumulation. Glöckner F, Ohm TG. J Neuropathol Exp Neurol. 2014 Sep;73(9):846-54.

[116] Tau overexpression impacts a neuroinflammation gene expression network perturbed in Alzheimer's disease. Wes PD, Easton A, Corradi J, Barten DM, Devidze N, DeCarr LB, Truong A, He A, Barrezueta NX, Polson C, Bourin C, Flynn ME, Keenan S, Lidge R, Meredith J, Natale J, Sankaranarayanan S, Cadelina GW, Albright CF, Cacace AM. PLoS One. 2014 Aug 25;9(8):e106050.

[117] TDP-43 pathology in the population: prevalence and associations with dementia and age. Keage HA[1], Hunter S[2], Matthews FE[3], Ince PG[4], Hodges J[5], Hokkanen SR[2], Highley JR[4], Dening T[6], Brayne C[2]. J Alzheimers Dis. 2014;42(2):641-50.

[118] High Levels of Homocysteine Results in Cerebral Amyloid Angiopathy in Mice. Li JG, Praticò D. J Alzheimers Dis. 2014 Jul 24.

[119] Neuroprotection by spice-derived nutraceuticals: you are what you eat! Kannappan R, Gupta SC, Kim JH, Reuter S, Aggarwal BB. Mol Neurobiol. 2011 Oct;44(2):142-59.

[120] Neuroinflammation in Alzheimer's disease; A source of heterogeneity and target for personalized therapy. Latta CH, Brothers HM, Wilcock DM. Neuroscience. 2014 Oct 5. pii: S0306-4522(14)00820-3.

[121] Astrocytes and neuroinflammation in Alzheimer's disease. Phillips EC, Croft CL, Kurbatskaya K, O'Neill MJ, Hutton ML, Hanger DP, Garwood CJ, Noble W. Biochem Soc Trans. 2014 Oct;42(5):1321-5.

[122] When astrocytes become harmful: Functional and inflammatory responses that contribute to Alzheimer's disease. Avila-Muñoz E, Arias C. Ageing Res Rev. 2014 Nov;18C:29-40.

[123] Systemic inflammation, blood-brain barrier vulnerability and cognitive/non-cognitive symptoms in Alzheimer disease: relevance to pathogenesis and therapy. Takeda S, Sato N, Morishita R. Front Aging Neurosci. 2014 Jul 29;6:171.

[124] Cerebral inflammation is an underlying mechanism of early death in Alzheimer's disease: a 13-year cause-specific multivariate mortality study. Nägga K, Wattmo C, Zhang Y, Wahlund LO, Palmqvist S. Alzheimers Res Ther. 2014 Jul 7;6(4):41.

[125] Cerebrospinal fluid cortisol and clinical disease progression in MCI and dementia of Alzheimer'stype. Popp J, Wolfsgruber S, Heuser I, Peters O, Hüll M, Schröder J, Möller HJ, Lewczuk P, Schneider A, Jahn H, Luckhaus C, Perneczky R, Frölich L, Wagner M, Maier W, Wiltfang J, Kornhuber J, Jessen F. Neurobiol Aging. 2014 Oct 31. pii: S0197-4580(14)00691-5.

[126] Immune responses in rapidly progressive dementia: a comparative study of neuroinflammatory markers in Creutzfeldt-Jakob disease, Alzheimer¿s disease and multiple sclerosis. Stoeck K, Schmitz M, Ebert E, Schmidt C, Zerr I. J Neuroinflammation. 2014 Oct 15;11(1):170.

[127] Mitochondrial dysfunction: different routes to Alzheimer's disease therapy. Picone P, Nuzzo D, Caruana L, Scafidi V, Di Carlo M. Oxid Med Cell Longev. 2014;2014:780179.

[128] Quantitative changes in the mitochondrial proteome from subjects with mild cognitive impairment, early stage, and late stage Alzheimer's disease. Lynn BC, Wang J, Markesbery WR, Lovell MA. J Alzheimers Dis. 2010;19(1):325-39.

[129] The mitochondrial O-linked N-acetylglucosamine transferase (mOGT) in the diabetic patient could be the initial trigger to develop Alzheimer disease. Lozano L[1], Lara-Lemus R[2], Zenteno E[1], Alvarado-Vásquez N[3]. Exp Gerontol. 2014 Oct;58:198-202.

[130] Insulin as a Bridge between Type 2 Diabetes and Alzheimer Disease - How Anti-Diabetics Could be a Solution for Dementia. Sebastião I[1], Candeias E[2], Santos MS[1],

de Oliveira CR[3], Moreira PI[4], Duarte AI[2]. <u>Front Endocrinol (Lausanne).</u> 2014 Jul 8;5:110.

[131] Biological mechanisms linking Alzheimer's disease and type-2 diabetes mellitus. Mushtaq G, Khan JA, Kamal MA[1]. <u>CNS Neurol Disord Drug Targets.</u> 2014;13(7):1192-201.

[132] Higher serum glucose levels are associated with cerebral hypometabolism in Alzheimer regions. Burns CM[1], Chen K, Kaszniak AW, Lee W, Alexander GE, Bandy D, Fleisher AS, Caselli RJ, Reiman EM. <u>Neurology.</u> 2013 Apr 23;80(17):1557-64.

[133] Type 2 Diabetes Aggravates Alzheimer's disease-Associated Vascular Alterations of the Aorta in Mice. Sena CM[1], Pereira AM[1], Carvalho C[2], Fernandes R[3], Seiça RM[1], Oliveira CR[4], Moreira PI[5]. <u>J Alzheimers Dis.</u> 2014 Dec 2.

[134] Vascular dysfunction associated with type 2 diabetes and Alzheimer's disease: a potential etiological linkage. Wang F[1], Guo X[2], Shen X[3], Kream RM[4], Mantione KJ[4], Stefano GB[4]. <u>Med Sci Monit Basic Res.</u> 2014 Aug 1;20:118-29.

[135] Brain alterations and clinical symptoms of dementia in diabetes: aβ/tau-dependent and independent mechanisms. Sato N[1], Morishita R[2.] <u>Front Endocrinol (Lausanne).</u> 2014 Sep 5;5:143.

[136] Food for thought: Regulation of synaptic function by metabolic hormones. McGregor G[1], Malekizadeh Y, Harvey J. <u>Mol Endocrinol.</u> 2014 Dec 3:me20141328.

[137] Insulin resistance in Alzheimer's disease. Dineley KT[1], Jahrling JB[1], Denner L[2]. <u>Neurobiol Dis.</u> 2014 Dec;72PA:92-103.

[138] Role of insulin resistance in Alzheimer's disease. Cai Z[1], Xiao M, Chang L, Yan LJ. <u>Metab Brain Dis.</u> 2014 Nov 16.

[139] Dysfunction in Executive Functioning in an Elderly Population with Diabetes Mellitus. Consbruck F, Vagt D, Mazur L, Page C, Mulligan K, Webbe F. <u>Arch Clin Neuropsychol.</u> 2014 Sep;29(6):533-4.

[140] Conversion of Mild Cognitive Impairment to Dementia among Subjects with Diabetes: A Population-Based Study of Incidence and Risk Factors with Five Years of Follow-up. Ma F[1], Wu T[2], Miao R[1], Xiao YY[2], Zhang W[1], Huang G[2]. <u>J Alzheimers Dis.</u> 2014 Aug 26.

[141] Is Brain Copper Deficiency in Alzheimer's, Lewy Body, and Creutzfeldt Jakob Diseases the Common Key for a Free Radical Mechanism and Oxidative Stress-Induced Damage? Deloncle R, Guillard O. J Alzheimers Dis. 2014 Aug 13.

[142] Copper subtype of Alzheimer's disease (AD): Meta-analyses, genetic studies and predictive value of non-ceruloplasmim copper in mild cognitive impairment conversion to full AD. Squitti R. J Trace Elem Med Biol. 2014 Oct;28(4):482-5.

[143] Preventive effects of ramelteon on delirium: a randomized placebo-controlled trial. Hatta K[1], Kishi Y[2], Wada K[3], Takeuchi T[4], Odawara T[5], Usui C[1], Nakamura H[6]; DELIRIA-J Group. JAMA Psychiatry. 2014 Apr;71(4):397-403.

[144] Contrastive conversational analysis of language production by Alzheimer's and control people. Boyé M, Grabar N, Thi Tran M. Stud Health Technol Inform. 2014;205:682-6.

[145] Assessing cognition and function in Alzheimer's disease clinical trials: Do we have the right tools? Snyder PJ, Kahle-Wrobleski K, Brannan S, Miller DS, Schindler RJ, DeSanti S, Ryan JM, Morrison G, Grundman M, Chandler J, Caselli RJ, Isaac M, Bain L, Carrillo MC. Alzheimers Dement. 2014 Nov;10(6):853-60.

[146] Functional disorganization of small-world brain networks in mild Alzheimer's disease and amnestic Mild Cognitive Impairment: an EEG study using Relative Wavelet Entropy (RWE). Frantzidis CA, Vivas AB, Tsolaki A, Klados MA, Tsolaki M, Bamidis PD. Front Aging Neurosci. 2014 Aug 26;6:224.

[147] Early neuropsychological detection of Alzheimer's disease. Bastin C, Salmon E. Eur J Clin Nutr. 2014 Nov;68(11):1192-1199.

[148] Dementia in the USA: state variation in prevalence. Koller D, Bynum JP. J Public Health (Oxf). 2014 Oct 20.

[149] Screening for cognitive impairment in older adults: U.S. Preventive Services Task Force recommendation statement. Moyer VA; U.S. Preventive Services Task Force. Ann Intern Med. 2014 Jun 3;160(11):791-7.

[150] USPSTF: No to Routine Screening for Cognitive Impairment. Sue Hughes http://www.medscape.com/viewarticle/822581. March 26, 2014.

[151] Factors associated with cognitive evaluations in the United States. Kotagal V, Langa KM, Plassman BL, Fisher GG, Giordani BJ, Wallace RB, Burke JR, Steffens DC, Kabeto M, Albin RL, Foster NL. Neurology. 2015 Jan 6;84(1):64-71.

[152] Public perceptions of presymptomatic testing for Alzheimer disease. Caselli RJ, Langbaum J, Marchant GE, Lindor RA, Hunt KS, Henslin BR, Dueck AC, Robert JS. Mayo Clin Proc. 2014 Oct;89(10):1389-96.

[153] Preferences of older people for early diagnosis and disclosure of Alzheimer's disease (AD) before and after considering potential risks and benefits. Robinson SM, Canavan M, O'Keeffe ST. Arch Gerontol Geriatr. 2014 Nov-Dec;59(3):607-12.

[154] The preclinical Alzheimer cognitive composite: measuring amyloid-related decline. Donohue MC[1], Sperling RA[2], Salmon DP[3], Rentz DM[2], Raman R[1], Thomas RG[3], Weiner M[4], Aisen PS[3]; Australian Imaging, Biomarkers, and Lifestyle Flagship Study of Ageing; Alzheimer's disease Neuroimaging Initiative; Alzheimer's disease Cooperative Study. JAMA Neurol. 2014 Aug;71(8):961-70.

[155] Cut-off values of blessed dementia rating scale and its clinical application in elderly Taiwanese. Yang YH[1], Lai CL, Lin RT, Tai CT, Liu CK. Kaohsiung J Med Sci. 2006 Aug;22(8):377-84.

[156] Simple Tool Helps Track Memory, Will Aid AD Trials. Megan Brooks. Reuters Health, February 26, 2015. http://www.medscape.com/viewarticle/840406_print.

[157] Charting the decline in spontaneous writing in Alzheimer's disease: a longitudinal study. Forbes-McKay K[1], Shanks M[2], Venneri A[2]. Acta Neuropsychiatr. 2014 Aug;26(4):246-52.

[158] The use of the Clock Drawing Test in bipolar disorder with or without dementia of Alzheimer's type. Aprahamian I, Radanovic M, Nunes PV, Ladeira RB, Forlenza OV. Arq Neuropsiquiatr. 2014 Dec 2.

[159] Everyday Cognition Scale Items that Best Discriminate Between and Predict Progression From Clinically Normal to Mild Cognitive Impairment. Marshall GA, Zoller AS, Kelly KE, Amariglio RE, Locascio JJ, Johnson KA, Sperling RA, Rentz DM, For The Alzheimer's disease Neuroimaging Initiative[1]. Curr Alzheimer Res. 2014;11(9):853-61.

[160] SIST-M-IR activities of daily living items that best discriminate clinically normal elderly from those with mild cognitive impairment. Zoller AS, Gaal IM, Royer CA, Locascio JJ, Amariglio RE, Blacker D, Okereke OI, Johnson KA, Sperling RA, Rentz DM, Marshall GA[1]. Curr Alzheimer Res. 2014;11(8):785-91.

[161] Differentiating normal from pathological brain ageing using standard neuropsychological tests. Wakefield SJ, McGeown WJ, Shanks MF, Venneri A. Curr Alzheimer Res. 2014;11(8):765-72.

¹⁶² Single neuropsychological test scores associated with rate of cognitive decline in early Alzheimer disease. Parikh M[1], Hynan LS, Weiner MF, Lacritz L, Ringe W, Cullum CM. Clin Neuropsychol. 2014;28(6):926-40.

¹⁶³ Innovative diagnostic tools for early detection of Alzheimer's disease. Laske C[1], Sohrabi HR[2], Frost SM[3], López-de-Ipiña K[4], Garrard P[5], Buscema M[6], Dauwels J[7], Soekadar SR[8], Mueller S[8], Linnemann C[8], Bridenbaugh SA[9], Kanagasingam Y[3], Martins RN[2], O'Bryant SE[10]. Alzheimers Dement. 2014 Nov 15. pii: S1552-5260(14)02463-7.

¹⁶⁴ Awareness of memory deficits in subjective cognitive decline, mild cognitive impairment, Alzheimer's disease and Parkinson's disease. Lehrner J[1], Kogler S[2], Lamm C[2], Moser D[1], Klug S[1], Pusswald G[1], Dal-Bianco P[1], Pirker W[1], Auff E[1]. Int Psychogeriatr. 2014 Nov 10:1-10.

¹⁶⁵ The clinical utility of informants' appraisals on prospective and retrospective memory in patients with early Alzheimer's disease. Hsu YH[1], Huang CF[2], Tu MC[2], Hua MS[3]. PLoS One. 2014 Nov 10;9(11):e112210.

¹⁶⁶Relationship of dementia screening tests with biomarkers of Alzheimer's disease. Galvin JE[1], Fagan AM, Holtzman DM, Mintun MA, Morris JC. Brain. 2010 Nov;133(11):3290-300.

¹⁶⁷ Longitudinal Association of Dementia and Depression. Snowden MB[1], Atkins DC[2], Steinman LE[3], Bell JF[4], Bryant LL[5], Copeland C[3], Fitzpatrick AL[6]. Am J Geriatr Psychiatry. 2014 Sep 21. pii: S1064-7481(14)00260-7.

¹⁶⁸ Prevalence and covariates of elevated depressive symptoms in rural memory clinic patients with mild cognitive impairment or dementia. Kosteniuk JG[1], Morgan DG[1], O'Connell ME[2], Crossley M[2], Kirk A[3], Stewart NJ[4], Karunanayake CP. Dement Geriatr Cogn Dis Extra. 2014 Jul 1;4(2):209-20.

¹⁶⁹ Examining the association between late-life depressive symptoms, cognitive function, and brain volumes in the context of cognitive reserve. O'Shea DM[1], Fieo RA, Hamilton JL, Zahodne LB, Manly JJ, Stern Y. Int J Geriatr Psychiatry. 2014 Aug 22.

¹⁷⁰Depressive symptoms are more strongly related to executive functioning and episodic memory among African American compared with non-Hispanic White older adults. Zahodne LB[1], Nowinski CJ[2], Gershon RC[3], Manly JJ[4]. Arch Clin Neuropsychol. 2014 Nov;29(7):663-9.

[171] Neuropathology of Depression in Alzheimer's disease: Current Knowledge and the Potential for New Treatments. Khundakar AA, Thomas AJ. J Alzheimers Dis. 2014 Sep 10.

[172] The Geriatric Depression Scale and the Cornell Scale for Depression in Dementia. A validity study. Kørner A[1], Lauritzen L, Abelskov K, Gulmann N, Marie Brodersen A, Wedervang-Jensen T, Marie Kjeldgaard K. Nord J Psychiatry. 2006;60(5):360-4.

[173] Decline in renal functioning is associated with longitudinal decline in global cognitive functioning, abstract reasoning and verbal memory. Davey A[1], Elias MF, Robbins MA, Seliger SL, Dore GA. Nephrol Dial Transplant. 2013 Jul;28(7):1810-9.

[174] Hemoglobin level in older persons and incident Alzheimer disease: prospective cohort analysis. Shah RC[1], Buchman AS, Wilson RS, Leurgans SE, Bennett DA. Neurology. 2011 Jul 19;77(3):219-26.

[175] Cerebral and blood correlates of reduced functional connectivity in mild cognitive impairment. Gonzalez-Escamilla G[1], Atienza M, Garcia-Solis D, Cantero JL. Brain Struct Funct. 2014 Nov 1.

[176] Homocysteine: a biomarker in neurodegenerative diseases. Herrmann W[1], Obeid R. Clin Chem Lab Med. 2011 Mar;49(3):435-41.

[177] The relationship between cholesterol and cognitive function is homocysteine-dependent. Cheng Y[1], Jin Y[1], Unverzagt FW[2], Su L[1], Yang L[3], Ma F[1], Hake AM[4], Kettler C[3], Chen C[1], Liu J[1], Bian J[5], Li P[6], Murrell JR[7], Hendrie HC[8], Gao S.[3] Clin Interv Aging. 2014 Oct 23;9:1823-9.

[178] Serum brain-derived neurotrophic factor and the risk for dementia: the Framingham Heart Study. Weinstein G[1], Beiser AS[2], Choi SH[3], Preis SR[4], Chen TC[5], Vorgas D[5], Au R[1], Pikula A[1], Wolf PA[1], DeStefano AL[2], Vasan RS[1], Seshadri S[1]. JAMA Neurol. 2014 Jan;71(1):55-61.

[179] Biomarkers in the diagnosis and management of Alzheimer's disease. Wurtman R. Metabolism. 2014 Oct 30. pii: S0026-0495(14)00343-6.

[180] FDA Approves Blood Test That Gauges Heart Attack Risk. E.J. Mundell. Dec. 15, 2014, new release, U.S. Food and Drug Administration. http://www.nlm.nih.gov/medlineplus/news/fullstory_149968.html. (*this news item will not be available after 03/15/2015).

[181] Peripheral Biomarkers of Alzheimer's disease. Khan TK, Alkon DL J Alzheimers Dis. 2014 Nov 5.

[182] Brain Insulin Resistance Marker May Diagnose Alzheimer's. Megan Brooks. November 25, 2014. Dimitrios Kapogiannis. Society for Neuroscience 2014 Annual Meeting: Poster 197.03. Presented November 16, 2014. http://www.medscape.com/viewarticle/835489_print.

[183] A platelet protein biochip rapidly detects an Alzheimer's disease-specific phenotype. Veitinger M[1], Oehler R, Umlauf E, Baumgartner R, Schmidt G, Gerner C, Babeluk R, Attems J, Mitulovic G, Rappold E, Lamont J, Zellner M. Acta Neuropathol. 2014 Nov;128(5):665-77.

[184] Serum coenzyme Q10 levels as a predictor of dementia in a Japanese general populat. Momiyama Y. Atherosclerosis. 2014 Oct 2;237(2):433-434.

[185] NT-proBNP and the Risk of Dementia: A Prospective Cohort Study with 14 Years of Follow-Up. Tynkkynen J[1], Laatikainen T[2], Salomaa V[3], Havulinna AS[3], Blankenberg S[4], Zeller T[4], Hernesniemi JA[1]. J Alzheimers Dis. 2014 Nov 14.

[186] Novel plasma biomarker surrogating cerebral amyloid deposition. Kaneko N[1], Nakamura A, Washimi Y, Kato T, Sakurai T, Arahata Y, Bundo M, Takeda A, Niida S, Ito K, Toba K, Tanaka K, Yanagisawa K. Proc Jpn Acad Ser B Phys Biol Sci. 2014;90(9):353-64..

[187] Plasma amyloid-β and risk of Alzheimer's disease in the Framingham Heart Study. Chouraki V[1], Beiser A[2], Younkin L[3], Preis SR[4], Weinstein G[5], Hansson O[6], Skoog I[7], Lambert JC[8], Au R[5], Launer L[9], Wolf PA[5], Younkin S[3], Seshadri S[5]. Alzheimers Dement. 2014 Sep 9. pii: S1552-5260(14)02496-0.

[188] Identification of preclinical Alzheimer's disease by a profile of pathogenic proteins in neurally derived blood exosomes: A case-control study. Fiandaca MS[1], Kapogiannis D[2], Mapstone M[3], Boxer A[4], Eitan E[2], Schwartz JB[5], Abner EL[6], Petersen RC[7], Federoff HJ[1], Miller BL[4], Goetzl EJ[8]. Alzheimers Dement. 2014 Aug 14. pii: S1552-5260(14)02469-8.

[189] Relationship between Serum Levels of Tau Fragments and Clinical Progression of Alzheimer's disease. Henriksen K, Byrjalsen I, Christiansen C, Karsdal MA. J Alzheimers Dis. 2014 Aug 28.

[190] A Global Immune Deficit in Alzheimer's disease and Mild Cognitive Impairment Disclosed by a Novel Data Mining Process. Gironi M[1], Borgiani B[1], Farina E[2], Mariani E[3], Cursano C[3], Alberoni M[2], Nemni R[2], Comi G[4], Buscema M[5], Furlan R[4], Grossi E[5]. J Alzheimers Dis. 2014 Sep 8.

[191] A Blood-Based, 7-Metabolite Signature for the Early Diagnosis of Alzheimer's disease. Olazarán J[1], Gil-de-Gómez L[2], Rodríguez-Martín A[2], Valentí-Soler M[3], Frades-Payo B[3], Marín-Muñoz J[4], Antúnez C[4], Frank-García A[5], Jiménez CA[5], Gracia LM[6], Torregrossa RP[6], Guisasola MC[7], Bermejo-Pareja F[8], Sánchez-Ferro Á[9], Pérez-Martínez DA[10], Palomo SM[10], Farquhar R[11], Rábano A[12], Calero M[13]. J Alzheimers Dis. 2015 Feb 3.

[192] Serum metabolomic biomarkers of dementia. Mousavi M[1], Jonsson P[2], Antti H[2], Adolfsson R[3], Nordin A[3], Bergdahl J[4], Eriksson K[5], Moritz T[6], Nilsson LG[7], Nyberg L[8]. Dement Geriatr Cogn Dis Extra. 2014 Jul 11;4(2):252-62.

[193] Predicative genetic testing for Alzheimer's disease. Lee T. Ann Acad Med Singapore. 2014 Sep;43(9):437-8.

[194] Genetics of Alzheimer's disease. Chouraki V, Seshadri S. Adv Genet. 2014;87:245-94.

[195] AlzBase: an Integrative Database for Gene Dysregulation in Alzheimer's disease. Bai Z[1], Han G, Xie B, Wang J, Song F, Peng X, Lei H. Mol Neurobiol. 2014 Nov 29.

[196] Plasma levels of apolipoprotein E and risk of dementia in the general population. Rasmussen KL[1], Tybjaerg-Hansen A, Nordestgaard BG, Frikke-Schmidt R. Ann Neurol. 2014 Dec 3.

[197] The ApoE gene is related with exceptional longevity: a systematic review and meta-analysis. Garatachea N[1], Marín PJ, Santos-Lozano A, Sanchis-Gomar F, Emanuele E, Lucia A. Rejuvenation Res. 2014 Nov 10.

[198] Women with the Alzheimer's risk marker ApoE4 lose Aβ-specific CD4⁺ T cells 10-20 years before men. Begum AN[1], Cunha C[1], Sidhu H[2], Alkam T[1], Scolnick J[3], Rosario ER[4], Ethell DW[1]. Transl Psychiatry. 2014 Jul 29;4:e414.

[199] The role of TREM2 R47H as a risk factor for Alzheimer's disease, frontotemporal lobar degeneration, amyotrophic lateral sclerosis, and Parkinson's disease. Lill CM[1], Rengmark A[2], Pihlstrøm L[2], Fogh I[3], Shatunov A[3], Sleiman PM[4], Wang LS[5], Liu T[6], Lassen CF[7], Meissner E[8], Alexopoulos P[9], Calvo A[10], Chio A[11], Dizdar N[12], Faltraco F[13], Forsgren L[14], Kirchheiner J[15], Kurz A[9], Larsen JP[16], Liebsch M[8], Linder J[14], Morrison KE[17], Nissbrandt H[18], Otto M[15], Pahnke J[19], Partch A[5], Restagno G[20], Rujescu D[21], Schnack C[15], Shaw CE[3], Shaw PJ[22], Tumani H[15], Tysnes OB[23], Valladares O[5], Silani V[24], van den Berg LH[25], van Rheenen W[25], Veldink JH[25], Lindenberger U[6], Steinhagen-Thiessen E[26]; SLAGEN Consortium, Teipel S[27], Perneczky R[28], Hakonarson H[4], Hampel H[29], von Arnim CA[15], Olsen JH[7], Van Deerlin VM[5], Al-

Chalabi A³, Toft M², Ritz B³⁰, Bertram L³¹. Alzheimers Dement. 2015 Apr 30. pii: S1552-5260(15)00122-3.

²⁰⁰ Comparison of brief cognitive tests and CSF biomarkers in predicting Alzheimer's disease in mild cognitive impairment: six-year follow-up study. Palmqvist S¹, Hertze J, Minthon L, Wattmo C, Zetterberg H, Blennow K, Londos E, Hansson O. PLoS One. 2012;7(6):e38639.

²⁰¹Biomarkers in the Diagnosis and Prognosis of Alzheimer's disease. Schaffer C¹, Sarad N¹, DeCrumpe A¹, Goswami D¹, Herrmann S¹, Morales J¹, Patel P¹, Osborne J². J Lab Autom. 2014 Nov 25.

²⁰² Plasma and cerebrospinal fluid amyloid beta for the diagnosis of Alzheimer's disease dementia and other dementias in people with mild cognitive impairment (MCI). Ritchie C¹, Smailagic N, Noel-Storr AH, Takwoingi Y, Flicker L, Mason SE, McShane R. Cochrane Database Syst Rev. 2014 Jun 10;6:CD008782.

²⁰³ Accuracy of brain amyloid detection in clinical practice using cerebrospinal fluid β-amyloid 42: a cross-validation study against amyloid positron emission tomography. Palmqvist S¹, Zetterberg H², Blennow K², Vestberg S³, Andreasson U², Brooks DJ⁴, Owenius R⁵, Hägerström D⁶, Wollmer P⁷, Minthon L⁸, Hansson O⁸. JAMA Neurol. 2014 Oct;71(10):1282-9.

²⁰⁴ Role of cerebrospinal fluid biomarkers to predict conversion to dementia in patients with mild cognitive impairment: a clinical cohort study. Tondelli M, Bedin R, Chiari A, Molinari MA, Bonifacio G, Lelli N, Trenti T, Nichelli P. Clin Chem Lab Med. 2014 Oct 2.

²⁰⁵ Cerebrospinal Fluid Biomarkers Distinguish Postmortem-Confirmed Alzheimer's disease from Other Dementias and Healthy Controls in the OPTIMA Cohort. Seeburger JL¹, Holder DJ¹, Combrinck M², Joachim C³, Laterza O¹, Tanen M¹, Dallob A¹, Chappell D¹, Snyder K¹, Flynn M¹, Simon A¹, Modur V¹, Potter WZ¹, Wilcock G³, Savage MJ¹, Smith AD³. J Alzheimers Dis. 2014 Nov 12.

²⁰⁶ Assessment of CSF Aβ42 as an aid to discriminating Alzheimer's disease from other dementias and mild cognitive impairment: a meta-analysis of 50 studies. Tang W¹, Huang Q², Wang Y³, Wang ZY¹, Yao YY⁴. J Neurol Sci. 2014 Oct 15;345(1-2):26-36.

²⁰⁷The clinical use of cerebrospinal fluid biomarker testing for Alzheimer's disease diagnosis: A consensus paper from the Alzheimer'sBiomarkers Standardization Initiative. Molinuevo JL¹, Blennow K², Dubois B³, Engelborghs S⁴, Lewczuk P⁵, Perret-

Liaudet A[6], Teunissen CE[7], Parnetti L[8]. Alzheimers Dement. 2014 Nov;10(6):808-817.

[208] Cerebrospinal Fluid Apolipoprotein E Concentration and Progression of Alzheimer's disease. Schmidt C[1], Gerlach N[1], Peter C[1], Gherib K[1], Lange K[2], Fride T[2], Zerr I[3]. J Alzheimers Dis. 2014 Aug 13.

[209] Apolipoprotein E genotype and the diagnostic accuracy of cerebrospinal fluid biomarkers for Alzheimer disease. Lautner R[1], Palmqvist S[2], Mattsson N[3], Andreasson U[1], Wallin A[1], Pålsson E[1], Jakobsson J[1], Herukka SK[4], Owenius R[5], Olsson B[1], Hampel H[6], Rujescu D[7], Ewers M[8], Landén M[9], Minthon L[2], Blennow K[1], Zetterberg H[10], Hansson O[2]; Alzheimer's disease Neuroimaging Initiative. JAMA Psychiatry. 2014 Oct;71(10):1183-91.

[210] Endostatin Level in Cerebrospinal Fluid of Patients with Alzheimer's disease. Salza R[1], Oudart JB[2], Ramont L[2], Maquart FX[2], Bakchine S[3], Thoannès H[4], Ricard-Blum S[1]. J Alzheimers Dis. 2014 Nov 18.

[211] Diagnostic impact of CSF biomarkers for Alzheimer's disease in a tertiary memory clinic. Duits FH[1], Prins ND[2], Lemstra AW[2], Pijnenburg YA[2], Bouwman FH[2], Teunissen CE[3], Scheltens P[2], van der Flier WM[4]. Alzheimers Dement. 2014 Aug 21.

[212] [Imaging diagnosis of dementia]. Ishii K. Nihon Rinsho. 2014 Apr;72(4):681-6. [Article in Japanese].

[213] The appropriate use of neuroimaging in the diagnostic work-up of dementia: an evidence-based analysis. Health Quality Ontario. Ont Health Technol Assess Ser. 2014 Feb 1;14(1):1-64.

[214] Alzheimer disease: focus on computed tomography. Reynolds A. Radiol Technol. 2013 Nov-Dec;85(2):187CT-211CT.

[215] Comparison between brain CT and MRI for voxel-based morphometry of Alzheimer's disease. Imabayashi E[1], Matsuda H[2], Tabira T[3], Arima K[4], Araki N[5], Ishii K[6], Yamashita F[7], Iwatsubo T[8]; Japanese Alzheimer's disease Neuroimaging Initiative. Brain Behav. 2013 Jul;3(4):487-93.

[216] Advances in MRI biomarkers for the diagnosis of Alzheimer's disease. Kehoe EG[1], McNulty JP, Mullins PG, Bokde AL. Biomark Med. 2014 Oct;8(9):1151-69.

[217] Loss of fornix white matter volume as a predictor of cognitive impairment in cognitively normal elderly individuals. Fletcher E[1], Raman M, Huebner P, Liu A, Mungas D, Carmichael O, DeCarli C. JAMA Neurol. 2013 Nov;70(11):1389-95.

[218] Lobar Microbleeds Are Associated with a Decline in Executive Functioning in Older Adults. Meier IB[1], Gu Y, Guzaman VA, Wiegman AF, Schupf N, Manly JJ, Luchsinger JA, Viswanathan A, Martinez-Ramirez S, Greenberg SM, Mayeux R, Brickman AM. Cerebrovasc Dis. 2014 Nov 25;38(5):377-383.

[219] White matter hyperintensities as early and independent predictors of Alzheimer's disease risk. Mortamais M[1], Artero S[1], Ritchie K[2]. J Alzheimers Dis. 2014 Jan 1;42(0):S393-400.

[220] Reconsidering harbingers of dementia: progression of parietal lobe white matter hyperintensities predicts Alzheimer's disease incidence. Brickman AM[1], Zahodne LB[2], Guzman VA[3], Narkhede A[3], Meier IB[3], Griffith EY[3], Provenzano FA[3], Schupf N[4], Manly JJ[5], Stern Y[5], Luchsinger JA[6], Mayeux R[7]. Neurobiol Aging. 2014 Jul 21. pii: S0197-4580(14)00488-6.

[221] A 10-year follow-up of hippocampal volume on magnetic resonance imaging in early dementia and cognitive decline. den Heijer T[1], van der Lijn F, Koudstaal PJ, Hofman A, van der Lugt A, Krestin GP, Niessen WJ, Breteler MM. Brain. 2010 Apr;133(Pt 4):1163-72.

[222] Cerebral blood flow measured by arterial spin labeling MRI as a preclinical marker of Alzheimer's disease. Wierenga CE[1], Hays CC[2], Zlatar ZZ[1]. J Alzheimers Dis. 2014 Jan 1;42(0):S411-9.

[223] Amyloid imaging in Alzheimer's disease: a literature review. Saidlitz P[1], Voisin T, Vellas B, Payoux P, Gabelle A, Formaglio M, Delrieu J. J Nutr Health Aging. 2014 Jul;18(7):723-40.

[224] Regional functional connectivity predicts distinct cognitive impairments in Alzheimer's disease spectrum. Ranasinghe KG[1], Hinkley LB[2], Beagle AJ[1], Mizuiri D[2], Dowling AF[2], Honma SM[2], Finucane MM[3], Scherling C[1], Miller BL[1], Nagarajan SS[2], Vossel KA[4]. Neuroimage Clin. 2014 Jul 23;5:385-95.

[225] Slowing of EEG Background Activity in Parkinson's and Alzheimer's disease with Early Cognitive Dysfunction. Benz N[1], Hatz F[1], Bousleiman H[2], Ehrensperger MM[3], Gschwandtner U[1], Hardmeier M[1], Ruegg S[1], Schindler C[4], Zimmermann R[1], Monsch AU[3], Fuhr P[1]. Front Aging Neurosci. 2014 Nov 18;6:314.

[226] The Acetylcholine Index: An Electroencephalographic Marker of Cholinergic Activity in the Living Human Brain Applied to Alzheimer's disease and Other Dementias. Johannsson M[1], Snaedal J, Johannesson GH, Gudmundsson TE, Johnsen K. Dement Geriatr Cogn Disord. 2014 Nov 27;39(3-4):132-142.

[227] Olfactory Deprivation Hastens Alzheimer-Like Pathologies in a Human Tau-Overexpressed Mouse Model via Activation of cdk5. Li K[1], Liu FF, He CX, Huang HZ, Xie AJ, Hu F, Liu D, Wang JZ, Zhu LQ. Mol Neurobiol. 2014 Dec 3.

[228] Olfaction and the 5-year incidence of cognitive impairment in an epidemiological study of older adults. Schubert CR[1], Carmichael LL, Murphy C, Klein BE, Klein R, Cruickshanks KJ. J Am Geriatr Soc. 2008 Aug;56(8):1517-21.

[229] Olfactory deficits predict cognitive decline and Alzheimer dementia in an urban community. Devanand DP[1], Lee S[2], Manly J[2], Andrews H[2], Schupf N[2], Doty RL[2], Stern Y[2], Zahodne LB[2], Louis ED[2], Mayeux R[2]. Neurology. 2014 Dec 3.

[230] The brain structural and cognitive basis of odor identification deficits in mild cognitive impairment and Alzheimer's disease. Kjelvik G, Saltvedt I, White LR, Stenumgård P, Sletvold O, Engedal K, Skåtun K, Lyngvær AK, Steffenach HA, Håberg AK[1]. BMC Neurol. 2014 Aug 26;14:168.

[231] Olfactory impairment and subjective olfactory complaints independently predict conversion to dementia: a longitudinal, population-based study. Stanciu I[1], Larsson M[1], Nordin S[2], Adolfsson R[3], Nilsson LG[4], Olofsson JK[1]. J Int Neuropsychol Soc. 2014 Feb;20(2):209-17.

[232] Odor identification and Alzheimer disease biomarkers in clinically normal elderly. Growdon ME[1], Schultz AP[1], Dagley AS[1], Amariglio RE[1], Hedden T[1], Rentz DM[1], Johnson KA[1], Sperling RA[1], Albers MW[1], Marshall GA[2]. Neurology. 2015 May 1. pii: 10.1212/WNL.0000000000001614.

[233] Can a Virtual Reality Cognitive Training Application Fulfill a Dual Role? Using the Virtual Supermarket Cognitive Training Application as a Screening Tool for Mild Cognitive Impairment. Zygouris S[1], Giakoumis D[2], Votis K[2], Doumpoulakis S[2], Konstantinos N[1], Segkouli S[3], Charalampos K[4], Tzovaras D[2], Tsolaki M[1]. J Alzheimers Dis. 2014 Nov 25.

[234] Everyday memory deficits in very mild Alzheimer's disease. Widmann CN[1], Beinhoff U, Riepe MW. Neurobiol Aging. 2012 Feb;33(2):297-303.

[235] Gait and balance analysis for patients with Alzheimer's disease using an inertial-sensor-based wearable instrument. Hsu YL, Chung PC, Wang WH, Pai MC, Wang CY, Lin CW, Wu HL, Wang JS. IEEE J Biomed Health Inform. 2014 Nov;18(6):1822-30.

[236] Measuring life space in older adults with mild-to-moderate Alzheimer's disease using mobile phone GPS. Tung JY[1], Rose RV, Gammada E, Lam I, Roy EA, Black SE, Poupart P. Gerontology. 2014;60(2):154-62.

[237] Topography of primitive reflexes in dementia: an F-18 fluorodeoxyglucose positron emission tomography study. Matias-Guiu JA[1], Cabrera-Martín MN, Fernádez-Matarrubia M, Moreno-Ramos T, Valles-Salgado M, Porta-Etessam J, Carreras JL, Matias-Guiu J. Eur J Neurol. 2015 Apr 29.

[238] Pulse wave velocity as a marker of cognitive impairment in the elderly. Scuteri A[1], Wang H[2]. J Alzheimers Dis. 2014 Jan 1;42(0):S401-10.

[239] Taking the pulse of aging: mapping pulse pressure and elasticity in cerebral arteries with optical methods. Fabiani M[1], Low KA, Tan CH, Zimmerman B, Fletcher MA, Schneider-Garces N, Maclin EL, Chiarelli AM, Sutton BP, Gratton G. Psychophysiology. 2014 Nov;51(11):1072-88.

[240] Retinal microvasculature in Alzheimer's disease. Cheung CY[1], Ong YT[2], Ikram MK[1], Chen C[3], Wong TY[4].
J Alzheimers Dis. 2014 Jan 1;42(0):S339-52.

[241] Eye Movements in Alzheimer's disease. Molitor RJ[1], Ko PC[1], Ally BA[2]. J Alzheimers Dis. 2014 Sep 2.

[242] Volatile organic compounds (VOCs) fingerprint of Alzheimer's disease. Mazzatenta A[1], Pokorski M[2], Sartucci F[3], Domenici L[4], Di Giulio C[5]. Respir Physiol Neurobiol. 2014 Oct 13.

[243] Utility of transcranial ultrasound in predicting Alzheimer's disease risk. Tomek A, Urbanová B, Hort J.
J Alzheimers Dis. 2014 Jan 1;42(0):S365-74.

[244] Attention capacity and self-report of subjective cognitive decline: A P3 ERP study. Smart CM[1], Segalowitz SJ[2], Mulligan BP[3], MacDonald SW[4]. Biol Psychol. 2014 Dec;103:144-51.

[245] Potential therapeutic strategies for Alzheimer's disease targeting or beyond β-amyloid: insights from clinical trials. Jia Q[1], Deng Y[1], Qing H[1]. Biomed Res Int. 2014;2014:837157.

[246] Role of nanomedicines in delivery of anti-acetylcholinesterase compounds to the brain in Alzheimer's disease. Ahmad MZ, Ahmad J, Amin S, Rahman M, Anwar M,

Mallick N, Ahmad FJ, Rahman Z, Kamal MA, Akhter S[1]. CNS Neurol Disord Drug Targets. 2014;13(8):1315-24.

[247]Intranasal therapeutic strategies for management of Alzheimer's disease. Sood S[1], Jain K, Gowthamarajan K. J Drug Target. 2014 May;22(4):279-94.

[248] Modeling test and treatment strategies for presymptomatic Alzheimer disease. Burke JF[1], Langa KM[2], Hayward RA[3], Albin RL[4]. PLoS One. 2014 Dec 4;9(12):e114339.

[249] Effectiveness and cost-effectiveness of the pharmacological treatment of Alzheimer's disease and vascular dementia. Versijpt J. J Alzheimers Dis. 2014;42 Suppl 3:S19-25.

[250]Response to cholinesterase inhibitors affects lifespan in Alzheimer's disease. Wattmo C, Londos E, Minthon L. BMC Neurol. 2014 Sep 10;14:173.

[251]Duration of therapy with acetylcholinesterase inhibitors in patients with mild-to-moderate Alzheimer's disease as reported in the literature. El Melik R[1], Dubil A, Pound MW. Consult Pharm. 2014 Jun;29(6):400-7.

[252] Acetylcholinesterase Inhibitors in Advanced AD: Stop or Go? Tan, ZS. February 24, 2015. http://www.medscape.com/viewarticle/840020_print.

[253] The use of medications approved for Alzheimer's disease in autism spectrum disorder: a systematic review. Rossignol DA[1], Frye RE[2] Front Pediatr. 2014 Aug 22;2:87.

[254] New tetracyclic tacrine analogs containing pyrano[2,3-c]pyrazole: Efficient synthesis, biological assessment and docking simulation study. Khoobi M[1], Ghanoni F[2], Nadri H[3], Moradi A[3], Pirali Hamedani M[1], Homayouni Moghadam F[4], Emami S[5], Vosooghi M[1], Zadmard R[2], Foroumadi A[1], Shafiee A[6]. Eur J Med Chem. 2014 Oct 18;89C:296-303.

[255] Syntheses of coumarin-tacrine hybrids as dual-site acetylcholinesterase inhibitors and their activity against butylcholinesterase, Aβ aggregation, and β-secretase. Sun Q[1], Peng DY[1], Yang SG[1], Zhu XL[1], Yang WC[2], Yang GF[3]. Bioorg Med Chem. 2014 Sep 1;22(17):4784-91.

[256]Donepezil Improves Gait Performance in Older Adults with Mild Alzheimer's disease: A Phase II Clinical Trial. Montero-Odasso M[1], Muir-Hunter SW[2], Oteng-Amoako A[3], Gopaul K[3], Islam A[3], Borrie M[4], Wells J[4], Speechley M[5]. J Alzheimers Dis. 2014 Jul 30.

[257] Donepezil decreases annual rate of hippocampal atrophy in suspected prodromal Alzheimer's disease. Dubois B, Chupin M, Hampel H, Lista S, Cavedo E, Croisile B, Tisserand GL, Touchon J, Bonafe A, Ousset PJ, Ameur AA, Rouaud O, Ricolfi F, Vighetto A, Pasquier F, Delmaire C, Ceccaldi M, Girard N, Dufouil C, Lehericy S, Tonelli I, Duveau F, Colliot O, Garnero L, Sarazin M, Dormont D, and the Hippocamus Study Group. Science Direct. http://dx.doi.org/10.1016/j.jalz.2014.10.003. Januray 14, 2015.

[258] The effect of galantamine on brain atrophy rate in subjects with mild cognitive impairment is modified by apolipoprotein E genotype: post-hoc analysis of data from a randomized controlled trial. Prins ND[1], van der Flier WA[1], Knol DL[2], Fox NC[3], Brashear HR[4], Nye JS[5], Barkhof F[6], Scheltens P[7]. Alzheimers Res Ther. 2014 Jul 21;6(4):47.

[259] Nasal Application of the Galantamine Pro-drug Memogain Slows Down Plaque Deposition and Ameliorates Behavior in 5X Familial Alzheimer's disease Mice. Bhattacharya S[1], Maelicke A[2], Montag D[1]. J Alzheimers Dis. 2015 Feb 26.

[260] Effect of Rivastigmine or Memantine Add-on Therapy Is Affected by Butyrylcholinesterase Genotype in Patients with Probable Alzheimer's disease. Han HJ[1], Kwon JC, Kim JE, Kim SG, Park JM, Park KW, Park KC, Park KH, Moon SY, Seo SW, Choi SH, Cho SJ. Eur Neurol. 2014 Nov 1;73(1-2):23-28.

[261] Memantine may affect pseudobulbar affect in patients with Alzheimer's disease. Prokšelj T[1], Jerin A[2], Kogoj A[3]. Acta Neuropsychiatr. 2013 Dec;25(6):361-6.

[262] Pharmacological treatment of neuropsychiatric symptoms in Alzheimer's disease: a systematic review and meta-analysis. Wang J[1], Yu JT[2], Wang HF[3], Meng XF[1], Wang C[1], Tan CC[1], Tan L[2]. J Neurol Neurosurg Psychiatry. 2015 Jan;86(1):101-9.

[263] Mood stabilizers for the treatment of behavioral and psychological symptoms of dementia: an update review. Yeh YC, Ouyang WC. Kaohsiung J Med Sci. 2012 Apr;28(4):185-93.

[264] [Recognition and treatment of behavioral and psychological symptoms of dementias: lessons from the CATIE-AD study]. Kálmán J[1], Kálmán S, Pákáski M. Neuropsychopharmacol Hung. 2008 Oct;10(4):233-49.
[Article in Hungarian].

[265] Atypical antipsychotics for the treatment of behavioral and psychological symptoms in dementia, with a particular focus on longer term outcomes and mortality. Bal-

lard C[1], Creese B, Corbett A, Aarsland D. Expert Opin Drug Saf. 2011 Jan;10(1):35-43.

[266] Aripiprazole in the treatment of Alzheimer's disease. De Deyn PP[1], Drenth AF, Kremer BP, Oude Voshaar RC, Van Dam D. Expert Opin Pharmacother. 2013 Mar;14(4):459-74.

[267] Therapeutic effects of quetiapine on memory deficit and brain β-amyloid plaque pathology in a transgenic mouse model of Alzheimer's disease. Zhu S, He J, Zhang R, Kong L, Tempier A, Kong J, Li XM. Curr Alzheimer Res. 2013 Mar;10(3):270-8.

[268] Agitation and aggression in Alzheimer's disease: an update on pharmacological and psychosocial approaches to care. Gallagher D[1], Herrmann N. Neurodegener Dis Manag. 2015 Feb;5(1):77-83.

[269] Role of citalopram in the treatment of agitation in Alzheimer's disease. Porsteinsson AP[1], Keltz MA, Smith JS. Neurodegener Dis Manag. 2014;4(5):345-9.

[270] Sertraline-induced potentiation of the CYP3A4-dependent neurotoxicity of carbamazepine: An in vitro study. Ghosh C[1], Hossain M, Spriggs A, Ghosh A, Grant GA, Marchi N, Perucca E, Janigro D. Epilepsia. 2015 Feb 5.

[271] Major depressive disorder in breast cancer: a critical systematic review of pharmacological and psychotherapeutic clinical trials. Carvalho AF, Hyphantis T, Sales PM, Soeiro-de-Souza MG, Macêdo DS, Cha DS, McIntyre RS, Pavlidis N. Cancer Treat Rev. 2014 Apr;40(3):349-55.

[272] Unjustified prescribing of CYP2D6 inhibiting SSRIs in women treated with tamoxifen. Binkhorst L, Mathijssen RH, van Herk-Sukel MP, Bannink M, Jager A, Wiemer EA, van Gelder T. Breast Cancer Res Treat. 2013 Jun;139(3):923-9.

[273] Use of paroxetine during tamoxifen therapy for breast cancer was associated with increased breast-cancer and all-cause mortality. Hillner BE Ann Intern Med. 2010 Jun 15;152(12):JC6-13.

[274] Selective serotonin reuptake inhibitors and breast cancer mortality in women receiving tamoxifen: a population based cohort study. Kelly CM, Juurlink DN, Gomes T, Duong-Hua M, Pritchard KI, Austin PC, Paszat LF. BMJ. 2010 Feb 8;340:c693.

[275] Escitalopram versus risperidone for the treatment of behavioral and psychotic symptoms associated with Alzheimer's disease: a randomized double-blind pilot study. Barak Y[1], Plopski I, Tadger S, Paleacu D. Int Psychogeriatr. 2011 Nov;23(9):1515-9.

[276] Benzodiazepine use and risk of Alzheimer's disease: case-control study. Billioti de Gage S[1], Moride Y[2], Ducruet T[3], Kurth T[4], Verdoux H[5], Tournier M[5], Pariente A[6], Bégaud B[6]. BMJ. 2014 Sep 9;349:g5205.

[277] Inappropriate sexual behavior in a geriatric population. Bardell A[1], Lau T, Fedoroff JP. Int Psychogeriatr. 2011 Sep;23(7):1182-8.

[278] Inappropriate sexual behaviors in cognitively impaired older individuals. Guay DR[1]. Am J Geriatr Pharmacother. 2008 Dec;6(5):269-88.

[279] The use of medroxyprogesterone acetate for the treatment of sexually inappropriate behavior in patients with dementia. Light SA[1], Holroyd S. J Psychiatry Neurosci. 2006 Mar;31(2):132-4.

[280] Cognitively-Based Methods of Enhancing and Maintaining Functioning in those at Risk of Alzheimer's disease. Hampstead BM[1], Mosti CB[2], Swirsky-Sacchetti T[3]. J Alzheimers Dis. 2014 Jan 1;42(0):S483-93.

[281] Is cognitive training an effective treatment for preclinical and early Alzheimer's disease? Gates NJ, Sachdev P. J Alzheimers Dis. 2014 Jan 1;42(0):S551-9.

[282] A rehabilitation program for Alzheimer's disease. Serdà i Ferrer BC[1], del Valle A. J Nurs Res. 2014 Sep;22(3):192-9.

[283] Effect of unawareness on rehabilitation outcome in a randomised controlled trial of multicomponent intervention for patients with mild Alzheimer's disease. Fernández-Calvo B[1], Contador I, Ramos F, Olazarán J, Mograbi DC, Morris RG. Neuropsychol Rehabil. 2014 Aug 14:1-30.

[284] Can education rescue genetic liability for cognitive decline? Cook CJ[1], Fletcher JM. Soc Sci Med. 2014 Jul 7. pii: S0277-9536(14)00417-1.

[285] Brain Training to Keep Dementia at Bay: Buyer Beware. Deborah Brauser. PLoS Med. November 18, 2014. http://www.medscape.com/viewarticle/835296_print.

[286] Alzheimer's disease: The role for neurosurgery. Pereira JL[1], Downes A[1], Gorgulho A[2], Patel V[1], Malkasian D[1], De Salles A[2]. Surg Neurol Int. 2014 Sep 5;5(Suppl 8):S385-90.

[287] The neurosurgical treatment of Alzheimer's disease: a review. Laxton AW[1], Stone S, Lozano AM. Stereotact Funct Neurosurg. 2014;92(5):269-81.

[288] What aspects of social network are protective for dementia? Not the quantity but the quality of social interactions is protective up to 15 years later. Amieva H[1], Stoykova R, Matharan F, Helmer C, Antonucci TC, Dartigues JF. Psychosom Med. 2010 Nov;72(9):905-11.

[289] Social Interaction Rescues Memory Deficit in an Animal Model of Alzheimer's disease by Increasing BDNF-Dependent Hippocampal Neurogenesis. Hsiao YH[1], Hung HC[2], Chen SH[3], Gean PW[4]. J Neurosci. 2014 Dec 3;34(49):16207-19.

[290] Maintaining health and wellness in the face of dementia: an exploratory analysis of individuals attending a rural and remote memory clinic. Dal Bello-Haas VP[1], O'Connell ME[2], Morgan DG[3]. Rural Remote Health. 2014 Jul-Sep;14(3):2722.

[291] Tailored lighting intervention improves measures of sleep, depression, and agitation in persons with Alzheimer's disease and related dementia living in long-term care facilities. Figueiro MG[1], Plitnick BA[1], Lok A[1], Jones GE[1], Higgins P[2], Hornick TR[3], Rea MS[1]. Clin Interv Aging. 2014 Sep 12;9:1527-37.

[292] The effects of transcranial LED therapy (TCLT) on cerebral blood flow in the elderly women. Salgado AS[1], Zângaro RA, Parreira RB, Kerppers II. Lasers Med Sci. 2014 Oct 3.

[293] Non-invasive brain stimulation of the right inferior frontal gyrus may improve attention in early Alzheimer's disease: A pilot study. Eliasova I[1], Anderkova L[1], Marecek R[1], Rektorova I[2]. J Neurol Sci. 2014 Nov 15;346(1-2):318-22.

[294] "The Castle of Remembrance": New insights from a cognitive training programme for autobiographical memory in Alzheimer's disease. Lalanne J[1], Gallarda T, Piolino P. Neuropsychol Rehabil. 2014 Aug 14:1-29.

[295] A computer-aided program for helping patients with moderate Alzheimer's disease engage in verbal reminiscence. Lancioni GE[1], Singh NN[2], O'Reilly MF[3], Sigafoos J[4], Ferlisi G[5], Zullo V[5], Schirone S[6], Prisco R[6], Denitto F[7] Res Dev Disabil. 2014 Nov;35(11):3026-33.

[296] Amyloid beta peptide immunotherapy in Alzheimer disease. Delrieu J[1], Ousset PJ[2], Voisin T[2], Vellas B[2]. Rev Neurol (Paris). 2014 Nov 6.

[297] Identification of structural determinants on tau protein essential for its pathological function: novel therapeutic target for tau immunotherapy in Alzheimer's disease. Kontsekova E[1], Zilka N[1], Kovacech B[2], Skrabana R[1], Novak M[1]. Alzheimers Res Ther. 2014 Aug 1;6(4):45.

[298] Efficacy and safety studies of gantenerumab in patients with Alzheimer's disease. Panza F[1], Solfrizzi V, Imbimbo BP, Giannini M, Santamato A, Seripa D, Logroscino G. Expert Rev Neurother. 2014 Sep;14(9):973-86.

[299] Intravenous immunoglobulins for Alzheimer's disease. Puli L, Tanila H, Relkin N[1]. Curr Alzheimer Res. 2014;11(7):626-36.

[300] Configuration-specific immunotherapy targeting cis pThr231-Pro232 tau for Alzheimer disease. Wang JZ[1], Zhang Y[2]. J Neurol Sci. 2014 Nov 13. pii: S0022-510X(14)00725-4.

[301] Long-acting intranasal insulin detemir improves cognition for adults with mild cognitive impairment or early-stage Alzheimer's disease dementia. Claxton A[1], Baker LD[2], Hanson A[1], Trittschuh EH[1], Cholerton B[3], Morgan A[1], Callaghan M[1], Arbuckle M[4], Behl C[1], Craft S[2]. J Alzheimers Dis. 2015 Jan 1;44(3):897-906.

[302] The potential of epigenetic therapies in neurodegenerative diseases. Coppedè F. Front Genet. 2014 Jul 14;5:220.

[303] A new way to produce hyperketonemia: Use of ketone ester in a case of Alzheimer's disease. Newport MT[1], VanItallie TB[2], Kashiwaya Y[3], King MT[4], Veech RL[5]. Alzheimers Dement. 2014 Oct 7. pii: S1552-5260(14)00032-6.

[304] A physically-modified saline suppresses neuronal apoptosis, attenuates tau phosphorylation and protects memory in an animal model of Alzheimer's disease. Modi KK[1], Jana A[1], Ghosh S[2], Watson R[2], Pahan K[1]. PLoS One. 2014 Aug 4;9(8):e103606.

[305] Single-walled carbon nanotubes alleviate autophagic/lysosomal defects in primary glia from a mouse model of Alzheimer's disease. Xue X[1], Wang LR, Sato Y, Jiang Y, Berg M, Yang DS, Nixon RA, Liang XJ. Nano Lett. 2014 Sep 10;14(9):5110-7.

[306] A brief review of recent advances in stem cell biology. Chen J[1], Zhou L[2], Pan SY[3]. Neural Regen Res. 2014 Apr 1;9(7):684-7.

[307] Developing neural stem cell-based treatments for neurodegenerative diseases. Byrne JA. Stem Cell Res Ther. 2014 May 30;5(3):72.

[308] Degradation of amyloid beta by human induced pluripotent stem cell-derived macrophages expressing Neprilysin-2. Takamatsu K[1], Ikeda T[2], Haruta M[3], Matsumura K[3], Ogi Y[4], Nakagata N[5], Uchino M[6], Ando Y[4], Nishimura Y[7], Senju S[3]. Stem Cell Res. 2014 Oct 12;13(3PA):442-453.

[309] Scanning ultrasound removes amyloid-β and restores memory in an Alzheimer's disease mouse model. Leinenga G[1], Götz J[2]. Sci Transl Med. 2015 Mar 11;7(278):278ra33.

[310] First-in-man tau vaccine targeting structural determinants essential for pathological tau-tau interaction reduces tau oligomerisation and neurofibrillary degeneration in an Alzheimer's disease model. Kontsekova E[1], Zilka N[1], Kovacech B[2], Novak P[1], Novak M[1]. Alzheimers Res Ther. 2014 Aug 1;6(4):44.

[311] J&J Strikes Alzheimer's Deal With AC Immune Worth Up to $509 Million. By Reuters Staff. Reuters. January 13, 2015. http://www.medscape.com/viewarticle/837938_print.

[312] Overcoming obstacles to repurposing for neurodegenerative disease. Shineman DW, Alam J, Anderson M, Black SE, Carman AJ, Cummings JL, Dacks PA, Dudley JT, Frail DE, Green A, Lane RF, Lappin D, Simuni T, Stefanacci RG, Sherer T, Fillit HM. Ann Clin Transl Neurol. 2014 Jul;1(7):512-8.

[313] Pharmacological strategies for the prevention of Alzheimer's disease. Doraiswamy PM[1], Xiong GL. Expert Opin Pharmacother. 2006 Jan;7(1):1-10.

[314] Discovering new treatments for Alzheimer's disease by repurposing approved medications. Appleby BS, Cummings JL. Curr Top Med Chem. 2013;13(18):2306-27.

[315] Psychotropic drug effects on gene transcriptomics relevant to Alzheimer disease. Lauterbach EC. Alzheimer Dis Assoc Disord. 2012 Jan-Mar;26(1):1-7.

[316] Use of antidepressants among community-dwelling persons with Alzheimer's disease: a nationwide register-based study. Laitinen ML, Lönnroos E, Bell JS, Lavikainen P, Sulkava R, Hartikainen S. Int Psychogeriatr. 2014 Nov 21:1-4.

[317] Imipramine and citalopram facilitate amyloid precursor protein secretion in vitro. Pákáski M, Bjelik A, Hugyecz M, Kása P, Janka Z, Kálmán J. Neurochem Int. 2005 Aug;47(3):190-5.

[318] Citalopram Attenuates Tau Hyperphosphorylation and Spatial Memory Deficit Induced by Social Isolation Rearing in Middle-Aged Rats. Ren QG, Gong WG, Wang YJ, Zhou QD, Zhang ZJ. J Mol Neurosci. 2014 Dec 5.

[319] An antidepressant decreases CSF Aβ production in healthy individuals and in transgenic AD mice. Sheline YI, West T, Yarasheski K, Swarm R, Jasielec MS, Fisher JR, Ficker WD, Yan P, Xiong C, Frederiksen C, Grzelak MV, Chott R, Bateman

RJ, Morris JC, Mintun MA, Lee JM, Cirrito JR. Sci Transl Med. 2014 May 14;6(236):236re4.

[320] P Serotonin signaling is associated with lower amyloid-β levels and plaques in transgenic mice and humans. Cirrito JR[1], Disabato BM, Restivo JL, Verges DK, Goebel WD, Sathyan A, Hayreh D, D'Angelo G, Benzinger T, Yoon H, Kim J, Morris JC, Mintun MA, Sheline YI. roc Natl Acad Sci U S A. 2011 Sep 6;108(36):14968-73.

[321] Synergistic inhibition of butyrylcholinesterase by galantamine and citalopram. Walsh R, Rockwood K, Martin E, Darvesh S. Biochim Biophys Acta. 2011 Dec;1810(12):1230-5.

[322] Distinct functional networks associated with improvement of affective symptoms and cognitive function during citalopram treatment in geriatric depression. Diaconescu AO, Kramer E, Hermann C, Ma Y, Dhawan V, Chaly T, Eidelberg D, McIntosh AR, Smith GS. Hum Brain Mapp. 2011 Oct;32(10):1677-91.

[323] Fluoxetine improves behavioral performance by suppressing the production of soluble β-amyloid in APP/PS1 mice. Wang J, Zhang Y, Xu H, Zhu S, Wang H, He J, Zhang H, Guo H, Kong J, Huang Q, Li XM. Curr Alzheimer Res. 2014;11(7):672-80.

[324] Therapeutic potentials of neural stem cells treated with fluoxetine in Alzheimer's disease. Chang KA, Kim JA, Kim S, Joo Y, Shin KY, Kim S, Kim HS, Suh YH. Neurochem Int. 2012 Nov;61(6):885-91.

[325] A Cognitive outcomes after sertaline treatment in patients with depression of Alzheimer disease. Munro CA[1], Longmire CF, Drye LT, Martin BK, Frangakis CE, Meinert CL, Mintzer JE, Porsteinsson AP, Rabins PV, Rosenberg PB, Schneider LS, Weintraub D, Lyketsos CG; Depression in Alzheimer's disease Study–2 Research Group (65 collaborators); Lyketsos C, Martin B, Niederehe G, Rosenberg P, Mintzer J, Weintraub D, Porsteinsson AP, Schneider L, Casper AS, Drye L, Meinert C, Evans C, Munro C, Rabins P, Lyketsos C, Evans C, Munro C, Rabins P, Boehmer K, Mosely A, Avramopoulos D, Meinert C, Martin B, Drye L, Frangakis C, Casper AS, Vaidya V, Meinert J, Niederehe G, Evans J, Chisar J, Ritz L, Zachariah E, Rosenberg P, Morrison A, Evans C, Rastogi P, Boehner K, Onyike C, Mintzer J, Longmire C, Faison WE, Hatchell M, Stuckey M, Weintraub D, Katz I, Stump T, Streim J, DiFilippo S, O'Neill K, Porsteinsson AP, Goldstein B, LaFountain J, McCallum C, Jakimovich L, Martin K, McGrath M, Cosman KM, Schneider LS, Pawluczyk S, Dagerman K, Sanabria R, Teodoro L, Wang Y, Zhang J. m J Geriatr Psychiatry. 2012 Dec;20(12):1036-44.

[326] Fetzima (levomilnacipran), a Drug for Major Depressive Disorder as a Dual Inhibitor for Human Serotonin Transporters and Beta-Site Amyloid Precursor Protein

Cleaving Enzyme-1. Rizvi SM, Shaikh S, Khan M, Biswas D, Hameed N, Shakil S. CNS Neurol Disord Drug Targets. 2014;13(8):1427-31.

[327]Norepinephrine Protects against Amyloid-β Toxicity via TrkB. Liu X, Ye K, Weinshenker D. J Alzheimers Dis. 2014 Sep 10.

[328] Molecular investigations of protriptyline as a multi-target directed ligand in Alzheimer's disease. Bansode SB, Jana AK, Batkulwar KB, Warkad SD, Joshi RS, Sengupta N, Kulkarni MJ. PLoS One. 2014 Aug 20;9(8):e105196.

[329] Response of the medial temporal lobe network in amnestic mild cognitive impairment to therapeutic intervention assessed by fMRI and memory task performance. Bakker A[1], Albert MS[2], Krauss G[2], Speck CL[1], Gallagher M[3]. Neuroimage Clin. 2015 Feb 21;7:688-98.

[330]Long-Term Lithium Treatment Reduces Glucose Metabolism in the Cerebellum and Hippocampus of Nondemented Older Adults: An [18F]FDG-PET Study. Forlenza OV, Coutinho AM, Aprahamian I, Prando S, Mendes LL, Diniz BS, Gattaz WF, Buchpiguel CA. ACS Chem Neurosci. 2014 Apr 29.

[331] Lithium, a common drug for bipolar disorder treatment, regulates amyloid-beta precursor protein processing. Su Y, Ryder J, Li B, Wu X, Fox N, Solenberg P, Brune K, Paul S, Zhou Y, Liu F, Ni B. Biochemistry. 2004 Jun 8;43(22):6899-908.

[332] Implications of the neuroprotective effects of lithium for the treatment of bipolar and neurodegenerative disorders. Bauer M, Alda M, Priller J, Young LT; International Group For The Study Of Lithium Treated Patients (IGSLI). Pharmacopsychiatry. 2003 Nov;36 Suppl 3:S250-4.

[333]Neuroprotective and neurotrophic actions of the mood stabilizer lithium: can it be used to treat neurodegenerative diseases? Chuang DM. Crit Rev Neurobiol. 2004;16(1-2):83-90.

[334]Does lithium prevent Alzheimer's disease? Forlenza OV, de Paula VJ, Machado-Vieira R, Diniz BS, Gattaz WF. Drugs Aging. 2012 May 1;29(5):335-42.

[335]Standard and trace-dose lithium: a systematic review of dementia prevention and other behavioral benefits. Mauer S1, Vergne D2, Ghaemi SN3. Aust N Z J Psychiatry. 2014 Sep;48(9):809-18.

[336]Microdose lithium treatment stabilized cognitive impairment in patients with Alzheimer's disease. Nunes MA, Viel TA, Buck HS. Curr Alzheimer Res. 2013 Jan;10(1):104-7.

[337] Long-term treatment with lithium alleviates memory deficits and reduces amyloid-β production in an aged Alzheimer's disease transgenic mouse model. Zhang X, Heng X, Li T, Li L, Yang D, Zhang X, Du Y, Doody RS, Le W. J Alzheimers Dis. 2011;24(4):739-49.

[338] Disease-modifying properties of long-term lithium treatment for amnestic mild cognitive impairment: randomised controlled trial. Forlenza OV, Diniz BS, Radanovic M, Santos FS, Talib LL, Gattaz WF. Br J Psychiatry. 2011 May;198(5):351-6.

[339] Does lithium protect against dementia? Kessing LV, Forman JL, Andersen PK. Bipolar Disord. 2010 Feb;12(1):87-94.

[340] Calcium dysregulation, and lithium treatment to forestall Alzheimer's disease - a merging of hypotheses. Wallace J. Cell Calcium. 2014 Mar;55(3):175-81.

[341] Long-term, low-dose lithium treatment does not impair renal function in the elderly: a 2-year randomized, placebo-controlled trial followed by single-blind extension. Aprahamian I, Santos FS, dos Santos B, Talib L, Diniz BS, Radanovic M, Gattaz WF, Forlenza OV[1]. J Clin Psychiatry. 2014 Jul;75(7):e672-8.

[342] GSK3 and tau: two convergence points in Alzheimer's disease. Hernandez F, Lucas JJ, Avila J. J Alzheimers Dis. 2013;33 Suppl 1:S141-4.

[343] A feasibility and tolerability study of lithium in Alzheimer's disease. Macdonald A, Briggs K, Poppe M, Higgins A, Velayudhan L, Lovestone S. Int J Geriatr Psychiatry. 2008 Jul;23(7):704-11.

[344] Lithium trial in Alzheimer's disease: a randomized, single-blind, placebo-controlled, multicenter 10-week study. Hampel H, Ewers M, Bürger K, Annas P, Mörtberg A, Bogstedt A, Frölich L, Schröder J, Schönknecht P, Riepe MW, Kraft I, Gasser T, Leyhe T, Möller HJ, Kurz A, Basun H. J Clin Psychiatry. 2009 Jun;70(6):922-31.

[345] Does lithium therapy protect against the onset of dementia? Dunn N, Holmes C, Mullee M. Alzheimer Dis Assoc Disord. 2005 Jan-Mar;19(1):20-2.

[346] Brain intraventricular injection of amyloid-β in zebrafish embryo impairs cognition and increases tau phosphorylation, effects reversed by lithium. Nery LR, Eltz NS, Hackman C, Fonseca R, Altenhofen S, Guerra HN, Freitas VM, Bonan CD, Vianna MR. PLoS One. 2014 Sep 4;9(9):e105862.

[347]Lithium suppresses Aβ pathology by inhibiting translation in an adult Drosophila model of Alzheimer's disease. Sofola-Adesakin O, Castillo-Quan JI, Rallis C, Tain LS, Bjedov I, Rogers I, Li L, Martinez P, Khericha M, Cabecinha M, Bähler J, Partridge L. Front Aging Neurosci. 2014 Jul 30;6:190.

[348]Statin use and cognitive changes in elderly patients with dementia. Raley KA, Hutchison AM. Consult Pharm. 2014 Jul;29(7):487-9.

[349]The Complex Actions of Statins in Brain and their Relevance for Alzheimer's disease Treatment: An Analytical Review. Mendoza-Oliva A, Zepeda A, Arias C. Curr Alzheimer Res. 2014;11(9):817-33.

[350] Simvastatin promotes adult hippocampal neurogenesis by enhancing Wnt/β-catenin signaling. Robin NC, Agoston Z, Biechele TL, James RG, Berndt JD, Moon RT. Stem Cell Reports. 2013 Dec 26;2(1):9-17.

[351] Hypercholesterolaemia-induced oxidative stress at the blood-brain barrier. Dias IH, Polidori MC, Griffiths HR. Biochem Soc Trans. 2014 Aug;42(4):1001-5.

[352] Statins, risk of dementia, and cognitive function: secondary analysis of the ginkgo evaluation of memory study. Bettermann K[1], Arnold AM, Williamson J, Rapp S, Sink K, Toole JF, Carlson MC, Yasar S, Dekosky S, Burke GL. J Stroke Cerebrovasc Dis. 2012 Aug;21(6):436-44.

[353] Exploring new indications for statins beyond atherosclerosis: Successes and setbacks. Waters DD[1]. J Cardiol. 2010 Mar;55(2):155-62.

[354] Statins in the prevention of dementia and Alzheimer's disease: a meta-analysis of observational studies and an assessment of confounding. Wong WB, Lin VW, Boudreau D, Devine EB. Pharmacoepidemiol Drug Saf. 2013 Apr;22(4):345-58.

[355]Insulin in the brain: its pathophysiological implications for States related with central insulin resistance, type 2 diabetes and Alzheimer's disease. Blázquez E, Velázquez E, Hurtado-Carneiro V, Ruiz-Albusac JM. Front Endocrinol (Lausanne). 2014 Oct 9;5:161.

[356]Insulin as a Bridge between Type 2 Diabetes and Alzheimer Disease - How Anti-Diabetics Could be a Solution for Dementia. Sebastião I, Candeias E, Santos MS, de Oliveira CR, Moreira PI, Duarte AI. Front Endocrinol (Lausanne). 2014 Jul 8;5:110.

[357]Does Insulin Therapy for Type 1 Diabetes Mellitus Protect Against Alzheimer's disease? Rdzak GM[1], Abdelghany O. Pharmacotherapy. 2014 Oct 3.

[358] Drugs developed for treatment of diabetes show protective effects in Alzheimer's and Parkinson's diseases. Hölscher C. Sheng Li Xue Bao. 2014 Oct 25;66(5):497-510.

[359] Long-acting intranasal insulin detemir improves cognition for adults with mild cognitive impairment or early-stage Alzheimer's disease dementia. Claxton A[1], Baker LD[2], Hanson A[1], Trittschuh EH[1], Cholerton B[3], Morgan A[1], Callaghan M[1], Arbuckle M[4], Behl C[1], Craft S[2]. J Alzheimers Dis. 2015 Jan 1;44(3):897-906.

[360] A single-dose pilot trial of intranasal rapid-acting insulin in apolipoprotein e4 carriers with mild-moderate Alzheimer's disease. Rosenbloom MH[1], Barclay TR, Pyle M, Owens BL, Cagan AB, Anderson CP, Frey WH 2nd, Hanson LR. CNS Drugs. 2014 Dec;28(12):1185-9.

[361] Metformin Treatment Alters Memory Function in a Mouse Model of Alzheimer's disease. DiTacchio KA, Heinemann SF, Dziewczapolski G. J Alzheimers Dis. 2014 Sep 3.

[362] Increased risk of cognitive impairment in patients with diabetes is associated with metformin. Moore EM, Mander AG, Ames D, Kotowicz MA, Carne RP, Brodaty H, Woodward M, Boundy K, Ellis KA, Bush AI, Faux NG, Martins R, Szoeke C, Rowe C, Watters DA; AIBL Investigators (150). Diabetes Care. 2013 Oct;36(10):2981-7.

[363] Diet modification and metformin have a beneficial effect in a fly model of obesity and mucormycosis. Shirazi F, Farmakiotis D, Yan Y, Albert N, Kim-Anh D, Kontoyiannis DP. PLoS One. 2014 Sep 30;9(9):e108635.

[364] Peripheral insulin-sensitizer drug metformin ameliorates neuronal insulin resistance and Alzheimer's-like changes. Gupta A, Bisht B, Dey CS. Neuropharmacology. 2011 May;60(6):910-20.

[365] NSAID prescribing precautions. Risser A[1], Donovan D, Heintzman J, Page T. Am Fam Physician. 2009 Dec 15;80(12):1371-8.

[366] Study Casts Doubt on Low-Dose Aspirin for Women Under 65. HealthDay News. http://www.nlm.nih.gov/medlineplus/news/fullstory_149798.html (*this news item will not be available after 03/05/2015). December 5, 2014.

[367] Is Alzheimer's disease Autoimmune Inflammation of the Brain That Can be Treated With Nasal Nonsteroidal Anti-Inflammatory Drugs? Lehrer S, Rheinstein PH. Am J Alzheimers Dis Other Demen. 2014 Aug 5.

[368] β-Amyloid induced effects on cholinergic, serotonergic, and dopaminergic neurons is differentially counteracted by anti-inflammatory drugs. Hochstrasser T[1], Hohsfield LA, Sperner-Unterweger B, Humpel C. J Neurosci Res. 2013 Jan;91(1):83-94.

[369] NOSH aspirin may have a protective role in Alzheimer's disease. Drochioiu G[1], Tudorachi L[1], Murariu M[2]. Med Hypotheses. 2015 Jan 14.

[370] FDA approved asthma therapeutic agent impacts amyloid β in the brain in a transgenic model of Alzheimer's disease. Hori Y, Takeda S, Cho H, Wegmann S, Shoup TM, Takahashi K, Irimia D, Elmaleh DR, Hyman BT, Hudry E. J Biol Chem. 2014 Dec 2. pii: jbc.M114.586602.

[371] Renin Angiotensin aldosterone system inhibition in controlling dementia-related cognitive decline. O'Caoimh R[1], Kehoe PG[2], Molloy DW[1]. J Alzheimers Dis. 2014 Jan 1;42(0):S575-86.

[372] Neuroprotective Effects of Angiotensin Receptor Blockers. Villapol S[1], Saavedra JM[2] Am J Hypertens. 2014 Oct 31.

[373] Do angiotensin receptor blockers protect against Alzheimer's disease? Kurinami H[1], Shimamura M, Sato N, Nakagami H, Morishita R. Drugs Aging. 2013 Jun;30(6):367-72.

[374] Angiotensin-Converting Enzyme in Cerebrospinal Fluid and Risk of Brain Atrophy. Jochemsen HM[1], van der Flier WM[2], Ashby EL[3], Teunissen CE[4], Jones RE[3], Wattjes MP[5], Scheltens P[6], Geerlings MI[7], Kehoe PG[3], Muller M[8]. J Alzheimers Dis. 2014 Sep 8.

[375] Medical genetics-based drug repurposing for Alzheimer's disease. Zhang XZ, Quan Y, Tang GY. Brain Res Bull. 2014 Nov 22;110C:26-29.

[376] Apolipoprotein E genotype-specific short-term cognitive benefits of treatment with the antihypertensive nilvadipine in Alzheimer's patients--an open-label trial. Kennelly S[1], Abdullah L, Kenny RA, Mathura V, Luis CA, Mouzon B, Crawford F, Mullan M, Lawlor B. Int J Geriatr Psychiatry. 2012 Apr;27(4):415-22.

[377] The Spleen Tyrosine Kinase (Syk) Regulates Alzheimer Amyloid-β Production and Tau Hyperphosphorylation. Paris D[1], Ait-Ghezala G[2], Bachmeier C[2], Laco G[2], Beaulieu-Abdelahad D[2], Lin Y[2], Jin C[2], Crawford F[2], Mullan M[2]. J Biol Chem. 2014 Dec 5;289(49):33927-44.

[378] A systematic review of calcium channel blocker use and cognitive decline/dementia in the elderly. Peters R[1], Booth A, Peters J. J Hypertens. 2014 Oct;32(10):1945-57; discussion 1957-8.

[379] Memory Impairment in Estrogen Receptor α Knockout Mice Through Accumulation of Amyloid-β Peptides. Hwang CJ[1], Yun HM, Park KR, Song JK, Seo HO, Hyun BK, Choi DY, Yoo HS, Oh KW, Hwang DY, Han SB, Hong JT. Mol Neurobiol. 2014 Aug 17.

[380] Estrogen receptors' neuroprotective effect against glutamate-induced neurotoxicity. Lan YL[1], Zhao J, Li S. Neurol Sci. 2014 Nov;35(11):1657-62.

[381] Estrogen intake and copper depositions: implications for Alzheimer's disease? Amtage F[1], Birnbaum D[2], Reinhard T[2], Niesen WD[1], Weiller C[1], Mader I[3], Meyer PT[4], Rijntjes M[1]. Case Rep Neurol. 2014 Jun 19;6(2):181-7.

[382] Sildenafil Decreases BACE1 and Cathepsin B Levels and Reduces APP Amyloidogenic Processing in the SAMP8 Mouse. Orejana L, Barros-Miñones L, Jordan J, Cedazo-Minguez A, Tordera RM, Aguirre N, Puerta E. Gerontol A Biol Sci Med Sci. 2014 Jul 25. pii: glu106.

[383] Nutrition and prevention of Alzheimer's dementia. Swaminathan A[1], Jicha GA[1]. Front Aging Neurosci. 2014 Oct 20;6:282.

[384] Dietary patterns as predictors of successful ageing. Hodge AM[1], O'Dea K, English DR, Giles GG, Flicker L. J Nutr Health Aging. 2014 Mar;18(3):221-7.

[385] Heme of consumed red meat can act as a catalyst of oxidative damage and could initiate colon, breast and prostate cancers, heart disease and other diseases. Tappel A. Med Hypotheses. 2007;68(3):562-4.

[386] Intestinal microbiota metabolism of L-carnitine, a nutrient in red meat, promotes atherosclerosis. Koeth RA[1], Wang Z, Levison BS, Buffa JA, Org E, Sheehy BT, Britt EB, Fu X, Wu Y, Li L, Smith JD, DiDonato JA, Chen J, Li H, Wu GD, Lewis JD, Warrier M, Brown JM, Krauss RM, Tang WH, Bushman FD, Lusis AJ, Hazen SL. Nat Med. 2013 May;19(5):576-85.

[387] Observational and ecological studies of dietary advanced glycation end products in national diets and Alzheimer's disease incidence and prevalence. Perrone L[1], Grant WB[2]. J Alzheimers Dis. 2015 Jan 1;45(3):965-79.

[388] Potential benefits of adherence to the Mediterranean diet on cognitive health. Féart C[1], Samieri C, Allès B, Barberger-Gateau P. Proc Nutr Soc. 2013 Feb;72(1):140-52.

[389] Diet and Alzheimer's disease risk factors or prevention: the current evidence. Solfrizzi V[1], Panza F, Frisardi V, Seripa D, Logroscino G, Imbimbo BP, Pilotto A. Expert Rev Neurother. 2011 May;11(5):677-708.

[390] Dietary Patterns and Cognitive Dysfunction in a 12-Year Follow-up Study of 70-Year-Old Men. Olsson E[1], Karlström B[1], Kilander L[2], Byberg L[3], Cederholm T[1], Sjögren P[1]. J Alzheimers Dis. 2014 Jul 25.

[391] Mediterranean Diet and Magnetic Resonance Imaging-Assessed Brain Atrophy in Cognitively Normal Individuals at Risk for Alzheimer's disease. Mosconi L, Murray J, Tsui WH, Li Y, Davies M, Williams S, Pirraglia E, Spector N, Osorio RS, Glodzik L, McHugh P, de Leon MJ. J Prev Alzheimers Dis. 2014 Jun;1(1):23-32.

[392] Prospective study of Dietary Approaches to Stop Hypertension- and Mediterranean-style dietary patterns and age-related cognitive change: the Cache County Study on Memory, Health and Aging. Wengreen H[1], Munger RG, Cutler A, Quach A, Bowles A, Corcoran C, Tschanz JT, Norton MC, Welsh-Bohmer KA. Am J Clin Nutr. 2013 Nov;98(5):1263-71.

[393] Relation of DASH- and Mediterranean-like dietary patterns to cognitive decline in older persons. Tangney CC[1], Li H[2], Wang Y[2], Barnes L[2], Schneider JA[2], Bennett DA[2], Morris MC[2]. Neurology. 2014 Oct 14;83(16):1410-6.

[394] Mediterranean diet habits in older individuals: associations with cognitive functioning and brain volumes. Titova OE[1], Ax E, Brooks SJ, Sjögren P, Cederholm T, Kilander L, Kullberg J, Larsson EM, Johansson L, Ahlström H, Lind L, Schiöth HB, Benedict C. Exp Gerontol. 2013 Dec;48(12):1443-8.

[395] Dietary patterns in Alzheimer's disease and cognitive aging. Gu Y[1], Scarmeas N. Curr Alzheimer Res. 2011 Aug;8(5):510-9.

[396] A Mediterranean diet improves HbA1c but not fasting blood glucose compared to alternative dietary strategies: a network meta-analysis. Carter P[1], Achana F, Troughton J, Gray LJ, Khunti K, Davies MJ. J Hum Nutr Diet. 2014 Jun;27(3):280-97.

[397] Medicinal chemistry of the epigenetic diet and caloric restriction. Martin SL[1], Hardy TM, Tollefsbol TO. Curr Med Chem. 2013;20(32):4050-9.

[398] Alzheimer's disease and epigenetic diet. Sezgin Z[1], Dincer Y[2]. Neurochem Int. 2014 Oct 5;78C:105-116.

[399] Nutrition, the brain and cognitive decline: insights from epigenetics. Dauncey MJ. Eur J Clin Nutr. 2014 Nov;68(11):1179-1185.

[400] Whole-food diet worsened cognitive dysfunction in an Alzheimer's disease mouse model. Parrott MD[1], Winocur G[2], Bazinet RP[3], Ma DW[4], Greenwood CE[5]. Neurobiol Aging. 2014 Aug 16. pii: S0197-4580(14)00526-0.

[401] Ketogenic diet in neuromuscular and neurodegenerative diseases. Paoli A[1], Bianco A[2], Damiani E[1], Bosco G[1]. Biomed Res Int. 2014;2014:474296.

[402] Regular fish consumption and age-related brain gray matter loss. Raji CA[1], Erickson KI[2], Lopez OL[3], Kuller LH[4], Gach HM[2], Thompson PM[5], Riverol M[6], Becker JT[7]. Am J Prev Med. 2014 Oct;47(4):444-51.

[403] MIND diet associated with reduced incidence of Alzheimer's disease. Morris MC[1], Tangney CC[2], Wang Y[3], Sacks FM[4], Bennett DA[5], Aggarwal NT[5]. Alzheimers Dement. 2015 Feb 11. pii: S1552-5260(15)00017-5.

[404] New 'MIND' diet may significantly protect against Alzheimer's disease. March 20, 2015. http://www.kurzweilai.net/new-mind-diet-may-significantly-protect-against-alzheimers-disease.

[405] Lower Risk of Alzheimer's disease Mortality with Exercise, Statin, and Fruit Intake. Williams PT.
J Alzheimers Dis. 2014 Nov 14.

[406] Life space and risk of Alzheimer disease, mild cognitive impairment, and cognitive decline in old age. James BD, Boyle PA, Buchman AS, Barnes LL, Bennett DA. Am J Geriatr Psychiatry. 2011 Nov;19(11):961-9.

[407] Neural correlates of cognitive intervention in persons at risk of developing Alzheimer's disease. Hosseini SM[1], Kramer JH[2], Kesler SR[3]. Front Aging Neurosci. 2014 Aug 26;6:231.

[408] Participation in cognitively stimulating activities and risk of incident Alzheimer disease. Wilson RS[1], Mendes De Leon CF, Barnes LL, Schneider JA, Bienias JL, Evans DA, Bennett DA. JAMA. 2002 Feb 13;287(6):742-8.

[409] Cognitive activities delay onset of memory decline in persons who develop dementia. Hall CB[1], Lipton RB, Sliwinski M, Katz MJ, Derby CA, Verghese J. Neurology. 2009 Aug 4;73(5):356-61.

[410] Participation in cognitively-stimulating activities is associated with brain structure and cognitive function in preclinical Alzheimer's disease. Schultz SA[1], Larson J, Oh J, Koscik R, Dowling MN, Gallagher CL, Carlsson CM, Rowley HA, Bendlin BB, Asthana S, Hermann BP, Johnson SC, Sager M, LaRue A, Okonkwo OC. Brain Imaging Behav. 2014 Oct 31.

[411] Higher education affects accelerated cortical thinning in Alzheimer's disease: a 5-year preliminary longitudinal study. Cho H[1], Jeon S[2], Kim C[3], Ye BS[4], Kim GH[5], Noh Y[6], Kim HJ[1], Yoon CW[7], Kim YJ[1], Kim JH[1], Park SE[1], Kim ST[8], Lee JM[2], Kang SJ[1], Suh MK[1], Chin J[1], Na DL[1], Kang DR[9], Seo SW[1]. Int Psychogeriatr. 2014 Sep 16:1-10.

[412] Education delays accelerated decline on a memory test in persons who develop dementia. Hall CB[1], Derby C, LeValley A, Katz MJ, Verghese J, Lipton RB. Neurology. 2007 Oct 23;69(17):1657-64.

[413] Effects of education on the progression of early- versus late-stage mild cognitive impairment. Ye BS[1], Seo SW, Cho H, Kim SY, Lee JS, Kim EJ, Lee Y, Back JH, Hong CH, Choi SH, Park KW, Ku BD, Moon SY, Kim S, Han SH, Lee JH, Cheong HK, Na DL. Int Psychogeriatr. 2013 Apr;25(4):597-606.

[414] Deconstructing Racial Differences: The Effects of Quality of Education and Cerebrovascular Risk Factors. Carvalho JO[1], Tommet D[2], Crane PK[3], Thomas ML[4], Claxton A[5], Habeck C[6], J Manly J[6], Romero HR[7]. J Gerontol B Psychol Sci Soc Sci. 2014 Aug 5.

[415] Bilingualism delays age at onset of dementia, independent of education and immigration status. Suvarna A, Bak TH, Duggirala V, Surampudi B, Shailaja M, Shukla AK, Chaudhuri JR, Subhash K. Neurology. November 6, 2013.

[416] The Babylonian benefit: Neurological research shows that being bilingual enhances mental performance and may protect from Alzheimer's disease. Weigmann K. EMBO Rep. 2014 Oct;15(10):1015-8.

[417] Meditation and neurodegenerative diseases. Newberg AB[1], Serruya M, Wintering N, Moss AS, Reibel D, Monti DA. Ann N Y Acad Sci. 2014 Jan;1307:112-23.

[418] Forever young: Meditation might slow the age-related loss of gray matter in the brain. U of California, Los Angeles. February 5th, 2015. http://medicalxpress.com/news/2015-02-young-meditation-age-related-loss-gray.html.

[419] Meditation's impact on default mode network and hippocampus in mild cognitive impairment: a pilot study. Wells RE[1], Yeh GY, Kerr CE, Wolkin J, Davis RB, Tan Y, Spaeth R, Wall RB, Walsh J, Kaptchuk TJ, Press D, Phillips RS, Kong J. Neurosci Lett. 2013 Nov 27;556:15-9.

[420] Exercise Increases the Dynamics of Diurnal Cortisol Secretion and Executive Function in People With Amnestic Mild Cognitive Impairment. Tortosa-Martínez J[1], Clow A, Caus-Pertegaz N, González-Caballero G, Abellán-Miralles I, Saenz MJ. J Aging Phys Act. 2014 Dec 2.

[421] mTOR and the health benefits of exercise. Watson K[1], Baar K[2]. Semin Cell Dev Biol. 2014 Dec;36C:130-139.

[422] Physical activity and risk of cognitive impairment and dementia in elderly persons. Laurin D[1], Verreault R, Lindsay J, MacPherson K, Rockwood K. Arch Neurol. 2001 Mar;58(3):498-504.

[423] Performance-based physical function and future dementia in older people. Wang L[1], Larson EB, Bowen JD, van Belle G. Arch Intern Med. 2006 May 22;166(10):1115-20.

[424] A systematic review of the evidence that brain structure is related to muscle structure and their relationship to brain and muscle function in humans over the lifecourse. Kilgour AH[1], Todd OM, Starr JM. BMC Geriatr. 2014 Jul 10;14:85.

[425] Physical activity, body mass index, and brain atrophy in Alzheimer's disease. Boyle CP[1], Raji CA[2], Erickson KI[3], Lopez OL[4], Becker JT[5], Gach HM[6], Longstreth WT Jr[7], Teverovskiy L[8], Kuller LH[9], Carmichael OT[10], Thompson PM[11]. Neurobiol Aging. 2014 Aug 27. pii: S0197-4580(14)00541-7.

[426] Exercise is more effective than diet control in preventing high fat diet-induced β-amyloid deposition and memory deficit in amyloid precursor protein transgenic mice. Maesako M[1], Uemura K, Kubota M, Kuzuya A, Sasaki K, Hayashida N, Asada-Utsugi M, Watanabe K, Uemura M, Kihara T, Takahashi R, Shimohama S, Kinoshita A. J Biol Chem. 2012 Jun 29;287(27):23024-33.

[427] Long-term treadmill exercise attenuates tau pathology in P301S tau transgenic mice. Ohia-Nwoko O, Montazari S, Lau YS, Eriksen JL. Mol Neurodegener. 2014 Nov 28;9(1):54.

[428] A combination of physical activity and computerized brain training improves verbal memory and increases cerebral glucose metabolism in the elderly. Shah T[1], Verdile G[2], Sohrabi H[1], Campbell A[3], Putland E[4], Cheetham C[5], Dhaliwal S[6],

Weinborn M[7], Maruff P[8], Darby D[9], Martins RN[1]. Transl Psychiatry. 2014 Dec 2;4:e487.

[429] Cardiorespiratory fitness is associated with brain structure, cognition, and mood in a middle-aged cohort at risk for Alzheimer's disease. Boots EA[1], Schultz SA, Oh JM, Larson J, Edwards D, Cook D, Koscik RL, Dowling MN, Gallagher CL, Carlsson CM, Rowley HA, Bendlin BB, LaRue A, Asthana S, Hermann BP, Sager MA, Johnson SC, Okonkwo OC. Brain Imaging Behav. 2014 Oct 16.

[430] Influence of BDNF Val66Met on the relationship between physical activity and brain volume. Brown BM[1], Bourgeat P[1], Peiffer JJ[1], Burnham S[1], Laws SM[1], Rainey-Smith SR[1], Bartrés-Faz D[1], Villemagne VL[1], Taddei K[1], Rembach A[1], Bush A[1], Ellis KA[1], Macaulay SL[1], Rowe CC[1], Ames D[1], Masters CL[1], Maruff P[1], Martins RN[2]; AIBL Research Group. Neurology. 2014 Oct 7;83(15):1345-52.

[431] Not only cardiovascular, but also coordinative exercise increases hippocampal volume in older adults. Niemann C[1], Godde B[2], Voelcker-Rehage C[2]. Front Aging Neurosci. 2014 Aug 4;6:170.

[432] Leisure activities, apolipoprotein E e4 status, and the risk of dementia. Yang SY[1], Weng PH[2], Chen JH[3], Chiou JM[4], Lew-Ting CY[5], Chen TF[6], Sun Y[7], Wen LL[8], Yip PK[9], Chu YM[10], Chen YC[11]. J Formos Med Assoc. 2014 Nov 4. pii: S0929-6646(14)00269-1.

[433] The Study of Mental and Resistance Training (SMART) Study-Resistance Training and/or Cognitive Training in Mild Cognitive Impairment: A Randomized, Double-Blind, Double-Sham Controlled Trial. Fiatarone Singh MA[1], Gates N[2], Saigal N[3], Wilson GC[3], Meiklejohn J[3], Brodaty H[4], Wen W[5], Singh N[6], Baune BT[7], Suo C[8], Baker MK[9], Foroughi N[10], Wang Y[11], Sachdev PS[5], Valenzuela M[12]. J Am Med Dir Assoc. 2014 Dec;15(12):873-80.

[434] What are the Benefits of Exercise for Alzheimer´s Disease? A Systematic Review of Past 10 Years. Hernández SS[1], Sandreschi PF, Silva FC, Arancibia BA, da Silva R, Gutierres PJ, Andrade A. J Aging Phys Act. 2014 Nov 21.

[435] Physical activity attenuates age-related biomarker alterations in preclinical AD. Okonkwo OC[1], Schultz SA[2], Oh JM[2], Larson J[2], Edwards D[2], Cook D[2], Koscik R[2], Gallagher CL[2], Dowling NM[2], Carlsson CM[2], Bendlin BB[2], LaRue A[2], Rowley HA[2], Christian BT[2], Asthana S[2], Hermann BP[2], Johnson SC[2], Sager MA[2]. Neurology. 2014 Nov 4;83(19):1753-60.

[436] Resistance Training Does not have an Effect on Cognition or Related Serum Biomarkers in Nonagenarians: A Randomized Controlled Trial. Ruiz JR[1], Gil-Bea F[2],

Bustamante-Ara N[3], Rodríguez-Romo G[4], Fiuza-Luces C[3], Serra-Rexach JA[5], Cedazo-Minguez A[6], Lucia A[7]. Int J Sports Med. 2014 Oct 20.

[437] Maintaining well-being and selfhood through physical activity: experiences of people with mild Alzheimer's disease. Cedervall Y[1], Torres S, Aberg AC. Aging Ment Health. 2014 Sep 30:1-10.

[438] Part 1: Potential Dangers of Extreme Endurance Exercise: How Much is Too Much? Part 2: Screening of School-age Athletes. O'Keefe JH[1], Lavie CJ[2], Guazzi M[3] Prog Cardiovasc Dis. 2014 Nov 15. pii: S0033-0620(14)00172-8.

[439] It is time to bust the myth of physical inactivity and obesity: you cannot outrun a bad diet. A Malhotra, T Noakes, S Phinney. Br J Sports Med. Editorial. 22 April 2015.

[440] Review: Best Fitness Trackers to Get You Up Off the Couch. Joanna Stern. December 16, 2014. Wall Street Journal. http://www.wsj.com/articles/review-best-fitness-trackers-to-get-you-up-off-the-couch-1418760813?mod=ST1.

[441] The Best Activity Trackers for Fitness. Jill Duffy. PC Magazine. December 23, 2014. http://www.pcmag.com/article2/0,2817,2404445,00.asp.

[442] FDA: Supplements, Meds Can Be Dangerous Mix. Mary Elizabeth Dallas. HealthDay News. http://www.nlm.nih.gov/medlineplus/news/fullstory_149275.html (*this news item will not be available after 02/02/2015). November 4, 2014.

[443] A Comprehensive Review of Potential Warfarin-Fruit Interactions. Norwood DA[1], Parke CK[2], Rappa LR[3]. J Pharm Pract. 2014 Aug 11.

[444] Is pomegranate juice a potential perpetrator of clinical drug-drug interactions? Review of the in vitro, preclinical and clinical evidence. Srinivas NR[1]. Eur J Drug Metab Pharmacokinet. 2013 Dec;38(4):223-9.

[445] NY Attorney General Eric Schneiderman Targets Popular Herbal Supplements. Mary Esch. Feb 3, 2015.
http://www.nbcnewyork.com/news/local/Eric-Schneiderman-Herbal-Supplements-New-York-Walmart-GNC-Walgreens-290640551.html;
http://www.nbcnewyork.com/news/local/Herbal-Supplement-Labels-DNA-Test-New-York--290680591.html.

[446] Eric Schneiderman leads state attorneys general in push for 'comprehensive inquiry' into herbal supplement industry. Michael O'keeffe. New York Daily News.

April 2, 2015. http://www.nydailynews.com/sports/i-team/state-attorney-generals-fed-up-supplements-article-1.2170570.

[447] Supplement industry leaders are unhappy with AGs' request for congressional inquiry. Michael O'keeffe. New York Daily News. April 2, 2015.http://www.nydailynews.com/blogs/iteam/supplement-industry-responds-request-inquiry-blog-entry-1.2171734.

[448] Nutrition and prevention of Alzheimer's dementia. Swaminathan A, Jicha GA. Front Aging Neurosci. 2014 Oct 20;6:282.

[449] Plasma nutrient status of patients with Alzheimer's disease: Systematic review and meta-analysis. Lopes da Silva S[1], Vellas B[2], Elemans S[3], Luchsinger J[4], Kamphuis P[1], Yaffe K[5], Sijben J[6], Groenendijk M[3], Stijnen T[7]. Alzheimers Dement. 2014 Jul;10(4):485-502.

[450] Differences in nutritional status between very mild Alzheimer's disease patients and healthy controls. Olde Rikkert MG[1], Verhey FR[2], Sijben JW[3], Bouwman FH[4], Dautzenberg PL[5], Lansink M[3], Sipers WM[6], van Asselt DZ[7], van Hees AM[3], Stevens M[8], Vellas B[9], Scheltens P[10] J Alzheimers Dis. 2014;41(1):261-71.

[451] Inhibition of early upstream events in prodromal Alzheimer's disease by use of targeted antioxidants. Prasad KN, Bondy SC[1]. Curr Aging Sci. 2014;7(2):77-90.

[452] Natural compounds and plant extracts as therapeutics against chronic inflammation in Alzheimer's disease - a translational perspective. Apetz N, Munch G, Govindaraghavan S, Gyengesi E[1]. CNS Neurol Disord Drug Targets. 2014;13(7):1175-91.

[453] Multiple dietary supplements do not affect metabolic and cardio-vascular health. Soare A[1], Weiss EP, Holloszy JO, Fontana L. Aging (Albany NY). 2014 Feb;6(2):149-57.

[454] Alzheimer's disease and antioxidant therapy: how long how far? Teixeira J[1], Silva T, Andrade PB, Borges F. Curr Med Chem. 2013;20(24):2939-52.

[455] Antioxidants for Alzheimer disease: a randomized clinical trial with cerebrospinal fluid biomarker measures. Galasko DR[1], Peskind E, Clark CM, Quinn JF, Ringman JM, Jicha GA, Cotman C, Cottrell B, Montine TJ, Thomas RG, Aisen P; Collaborators (20) Weisman D, Pay MM, Lerner A, Ziol E, Quinn J, Mulnard R, McAdams-Ortiz C, Ringman J, Bardens J, Jicha G, Clark CM, Pham C, Peskind E, Mandelco L, Walker A, Kirbach S, DeKosky S, Mishler-Rickard C, Kittur S, Mirje S. Alzheimer's Disease Cooperative Study. Arch Neurol. 2012 Jul;69(7):836-41.

[456] Dietary antioxidants, cognitive function and dementia--a systematic review. Crichton GE[1], Bryan J, Murphy KJ. Plant Foods Hum Nutr. 2013 Sep;68(3):279-92.

[457] Plasma nutrient status of patients with Alzheimer's disease: Systematic review and meta-analysis. Lopes da Silva S[1], Vellas B[2], Elemans S[3], Luchsinger J[4], Kamphuis P[1], Yaffe K[5], Sijben J[6], Groenendijk M[3], Stijnen T[7]. Alzheimers Dement. 2014 Jul;10(4):485-502.

[458] Nutrient intake and brain biomarkers of Alzheimer's disease in at-risk cognitively normal individuals: a cross-sectional neuroimaging pilot study. Mosconi L[1], Murray J[1], Davies M[1], Williams S[1], Pirraglia E[1], Spector N[1], Tsui WH[1], Li Y[1], Butler T[1], Osorio RS[1], Glodzik L[1], Vallabhajosula S[2], McHugh P[1], Marmar CR[3], de Leon MJ[1]. BMJ Open. 2014 Jun 24;4(6):e004850.

[459] Supplemental substances derived from foods as adjunctive therapeutic agents for treatment of neurodegenerative diseases and disorders. Bigford GE[1], Del Rossi G[2]. Adv Nutr. 2014 Jul 14;5(4):394-403.

[460] A Phase II Randomized Clinical Trial of a Nutritional Formulation for Cognition and Mood in Alzheimer's Disease. Remington R[1], Bechtel C[2], Larsen D[3], Samar A[4], Doshanjh L[5], Fishman P[6], Luo Y[6], Smyers K[1], Page R[2], Morrell C[5], Shea TB.[1] J Alzheimers Dis. 2015 Jan 1;45(2):395-405.

[461] Mitochondrial biogenesis: pharmacological approaches. Valero T[1]. Curr Pharm Des. 2014;20(35):5507-9.

[462] In vitro mitochondrial failure and oxidative stress mimic biochemical features of Alzheimer disease. Selvatici R[1], Marani L, Marino S, Siniscalchi A. Neurochem Int. 2013 Aug;63(2):112-20.

[463] Vitamin A and Alzheimer's disease. Ono K[1], Yamada M. Geriatr Gerontol Int. 2012 Apr;12(2):180-8.

[464] Retinoids for treatment of Alzheimer's disease. Lerner AJ[1], Gustaw-Rothenberg K, Smyth S, Casadesus G. Biofactors. 2012 Mar-Apr;38(2):84-9.

[465] Retinoic acid attenuates beta-amyloid deposition and rescues memory deficits in an Alzheimer's disease transgenic mouse model. Ding Y[1], Qiao A, Wang Z, Goodwin JS, Lee ES, Block ML, Allsbrook M, McDonald MP, Fan GH. J Neurosci. 2008 Nov 5;28(45):11622-34.

[466] Retinoids as potential targets for Alzheimer's disease. Sodhi RK[1], Singh N[2]. Pharmacol Biochem Behav. 2014 May;120:117-23.

[467] Mitochondrion-specific antioxidants as drug treatments for Alzheimer disease. Palacios HH[1], Yendluri BB, Parvathaneni K, Shadlinski VB, Obrenovich ME, Leszek J, Gokhman D, Gąsiorowski K, Bragin V, Aliev G. CNS Neurol Disord Drug Targets. 2011 Mar;10(2):149-62.

[468] [Acetyl-L-carnitine (carnicetine) in the treatment of early stages of Alzheimer's disease and vascular dementia]. [Article in Russian]. Gavrilova SI, Kalyn IaB, Kolykhalov IV, Roshchina IF, Selezneva ND. Zh Nevrol Psikhiatr Im S S Korsakova. 2011;111(9):16-22.

[469] Alpha-lipoic acid as a pleiotropic compound with potential therapeutic use in diabetes and other chronic diseases. Gomes MB, Negrato CA. Diabetol Metab Syndr. 2014 Jul 28;6(1):80.

[470] Reversal of metabolic deficits by lipoic acid in a triple transgenic mouse model of Alzheimer's disease: a 13C NMR study. Sancheti H, Kanamori K, Patil I, Díaz Brinton R, Ross BD, Cadenas E. J Cereb Blood Flow Metab. 2014 Feb;34(2):288-96.

[471] A randomized placebo-controlled pilot trial of omega-3 fatty acids and alpha lipoic acid in Alzheimer's disease. Shinto L, Quinn J, Montine T, Dodge HH, Woodward W, Baldauf-Wagner S, Waichunas D, Bumgarner L, Bourdette D, Silbert L, Kaye J. J Alzheimers Dis. 2014;38(1):111-20.

[472] Oxidative modification of lipoic acid by HNE in Alzheimer disease brain. Hardas SS, Sultana R, Clark AM, Beckett TL, Szweda LI, Murphy MP, Butterfield DA. Redox Biol. 2013 Jan 30;1(1):80-5.

[473] The possible role of antioxidant vitamin C in Alzheimer's disease treatment and prevention. Heo JH, Hyon-Lee, Lee KM. Am J Alzheimers Dis Other Demen. 2013 Mar;28(2):120-5.

[474] Effect of one-year vitamin C- and E-supplementation on cerebrospinal fluid oxidation parameters and clinical course in Alzheimer's disease. Arlt S, Müller-Thomsen T, Beisiegel U, Kontush A. Neurochem Res. 2012 Dec;37(12):2706-14.

[475] High-dose of vitamin C supplementation reduces amyloid plaque burden and ameliorates pathological changes in the brain of 5XFAD mice. Kook SY, Lee KM, Kim Y, Cha MY, Kang S, Baik SH, Lee H, Park R, Mook-Jung I. Cell Death Dis. 2014 Feb 27;5:e1083.

[476] Effects of Ashwagandha (roots of Withania somnifera) on neurodegenerative diseases. Kuboyama T[1], Tohda C, Komatsu K. Biol Pharm Bull. 2014;37(6):892-7.

[477] Blood-brain barrier permeability of bioactive withanamides present in Withania somnifera fruit extract. Vareed SK[1], Bauer AK, Nair KM, Liu Y, Jayaprakasam B, Nair MG. Phytother Res. 2014 Aug;28(8):1260-4.

[478] Withania somnifera reverses Alzheimer's disease pathology by enhancing low-density lipoprotein receptor-related protein in liver. Sehgal N[1], Gupta A, Valli RK, Joshi SD, Mills JT, Hamel E, Khanna P, Jain SC, Thakur SS, Ravindranath V. Proc Natl Acad Sci U S A. 2012 Feb 28;109(9):3510-5.

[479] Computational evidence to inhibition of human acetyl cholinesterase by withanolide a for Alzheimer treatment. Grover A[1], Shandilya A, Agrawal V, Bisaria VS, Sundar D. J Biomol Struct Dyn. 2012;29(4):651-62.

[480] Withanamides in Withania somnifera fruit protect PC-12 cells from beta-amyloid responsible for Alzheimer's disease. Jayaprakasam B[1], Padmanabhan K, Nair MG. Phytother Res. 2010 Jun;24(6):859-63.

[481] Efficacy of vitamins B supplementation on mild cognitive impairment and Alzheimer's disease: a systematic review and meta-analysis. Li MM, Yu JT, Wang HF, Jiang T, Wang J, Meng XF, Tan CC, Wang C, Tan L. Curr Alzheimer Res. 2014;11(9):844-52.

[482] Critical levels of brain atrophy associated with homocysteine and cognitive decline. de Jager CA. Neurobiol Aging. 2014 Sep;35 Suppl 2:S35-9.

[483] Acceleration of brain amyloidosis in an Alzheimer's disease mouse model by a folate, vitamin B6 and B12-deficient diet. Zhuo JM, Praticò D. Exp Gerontol. 2010 Mar;45(3):195-201.

[484] Serum homocysteine levels are correlated with behavioral and psychological symptoms of Alzheimer's disease. Kim H, Lee KJ. Neuropsychiatr Dis Treat. 2014 Oct 3;10:1887-96.

[485] Higher homocysteine associated with thinner cortical gray matter in 803 participants from the Alzheimer's disease Neuroimaging Initiative. Madsen SK[1], Rajagopalan P[1], Joshi SH[2], Toga AW[1], Thompson PM[3]; the Alzheimer's disease Neuroimaging Initiative (ADNI). Neurobiol Aging. 2014 Aug 30. pii: S0197-4580(14)00562-4.

[486] Cognitive and clinical outcomes of homocysteine-lowering B-vitamin treatment in mild cognitive impairment: a randomized controlled trial. de Jager CA, Oulhaj A, Jacoby R, Refsum H, Smith AD. Int J Geriatr Psychiatry. 2012 Jun;27(6):592-600.

[487] Update on vitamin B12 deficiency. Langan RC[1], Zawistoski KJ. Am Fam Physician. 2011 Jun 15;83(12):1425-30.

[488] Vitamin B12 in neurology and ageing; clinical and genetic aspects. McCaddon A. Biochimie. 2013 May;95(5):1066-76.

[489] Among vitamin B12 deficient older people, high folate levels are associated with worse cognitive function: combined data from three cohorts. Moore EM[1], Ames D[2], Mander AG[3], Carne RP[4], Brodaty H[5], Woodward MC[6], Boundy K[7], Ellis KA[8], Bush AI[9], Faux NG[10], Martins RN[11], Masters CL[12], Rowe CC[13], Szoeke C[14], Watters DA[4]. J Alzheimers Dis. 2014;39(3):661-8.

[490] High-dose B vitamin supplementation and cognitive decline in Alzheimer disease: a randomized controlled trial. Aisen PS[1], Schneider LS, Sano M, Diaz-Arrastia R, van Dyck CH, Weiner MF, Bottiglieri T, Jin S, Stokes KT, Thomas RG, Thal LJ; Alzheimer Disease Cooperative Study. JAMA. 2008 Oct 15;300(15):1774-83.

[491] Cognitive impairment and vitamin B12: a review. Moore E[1], Mander A, Ames D, Carne R, Sanders K, Watters D. Int Psychogeriatr. 2012 Apr;24(4):541-56.

[492] Berberine attenuates axonal transport impairment and axonopathy induced by Calyculin A in N2a cells. Liu X[1], Zhou J[1], Abid MD[2], Yan H[1], Huang H[1], Wan L[1], Feng Z[1], Chen J[1]. PLoS One. 2014 Apr 8;9(4):e93974.

[493] Berberine suppresses amyloid-beta-induced inflammatory response in microglia by inhibiting nuclear factor-kappaB and mitogen-activated protein kinase signalling pathways. Jia L[1], Liu J, Song Z, Pan X, Chen L, Cui X, Wang M. J Pharm Pharmacol. 2012 Oct;64(10):1510-21.

[494] Piperine, the main alkaloid of Thai black pepper, protects against neurodegeneration and cognitive impairment in animal model of cognitive deficit like condition of Alzheimer's disease. Chonpathompikunlert P[1], Wattanathorn J, Muchimapura S. Food Chem Toxicol. 2010 Mar;48(3):798-802.

[495] Lycopene attenuates insulin signaling deficits, oxidative stress, neuroinflammation, and cognitive impairment in fructose-drinking insulin resistant rats. Yin Q[1], Ma Y[1], Hong Y[1], Hou X[1], Chen J[1], Shen C[2], Sun M[1], Shang Y[1], Dong S[1], Zeng Z[3], Pei JJ[4], Liu X[5]. Neuropharmacology. 2014 Nov;86:389-96.

[496] Serum lycopene, lutein and zeaxanthin, and the risk of Alzheimer's disease mortality in older adults. Min JY[1], Min KB. Dement Geriatr Cogn Disord. 2014;37(3-4):246-56.

[497] Serum lycopene, lutein and zeaxanthin, and the risk of Alzheimer's disease mortality in older adults. Min JY[1], Min KB. Dement Geriatr Cogn Disord. 2014;37(3-4):246-56.

[500] Chia (Salvia hispanica L.) enhances HSP, PGC-1α expressions and improves glucose tolerance in diet-induced obese rats. Marineli Rda S[1], Moura CS[1], Moraes ÉA[1], Lenquiste SA[1], Lollo PC[1], Morato PN[1], Amaya-Farfan J[1], Maróstica MR Jr[2]. Nutrition. 2015 May;31(5):740-8.

[501] Chia flour supplementation reduces blood pressure in hypertensive subjects. Toscano LT[1], da Silva CS, Toscano LT, de Almeida AE, Santos Ada C, Silva AS. Plant Foods Hum Nutr. 2014 Dec;69(4):392-8.

[502] Reduction in postprandial glucose excursion and prolongation of satiety: possible explanation of the long-term effects of whole grain Salba (Salvia Hispanica L.). Vuksan V[1], Jenkins AL, Dias AG, Lee AS, Jovanovski E, Rogovik AL, Hanna A. Eur J Clin Nutr. 2010 Apr;64(4):436-8.

[503] An in vitro study of neuroprotective properties of traditional Chinese herbal medicines thought to promote healthy aging and longevity. Shen B, Truong J, Helliwell R, Govindaraghavan S, Sucher NJ[1]. BMC Complement Altern Med. 2013 Dec 27;13:373.

[504] Smart soup, a traditional Chinese medicine formula, ameliorates amyloid pathology and related cognitive deficits. Hou Y[1], Wang Y[2], Zhao J[1], Li X[1], Cui J[1], Ding J[2], Wang Y[3], Zeng X[1], Ling Y[4], Shen X[5], Chen S[2], Huang C[4], Pei G[6]. PLoS One. 2014 Nov 11;9(11):e111215.

[505] Treating Alzheimer's disease with Yizhijiannao granules by regulating expression of multiple proteins in temporal lobe. Zhu H[1], Luo L[2], Hu S[1], Dong K[1], Li G[1], Zhang T[1]. Neural Regen Res. 2014 Jul 1;9(13):1283-7.

[506] Virgin coconut oil and its potential cardioprotective effects. Babu AS, Veluswamy SK, Arena R, Guazzi M, Lavie CJ. Postgrad Med. 2014 Nov;126(7):76-83.

[507] Antistress and antioxidant effects of virgin coconut oil in vivo. Yeap SK, Beh BK, Ali NM, Yusof HM, Ho WY, Koh SP, Alitheen NB, Long K. Exp Ther Med. 2015 Jan;9(1):39-42.

[508] Coconut oil attenuates the effects of amyloid-β on cortical neurons in vitro. Nafar F, Mearow KM. J Alzheimers Dis. 2014;39(2):233-7. doi: 10.3233/JAD-131436.

[509] Young coconut juice, a potential therapeutic agent that could significantly reduce some pathologies associated with Alzheimer's disease: novel findings. Radenahmad N, Saleh F, Sawangjaroen K, Vongvatcharanon U, Subhadhirasakul P, Rundorn W, Withyachumnarnkul B, Connor JR. Br J Nutr. 2011 Mar;105(5):738-46.

[510] Caffeine suppresses amyloid-beta levels in plasma and brain of Alzheimer's disease transgenic mice. Cao C, Cirrito JR, Lin X, Wang L, Verges DK, Dickson A, Mamcarz M, Zhang C, Mori T, Arendash GW, Holtzman DM, Potter H. J Alzheimers Dis. 2009;17(3):681-97.

[511] Coffee intake in midlife and risk of dementia and its neuropathologic correlates. Gelber RP, Petrovitch H, Masaki KH, Ross GW, White LR. J Alzheimers Dis. 2011;23(4):607-15.

[512] Possible health effects of caffeinated coffee consumption on Alzheimer's disease and cardiovascular disease. You DC¹, Kim YS, Ha AW, Lee YN, Kim SM, Kim CH, Lee SH, Choi D, Lee JM. Toxicol Res. 2011 Mar;27(1):7-10.

[513] Does coenzyme-Q have a protective effect against atorvastatin induced myopathy? A histopathological and immunohistochemical study in albino rats. Khalil MS, Khamis N, Al-Drees A, Abdulghani HM. Histol Histopathol. 2014 Nov 4.

[514] The Hypothalamus in Alzheimer's disease: A Golgi and Electron Microscope Study. Baloyannis SJ, Mavroudis I, Mitilineos D, Baloyannis IS, Costa VG. Am J Alzheimers Dis Other Demen. 2014 Nov 7. pii: 1533317514556876.

[515] Coenzyme Q10 protects human endothelial cells from β-amyloid uptake and oxidative stress-induced injury. Durán-Prado M, Frontiñán J, Santiago-Mora R, Peinado JR, Parrado-Fernández C, Gómez-Almagro MV, Moreno M, López-Domínguez JA, Villalba JM, Alcaín FJ. PLoS One. 2014 Oct 1;9(10):e109223.

[516] Coenzyme Q10 and α-tocopherol reversed age-associated functional impairments in mice. Shetty RA, Ikonne US, Forster MJ, Sumien N. Exp Gerontol. 2014 Oct;58:208-18.

[517] Cooking enhances curcumin anti-cancerogenic activity through pyrolytic formation of "deketene curcumin." Dahmke IN, Boettcher SP, Groh M, Mahlknecht U. Food Chem. 2014 May 15;151:514-9.

[518] Therapeutic potential of turmeric in Alzheimer's disease: curcumin or curcuminoids? Ahmed T[1], Gilani AH. Phytother Res. 2014 Apr;28(4):517-25.

[519] Molecular Chaperone Dysfunction in Neurodegenerative Diseases and Effects of Curcumin. Maiti P[1], Manna J[2], Veleri S[3], Frautschy S[4]. Biomed Res Int. 2014;2014:495091.

[520] Structure activity relationship study of curcumin analogues toward the amyloid-beta aggregation inhibitor. Endo H, Nikaido Y, Nakadate M, Ise S, Konno H. Bioorg Med Chem Lett. 2014 Dec 15;24(24):5621-6.

[521] Curcumin derivative with the substitution at C-4 position, but not curcumin, is effective against amyloid pathology in APP/PS1 mice. Yanagisawa D, Ibrahim NF, Taguchi H, Morikawa S, Hirao K, Shirai N, Sogabe T, Tooyama I. Neurobiol Aging. 2014 Aug 2. pii: S0197-4580(14)00510-7.

[522] Amelioration of cognitive deficits and neurodegeneration by curcumin in rat model of sporadic dementia of Alzheimer's type (SDAT). Ishrat T, Hoda MN, Khan MB, Yousuf S, Ahmad M, Khan MM, Ahmad A, Islam F. Eur Neuropsychopharmacol. 2009 Sep;19(9):636-47.

[523] Effects of turmeric on Alzheimer's disease with behavioral and psychological symptoms of dementia. Hishikawa N[1], Takahashi Y, Amakusa Y, Tanno Y, Tuji Y, Niwa H, Murakami N, Krishna UK. Ayu. 2012 Oct;33(4):499-504. doi: 10.4103/0974-8520.110524.

[524] Oral curcumin for Alzheimer's disease: tolerability and efficacy in a 24-week randomized, double blind, placebo-controlled study. Ringman JM[1], Frautschy SA[2], Teng E[2], Begum AN[3], Bardens J[1], Beigi M[4], Gylys KH[5], Badmaev V[6], Heath DD[7], Apostolova LG[1], Porter V[8], Vanek Z[8], Marshall GA[9], Hellemann G[10], Sugar C[10], Masterman DL[11], Montine TJ[12], Cummings JL[13], Cole GM[2]. Alzheimers Res Ther. 2012 Oct 29;4(5):43.

[525] Vitamin D deficiency predicts cognitive decline in older men and women: The Pro.V.A. Study. Toffanello ED[1], Coin A[2], Perissinotto E[2], Zambon S[2], Sarti S[2], Veronese N[2], De Rui M[2], Bolzetta F[2], Corti MC[2], Crepaldi G[2], Manzato E[2], Sergi G[2]. Neurology. 2014 Nov 5.

[526] [Treatment with vitamin D and slowing of progression to severe stage of Alzheimer's disease].
[Article in Spanish]. Chaves M[1], Toral A, Bisonni A, Rojas JI, Fernández C, Basallo MJ, Matusevich D, Cristiano E, Golimstok A. Vertex. 2014 Mar-Apr;25(114):85-91.

[527] Vitamin D and the risk of dementia and Alzheimer disease. Littlejohns TJ[1], Henley WE[1], Lang IA[1], Annweiler C[1], Beauchet O[1], Chaves PH[1], Fried L[1], Kestenbaum BR[1], Kuller LH[1], Langa KM[1], Lopez OL[1], Kos K[1], Soni M[1], Llewellyn DJ[2]. Neurology. 2014 Sep 2;83(10):920-8.

[528] Vitamin D and white matter abnormalities in older adults: a quantitative volumetric analysis of brain MRI. Annweiler C[1], Bartha R[2], Karras SN[3], Gautier J[4], Roche F[5], Beauchet O[6]. Exp Gerontol. 2015 Mar;63:41-7.

[529] Effects of Vitamin E on Cognitive Performance during Aging and in Alzheimer's disease. Fata GL[1], Weber P[2], Mohajeri MH[3]. Nutrients. 2014 Nov 28;6(12):5453-5472.

[530] Vitamin E for Alzheimer's dementia and mild cognitive impairment. Farina N[1], Isaac MG, Clark AR, Rusted J, Tabet N. Cochrane Database Syst Rev. 2012 Nov 14;11:CD002854.

[531] Dietary intakes of vitamin E, vitamin C, and β-carotene and risk of Alzheimer's disease: a meta-analysis. Li FJ[1], Shen L, Ji HF. J Alzheimers Dis. 2012;31(2):253-8.

[532] Aβ and tau toxicities in Alzheimer's are linked via oxidative stress-induced p38 activation: protective role of vitamin E. Giraldo E[1], Lloret A[1], Fuchsberger T[1], Viña J[1]. Redox Biol. 2014 Mar 10;2:873-7.

[533] Lymphocytic mitochondrial aconitase activity is reduced in Alzheimer's disease and mild cognitive impairment. Mangialasche F[1], Baglioni M[2], Cecchetti R[2], Kivipelto M[3], Ruggiero C[2], Piobbico D[4], Kussmaul L[5], Monastero R[6], Brancorsini S[4], Mecocci P[2]. J Alzheimers Dis. 2015;44(2):649-60.

[534] A Phase II Randomized Clinical Trial of a Nutritional Formulation for Cognition and Mood in Alzheimer's Disease. Remington R[1], Bechtel C[2], Larsen D[3], Samar A[4], Doshanjh L[5], Fishman P[6], Luo Y[6], Smyers K[1], Page R[2], Morrell C[5], Shea TB[1]. J Alzheimers Dis. 2015 Jan 1;45(2):395-405.

[535] Possible protective action of neurotrophic factors and natural compounds against common neurodegenerative diseases. Numakawa T. Neural Regen Res. 2014 Aug 15;9(16):1506-8.

[536] Natural polyphenols binding to amyloid: A broad class of compounds to treat different human amyloid diseases. Ngoungoure VL[1], Schluesener J, Moundipa PF, Schluesener H. Mol Nutr Food Res. 2014 Aug 28.

[537]Dietary polyphenol-derived protection against neurotoxic β-amyloid protein: from molecular to clinical. Smid SD[1], Maag JL, Musgrave IF. Food Funct. 2012 Dec;3(12):1242-50.

[538]The role of polyphenols in the modulation of sirtuins and other pathways involved in Alzheimer's disease. Jayasena T[1], Poljak A, Smythe G, Braidy N, Münch G, Sachdev P. Ageing Res Rev. 2013 Sep;12(4):867-83.

[539] Flavonoids, cognition, and dementia: actions, mechanisms, and potential therapeutic utility for Alzheimer disease. Williams RJ[1], Spencer JP. Free Radic Biol Med. 2012 Jan 1;52(1):35-45.

[540]Neuroprotective effects of berry fruits on neurodegenerative diseases. Subash S[1], Essa MM[1], Al-Adawi S[2], Memon MA[3], Manivasagam T[4], Akbar M[5]. Neural Regen Res. 2014 Aug 15;9(16):1557-66.

[541]Consumption of fig fruits grown in Oman can improve memory, anxiety, and learning skills in a transgenic mice model of Alzheimer's disease. Subash S, Essa MM, Braidy N, Al-Jabri A, Vaishnav R, Al-Adawi S, Al-Asmi A, Guillemin GJ. Nutr Neurosci. 2014 Jun 18.

[542]Total polyphenols and antioxidant activity in different species of apples grown in Georgia. Gogia N, Gongadze M, Bukia Z, Esaiashvili M, Chkhikvishvili I. Georgian Med News. 2014 Jul-Aug;(232-233):107-12.

[543] Anti-dementia Activity of Nobiletin, a Citrus Flavonoid: A Review of Animal Studies. Nakajima A[1], Ohizumi Y[2], Yamada K[1]. Clin Psychopharmacol Neurosci. 2014 Aug;12(2):75-82.

[544]Folic acid with or without vitamin B12 for cognition and dementia. Malouf M[1], Grimley EJ, Areosa SA. Cochrane Database Syst Rev. 2003;(4):CD004514.

[545] Results of 2-year vitamin B treatment on cognitive performance: secondary data from an RCT. van der Zwaluw NL[1], Dhonukshe-Rutten RA[2], van Wijngaarden JP[1], Brouwer-Brolsma EM[1], van de Rest O[1], In 't Veld PH[1], Enneman AW[1], van Dijk SC[1], Ham AC[1], Swart KM[1], van der Velde N[1], van Schoor NM[1], van der Cammen TJ[1], Uitterlinden AG[1], Lips P[1], Kessels RP[1], de Groot LC[1]. Neurology. 2014 Dec 2;83(23):2158-66.

[546] Brain atrophy in cognitively impaired elderly: the importance of long-chain ω-3 fatty acids and B vitamin status in a randomized controlled trial. Jernerén F[1], Elshorbagy AK[1], Oulhaj A[1], Smith SM[1], Refsum H[1], Smith AD[1]. Am J Clin Nutr. 2015 Apr 15.

[547] Associations between Homocysteine, Folic Acid, Vitamin B12 and Alzheimer's Disease: Insights from Meta-Analyses. Shen L[1], Ji HF[1]. J Alzheimers Dis. 2015 Apr 8.

[548] Potential Therapeutic Implications of Gelsolin in Alzheimer's disease. Ji L[1], Zhao X[2], Hua Z[2]. J Alzheimers Dis. 2014 Sep 10.

[549] Efficacy and adverse effects of ginkgo biloba for cognitive impairment and dementia: a systematic review and meta-analysis. Tan MS, Yu JT, Tan CC, Wang HF, Meng XF, Wang C, Jiang T, Zhu XC, Tan L. J Alzheimers Dis. 2015 Jan 1;43(2):589-603.

[550] A systematic review on natural medicines for the prevention and treatment of Alzheimer's disease with meta-analyses of intervention effect of ginkgo. Yang M, Xu DD, Zhang Y, Liu X, Hoeven R, Cho WC. Am J Chin Med. 2014;42(3):505-21.

[551] Effects of Gingko biloba supplementation in Alzheimer's disease patients receiving cholinesterase inhibitors: data from the ICTUS study. Canevelli M, Adali N, Kelaiditi E, Cantet C, Ousset PJ, Cesari M; ICTUS/DSA Group (42 collaborators). Phytomedicine. 2014 May 15;21(6):888-92.

[552] EGb761 Provides a Protective Effect against Aβ1-42 Oligomer-Induced Cell Damage and Blood-Brain Barrier Disruption in an In Vitro bEnd.3 Endothelial Model. Wan WB, Cao L, Liu LM, Kalionis B, Chen C, Tai XT, Li YM, Xia SJ. PLoS One. 2014 Nov 26;9(11):e113126.

[553] Effect of Memo®, a natural formula combination, on Mini-Mental State Examination scores in patients with mild cognitive impairment. Yakoot M, Salem A, Helmy S. Clin Interv Aging. 2013;8:975-81.

[554] Efficacy of rivastigmine in comparison to ginkgo for treating Alzheimer'sdementia. Nasab NM, Bahrammi MA, Nikpour MR, Rahim F, Naghibis SN. J Pak Med Assoc. 2012 Jul;62(7):677-80.

[555] Ginkgo biloba extract EGb 761 in the treatment of dementia: a pharmacoeconomic analysis of the Austrian setting. Wien KRainer M, Mucke H, Schlaefke S. lin Wochenschr. 2013 Jan;125(1-2):8-15.

[556] Mitochondrial effects of Ginkgo biloba extract. Eckert A[1]. Int Psychogeriatr. 2012 Aug;24 Suppl 1:S18-20.

[557] Ginkgo biloba extract EGb 761® in dementia with neuropsychiatric features: a randomised, placebo-controlled trial to confirm the efficacy and safety of a daily dose of 240 mg. Herrschaft H, Nacu A, Likhachev S, Sholomov I, Hoerr R, Schlaefke S. J Psychiatr Res. 2012 Jun;46(6):716-23.

[558] Ginkgo biloba for preventing cognitive decline in older adults: a randomized trial. Snitz BE[1], O'Meara ES, Carlson MC, Arnold AM, Ives DG, Rapp SR, Saxton J, Lopez OL, Dunn LO, Sink KM, DeKosky ST; Ginkgo Evaluation of Memory (GEM) Study Investigators (Collaborators (55). JAMA. 2009 Dec 23;302(24):2663-70.

[559] Ginkgolide B revamps neuroprotective role of apurinic/apyrimidinic endonuclease 1 and mitochondrial oxidative phosphorylation against Aβ25-35 -induced neurotoxicity in human neuroblastoma cells. Kaur N[1], Dhiman M, Perez-Polo JR, Mantha AK. J Neurosci Res. 2015 Jun;93(6):938-47.

[560] A combination of supplements may reduce the risk of Alzheimer's disease in elderly Japanese with normal cognition. Bun S[1], Ikejima C[2], Kida J[1], Yoshimura A[1], Lebowitz AJ[1], Kakuma T[3], Asada T[4]. J Alzheimers Dis. 2015 Jan 1;45(1):15-25.

[561] Efficacy and tolerability of Ginkgo biloba extract EGb 761® in dementia: a systematic review and meta-analysis of randomized placebo-controlled trials. Gauthier S[1], Schlaefke S[2]. Clin Interv Aging. 2014 Nov 28;9:2065-77.

[562] In vitro evaluation of anti-Alzheimer effects of dry ginger (Zingiber officinale Roscoe) extract. Mathew M, Subramanian S. Indian J Exp Biol. 2014 Jun;52(6):606-12.

[563] 6-Shogaol, an active constituent of ginger, attenuates neuroinflammation and cognitive deficits in animal models of dementia. Moon M[1], Kim HG[2], Choi JG[3], Oh H[4], Lee PK[5], Ha SK[6], Kim SY[7], Park Y[7], Huh Y[8], Oh MS[9].
Biochem Biophys Res Commun. 2014 Jun 20;449(1):8-13.

[564] Protective effects of ginger root extract on Alzheimer disease-induced behavioral dysfunction in rats. Zeng GF[1], Zhang ZY, Lu L, Xiao DQ, Zong SH, He JM. Rejuvenation Res. 2013 Apr;16(2):124-33.

[565] Ginsenoside Rd attenuates tau protein phosphorylation via the PI3K/AKT/GSK-3β pathway after transient forebrain ischemia. Zhang X, Shi M, Ye R, Wang W, Liu X, Zhang G, Han J, Zhang Y, Wang B, Zhao J, Hui J, Xiong L, Zhao G. Neurochem Res. 2014 Jul;39(7):1363-73.

[566] Protective effects of ginsenoside Rg1 on chronic restraint stress induced learning and memory impairments in male mice. Wang Y, Kan H, Yin Y, Wu W, Hu W, Wang M, Li W, Li W. Pharmacol Biochem Behav. 2014 May;120:73-81.

[567] Ginsenoside Rg5 improves cognitive dysfunction and beta-amyloid deposition in STZ-induced memory impaired rats via attenuating neuroinflammatory responses. Chu S, Gu J, Feng L, Liu J, Zhang M, Jia X, Liu M, Yao D. Int Immunopharmacol. 2014 Apr;19(2):317-26.

[568] Effects of Panax notoginseng saponin on α, β, and γ secretase involved in Aβ deposition in SAMP8 mice. Huang J[1], Wu D, Wang J, Li F, Lu L, Gao Y, Zhong Z. Neuroreport. 2014 Jan 22;25(2):89-93.

[569] An open-label trial of Korean red ginseng as an adjuvant treatment for cognitive impairment in patients with Alzheimer's disease. Heo JH[1], Lee ST, Chu K, Oh MJ, Park HJ, Shim JY, Kim M. Eur J Neurol. 2008 Aug;15(8):865-8.

[570] Panax ginseng enhances cognitive performance in Alzheimer disease. Lee ST, Chu K, Sim JY, Heo JH, Kim M. Alzheimer Dis Assoc Disord. 2008 Jul-Sep;22(3):222-6.

[571] Ginseng for cognitive function in Alzheimer's disease: a systematic review. Lee MS[1], Yang EJ, Kim JI, Ernst E. J Alzheimers Dis. 2009;18(2):339-44.

[572] Chemical investigation of commercial grape seed derived products to assess quality and detect adulteration. Villani TS[1], Reichert W[2], Ferruzzi MG[3], Pasinetti GM[4], Simon JE[5], Wu Q[6]. Food Chem. 2015 Mar 1;170:271-80.

[573] Effects of grape seed proanthocyanidin extract on renal injury in type 2 diabetic rats. Bao L, Zhang Z, Dai X, Ding Y, Jiang Y, Li Y, Li Y. Mol Med Rep. 2015 Jan;11(1):645-52.

[574] Grape seed extract has superior beneficial effects than vitamin E on oxidative stress and apoptosis in the hippocampus of streptozotocin induced diabetic rats. Yonguc GN, Dodurga Y, Adiguzel E, Gundogdu G, Kucukatay V, Ozbal S, Yilmaz I, Cankurt U, Yilmaz Y, Akdogan [3]. Gene. 2014 Oct 30. pii: S0378-1119(14)01227-X.

[575] Functional modification of adipocytes by grape seed extract impairs their pro-tumorigenic signaling on colon cancer stem cells and the daughter cancer cells. Kumar S, Kumar D, Raina K, Agarwal R, Agarwal C. Oncotarget. 2014 Oct 30;5(20):10151-69.

[576] Targeting multiple pathogenic mechanisms with polyphenols for the treatment of Alzheimer's disease-experimental approach and therapeutic implications. Wang J, Bi

W, Cheng A, Freire D, Vempati P, Zhao W, Gong B, Janle EM, Chen TY, Ferruzzi MG, Schmeidler J, Ho L, Pasinetti GM. Front Aging Neurosci. 2014 Mar 14;6:42.

[577] Gallic acid is the major component of grape seed extract that inhibits amyloid fibril formation. Liu Y, Pukala TL, Musgrave IF, Williams DM, Dehle FC, Carver JA. Bioorg Med Chem Lett. 2013 Dec 1;23(23):6336-40.

[578] Ultrastructural alterations of Alzheimer's disease paired helical filaments by grape seed-derived polyphenols. Ksiezak-Reding H, Ho L, Santa-Maria I, Diaz-Ruiz C, Wang J, Pasinetti GM. Neurobiol Aging. 2012 Jul;33(7):1427-39.

[579] Role of grape seed polyphenols in Alzheimer's disease neuropathology. Pasinetti GM, Ho L. Nutr Diet Suppl. 2010 Aug 1;2010(2):97-103.

[580] Bioavailability of gallic acid and catechins from grape seed polyphenol extract is improved by repeated dosing in rats: implications for treatment in Alzheimer's disease. Ferruzzi MG, Lobo JK, Janle EM, Cooper B, Simon JE, Wu QL, Welch C, Ho L, Weaver C, Pasinetti GM. J Alzheimers Dis. 2009;18(1):113-24.

[581] Green tea and theanine: health benefits. Cooper R. Int J Food Sci Nutr. 2012 Mar;63 Suppl 1:90-7.

[582] Black tea: chemical analysis and stability. Li S, Lo CY, Pan MH, Lai CS, Ho CT. Food Funct. 2013 Jan;4(1):10-8.

[583] The role of green tea extract and powder in mitigating metabolic syndromes with special reference to hyperglycemia and hypercholesterolemia. Yousaf S, Butt MS, Suleria HA, Iqbal MJ. Food Funct. 2014 Mar;5(3):545-56.

[584] Inhibition of acetylcholinesterase by green and white tea and their simulated intestinal metabolites. Okello EJ[1], Leylabi R, McDougall GJ. Food Funct. 2012 Jun;3(6):651-61.

[585] The benefits and risks of consuming brewed tea: beware of toxic element contamination. Schwalfenberg G, Genuis SJ, Rodushkin I. J Toxicol. 2013;2013:370460.

[586] Epigallocatechin-3-gallate (EGCG)-stabilized selenium nanoparticles coated with Tet-1 peptide to reduce amyloid-β aggregation and cytotoxicity. Zhang J[1], Zhou X, Yu Q, Yang L, Sun D, Zhou Y, Liu J. ACS Appl Mater Interfaces. 2014 Jun 11;6(11):8475-87.

[587] Effects of Flavonoid Compounds on β-amyloid-peptide-induced Neuronal Death in Cultured Mouse Cortical Neurons. Choi SM, Kim BC, Cho YH, Choi KH, Chang J, Park MS, Kim MK, Cho KH, Kim JK. Chonnam Med J. 2014 Aug;50(2):45-51.

[588] The green tea polyphenol (-)-epigallocatechin gallate prevents the aggregation of tau protein into toxic oligomers at substoichiometric ratios. Wobst HJ, Sharma A, Diamond MI, Wanker EE, Bieschke J. FEBS Lett. 2014 Nov 29.

[589] Dietary (-)-epicatechin as a potent inhibitor of βγ-secretase amyloid precursor protein processing. Cox CJ[1], Choudhry F[2], Peacey E[2], Perkinton MS[2], Richardson JC[3], Howlett DR[2], Lichtenthaler SF[4], Francis PT[2], Williams RJ[5]. Neurobiol Aging. 2014 Jul 30. pii: S0197-4580(14)00501-6.

[590] Neuroprotective effects of resveratrol and epigallocatechin gallate polyphenols are mediated by the activation of protein kinase C gamma. Menard C, Bastianetto S, Quirion R. Front Cell Neurosci. 2013 Dec 26;7:281.

[591] Serum cytokine profile in Alzheimer's disease patients after ingestion of an antioxidant beverage. Rubio-Perez JM, Morillas-Ruiz JM[1]. CNS Neurol Disord Drug Targets. 2013 Dec;12(8):1233-41.

[592] Green tea catechin leads to global improvement among Alzheimer's disease-related phenotypes in NSE/hAPP-C105 Tg mice. Lim HJ, Shim SB, Jee SW, Lee SH, Lim CJ, Hong JT, Sheen YY, Hwang DY. J Nutr Biochem. 2013 Jul;24(7):1302-13.

[593] Oolong, black and pu-erh tea suppresses adiposity in mice via activation of AMP-activated protein kinase. Yamashita Y, Wang L, Wang L, Tanaka Y, Zhang T, Ashida H. Food Funct. 2014 Oct 24;5(10):2420-9.

[594] Intake of green tea inhibited increase of salivary chromogranin A after mental task stress loads. Yoto A, Murao S, Nakamura Y, Yokogoshi H. J Physiol Anthropol. 2014 Jul 17;33:20.

[595] Coffee and tea consumption are inversely associated with mortality in a multiethnic urban population. Gardener H[1], Rundek T, Wright CB, Elkind MS, Sacco RL. J Nutr. 2013 Aug;143(8):1299-308.

[596] Antibacterial, antiadherence, antiprotease, and anti-inflammatory activities of various tea extracts: potential benefits for periodontal diseases. Zhao L, La VD, Grenier D. J Med Food. 2013 May;16(5):428-36.

[597] Effect of hesperidin on neurobehavioral, neuroinflammation, oxidative stress and lipid alteration in intracerebroventricular streptozotocin induced cognitive impairment

in mice. Javed H[1], Vaibhav K[1], Ahmed ME[1], Khan A[1], Tabassum R[1], Islam F[2], Safhi MM[3], Islam F[4]. J Neurol Sci. 2014 Nov 6. pii: S0022-510X(14)00714-X.

[598] Hesperidin alleviates cognitive impairment, mitochondrial dysfunction and oxidative stress in a mouse model of Alzheimer's disease. Wang D[1], Liu L, Zhu X, Wu W, Wang Y. Cell Mol Neurobiol. 2014 Nov;34(8):1209-21.

[599] Hesperidin ameliorates behavioral impairments and neuropathology of transgenic APP/PS1 mice. Li C[1], Zug C[1], Qu H[2], Schluesener H[1], Zhang Z[3]. Behav Brain Res. 2015 Mar 15;281:32-42.

[600] Huperzine A: Is it an Effective Disease-Modifying Drug for Alzheimer's disease? Qian ZM[1], Ke Y[2].
Front Aging Neurosci. 2014 Aug 19;6:216.

[601] Huperzine a in the treatment of Alzheimer's disease and vascular dementia: a meta-analysis. Xing SH[1], Zhu CX[2], Zhang R[1], An L[1]. Evid Based Complement Alternat Med. 2014;2014:363985.

[602] Reducing iron in the brain: a novel pharmacologic mechanism of huperzine A in the treatment of Alzheimer's disease. Huang XT[1], Qian ZM[2], He X[3], Gong Q[3], Wu KC[3], Jiang LR[4], Lu LN[3], Zhu ZJ[3], Zhang HY[5], Yung WH[3], Ke Y[6]. Neurobiol Aging. 2014 May;35(5):1045-54.

[603] Huperzine A for Alzheimer's disease: a systematic review and meta-analysis of randomized clinical trials. Yang G[1], Wang Y, Tian J, Liu JP. PLoS One. 2013 Sep 23;8(9):e74916.

[604] Comparison of the efficacy of four cholinesterase inhibitors in combination with memantine for the treatment of Alzheimer's disease. Shao ZQ[1]. Int J Clin Exp Med. 2015 Feb 15;8(2):2944-8.

[605] Composition and antioxidant activity of kale (Brassica oleracea L. var. acephala) raw and cooked. Sikora E[1], Bodziarczyk I. Acta Sci Pol Technol Aliment. 2012 Jul-Sep;11(3):239-48.

[606] Characterization and quantification of flavonoids and hydroxycinnamic acids in curly kale (Brassica oleracea L. Convar. acephala Var. sabellica) by HPLC-DAD-ESI-MSn. Olsen H[1], Aaby K, Borge GI. J Agric Food Chem. 2009 Apr 8;57(7):2816-25.

[607] Magnesium in disease prevention and overall health. Volpe SL. Adv Nutr. 2013 May 1;4(3):378S-83S.

[608] Dietary Mineral Intake and Risk of Mild Cognitive Impairment: The PATH through Life Project. Cherbuin N[1], Kumar R[2], Sachdev PS[3], Anstey KJ[1]. Front Aging Neurosci. 2014 Feb 4;6:4.

[609] Elevation of brain magnesium prevents and reverses cognitive deficits and synaptic loss in Alzheimer's disease mouse model. Li W[1], Yu J, Liu Y, Huang X, Abumaria N, Zhu Y, Huang X, Xiong W, Ren C, Liu XG, Chui D, Liu G. J Neurosci. 2013 May 8;33(19):8423-41.

[610] Magnesium protects cognitive functions and synaptic plasticity in streptozotocin-induced sporadic Alzheimer's model. Xu ZP[1], Li L[1], Bao J[1], Wang ZH[1], Zeng J[1], Liu EJ[1], Li XG[1], Huang RX[1], Gao D[1], Li MZ[1], Zhang Y[2], Liu GP[1], Wang JZ[1]. PLoS One. 2014 Sep 30;9(9):e108645.

[611] Local melatonin regulates inflammation resolution: a common factor in neurodegenerative, psychiatric and systemic inflammatory disorders. Anderson G, Maes M. CNS Neurol Disord Drug Targets. 2014;13(5):817-27.

[612] Melatonin and mitochondrial dysfunction in the central nervous system. Cardinali DP, Pagano ES, Scacchi Bernasconi PA, Reynoso R, Scacchi P. Horm Behav. 2013 Feb;63(2):322-30.

[613] Melatonin: functions and ligands. Singh M, Jadhav HR. Drug Discov Today. 2014 Sep;19(9):1410-8.

[614] Melatonin in aging and disease -multiple consequences of reduced secretion, options and limits of treatment. Hardeland R[1]. Aging Dis. 2012 Apr;3(2):194-225.

[615] Regional upregulation of hippocampal melatonin MT2 receptors by valproic acid: therapeutic implications for Alzheimer's disease. Bahna SG, Sathiyapalan A, Foster JA, Niles LP. Neurosci Lett. 2014 Jul 25;576:84-7.

[616] Melatonin and synthetic analogs as antioxidants. Suzen S. Curr Drug Deliv. 2013 Feb;10(1):71-5.

[617] Amyloid-β peptide induces mitochondrial dysfunction by inhibition of preprotein maturation. Mossmann D, Vögtle FN, Taskin AA, Teixeira PF, Ring J, Burkhart JM, Burger N, Pinho CM, Tadic J, Loreth D, Graff C, Metzger F, Sickmann A, Kretz O, Wiedemann N, Zahedi RP, Madeo F, Glaser E, Meisinger C. Cell Metab. 2014 Oct 7;20(4):662-9.

[618]Melatonin attenuates D-galactose-induced memory impairment, neuroinflmmation and neurodegeneration via RAGE/NF-K B/JNK signaling pathway in aging mouse model. Ali T, Badshah H, Kim TH, Kim MO. J Pineal Res. 2014 Nov 17. doi: 10.1111/jpi.12194.

[619]Melatonin-mediated β-catenin activation protects neuron cells against prion protein-induced neurotoxicity. Jeong JK, Lee JH, Moon JH, Lee YJ, Park SY. J Pineal Res. 2014 Nov;57(4):427-34.

[620]Melatonin stimulates the non amyloidogenic processing of βapp through the positive transcriptional regulation of adam10 and adam17. Shukla M, Htoo HH, Wintachai P, Hernandez JF, Dubois C, Postina R, Xu H, Checler F, Smith DR, Govitrapong P, Vincent B. J Pineal Res. 2014 Dec 9.

[621] The interaction between amyloid-β peptides and anionic lipid membranes containing cholesterol and melatonin. Dies H, Toppozini L, Rheinstädter MC PLoS One. 2014 Jun 10;9(6):e99124.

[622] Does melatonin ameliorate neurological changes associated with Alzheimer's disease in ovariectomized rat model? Ahmed HH, Estefan SF, Mohamd EM, Farrag AelR, Salah RS. Indian J Clin Biochem. 2013 Oct;28(4):381-9.

[623]Role of melatonin supplementation in neurodegenerative disorders. Polimeni G, Esposito E, Bevelacqua V, Guarneri C, Cuzzocrea S. Front Biosci (Landmark Ed). 2014 Jan 1;19:429-46.

[624]Melatonin protects against amyloid-β-induced impairments of hippocampal LTP and spatial learning in rat. Liu XJ, Yuan L, Yang D, Han WN, Li QS, Yang W, Liu QS, Qi JS. Synapse. 2013 Sep;67(9):626-36.

[625]Caffeine increases mitochondrial function and blocks melatonin signaling to mitochondria in Alzheimer's mice and cells. Dragicevic N, Delic V, Cao C, Copes N, Lin X, Mamcarz M, Wang L, Arendash GW, Bradshaw PC. Neuropharmacology. 2012 Dec;63(8):1368-79.

[626]Melatonin antioxidative defense: therapeutical implications for aging and neurodegenerative processes. Pandi-Perumal SR, BaHammam AS, Brown GM, Spence DW, Bharti VK, Kaur C, Hardeland R, Cardinali DP. Neurotox Res. 2013 Apr;23(3):267-300.

[627]Melatonin plus physical exercise are highly neuroprotective in the 3xTg-AD mouse. García-Mesa Y, Giménez-Llort L, López LC, Venegas C, Cristòfol R, Escames G, Acuña-Castroviejo D, Sanfeliu C. Neurobiol Aging. 2012 Jun;33(6):1124.e13-29.

[628] Add-on prolonged-release melatonin for cognitive function and sleep in mild to moderate Alzheimer's disease: a 6-month, randomized, placebo-controlled, multicenter trial. Wade AG, Farmer M, Harari G, Fund N, Laudon M, Nir T, Frydman-Marom A, Zisapel N. Clin Interv Aging. 2014 Jun 18;9:947-61.

[629] Melatonin in Alzheimer's disease. Lin L[1], Huang QX, Yang SS, Chu J, Wang JZ, Tian Q. Int J Mol Sci. 2013 Jul 12;14(7):14575-93.

[630] Therapeutic application of melatonin in mild cognitive impairment. Cardinali DP, Vigo DE, Olivar N, Vidal MF, Furio AM, Brusco LI. Am J Neurodegen Dis. 2012;1(3):280-91.

[631] Interaction of neurons and astrocytes underlies the mechanism of Aβ-induced neurotoxicity. Angelova PR, Abramov AY. Biochem Soc Trans. 2014 Oct;42(5):1286-90.

[632] N-acetyl cysteine prevents synergistic, severe toxicity from two hits of oxidative stress. Unnithan AS[1], Jiang Y[1], Rumble JL[1], Pulugulla SH[1], Posimo JM[1], Gleixner AM[1], Leak RK[2]. Neurosci Lett. 2014 Feb 7;560:71-6.

[633] Amelioration of social isolation-triggered onset of early Alzheimer's disease-related cognitive deficit by N-acetylcysteine in a transgenic mouse model. Hsiao YH[1], Kuo JR, Chen SH, Gean PW. Neurobiol Dis. 2012 Mar;45(3):1111-20.

[634] The effect of omega-3 Fatty acids on biomarkers of inflammation: a rapid evidence assessment of the literature. Khorsan R[1], Crawford C[2], Ives JA[2], Walter AR[2], Jonas WB[2]. Mil Med. 2014 Nov;179(11 Suppl):2-60.

[635] Omega-3 fatty acids intake and risks of dementia and Alzheimer's disease: A meta-analysis. Wu S[1], Ding Y[2], Wu F[3], Li R[1], Hou J[4], Mao P[5]. Neurosci Biobehav Rev. 2014 Nov 21;48C:1-9.

[636] Regular fish consumption and age-related brain gray matter loss. Raji CA[1], Erickson KI[2], Lopez OL[3], Kuller LH[4], Gach HM[2], Thompson PM[5], Riverol M[6], Becker JT[7]. Am J Prev Med. 2014 Oct;47(4):444-51.

[637] Omega-3 fatty acid supplementation and cognitive function: are smaller dosages more beneficial? Abubakari AR[1], Naderali MM[2], Naderali EK[3] Int J Gen Med. 2014 Sep 19;7:463-73.

[638] Omega-3 fatty acids: a growing ocean of choices. Fares H[1], Lavie CJ, DiNicolantonio JJ, O'Keefe JH, Milani RV. Curr Atheroscler Rep. 2014 Feb;16(2):389.

[639] Why fish oil fails: a comprehensive 21st century lipids-based physiologic analysis. Peskin BS. J Lipids. 2014;2014:495761.

[640] Nutrient intake and plasma β-amyloid. Gu Y[1], Schupf N, Cosentino SA, Luchsinger JA, Scarmeas N. Neurology. 2012 Jun 5;78(23):1832-40.

[641] [Contribution of omega-3 fatty acids for memory and cognitive function]. [Article in Spanish]
Waitzberg DL[1], Garla P[2]. Nutr Hosp. 2014 Sep 1;30(3):467-77.

[642] Association of fish oil supplement use with preservation of brain volume and cognitive function. Daiello LA[1], Gongvatana A[2], Dunsiger S[3], Cohen RA[2], Ott BR[4]; Alzheimer's disease Neuroimaging Initiative. Alzheimers Dement. 2014 Jun 18. pii: S1552-5260(14)00079-X.

[643] Effects of supplementation with omega-3 fatty acids on oxidative stress and inflammation in patients with Alzheimer's disease: the OmegAD study. Freund-Levi Y[1], Vedin I[2], Hjorth E[3], Basun H[4], Faxén Irving G[5], Schultzberg M[3], Eriksdotter M[1], Palmblad J[2], Vessby B[6], Wahlund LO[1], Cederholm T[6], Basu S[7] J Alzheimers Dis. 2014;42(3):823-31.

[644] Higher RBC EPA + DHA corresponds with larger total brain and hippocampal volumes: WHIMS-MRI study. Pottala JV1, Yaffe K, Robinson JG, Espeland MA, Wallace R, Harris WS. Neurology. 2014 Feb 4;82(5):435-42.

[645] Potent health effects of pomegranate. Zarfeshany A[1], Asgary S[2], Javanmard SH[1]. Adv Biomed Res. 2014 Mar 25;3:100.

[646] Preventive and prophylactic mechanisms of action of pomegranate bioactive constituents. Viladomiu M[1], Hontecillas R, Lu P, Bassaganya-Riera J. Evid Based Complement Alternat Med. 2013;2013:789764.

[647] The pharmacological use of ellagic acid-rich pomegranate fruit. Usta C[1], Ozdemir S, Schiariti M, Puddu PE. Int J Food Sci Nutr. 2013 Nov;64(7):907-13.

[648] Pomegranate phenolics inhibit formation of advanced glycation end products by scavenging reactive carbonyl species. Liu W[1], Ma H, Frost L, Yuan T, Dain JA, Seeram NP. Food Funct. 2014 Oct 22;5(11):2996-3004.

⁶⁴⁹ Pomegranate Extract Modulates Processing of Amyloid-β Precursor Protein in an Aged Alzheimer's disease Animal Model. Ahmed AH, Subaiea GM, Eid A, Li L, Seeram NP, Zawia NH[1]. Curr Alzheimer Res. 2014;11(9):834-43.

⁶⁵⁰Pomegranate polyphenols and extract inhibit nuclear factor of activated T-cell activity and microglial activation in vitro and in a transgenic mouse model of Alzheimer disease. Rojanathammanee L[1], Puig KL, Combs CK. J Nutr. 2013 May;143(5):597-605.

⁶⁵¹ Long-term (15 mo) dietary supplementation with pomegranates from Oman attenuates cognitive and behavioral deficits in a transgenic mice model of Alzheimer's disease. Subash S[1], Braidy N[2], Essa MM[3], Zayana AB[1], Ragini V[4], Al-Adawi S[4], Al-Asmi A[4], Guillemin GJ[5]. Nutrition. 2015 Jan;31(1):223-9.

⁶⁵² Pomegranate from Oman Alleviates the Brain Oxidative Damage in Transgenic Mouse Model of Alzheimer's disease. Subash S[1], Essa MM[2], Al-Asmi A[3], Al-Adawi S[3], Vaishnav R[4], Braidy N[5], Manivasagam T[6], Guillemin GJ[7]. J Tradit Complement Med. 2014 Oct;4(4):232-8.

⁶⁵³ Memory boosting effect of Citrus limon, Pomegranate and their combinations. Riaz A[1], Khan RA[2], Algahtani HA[3]. Pak J Pharm Sci. 2014 Nov;27(6):1837-40.

⁶⁵⁴Pomegranate fruit as a rich source of biologically active compounds. Sreekumar S[1], Sithul H[1], Muraleedharan P[1], Azeez JM[1], Sreeharshan S[1]. Biomed Res Int. 2014;2014:686921.

⁶⁵⁵ Neuroprotective effects of berry fruits on neurodegenerative diseases. Subash S[1], Essa MM[1], Al-Adawi S[2], Memon MA[3], Manivasagam T[4], Akbar M[5]. Neural Regen Res. 2014 Aug 15;9(16):1557-66.

⁶⁵⁶ The flavonoid quercetin ameliorates Alzheimer's disease pathology and protects cognitive and emotional function in aged triple transgenic Alzheimer's disease model mice. Sabogal-Guáqueta AM[1], Muñoz-Manco JI[1], Ramírez-Pineda JR[2], Lamprea-Rodriguez M[3], Osorio E[4], Cardona-Gómez GP[5]. Neuropharmacology. 2015 Feb 7;93C:134-145.

⁶⁵⁷ Amyloid-beta (Aβ(1-42))-induced paralysis in Caenorhabditis elegans is inhibited by the polyphenol quercetin through activation of protein degradation pathways. Regitz C[1], Dußling LM, Wenzel U. Mol Nutr Food Res. 2014 Oct;58(10):1931-40.

⁶⁵⁸In silico QSAR analysis of quercetin reveals its potential as therapeutic drug for Alzheimer's disease. Islam MR[1], Zaman A[2], Jahan I[3], Chakravorty R[4], Chakraborty S[5]. J Young Pharm. 2013 Dec;5(4):173-9.

[659] Differential protective effects of quercetin, resveratrol, rutin and epigallocatechin gallate against mitochondrial dysfunction induced by indomethacin in Caco-2 cells. Carrasco-Pozo C[1], Mizgier ML, Speisky H, Gotteland M. Chem Biol Interact. 2012 Feb 5;195(3):199-205.

[660] Inhibition of microglial activation by elderberry extracts and its phenolic components. Simonyi A[1], Chen Z[2], Jiang J[2], Zong Y[3], Chuang DY[3], Gu Z[4], Lu CH[5], Fritsche KL[5], Greenlief CM[6], Rottinghaus GE[7], Thomas AL[8], Lubahn DB[9], Sun GY[10]. Life Sci. 2015 Mar 2. pii: S0024-3205(15)00106-X.

[661] Resveratrol: French paradox revisited. Catalgol B, Batirel S, Taga Y, Ozer NK. Front Pharmacol. 2012 Jul 17;3:141.

[662] Neuroprotective action of resveratrol. Bastianetto S, Ménard C, Quirion R. Biochim Biophys Acta. 2014 Oct 2. pii: S0925-4439(14)00292-0.

[663] Resveratrol in peanuts. Sales JM, Resurreccion AV. Crit Rev Food Sci Nutr. 2014;54(6):734-70.

[664] Resveratrol in metabolic health: an overview of the current evidence and perspectives. Poulsen MM, Jørgensen JO, Jessen N, Richelsen B, Pedersen SB. Ann N Y Acad Sci. 2013 Jul;1290:74-82.

[665] Small molecule SIRT1 activators for the treatment of aging and age-related diseases. Hubbard BP[1], Sinclair DA[2]. Trends Pharmacol Sci. 2014 Mar;35(3):146-54.

[666] Resveratrol: Anti-Obesity Mechanisms of Action. Aguirre L, Fernández-Quintela A, Arias N, Portillo MP. Molecules. 2014 Nov 14;19(11):18632-18655.

[667] Roles of resveratrol and other grape-derived polyphenols in Alzheimer's disease prevention and treatment. Pasinetti GM, Wang J, Ho L, Zhao W, Dubner L. Biochim Biophys Acta. 2014 Oct 12. pii: S0925-4439(14)00312-3.

[668] Interaction of Aβ(25-35) fibrillation products with mitochondria: Effect of small-molecule natural products. Ghobeh M, Ahmadian S, Meratan AA, Ebrahim-Habibi A, Ghasemi A, Shafizadeh M, Nemat-Gorgani M. Biopolymers. 2014 Nov;102(6):473-86.

[669] Resveratrol improves cognition and reduces oxidative stress in rats with vascular dementia. Ma X[1], Sun Z[2], Liu Y[1], Jia Y[1], Zhang B[1], Zhang J[2]. Neural Regen Res. 2013 Aug 5;8(22):2050-9.

[670] Neuroprotective effects of resveratrol and epigallocatechin gallate polyphenols are mediated by the activation of protein kinase C gamma. Menard C, Bastianetto S, Quirion R. Front Cell Neurosci. 2013 Dec 26;7:281.

[671] Resveratrol improves learning and memory in normally aged mice through microRNA-CREB pathway. Zhao YN, Li WF, Li F, Zhang Z, Dai YD, Xu AL, Qi C, Gao JM, Gao J. Biochem Biophys Res Commun. 2013 Jun 14;435(4):597-602.

[672] Resveratrol inhibits β-amyloid-induced neuronal apoptosis through regulation of SIRT1-ROCK1 signaling pathway. Feng X[1], Liang N, Zhu D, Gao Q, Peng L, Dong H, Yue Q, Liu H, Bao L, Zhang J, Hao J, Gao Y, Yu X, Sun J. PLoS One. 2013;8(3):e59888.

[673] Resveratrol effects on astrocyte function: relevance to neurodegenerative diseases. Wight RD, Tull CA, Deel MW, Stroope BL, Eubanks AG, Chavis JA, Drew PD, Hensley LL. Biochem Biophys Res Commun. 2012 Sep 14;426(1):112-5.

[674] SIRT1 regulates dendritic development in hippocampal neurons. Codocedo JF, Allard C, Godoy JA, Varela-Nallar L, Inestrosa NC. PLoS One. 2012;7(10):e47073.

[675] Sirtuin modulators control reactive gliosis in an in vitro model of Alzheimer's disease. Scuderi C, Stecca C, Bronzuoli MR, Rotili D, Valente S, Mai A, Steardo L. Front Pharmacol. 2014 May 13;5:89.

[676] Roles of resveratrol and other grape-derived polyphenols in Alzheimer's disease prevention and treatment.
Pasinetti GM[1], Wang J[2], Ho L[2], Zhao W[2], Dubner L[3]. Biochim Biophys Acta. 2015 Jun;1852(6):1202-1208.

[677] Neuroprotective action of resveratrol. Bastianetto S[1], Ménard C[2], Quirion R[3]. Biochim Biophys Acta. 2015 Jun;1852(6):1195-1201.

[678] Neuroprotective effect of Rhodiola rosea Linn against MPTP induced cognitive impairment and oxidative stress. Jacob R[1], Nalini G[1], Chidambaranathan N[1]. Ann Neurosci. 2013 Apr;20(2):47-51.

[679] Salidroside attenuates beta amyloid-induced cognitive deficits via modulating oxidative stress and inflammatory mediators in rat hippocampus. Zhang J[1], Zhen YF, Pu-Bu-Ci-Ren, Song LG, Kong WN, Shao TM, Li X, Chai XQ. Behav Brain Res. 2013 May 1;244:70-81.

[680] Salidroside attenuates allergic airway inflammation through negative regulation of nuclear factor-kappa B and p38 mitogen-activated protein kinase. Yan GH[1], Choi YH. J Pharmacol Sci. 2014;126(2):126-35.

[681] Inhibitory effects of salidroside on nitric oxide and prostaglandin E_2 production in lipopolysaccharide-stimulated RAW 264.7 macrophages. Song B[1], Huang G, Xiong Y, Liu J, Xu L, Wang Z, Li G, Lu J, Guan S. J Med Food. 2013 Nov;16(11):997-1003.

[682] Antidepressant-like effects of salidroside on olfactory bulbectomy-induced pro-inflammatory cytokine production and hyperactivity of HPA axis in rats. Yang SJ[1], Yu HY[1], Kang DY[1], Ma ZQ[1], Qu R[2], Fu Q[3], Ma SP. Pharmacol Biochem Behav. 2014 Sep;124:451-7.

[683] Comparing the efficacy and safety of Crocus sativus L. with memantine in patients with moderate to severe Alzheimer's disease: a double-blind randomized clinical trial. Farokhnia M, Shafiee Sabet M, Iranpour N, Gougol A, Yekehtaz H, Alimardani R, Farsad F, Kamalipour M, Akhondzadeh S. Hum Psychopharmacol. 2014 Jul;29(4):351-9.

[684] Selenium status in elderly: Relation to cognitive decline. Rita Cardoso B[1], Silva Bandeira V[2], Jacob-Filho W[3], Franciscato Cozzolino SM[2]. J Trace Elem Med Biol. 2014 Oct;28(4):422-6.

[685] Selenium and selenoprotein function in brain disorders. Pillai R[1], Uyehara-Lock JH, Bellinger FP. IUBMB Life. 2014 Apr;66(4):229-39.

[686] Selenomethionine ameliorates cognitive decline, reduces tau hyperphosphorylation, and reverses synaptic deficit in the triple transgenic mouse model of Alzheimer's disease. Song G, Zhang Z, Wen L, Chen C, Shi Q, Zhang Y, Ni J, Liu Q. J Alzheimers Dis. 2014;41(1):85-99.

[687] Souvenaid®: a new approach to management of early Alzheimer's disease. Ritchie CW[1], Bajwa J, Coleman G, Hope K, Jones RW, Lawton M, Marven M, Passmore P. J Nutr Health Aging. 2014 Mar;18(3):291-9.

[688] The effect of souvenaid on functional brain network organisation in patients with mild Alzheimer's disease: a randomised controlled study. de Waal H[1], Stam CJ[2], Lansbergen MM[3], Wieggers RL[3], Kamphuis PJ[3], Scheltens P[1], Maestú F[4], van Straaten EC[5]. PLoS One. 2014 Jan 27;9(1):e86558.

[689] The S-Connect study: results from a randomized, controlled trial of Souvenaid in mild-to-moderate Alzheimer's disease. Shah RC[1], Kamphuis PJ[2], Leurgans S[1],

Swinkels SH³, Sadowsky CH⁴, Bongers A², Rappaport SA⁵, Quinn JF⁶, Wieggers RL², Scheltens P⁷, Bennett DA¹. Alzheimers Res Ther. 2013 Nov 26;5(6):59.

⁶⁹⁰ Cerebral ABC transporter-common mechanisms may modulate neurodegenerative diseases and depression in elderly subjects. Pahnke J¹, Fröhlich C², Paarmann K³, Krohn M³, Bogdanovic N⁴, Årsland D⁵, Winblad B⁶. Arch Med Res. 2014 Nov;45(8):738-43.

⁶⁹¹ Reduced Alzheimer's disease pathology by St. John's Wort treatment is independent of hyperforin and facilitated by ABCC1 and microglia activation in mice. Hofrichter J, Krohn M, Schumacher T, Lange C, Feistel B, Walbroel B, Heinze HJ, Crockett S, Sharbel TF, Pahnke J¹. Curr Alzheimer Res. 2013 Dec;10(10):1057-69.

⁶⁹²St. John's Wort reduces beta-amyloid accumulation in a double transgenic Alzheimer's disease mouse model-role of P-glycoprotein. Brenn A¹, Grube M, Jedlitschky G, Fischer A, Strohmeier B, Eiden M, Keller M, Groschup MH, Vogelgesang S. Brain Pathol. 2014 Jan;24(1):18-24.

⁶⁹³ The effects of walnut supplementation on hippocampal NMDA receptor subunits NR2A and NR2B of rats. Hicyilmaz H, Vural H, Delibas N, Sutcu R, Gultekin F, Yilmaz N. Nutr Neurosci. 2014 Dec 18.

⁶⁹⁴Inverse association between the frequency of nut consumption and obesity among Iranian population: Isfahan Healthy Heart Program. Mohammadifard N¹, Yazdekhasti N, Stangl GI, Sarrafzadegan N. Eur J Nutr. 2014 Oct 14.

⁶⁹⁵ Long-term associations of nut consumption with body weight and obesity. Jackson CL¹, Hu FB¹. Am J Clin Nutr. 2014 Jun 4;100 (Supplement 1):408S-411S.

⁶⁹⁶Cytotoxic effects of ellagitannins isolated from walnuts in human cancer cells. Le V¹, Esposito D, Grace MH, Ha D, Pham A, Bortolazzo A, Bevens Z, Kim J, Okuda R, Komarnytsky S, Lila MA, White JB. Nutr Cancer. 2014;66(8):1304-14.

⁶⁹⁷Walnut polyphenol metabolites, urolithins A and B, inhibit the expression of the prostate-specific antigen and the androgen receptor in prostate cancer cells. Sánchez-González C¹, Ciudad CJ, Noé V, Izquierdo-Pulido M. Food Funct. 2014 Nov;5(11):2922-30.

⁶⁹⁸ Walnuts have potential for cancer prevention and treatment in mice. Hardman WE¹. J Nutr. 2014 Apr;144(4 Suppl):555S-560S.

[699] Serum metabolites from walnut-fed aged rats attenuate stress-induced neurotoxicity in BV-2 microglial cells. Fisher DR, Poulose SM, Bielinski DF, Shukitt-Hale B. Nutr Neurosci. 2014 Aug 25.

[700] Dietary supplementation of walnuts improves memory deficits and learning skills in transgenic mouse model of Alzheimer's disease. Muthaiyah B[1], Essa MM[1], Lee M[1], Chauhan V[1], Kaur K[1], Chauhan A[1]. J Alzheimers Dis. 2014;42(4):1397-405.

[701] Role of walnuts in maintaining brain health with age. Poulose SM[1], Miller MG, Shukitt-Hale B. J Nutr. 2014 Apr;144(4 Suppl):561S-566S.

[702] Grape juice, berries, and walnuts affect brain aging and behavior. Joseph JA[1], Shukitt-Hale B, Willis LM.
J Nutr. 2009 Sep;139(9):1813S-7S.

[703] Walnuts decrease risk of cardiovascular disease: a summary of efficacy and biologic mechanisms. Kris-Etherton PM[1]. J Nutr. 2014 Apr;144(4 Suppl):547S-554S.

[704] Effects of Juglans regia L. leaf extract on hyperglycemia and lipid profiles in type two diabetic patients: a randomized double-blind, placebo-controlled clinical trial. Hosseini S[1], Jamshidi L[2], Mehrzadi S[3], Mohammad K[4], Najmizadeh AR[5], Alimoradi H[6], Huseini HF[7]. J Ethnopharmacol. 2014 Mar 28;152(3):451-6.

[705] Spatial memory deficits in a mouse model of late-onset Alzheimer's disease are caused by zinc supplementation and correlate with amyloid-beta levels. Flinn JM[1], Bozzelli PL[1], Adlard PA[2], Railey AM[1].
Front Aging Neurosci. 2014 Oct 22;6:174.

[706] The role of zinc in the pathogenesis and treatment of central nervous system (CNS) diseases. Implications of zinc homeostasis for proper CNS function. Tyszka-Czochara M, Grzywacz A, Gdula-Argasińska J, Librowski T, Wiliński B, Opoka W. Acta Pol Pharm. 2014 May-Jun;71(3):369-77.

[707] Zinc modulates aluminium-induced oxidative stress and cellular injury in rat brain. Singla N[1], Dhawan DK. Metallomics. 2014 Oct;6(10):1941-50.

[708] Alzheimer's Association Backs Three Nondrug Studies. Megan Brooks. November 4, 2014. http://www.medscape.com/viewarticle/834387_print.

[709] Posttraumatic stress disorder-like induction elevates β-amyloid levels, which directly activates corticotropin-releasing factor neurons to exacerbate stress responses. Justice NJ[1], Huang L[2], Tian JB[3], Cole A[4], Pruski M[5], Hunt AJ Jr[6], Flores R[5], Zhu MX[3], Arenkiel BR[2], Zheng H[7]. J Neurosci. 2015 Feb 11;35(6):2612-23.

[710] Chronic stress as a risk factor for Alzheimer's disease. Machado A, Herrera AJ, de Pablos RM, Espinosa-Oliva AM, Sarmiento M, Ayala A, Venero JL, Santiago M, Villarán RF, Delgado-Cortés MJ, Argüelles S, Cano J. Rev Neurosci. 2014;25(6):785-804.

[711] The presence of a dog attenuates cortisol and heart rate in the Trier Social Stress Test compared to human friends. Polheber JP[1], Matchock RL. J Behav Med. 2014 Oct;37(5):860-7.

[712] Prayer at midlife is associated with reduced risk of cognitive decline in Arabic women. Inzelberg R[1], Afgin AE, Massarwa M, Schechtman E, Israeli-Korn SD, Strugatsky R, Abuful A, Kravitz E, Farrer LA, Friedland RP. Curr Alzheimer Res. 2013 Mar;10(3):340-6.

[713] Lifestyle behavior pattern is associated with different levels of risk for incident dementia and Alzheimer's disease: the Cache County study. Norton MC[1], Dew J, Smith H, Fauth E, Piercy KW, Breitner JC, Tschanz J, Wengreen H, Welsh-Bohmer K; Cache County Investigators. J Am Geriatr Soc. 2012 Mar;60(3):405-12.

[714] Orexinergic system dysregulation, sleep impairment, and cognitive decline in Alzheimer disease. Liguori C[1], Romigi A[1], Nuccetelli M[2], Zannino S[1], Sancesario G[3], Martorana A[3], Albanese M[1], Mercuri NB[4], Izzi F[1], Bernardini S[2], Nitti A[1], Sancesario GM[5], Sica F[6], Marciani MG[6], Placidi F[1]. JAMA Neurol. 2014 Dec 1;71(12):1498-505.

[715] How E-books May Disrupt Your Sleep. Nicholas Bakalar. *http://well.blogs.nytimes.com/2014/12/22/e-books-may-interfere-with-sleep/?_r=0*.

[716] Associations between Dementia Outcomes and Depressive Symptoms, Leisure Activities, and Social Support. Heser K[1], Wagner M[2], Wiese B[3], Prokein J[3], Ernst A[4], König HH[5], Brettschneider C[5], Riedel-Heller SG[6], Luppa M[6], Weyerer S[7], Eifflaender-Gorfer S[7], Bickel H[8], Mösch E[8], Pentzek M[9], Fuchs A[9], Maier W[2], Scherer M[4], Eisele M[4]; AgeCoDe Study Group. Dement Geriatr Cogn Dis Extra. 2014 Dec 10;4(3):481-93.

[717] What aspects of social network are protective for dementia? Not the quantity but the quality of social interactions is protective up to 15 years later. Amieva H[1], Stoykova R, Matharan F, Helmer C, Antonucci TC, Dartigues JF. Psychosom Med. 2010 Nov;72(9):905-11.

[718] Life Expectancy Reaches Record High in United States. Troy Brown. October 08, 2014. http://www.medscape.com/viewarticle/832981.

[719] Future prospects for longevity. Leeson GW. Post Reprod Health. 2014 Mar 13;20(1):11-15.

[720] Drugs that modulate aging: the promising yet difficult path ahead. Kennedy BK[1], Pennypacker JK[2]. Transl Res. 2014 May;163(5):456-65.

[721] We are ageing. Kolovou GD, Kolovou V, Mavrogeni S. Biomed Res Int. 2014;2014:808307.

[722] How Silicon Valley is trying to cure aging. Josie Ensor. February 14, 2015. http://www.telegraph.co.uk/news/worldnews/northamerica/usa/11413041/How-Silicon-Valley-is-trying-to-cure-aging.html.

[723] [Reversal of aging and lifespan elongation. Current biomedical key publications and the implications for geriatrics] [Article in German]. Bollheimer LC[1], Volkert D, Bertsch T, Sieber CC, Büttner R. Z Gerontol Geriatr. 2013 Aug;46(6):563-8.

[724] Aging is not a disease: implications for intervention. Rattan SI[1]. Aging Dis. 2014 Jun 1;5(3):196-202.

[725] Defining Successful Aging: A Tangible or Elusive Concept? Martin P[1], Kelly N[2], Kahana B[3], Kahana E[4], J Willcox B[5], Willcox DC[6], Poon LW[7]. Gerontologist. 2014 May 18.

[726] The search for antiaging interventions: from elixirs to fasting regimens. de Cabo R[1], Carmona-Gutierrez D[2], Bernier M[3], Hall MN[4], Madeo F[5]. Cell. 2014 Jun 19;157(7):1515-26.

[727] Aging and energetics' 'Top 40' future research opportunities 2010-2013. Allison DB[1], Antoine LH[2], Ballinger SW[3], Bamman MM[4], Biga P[5], Darley-Usmar VM[6], Fisher G[7], Gohlke JM[8], Halade GV[9], Hartman JL[10], Hunter GR[7], Messina JL[11], Nagy TR[12], Plaisance EP[7], Powell ML[5], Roth KA[5], Sandel MW[13], Schwartz TS[14], Smith DL[15], Sweatt JD[16], Tollefsbol TO[5], Watts SA[5], Yang Y[17], Zhang J[18], Austad SN[19]. F1000Res. 2014 Sep 12;3:219.

[728] In search of antiaging modalities: evaluation of mTOR- and ROS/DNA damage-signaling by cytometry. Darzynkiewicz Z[1], Zhao H, Halicka HD, Li J, Lee YS, Hsieh TC, Wu JM. Cytometry A. 2014 May;85(5):386-99.

[729] Interventions to Slow Aging in Humans: Are We Ready? Longo VD[1], Antebi A, Bartke A, Barzilai N, Brown-Borg HM, Caruso C, Curiel TJ, de Cabo R, Franceschi C, Gems D, Ingram DK, Johnson TE, Kennedy BK, Kenyon C, Klein S, Kopchick JJ,

Lepperdinger G, Madeo F, Mirisola MG, Mitchell JR, Passarino G, Rudolph KL, Sedivy JM, Shadel GS, Sinclair DA, Spindler SR, Suh Y, Vijg J, Vinciguerra M, Fontana L. Aging Cell. 2015 Apr 22.

[730] Dietary restriction and the pursuit of effective mimetics. Selman C[1]. Proc Nutr Soc. 2014 May;73(2):260-70.

[731] Calorie restriction and dietary restriction mimetics: a strategy for improving healthy aging and longevity. Testa G, Biasi F, Poli G, Chiarpotto E[1]. Curr Pharm Des. 2014;20(18):2950-77.

[732] Medicinal chemistry of the epigenetic diet and caloric restriction. Martin SL[1], Hardy TM, Tollefsbol TO. Curr Med Chem. 2013;20(32):4050-9.

[733] Molecular Links between Caloric Restriction and Sir2/SIRT1 Activation. Wang Y[1] .Diabetes Metab J. 2014 Oct;38(5):321-9.

[734] Protein and amino acid restriction, aging and disease: from yeast to humans. Mirzaei H[1], Suarez JA[1], Longo VD[2]. Trends Endocrinol Metab. 2014 Nov;25(11):558-566.

[735] How Much Should We Weigh for a Long and Healthy Life Span? The Need to Reconcile Caloric Restriction versus Longevity with Body Mass Index versus Mortality Data. Lorenzini A[1]. Front Endocrinol (Lausanne). 2014 Jul 30;5:121.

[736] Of mice and men: the benefits of caloric restriction, exercise, and mimetics. Mercken EM[1], Carboneau BA, Krzysik-Walker SM, de Cabo R. Ageing Res Rev. 2012 Jul;11(3):390-8.

[737] Skeletal muscle as a regulator of the longevity protein, Klotho. Avin KG[1], Coen PM[2], Huang W[3], Stolz DB[4], Sowa GA[3], Dubé JJ[5], Goodpaster BH[5], O'Doherty RM[5], Ambrosio F[6]. Front Physiol. 2014 Jun 17;5:189.

[738] NFκB2 Gene as a Novel Candidate that Epigenetically Responds to Interval Walking Training. Zhang Y[1], Hashimoto S[1], Fujii C[1], Hida S[1], Ito K[1], Matsumura T[1], Sakaizawa T[1], Morikawa M[2], Masuki S[2], Nose H[2], Higuchi K[3], Nakajima K[4], Taniguchi S[1]. Int J Sports Med. 2015 Apr 22.

[739] Effect of antioxidants supplementation on aging and longevity. Sadowska-Bartosz I[1], Bartosz G[2]. Biomed Res Int. 2014;2014:404680.

[740] Evaluation of resveratrol, green tea extract, curcumin, oxaloacetic acid, and medium-chain triglyceride oil on life span of genetically heterogeneous mice. Strong R[1],

Miller RA, Astle CM, Baur JA, de Cabo R, Fernandez E, Guo W, Javors M, Kirkland JL, Nelson JF, Sinclair DA, Teter B, Williams D, Zaveri N, Nadon NL, Harrison DE. J Gerontol A Biol Sci Med Sci. 2013 Jan;68(1):6-16.

[741] The three genetics (nuclear DNA, mitochondrial DNA, and gut microbiome) of longevity in humans considered as metaorganisms. Garagnani P[1], Pirazzini C[2], Giuliani C[3], Candela M[4], Brigidi P[4], Sevini F[2], Luiselli D[3], Bacalini MG[2], Salvioli S[2], Capri M[2], Monti D[5], Mari D[6], Collino S[7], Delledonne M[8], Descombes P[9], Franceschi C[10]. Biomed Res Int. 2014;2014:560340.

[742] Identification of a prognostic signature for old-age mortality by integrating genome-wide transcriptomic data with the conventional predictors: the Vitality 90+ Study. Jylhävä J[1], Raitanen J, Marttila S, Hervonen A, Jylhä M, Hurme M. BMC Med Genomics. 2014 Sep 11;7:54.

[743] On the immunological theory of aging. Fulop T[1], Witkowski JM, Pawelec G, Alan C, Larbi A. Interdiscip Top Gerontol. 2014;39:163-76.

[744] Immunostimulatory activity of lifespan-extending agents. Bravo-San Pedro JM[1], Senovilla L. Aging (Albany NY). 2013 Nov;5(11):793-801.

[745] Life extension factor klotho prevents mortality and enhances cognition in hAPP transgenic mice. Dubal DB[1], Zhu L[2], Sanchez PE[2], Worden K[2], Broestl L[3], Johnson E[2], Ho K[4], Yu GQ[4], Kim D[4], Betourne A[3], Kuro-O M[5], Masliah E[6], Abraham CR[7], Mucke L[1]. J Neurosci. 2015 Feb 11;35(6):2358-71.

[746] Aging: A mitochondrial DNA perspective, critical analysis and an update. Shokolenko IN[1], Wilson GL[1], Alexeyev MF[1]. World J Exp Med. 2014 Nov 20;4(4):46-57.

[747] Mitochondrial stress signaling in longevity: a new role for mitochondrial function in aging. Hill S[1], Van Remmen H[2]. Redox Biol. 2014 Jul 27;2:936-44.

[748] Tipping the metabolic scales towards increased longevity in mammals. Riera CE[1], Dillin A[1]. Nat Cell Biol. 2015 Mar;17(3):196-203.

[749] Sirtuins: guardians of mammalian healthspan. Giblin W, Skinner ME, Lombard DB. Trends Genet. 2014 Jul;30(7):271-86.

[750] Small-molecule allosteric activators of sirtuins. Sinclair DA[1], Guarente L. Annu Rev Pharmacol Toxicol. 2014;54:363-80. doi: 10.1146/annurev-pharmtox-010611-134657.

[751] Activation of SIRT3 by resveratrol ameliorates cardiac fibrosis and improves cardiac function via the TGF-β/Smad3 pathway. Chen T[1], Li J[1], Liu J[2], Li N[1], Wang S[1], Liu H[1], Zeng M[1], Zhang Y[1], Bu P[3]. Am J Physiol Heart Circ Physiol. 2015 Mar 1;308(5):H424-34.

[752] Telomere Length Variations in Aging and Age-Related Diseases. Rizvi S, Raza ST[1], Mahdi F. Curr Aging Sci. 2015 Jan 22.

[753] Effect of comprehensive lifestyle changes on telomerase activity and telomere length in men with biopsy-proven low-risk prostate cancer: 5-year follow-up of a descriptive pilot study. Ornish D[1], Lin J, Chan JM, Epel E, Kemp C, Weidner G, Marlin R, Frenda SJ, Magbanua MJ, Daubenmier J, Estay I, Hills NK, Chainani-Wu N, Carroll PR, Blackburn EH. Lancet Oncol. 2013 Oct;14(11):1112-20. doi: 10.1016/S1470-2045(13)70366-8. Epub 2013 Sep 17.

[754] Artemisinin mimics calorie restriction to trigger mitochondrial biogenesis and compromise telomere shortening in mice. Wang DT[1], He J[1], Wu M[2], Li SM[3], Gao Q[1], Zeng QP[1]. PeerJ. 2015 Mar 5;3:e822.

[755] Mediterranean diet and telomere length in Nurses' Health Study: population based cohort study. Crous-Bou M[1], Fung TT[2], Prescott J[3], Julin B[1], Du M[4], Sun Q[5], Rexrode KM[6], Hu FB[7], De Vivo I[8]. BMJ. 2014 Dec 2;349:g6674.

[756] Factors responsible for mortality variation in the United States: A latent variable analysis. Tencza C[1], Stokes A[1], Preston S[1]. Demogr Res. 2014 Jul;21(2):27-70.

[757] Predictors of Exceptional Longevity: Effects of Early-Life Childhood Conditions, Midlife Environment and Parental Characteristics. Gavrilov LA, Gavrilova NS. Living 100 Monogr. 2014;2014:1-18.

[758] Genetic factors associated with longevity: A review of recent findings. Shadyab AH[1], LaCroix AZ[2]. Ageing Res Rev. 2014 Nov 5;19C:1-7.

[759] Serum dehydroepiandrosterone-sulfate reflects age better than health status, and may increase with cigarette smoking and alcohol drinking in middle-aged men. Nagaya T[1], Kondo Y, Okinaka T. Aging Clin Exp Res. 2012 Apr;24(2):134-8.

[760] 'Biological clock' can be watched by observing a process known as methylation, which happens to DNA. Andrew Griffin. January 30, 2015.
http://www.independent.co.uk/news/science/dna-clues-could-predict-when-people-will-die-10014400.html?printService=print.

[761] The ApoE gene is related with exceptional longevity: a systematic review and meta-analysis. Garatachea N[1], Marín PJ, Santos-Lozano A, Sanchis-Gomar F, Emanuele E, Lucia A. Rejuvenation Res. 2014 Nov 10.

[762] Early-life nutritional programming of longevity. Vaiserman AM[1]. J Dev Orig Health Dis. 2014 Jun 13:1-14.

[763] Treadmill performance predicts risk of death, researchers say. March 02, 2015. http://www.foxnews.com/health/2015/03/02/treadmill-performance-predicts-risk-death-researchers-say/.

[764] Study: Lack Of Exercise Causes Twice As Many Deaths As Obesity. ATLANTA (CBS Atlanta). http://atlanta.cbslocal.com/2015/01/15/study-lack-of-exercise-causes-twice-as-many-deaths-as-obesity/.

[765] Sedentary Time and Its Association With Risk for Disease Incidence, Mortality, and Hospitalization in Adults: A Systematic Review and Meta-analysisSedentary Time and Disease Incidence, Mortality, and Hospitalization. Aviroop Biswas, BSc; Paul I. Oh, MD, MSc; Guy E. Faulkner, PhD; Ravi R. Bajaj, MD; Michael A. Silver, BSc; Marc S. Mitchell, MSc; and David A. Alter, MD, PhD. Ann Intern Med. 2015;162(2):123-132.

[766] Elite athletes live longer than the general population: a meta-analysis. Garatachea N, Santos-Lozano A, Sanchis-Gomar F, Fiuza-Luces C, Pareja-Galeano H, Emanuele E, Lucia A. Mayo Clin Proc. 2014 Sep;89(9):1195-200.

[767] Short spurts of vigorous exercise helps prevent early death, says study. Steve Connor. April 6, 2015. http://www.independent.co.uk/life-style/health-and-families/health-news/short-spurts-of-vigorous-exercise-helps-prevent-early-death-says-study-10158073.html?printService=print.

[768] Dose of jogging and long-term mortality: the Copenhagen City Heart Study. Schnohr P[1], O'Keefe JH[2], Marott JL[3], Lange P[4], Jensen GB[5]. J Am Coll Cardiol. 2015 Feb 10;65(5):411-9.

[769] Face scans show how fast a person is aging. Dennis Thompson. HealthDay News. March 31, 2015. http://www.myfoxny.com/story/28663965/face-scans-show-how-fast-a-person-is-aging.

[770] Higher-fiber diet linked to lower risk of death. Shereen Lehman. Reuters. January 12, 2015. Source: *http://bit.ly/1zRqnHa American Journal of Epidemiology, online December 31, 2014.*

[771] Your Friends Know How Long You Will Live: A 75-Year Study of Peer-Rated Personality Traits. Jackson JJ, Connolly JJ, Garrison SM, Leveille MM, Connolly SL. Psychol Sci. 2015 Jan 12.

[772] Handshake strength could predict heart attack risk Laura Donnelly. The Telegraph. May 14, 2015. http://www.telegraph.co.uk/journalists/laura-donnelly/11603129/Handshake-strength-could-predict-heart-attack-risk.html.

[773] Adherence to a healthy diet according to the World Health Organization guidelines and all-cause mortality in elderly adults from Europe and the United States. Jankovic N, Geelen A, Streppel MT, de Groot LC, Orfanos P, van den Hooven EH, Pikhart H, Boffetta P, Trichopoulou A, Bobak M, Bueno-de-Mesquita HB, Kee F, Franco OH, Park Y, Hallmans G, Tjønneland A, May AM, Pajak A, Malyutina S, Kubinova R, Amiano P, Kampman E, Feskens EJ. Am J Epidemiol. 2014 Nov 15;180(10):978-88.

[774] Heart rate reduction and longevity in mice. Gent S, Kleinbongard P, Dammann P, Neuhäuser M, Heusch G.
Basic Res Cardiol. 2015 Mar;110(2):460.

[775] Resting Heart Rate: Risk Indicator and Emerging Risk Factor in Cardiovascular Disease. Böhm M^1, Reil JC^2, Deedwania P^3, Kim JB^4, Borer JS^5. Am J Med. 2014 Oct 15. pii: S0002-9343(14)00889-4.

[776] Being Alone As Bad As Smoking, Excessive Drinking. March 16, 2015.
http://minnesota.cbslocal.com/2015/03/16/study-being-alone-as-bad-as-smoking-excessive-drinking/.

[777] The Matthew effect in empirical data. Perc M^1. J R Soc Interface. 2014 Sep 6;11(98):20140378.

[778] New Developments in the Biodemography of Aging and Longevity. Gavrilov LA, Gavrilova NS. Gerontology. 2014 Dec 20.

[779] Mediterranean diet and telomere length in Nurses' Health Study: population based cohort study. Crous-Bou M, Fung TT, Prescott J, Julin B, Du M, Sun Q, Rexrode KM, Hu FB, De Vivo I. BMJ. 2014 Dec 2;349:g6674.

[780] Is Milk Your Friend or Foe? HealthDay. October 29, 2014. [Source: BMJ Online. October 28, 2014.] http://www.nlm.nih.gov/medlineplus/news/fullstory_149181.html (*this news item will not be available after 01/27/2015).

[781] Association of nut consumption with total and cause-specific mortality. Bao Y, Han J, Hu FB, Giovannucci EL, Stampfer MJ, Willett WC, Fuchs CS. N Engl J Med. 2013 Nov 21;369(21):2001-11.

[782] An oral health study of centenarians and children of centenarians. Kaufman LB, Setiono TK, Doros G, Andersen S, Silliman RA, Friedman PK, Perls TT. J Am Geriatr Soc. 2014 Jun;62(6):1168-73.

[783] Purpose in Life as a Predictor of Mortality Across Adulthood. Hill PL[1], Turiano NA[2]. Psychol Sci. 2014 May 8;25(7):1482-1486.

[784] Study found older people who felt life had meaning had better survival. Robert Preidt. HealthDay News November 7, 2014.
http://www.nlm.nih.gov/medlineplus/news/fullstory_149350.html (*this news item will not be available after 02/05/2015).

[785] In search of antiaging modalities: evaluation of mTOR- and ROS/DNA damage-signaling by cytometry. Darzynkiewicz Z[1], Zhao H, Halicka HD, Li J, Lee YS, Hsieh TC, Wu JM. Cytometry A. 2014 May;85(5):386-99.

[786] Progressive rise in red blood cell distribution width predicts mortality and cardio-vascular events in end-stage renal disease patients. Yoon HE[1], Kim SJ[1], Hwang HS[2], Chung S[2], Yang CW[2], Shin SJ[1]. PLoS One. 2015 May 11;10(5):e0126272.

[787] Change in Red Blood Cell Distribution width During the Last Years of Life in Geriatric Patients. Martínez-Velilla N[1], Cambra-Contin K, García-Baztán A, Alonso-Renedo J, Herce PA, Ibáñez-Beroiz B.
J Nutr Health Aging. 2015;19(5):590-4.

[788] Association of the dispersion in red blood cell volume with mortality. Horne BD[1,2], Muhlestein JB[1,3], Bennett ST[4,5], Muhlestein JB[3], Ronnow BS[1], May HT[1], Bair TL[1], Anderson JL[1,3]. Eur J Clin Invest. 2015 Mar 7.

[789] Real vs perceived age: A matter of life and death. December 15, 2014. [From a study published in JAMA Internal Medicine: REAL VS. PERCEIVED AGE.]
http://www.sunherald.com/2014/12/15/5970702_real-vs-perceived-age-a-matter.html?rh=1#storylink=cpy.

[790] Human longevity is associated with regular sleep patterns, maintenance of slow wave sleep, and favorable lipid profile. Mazzotti DR, Guindalini C, Moraes WA, Andersen ML, Cendoroglo MS, Ramos LR, Tufik S. Front Aging Neurosci. 2014 Jun 24;6:134.

[791] Childhood sleep duration and lifelong mortality risk. Duggan KA[1], Reynolds CA[1], Kern ML[2], Friedman HS. Health Psychol. 2014 Oct;33(10):1195-203.

[792] Sun may determine lifespan at birth: study. Mariette Le Roux. January 7, 2015. http://news.yahoo.com/sun-may-determine-lifespan-birth-study-003745386.html;_ylt=AwrSyCN8cq1UuCMAJ5vQtDMD.

[793] Real time analysis of volatile organic compounds (VOCs) in centenarians. Mazzatenta A[1], Pokorski M[2], Di Giulio C[3]. Respir Physiol Neurobiol. 2014 Dec 24. pii: S1569-9048(14)00346-2.

[794] Effects of antidepressants on longevity and dementia onset among adults with Down syndrome: a retrospective study. Tsiouris JA, Patti PJ, Flory MJ. J Clin Psychiatry. 2014 Jul;75(7):731-7.

[795] Angiotensin Ii Blockade: How Its Molecular Targets May Signal To Mitochondria And Slow Aging. Coincidences With Calorie Restriction And Mtor Inhibition. de Cavanagh EA[1], Inserra F[2], Ferder L[3]. Am J Physiol Heart Circ Physiol. 2015 May 1:ajpheart.00459.2014.

[796] A CHEAP over-the-counter painkiller may have astonishing powers to extend life, say researchers. Jo Willey. Express. December 19, 2014. [Based on: Enhanced longevity by ibuprofen, conserved in multiple species, occurs in yeast through inhibition of tryptophan import. He C[1], Tsuchiyama SK[1], Nguyen QT[2], Plyusnina EN[3], Terrill SR[2], Sahibzada S[2], Patel B[1], Faulkner AR[1], Shaposhnikov MV[3], Tian R[1], Tsuchiya M[1], Kaeberlein M[4], Moskalev AA[5], Kennedy BK[1], Polymenis M[2]. PLoS Genet. 2014 Dec 18;10(12):e1004860.].

[797] Longevity, aging and rapamycin. Ehninger D, Neff F, Xie K. Cell Mol Life Sci. 2014 Nov;71(22):4325-46.

[798] How longevity research can lead to therapies for Alzheimer's disease: The rapamycin story. Richardson A, Galvan V, Lin AL, Oddo S. Exp Gerontol. 2014 Dec 3. pii: S0531-5565(14)00349-0.

[799] The Achilles' Heel of Senescent Cells: From Transcriptome to Senolytic Drugs. Zhu Y[1], Tchkonia T, Pirtskhalava T, Gower A, Ding H, Giorgadze N, Palmer AK, Ikeno Y, Borden G, Lenburg M, O'Hara SP, LaRusso NF, Miller JD, Roos CM, Verzosa GC, LeBrasseur NK, Wren JD, Farr JN, Khosla S, Stout MB, McGowan SJ, Fuhrmann-Stroissnigg H, Gurkar AU, Zhao J, Colangelo D, Dorronsoro A, Ling YY, Barghouthy AS, Navarro DC, Sano T, Robbins PD, Niedernhofer LJ, Kirkland JL. Aging Cell. 2015 Mar 9.

[800] Impacts of metformin and aspirin on life history features and longevity of crickets: trade-offs versus cost-free life extension? Hans H[1], Lone A, Aksenov V, Rollo CD. Age (Dordr). 2015 Apr;37(2):31.

[801] Frailty Attenuates the Impact of Metformin on Reducing Mortality in Older Adults with Type 2 Diabetes. Wang CP[1], Lorenzo C[2], Espinoza SE[3]. J Endocrinol Diabetes Obes. 2014;2(2).

[802] Metformin promotes lifespan through mitohormesis via the peroxiredoxin PRDX-2. De Haes W[1], Frooninckx L[1], Van Assche R[1], Smolders A[2], Depuydt G[1], Billen J[3], Braeckman BP[2], Schoofs L[4], Temmerman L[1]. Proc Natl Acad Sci U S A. 2014 Jun 17;111(24):E2501-9.

[803] Consumption of polyphenol plants may slow aging and associated diseases. Uysal U[1], Seremet S, Lamping JW, Adams JM, Liu DY, Swerdlow RH, Aires DJ. Curr Pharm Des. 2013;19(34):6094-111.

[804] Effects of nutritional components on aging. Lee D[1], Hwang W, Artan M, Jeong DE, Lee SJ. Aging Cell. 2014 Oct 22.

[805] AMPK activation--protean potential for boosting healthspan. McCarty MF[1]. Age (Dordr). 2014 Apr;36(2):641-63.

[806] Significant longevity-extending effects of Alpinia zerumbet leaf extract on the life span of Caenorhabditis elegans. Upadhyay A[1], Chompoo J, Taira N, Fukuta M, Tawata S. Biosci Biotechnol Biochem. 2013;77(2):217-23.

[807] Involvement of the catecholaminergic system on the antidepressant-like effects of Alpinia zerumbet in mice. Bevilaqua F[1], Mocelin R, Grimm C Jr, da Silva Junior NS, Buzetto TL, Conterato GM, Roman WA Jr, Piato AL. Pharm Biol. 2015 Apr 17:1-6.

[808] Essential Oils from Fructus A. zerumbet Protect Human Aortic Endothelial Cells from Apoptosis Induced by Ox-LDL In Vitro. Chen Y[1], Li D[1], Xu Y[2], Zhang Y[2], Tao L[2], Li S[2], Jiang Y[2], Shen X[1]. Evid Based Complement Alternat Med. 2014;2014:956824.

[809] Anti-obesity effects of hispidin and Alpinia zerumbet bioactives in 3T3-L1 adipocytes. Tu PT[1], Tawata S[2]. Molecules. 2014 Oct 15;19(10):16656-71.

[810] Vitamin D and mortality: meta-analysis of individual participant data from a large consortium of cohort studies from Europe and the United States. Schöttker B, Jorde R, Peasey A, Thorand B, Jansen EH, Groot Ld, Streppel M, Gardiner J, Ordóñez-Mena JM, Perna L, Wilsgaard T, Rathmann W, Feskens E, Kampman E, Siganos G,

Njølstad I, Mathiesen EB, Kubínová R, Pająk A, Topor-Madry R, Tamosiunas A, Hughes M, Kee F, Bobak M, Trichopoulou A, Boffetta P, Brenner H; Consortium on Health and Ageing: Network of Cohorts in Europe and the United States. BMJ. 2014 Jun 17;348:g3656.

[811] Mediterranean diet and healthy aging: a Sicilian perspective. Vasto S[1], Buscemi S, Barera A, Di Carlo M, Accardi G, Caruso C. Gerontology. 2014;60(6):508-18.

[812] Xenohormetic and anti-aging activity of secoiridoid polyphenols present in extra virgin olive oil: a new family of gerosuppressant agents. Menendez JA[1], Joven J, Aragonès G, Barrajón-Catalán E, Beltrán-Debón R, Borrás-Linares I, Camps J, Corominas-Faja B, Cufí S, Fernández-Arroyo S, Garcia-Heredia A, Hernández-Aguilera A, Herranz-López M, Jiménez-Sánchez C, López-Bonet E, Lozano-Sánchez J, Luciano-Mateo F, Martin-Castillo B, Martin-Paredero V, Pérez-Sánchez A, Oliveras-Ferraros C, Riera-Borrull M, Rodríguez-Gallego E, Quirantes-Piné R, Rull A, Tomás-Menor L, Vazquez-Martin A, Alonso-Villaverde C, Micol V, Segura-Carretero A. Cell Cycle. 2013 Feb 15;12(4):555-78.

[813] Analysis of lifespan-promoting effect of garlic extract by an integrated metabolo-proteomics approach. Huang CH[1], Hsu FY[2], Wu YH[2], Zhong L[3], Tseng MY[4], Kuo CJ[2], Hsu AL[5], Liang SS[6], Chiou SH[7]. J Nutr Biochem. 2015 Apr 2. pii: S0955-2863(15)00071-6.

[814] The molecular targets of resveratrol. Kulkarni SS, Cantó C. Biochim Biophys Acta. 2014 Oct 12. pii: S0925-4439(14)00311-1.

[815] Diet and aging. Ribarič S.[1] Oxid Med Cell Longev. 2012;2012:741468.

[816] Lifespan and healthspan extension by resveratrol. Bhullar KS[1], Hubbard BP[2]. Biochim Biophys Acta. 2015 Jan 29. pii: S0925-4439(15)00021-6.

[817] Mediterranean way of drinking and longevity. Giacosa A, Barale R, Bavaresco L, Faliva MA, Gerbi V, La Vecchia C, Negri E, Opizzi A, Perna S, Pezzotti M, Rondanelli M. Crit Rev Food Sci Nutr. 2014 Sep 10.

[818] Sirtuins in cognitive aging and Alzheimer's disease. Braidy N, Jayasena T, Poljak A, Sachdev PS. Curr Opin Psychiatry. 2012 May;25(3):226-30.

[819] Resveratrol rescues SIRT1-dependent adult stem cell decline and alleviates progeroid features in laminopathy-based progeria. Liu B, Ghosh S, Yang X, Zheng H, Liu X, Wang Z, Jin G, Zheng B, Kennedy BK, Suh Y, Kaeberlein M, Tryggvason K, Zhou Z. Cell Metab. 2012 Dec 5;16(6):738-50.

[820] Antiaging properties of a grape-derived antioxidant are regulated by mitochondrial balance of fusion and fission leading to mitophagy triggered by a signaling network of Sirt1-Sirt3-Foxo3-PINK1-PARKIN. Das S, Mitrovsky G, Vasanthi HR, Das DK. Oxid Med Cell Longev. 2014;2014:345105.

[821] Dietary resveratrol prevents Alzheimer's markers and increases life span in SAMP8. Porquet D, Casadesús G, Bayod S, Vicente A, Canudas AM, Vilaplana J, Pelegrí C, Sanfeliu C, Camins A, Pallàs M, del Valle J. Age (Dordr). 2013 Oct;35(5):1851-65.

[822] Resveratrol levels and all-cause mortality in older community-dwelling adults. Semba RD[1], Ferrucci L[2], Bartali B[3], Urpí-Sarda M[4], Zamora-Ros R[4], Sun K[1], Cherubini A[5], Bandinelli S[6], Andres-Lacueva C[4]. JAMA Intern Med. 2014 Jul;174(7):1077-84.

[823] Resveratrol and food effects on lifespan and reproduction in the model crustacean Daphnia. Kim E, Ansell CM, Dudycha JL. J Exp Zool A Ecol Genet Physiol. 2014 Jan;321(1):48-56.

[824] Resveratrol in mammals: effects on aging biomarkers, age-related diseases, and life span. Marchal J, Pifferi F, Aujard F. Ann N Y Acad Sci. 2013 Jul;1290:67-73.

[825] Resveratrol vs. calorie restriction: data from rodents to humans. Lam YY, Peterson CM, Ravussin E. Exp Gerontol. 2013 Oct;48(10):1018-24.

[826] The lifespan extension effects of resveratrol are conserved in the honey bee and may be driven by a mechanism related to caloric restriction. Rascón B, Hubbard BP, Sinclair DA, Amdam GV. Aging (Albany NY). 2012 Jul;4(7):499-508.

[827] The effect of resveratrol on longevity across species: a meta-analysis. Hector KL, Lagisz M, Nakagawa S. Biol Lett. 2012 Oct 23;8(5):790-3.

[828] The impact of moderate wine consumption on health. Artero A[1], Artero A[2], Tarín JJ[3], Cano A[4]. Maturitas. 2014 Oct 2. pii: S0378-5122(14)00294-1.

[829] Pomegranate Juice Enhances Healthy Lifespan in Drosophila melanogaster: An Exploratory Study. Balasubramani SP, Mohan J, Chatterjee A, Patnaik E, Kukkupuni SK, Nongthomba U, Venkatasubramanian P. Front Public Health. 2014 Dec 16;2:245.

[830] Identification of longevity, fertility and growth-promoting properties of pomegranate in Caenorhabditis elegans. Kılıçgün H[1], Arda N[2], Uçar EÖ[2]. Pharmacogn Mag. 2015 Apr-Jun;11(42):356-9.

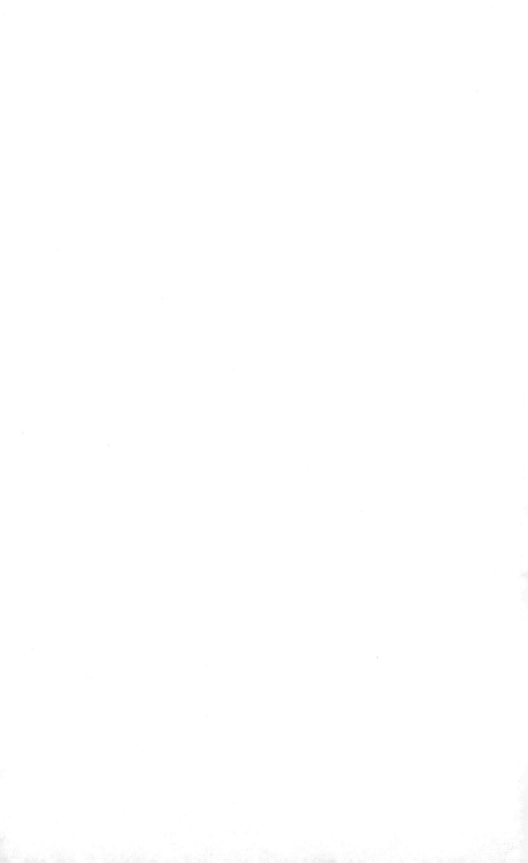

CPSIA information can be obtained
at www.ICGtesting.com
Printed in the USA
FSHW010119030122
87342FS